TYLMAN'S THEORY AND PRACTICE OF FIXED PROSTHODONTICS

TYLMAN'S
THEORY AND PRACTICE OF
FIXED PROSTHODONTICS

STANLEY D. TYLMAN
A.B., D.D.S., M.S., F.A.C.D.

WILLIAM F. P. MALONE
D.D.S., M.S., Ph.D., F.A.C.D.

Consulting editors

DAVID L. KOTH, D.D.S., M.S.
BOLESLAW MAZUR, D.D.S., M.S.
HOSEA F. SAWYER, D.D.S., M.S.

SEVENTH EDITION
with 1390 *illustrations and 2 color plates*

THE C. V. MOSBY COMPANY

Saint Louis   1978

The C. V. Mosby Company
11830 Westline Industrial Drive, St. Louis, Missouri 63141

Library of Congress Cataloging in Publication Data

Tylman, Stanley Daniel, 1893-
  Tylman's Theory and practice of fixed prosthodontics.

  Previous ed. published in 1970 under title: Theory and practice of crown and fixed partial prosthodontics (bridge)
  Bibliography: p.
  Includes index.
  1. Crowns (Dentistry) 2. Bridges (Dentistry)
I. Malone, William F., 1930-   joint author.
II. Title.
RK666.T9   1978   617.6'92   78-17821
ISBN 0-8016-5166-2

CB/CB/B   9   8   7   6   5   4   3   2   1

Contributors

Raoul H. Boitel, Dr. med. dent., D.D.S., F.I.C.D.
Instructor, Staff Education, Crown and Bridge Department, University of Zurich, Zurich, Switzerland

Gilbert I. Brinsden, B.D.Sc., L.D.S., M.S.D., F.R.A.C.D.S.
Professor and Chairman, Department of Fixed Prosthodontics, Northwestern University Dental School, Chicago, Illinois

Joseph L. Caruso, B.A., D.D.S.
Department of Fixed Prosthodontics, Loyola University, School of Dentistry, Maywood, Illinois

Gordon J. Christensen, D.D.S., M.S.D., Ph.D.
Co-Director, Clinical Research Associates, Private Practice of Prosthodontics, Adjunct Professor of Biologic Sciences, Brigham Young University, Post-Graduate Lecturer, Provo, Utah

Robert J. Crum, D.D.S., F.A.C.D.
Director, Prosthodontic Residency Program, Veterans Administration Hospital, Hines; Clinical Professor of Prosthodontics, Loyola University, School of Dentistry; Maywood; Clinical Associate Professor of Prosthodontics, University of Illinois, College of Dentistry, Chicago, Illinois

Paul D. Dinga, B.S., D.D.S.
Assistant Professor of Fixed Prosthodontics, Loyola University, School of Dentistry, Maywood, Illinois

John E. Flocken, B.S., D.M.D.
Clinical Professor of Restorative Dentistry, University of California at Los Angeles, School of Dentistry, Los Angeles, California

John K. Francis, D.D.S., F.A.C.S.S.
Clinical Associate Professor, Department of Periodontics, Loyola University, School of Dentistry, Maywood; President, Dental Staff, Hinsdale Hospital, Hinsdale; Guest Lecturer, Northwestern University, School of Dentistry, Diplomate, American Board of Periodontology, Chicago, Illinois

Daniel Frederickson, M.S., D.D.S.
Libby, Montana

Niles F. Guichet, D.D.S.
Anaheim, California

James D. Harrison, D.D.S., M.Sc., M.A.
Professor, Department of Restorative Dentistry, Southern Illinois University, School of Dental Medicine, Edwardsville, Illinois

Raymond F. Henneman, D.D.S.
Clinical Associate Professor, Department of Fixed Prosthodontics, Loyola University, School of Dentistry, Maywood, Illinois

Lee M. Jameson, B.S., D.D.S., M.S.
Associate Professor, Department of Fixed Prosthodontics, Loyola University, School of Dentistry, Maywood, Illinois

August J. Kaleta, D.D.S., M.S.
Assistant Professor of Fixed Prosthodontics, University of Illinois, College of Dentistry, Chicago, Illinois

William J. Kelly, Jr., D.D.S., M.S.D.

Clinical Professor, Department of Restorative Dentistry, University of Southern Illinois, School of Dental Medicine, Edwardsville, Illinois

David L. Koth, D.D.S., M.S.

Director, Fixed Prosthetics, Department of Restorative Dentistry, Medical College of Georgia, School of Dentistry, Augusta, Georgia

Alfred C. Long, D.D.S., F.A.C.D.

Professor and Chairman, Department of Fixed Prosthodontics, The Ohio State University, College of Dentistry, Columbus, Ohio

Parker E. Mahan, D.D.S., Ph.D., F.A.C.D.

Professor and Chairman, Department of Basic Dental Sciences, University of Florida, College of Dentistry, Gainesville, Florida

William F. P. Malone, D.D.S., M.S., Ph.D., F.A.C.D.

Professor of Fixed Prosthodontics, Loyola University, School of Dentistry, Maywood, Illinois; Director of Post-Graduate Prosthodontics; Certified Illinois State Board Specialist in Prosthodontics

Maury Massler, D.D.S., M.S., D.Sc.

Professor Emeritus, Tufts University, School of Dental Medicine, Boston, Massachusetts

Boleslaw Mazur, B.S., D.D.S., M.S.

Professor, Department of Fixed Prosthodontics, Loyola University, School of Dentistry, Maywood, Illinois

John W. McLean, O.B.E., D.Sc., M.D.S. (London), L.D.S., R.C.S.(England)

Clinical Consultant to the Laboratory of the Government Chemist, London, England

Gregory P. Miller, A.T., B.S., C.D.T.

Department of Post-Graduate Prosthodontics, Loyola University, School of Dentistry, Maywood, Illinois

Joseph C. Morganelli, D.D.S., M.Ed.

Chairman, Department of Fixed Prosthodontics, Loyola University, School of Dentistry, Maywood, Illinois

George H. Moulton, B.A., D.D.S., F.A.C.D.

Dean Emeritus, Professor and Former Chairman, Crown and Bridge Dentistry, Emory University, School of Dentistry, Atlanta, Georgia

Joachim Nordt, C.D.T.

Master Dental Technician
Highland Park, Illinois

Robert Pinkerton, B.S., D.D.S.

Assistant Professor, Department of Fixed Prosthodontics, University of Southern California, School of Dentistry, Los Angeles, California

Richard N. Pipia, B.S., D.D.S., F.A.C.D.

Clinical Associate Professor, Fixed Crown and Bridge Department, Loyola University, School of Dentistry, Maywood, Illinois

Zigmund C. Porter, B.S., D.D.S., F.A.C.D., F.I.C.D., F.A.C.S.S.

Associate Professor and Director of Postgraduate Periodontics, University of Illinois at the Medical Center, College of Dentistry, Chicago; Clinical Associate Professor, Department of Fixed Prosthetics, Loyola University, School of Dentistry, Maywood, Illinois; Visiting Professor, School of Continuing Medical Education, Dental Division, Ramat-Aviv, Tel-Aviv, Israel

J. Marvin Reynolds, D.D.S.

Professor, Department of Restorative Dentistry; Director, Fixed Prosthodontics Postdoctoral Program, School of Dentistry, Medical College of Georgia, Augusta, Georgia

James L. Sandrik, Ph.D.

Chairman, Department of Dental Materials, Loyola University, School of Dentistry, Maywood, Illinois

Hosea F. Sawyer, D.D.S., M.S.

Former Associate Professor and Chairman, Department of Operative Dentistry, Loyola University, School of Dentistry, Maywood, Illinois

Stanley D. Tylman, A.B., D.D.S., M.S., F.A.C.D.

Emeritus Professor of Prosthetic Dentistry, University of Illinois, College of Dentistry, Chicago, Illinois; Professor Honoris Causa, Universities of Brazil, Argentina, Venezuela, and Bolivia; Certified Illinois State Board Specialist in Prosthodontics

Anthony T. Young, D.D.S., M.S.

Assistant Professor of Dental Surgery, Head, Section of General Dentistry, University of Chicago, Walter G. Zoller Memorial Dental Clinic, Chicago, Illinois

Preface

Education and research are continuous processes. Innovative technical discoveries and new biological concepts in related sciences have affected the progress, objectives, and practice of prosthodontic dentistry. The interrelationship of periodontics, orthodontics, and endodontics with fixed prosthodontics has provided a climate for comprehensive patient treatment.

Dr. Tylman's efforts in the previous editions have offered the student and practitioner those concepts and methods that were based on 40 years of clinical experience and research of accepted leaders in biological and related sciences. The purpose of this edition remains the same: to provide a publication that stresses current methods of treatment in fixed prosthodontics. All advances in therapeutic techniques involve conflicts in opinion that are reflected intellectually as a form of controversy. There are even conflicting, if not diametrically opposed ideas, between authors of various chapters within this edition. However, innovative procedures, based upon scientific data, produce a healthy climate for the advancement of the profession of dentistry. This implies that the dentist must accept the responsibility to familiarize himself with newer methods of treatment, which may depart from traditional concepts. Imaginative prosthodontic procedures are impossible to implement if the dentist has no knowledge of their existence.

In any attempt to render service to the dental patient, a planned sequence of therapy is necessary to supply adequate oral health treatment. If prosthodontic procedures are initiated prior to the establishment of a sound, scholarly diagnosis or if the sequence is illogical, they could have an adverse effect on the dental health status of the patient. The development of a practical treatment plan must be flexible enough for alternate directions in therapy but relatively uncomplicated in its overall application.

Problem identification, oral diagnosis, problem solution, and treatment planning are dealt with in the text as complementary procedures. It is the object of this text to accentuate a programmed, intellectual review of all diagnostic tools prior to the initiation of any treatment.

We sincerely hope that this book not only presents the traditional fixed prosthodontic procedures in a comprehensive manner, but helps to elucidate the innovative and heroic dental procedures. One of the newer aspects of this book, when compared to the former editions, is more emphasis on periodontics, occlusion, and coverage of the fixed-removable type of prosthesis. We sincerely hope our illustrations are helpful in the identification of the new materials and improved techniques. This trend to combine fixed and removable prosthetics is a natural development in light of educational policies to combine restorative departments, economic pressures, and commitments to treat more patients in a comprehensive manner. A greater response of restorative dentistry to periodontics and occlusal dysfunction and how they affect fixed prosthodontics was considered of paramount importance.

The main theme of the book can be summarized in two axioms:

1. The dentist should perform as few dental procedures as necessary to achieve and maintain optimal dental health for the patient.
2. The dentist should prevent as much treatment as possible by early recognition of clinical conditions that deviate from the normal aging processes.

A fairly large contingent of authors have contributed to this new edition. We offer to them our heartfelt thanks. We are also thankful to those numerous dentists, journals, and dental manufacturers who so graciously assisted in furnishing material and illustrations. Research groups are too numerous to thank individually but are gratefully acknowledged by the authors of this book. We have all attempted to perpetuate the work of the senior author, Dr. Stanley Tylman, whose outstanding contributions to society as an author, researcher, dentist, and a man transcend time.

William F. P. Malone

Contents

COLOR PLATES

1

Considerations in oral diagnosis and treatment planning

Gilbert Brinsden

The definition of "diagnosis" as it applies to the patient seeking clinical dental treatment encompasses three major areas:
1. Recognition and identification of the abnormal conditions present in the mouth and their potential influence on the longevity of the dentition
2. Evaluation of the seriousness of these conditions
3. Determination of the etiological factors responsible

Establishing a diagnosis largely centers around the collection of "facts." These and the senses of sight, touch, and sound combined with dialog between the patient and dentist help establish the patient's symptoms, which, in turn, provide the basis for identification of the disease by the observance of the presenting clinical signs. Identification of a diseased condition is related directly to the dentist's understanding and evaluation of what constitutes a healthy state, and the seriousness of any abnormality is based upon its degree of deviation from the normal statistical range within a given random sample of patients.

The diagnosis of any dental condition in whatever area of clinical dentistry, regardless of specialty, requires the accumulation of certain preliminary information. This information can be divided into the following five basic categories:
1. Identification of the patient's essential statistics

2. Recording of the patient's medical and dental history
3. Examination and charting of the oral cavity
4. Analysis of the patient's chief complaint
5. A summary of the related facts

For further information in this area the reader should direct his attention to any of the recognized texts in oral diagnosis and treatment planning.

RECOGNITION AND IDENTIFICATION OF ABNORMAL CONDITIONS IN THE MOUTH

To obtain a comprehensive diagnosis in the particular area of fixed prosthodontics, the dentist should first recognize and identify the abnormal conditions present in the stomatognathic system. To accomplish this, he must perform a thorough examination of the conditions existing by establishing the facts that emerge from the following areas of information.

Patient medical and dental history

Medical history. In most dental offices and dental schools the medical history is accomplished through the use of a comprehensive health questionnaire form, which provides a general health profile of the patient. A patient seeking dental treatment may at the same time be under the care of a physician, and it is therefore important for the dentist to be aware of any medication that may have been prescribed. Most questionnaires are designed to highlight the relationship of drugs used in particular systemic diseases that may precipitate specific medical complications for the dentist during treatment. Adverse drug reactions and allergic reactions must also be recorded to safeguard the patient throughout his dental treatment. Factors emerging from such a questionnaire could relate directly to the diagnosis and subsequent treatment of the patient, and, if so, should be discussed thoroughly with the patient's physician.

Dental history. All students of dentistry and dental practitioners have been taught the principles of obtaining a good dental history, the repetition of which is not necessary here. It is however important to correct the attitude of a misinformed patient since patient cooperation is necessary if optimum dental health is to be attained. The role of patient education assumes a vitally important function in the treatment of a patient requiring fixed prosthodontics, as a well-informed patient is more likely to become a cooperative patient. During this early stage of case review, the dialog between the patient and the dentist should provide the dentist with an insight into the patient's interest and attitudes concerning dentistry. This will help the dentist evaluate the degree of cooperation he can expect during the course of further treatment.

Uppermost in the patient's mind during this preliminary dialog is the chief dental complaint that initiated his seeking dental treatment. The chief complaint is usually associated with pain or discomfort and may be directly related with one or more cariously involved teeth, the supporting tooth structures, or the temporomandibular joints. Whatever the nature of this complaint, it must be investigated immediately and the pain or discomfort eliminated prior to completion of the final diagnosis and development of the treatment plan.

Radiographic examination

A radiographic examination, though a necessary adjunct, does not supplant a thorough clinical examination and should include a set of 14 intraoral films as well as four bitewing films for the average adult patient. A panoramic film survey is also useful in diagnosis because it provides an overview of the calcified structures and sinuses and may eliminate needless diagnostic tests. Occasionally, extraoral films of the temporomandibular joints may be necessary for those patients experiencing pain and joint dysfunction.

At this stage it is advisable to take a series of clinical photographs. These will serve as a basis for assessing changes in the appearance of the soft tissues as well as providing a permanent record of the presenting esthetic condition. The following information can be provided from a good intraoral radiographic survey:

Intraoral radiographic examination

1. Degree of bone loss and overall remaining bone support (determination of crown-root ratio)
2. Presence or absence of residual roots and rarified areas underlying edentulous spaces
3. Root number and morphology (short, long, slender, bifurcated, hypercementosis)
4. Axial inclination of teeth and tooth roots (estimate degree of nonparallelism if present)
5. Presence of apical disease or root resorption
6. Overall quality of supporting bone, trabeculation patterns, and reaction to functional changes
7. Width of periodontal ligament—evidence of changes in occlusal or incisal function, or both
8. Continuity and integrity of the lamina dura
9. Specific identification of areas of vertical and horizontal bone loss, periodontal pockets, and root furcation involvement
10. Calculus deposits

11. Presence of caries and assessment of preexisting restorations and their relation to the dental pulp
12. Assessment of root fillings and pulpmorphology (particularly pulp stones)

From a radiographic examination, satisfactory abutment teeth would be those teeth whose length of root support within the bony alveolus is greater than the combined length of the tooth crown and root surface exposed beyond the alveolus. The abutment teeth would also have to possess good root form, a normal periodontal ligament width, minimal caries involvement, and no root abnormalities.

It is desirable that the divergence in parallelism between the long axis of acceptable abutment teeth does not exceed a range of 25 to 30 degrees, otherwise occlusal forces applied to the completed bridge may be directed in an axis other than the long axis of the abutment root. When this occurs, breakdown of the tissues with pocket development and subsequent bone loss are frequently observed and, if left untreated, will ultimately lead to the failure of the bridge.

Although the desirable crown-root ratio of a healthy abutment tooth is approximately 1:1½, a less favorable ratio can be accepted if the axial relationships of abutment teeth are similarly parallel, no periodontal disease is present, and the possibility of splinting together two or more abutments exists.

An unsatisfactory abutment tooth would be one whose root support within the alveolus was substantially less than the combined length of the tooth crown and root surface exposed beyond the alveolus. These teeth will almost certainly demonstrate extensive loss of supporting bone as the result of prolonged untreated periodontal disease. They may also demonstrate short malformed or tapered root forms, which together with supporting bone loss further compounds the unsatisfactory situation. Or the axial rela-

tionship of the abutment tooth may be greater than 25 to 30 degrees off parallelism with the remaining teeth, thereby disqualifying it as a suitable abutment, unless limited orthodontic treatment can be instituted to upright it in a more favorable axial inclination.

Fig. 1-1, *A*, illustrates a mandibular second molar with generalized bone loss and mesial crestal involvement together with an unfavorable axial inclination for bridge preparation. Fig. 1-1, *B*, shows the same second molar uprighted orthodontically to a more favorable axial relationship with some improvement in the mesial crestal involvement. Fig. 1-1, *C*, shows the placement of a temporary metal and acrylic bridge prior to the completion of periodontal treatment. Furcation involvement may frequently be present in patients experiencing periodontal disease and, depending on the degree of seriousness, may be untreatable from a periodontal viewpoint. Fig. 1-2 illustrates a class II furcation involvement where the clinical probings indicate that successful periodontal treatment cannot be instituted and the tooth should therefore be extracted. Many furcation involvements, however, can be treated successfully by skillful hemisection of one or more roots leaving the root or roots best supported by alveolar bone in situ. This procedure eliminates the furcation and is generally referred to as bicuspidization of the tooth. Fig. 1-3, *A*, shows a mandibular root-treated second molar tooth in which a class II furcation exists compounded by the presence of distal caries and a large portion of excess amalgam. Although the crown-root ratio is not ideal, hemisection of the distal root (bicuspidization) could allow the mesial root to remain as a healthy abutment for a posterior bridge. Fig. 1-3, *B*, illustrates the radiograph taken after periodontal treatment including hemisection and orthodontic treatment to upright the abutment teeth in a more favorable axial relationship. Fig. 1-3, *C*, shows the posterior abutments of

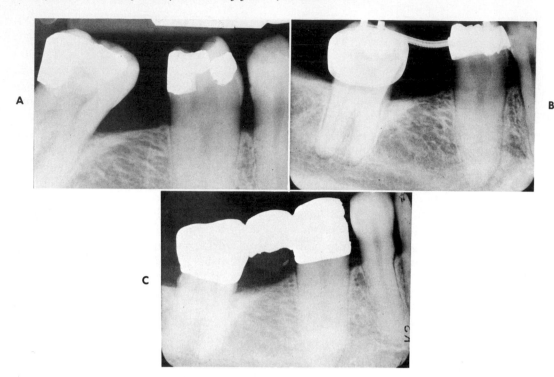

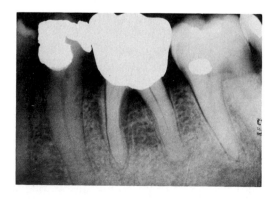

Fig. 1-1. A, Difference in long-axis parallelism between the mandibular second molar and second bicuspid is approximately 30 degrees. There has been generalized bone loss and mesial crestal involvement of molar. The success of bridge placement without uprighting of molar orthodontically is doubtful since the masticatory load would not be directed along the long axis of the molar tooth. Continued mesial crestal break-down might occur. **B,** Tooth in **A** uprighted to a more favorable axial relationship by use of simple orthodontic appliance. Note improvement in condition and level of mesial crestal bone of molar. Prognosis for bridge placement at this stage is greatly improved. **C,** Three-unit metal and acrylic treatment bridge has been placed prior to completion of the periodontal treatment. Mesial contact has been provided in acrylic resin. Note correction of occlusal plane and improvement of mesial crestal bone of molar. Placement of final bridge will take place after completion of periodontal treatment.

Fig. 1-2. Class II (through-and-through) furcation involvement of the mandibular first molar tooth on which a crown has been placed. Note progress of mesial root decalcification. Progress of disease process is not so evident on second bicuspid and second molar teeth.

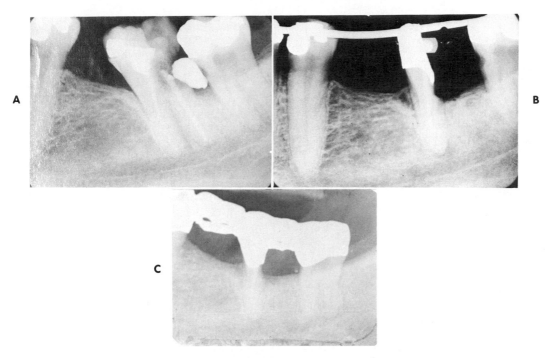

Fig. 1-3. A, Class II furcation involvement in this molar root filled tooth is not so visible as that in Fig. 1-2. Radiography clearly shows destruction of distal root of molar as well as some mesial crestal involvement. Hemisection of distal root followed by orthodontic treatment to make upright the remaining mesial root was performed to improve supporting bone picture and to direct masticatory load in long axis of abutment teeth. **B,** Improvement of supporting bone and axial inclination of mesial root of molar tooth approximately 16 weeks after placement of orthodontic appliance. **C,** Placement of five-tooth temporary metal and acrylic bridge (treatment bridge) prior to completion of periodontal treatment. Note improved axial relationship of the two posterior abutments and healing of alveolar bone after hemisection of distal root. Remaining molar abutment root now presents with a crown-root ratio of 1:1.

the completed bridge with the uprighted third and second molar-abutment tooth roots. The hemisected second molar now has the radiographic appearance of a bicuspid tooth and demonstrates a crown-root ratio of 1:1.

Information provided by diagnostic casts

Study casts in a good quality stone must be secured from accurate and well extended alginate impressions of the maxillary arch and hard palate and the mandibular arch. After trimming and removal of stone blebs, the casts are mounted in centric relation on a semiadjustable articulator by means of a face-bow and oc-

clusal wax records. Once accurately mounted on the articulator, the casts are usually referred to as "diagnostic casts." See Fig. 1-4 for the procedure.

EXAMINATION OF MOUNTED CASTS

Examination of the mounted casts will reveal information in the following areas:

Evidence of collapsed posterior arches. This is usually seen as a result of early extraction of the first molar teeth followed by other extractions at a later date (Fig. 1-5).

Evidence of supereruption of teeth beyond original occlusal plane. When an antagonist tooth is extracted, the remain-

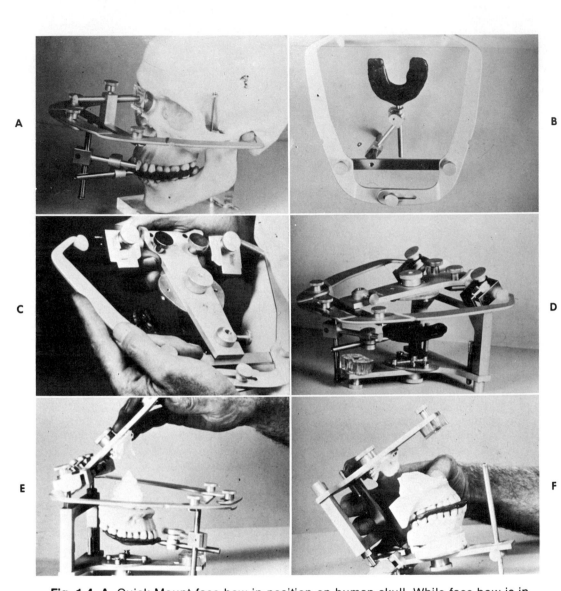

Fig. 1-4. A, Quick Mount face-bow in position on human skull. While face-bow is in place, the condylar width is recorded by markings on front of face-bow side arms. **B,** Quick Mount face-bow with registration of maxillary teeth locked in position. **C,** Face-bow registration is transferred to maxillary element of articulator. Holes in ear-pieces are placed onto pins extending from eminentia of articulator. **D,** Lower frame of articulator is used as a support for face-bow registration and upper frame of articulator while upper cast is mounted after mandibular condylar elements are moved to center holes of articulator frame to correspond to a medium registration. **E,** Upper cast is placed into registration of face-bow fork; fast-setting mounting stone is applied to the cast and mounting plate. **F,** With articulator inverted and with a centric relation registration, lower cast is positioned onto upper cast and mounting stone applied to cast and mounting plate.

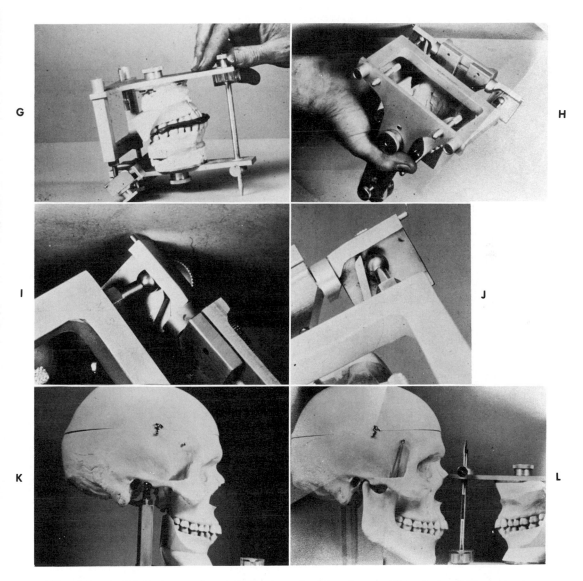

Fig. 1-4, cont'd. G, Lower frame is then pushed to place until incisal guide contacts guide pin. A permanent incisal guide registration may be obtained later by cutting of guide paths into plastic incisal guide block to accommodate lateral excursions of patients. **H,** Sideshift (Bennett movement) guide is moved laterally until it also contacts the right condyle element and locked into position. **I,** Close-up of this sideshift guide in position. **J,** Close-up of left condyle showing how it has moved away from its sideshift guide. (This system is repeated for opposite side). **K,** With lower cast mounted on articulator frame, it replaces mandible of skull. **L,** Side view of skull and articulated casts. *Continued.*

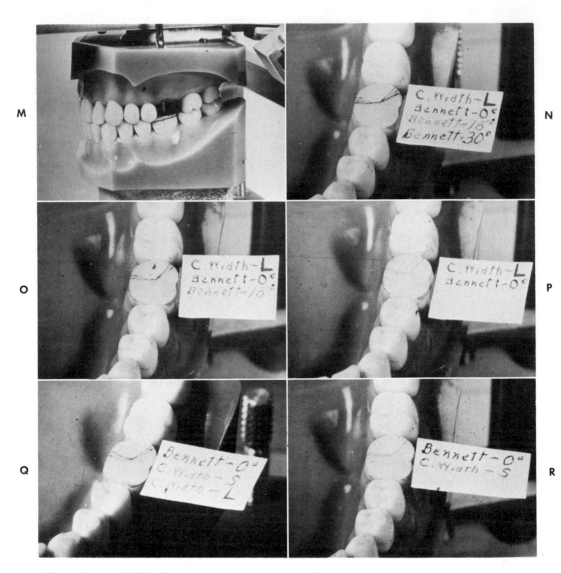

Fig. 1-4, cont'd. M, Side view of arrangement. Flat shim of fused procelain was luted to surface of ground-away lower molar tooth with tacky sticky wax to receive ink markings. With Dentoforms in centric relation, stylus rests on approximate center of lower left first molar tooth. Moving the articulator into right lateral excursion will draw a line from center to buccal surface of tooth. Left lateral excursion will mark from center to lingual surface of tooth. **N to P,** Various paths caused by change of only the amount of sideshift allowed, as indicated on individual slides. **Q and R,** With amount of sideshift constant, but changing of condylar width.

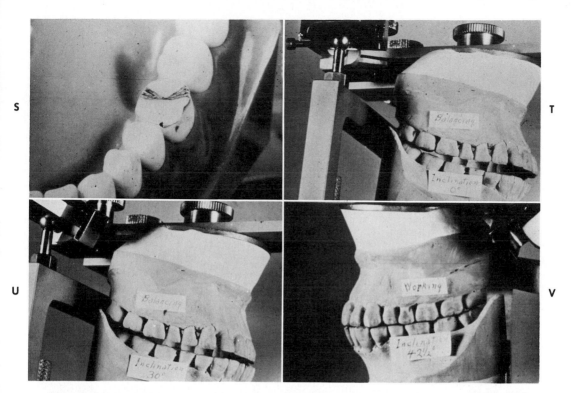

Fig. 1-4, cont'd. S, Composite of several paths caused by changing of condylar width and amount of sideshift in various combinations. **T,** With casts forced into left lateral excursion, but with no angle of eminentia, third molars on right side are in heavy contact. No other teeth come close to meeting. **U,** Setting the inclination to the "average" 30 degrees, with upper right second and third molar contacting right lower third molar. Teeth are much closer, but still no contact. **V,** Checkbite registration taken from skull set condylar guidance at inclination of 42.5 degrees. At this setting, the molar teeth come close or into very light contact.

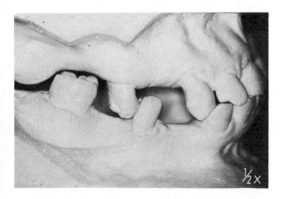

Fig. 1-5. Right side illustrates results of multiple extractions of posterior teeth without replacement. Loss of opposing occlusal surface contact contributes to an overall loss of vertical dimension. Remaining anterior tooth contact results in tooth separation and displacement of lower canine anteriorly.

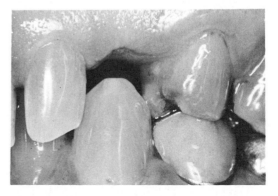

Fig. 1-6. Extraction of maxillary cuspid 12 months previously allows mandibular canine to erupt into newly created space. This situation will pose difficulties for placement of canine pontic in maxillary replacement bridge.

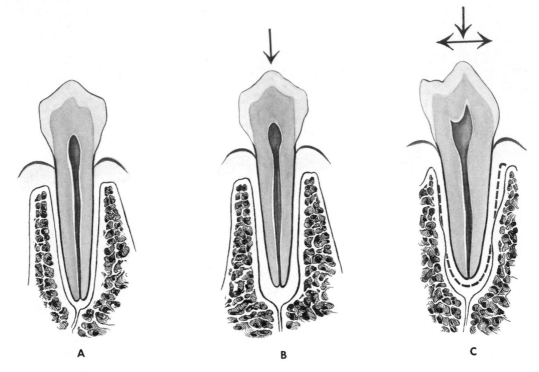

Fig. 1-7. A, Lower conic premolar in normal relationship with its supporting structure. **B,** Widening of periodontal ligament and bone modification periapically because of vertical stresses. **C,** Diagram showing result of inordinate vertical and horizontal stresses on periodontal ligament and supportive bone.

ing tooth or teeth may erupt beyond the normal occlusal plane, predisposing the patient to occlusal interferences. Abnormal wear facets may be seen on the occlusal surfaces of these teeth (Fig. 1-6).

Evidence of tooth movement. Once the mesiodistal integrity of the posterior arch is destroyed by the extraction of one or more teeth, the remaining teeth are free to move either by bodily movement or tipping. Tooth movement in any one direction can be accompanied by subtle changes in axial inclination (Fig. 1-7) and rotation attributable to occlusal forces that complicate the final location of the tooth and render it unsuitable for a bridge abutment.

Evidence of changes in axial inclination of the teeth. Although visible in radiographs, changes in axial inclination can best be studied on the diagnostic casts where the differences in parallelism of proposed abutment teeth can be directly measured. Discrepancies in parallelism exceeding a range of 25 to 30 degrees indicate doubtful abutment teeth unless orthodontic correction is proposed.

Evidence of present status of occlusion by observing wear-facet patterns. Some occlusal surfaces in relation to the patient's age may present excessive wear facets, which may indicate the presence of occlusal interferences. Movements of the articulator from centric relation position to centric occlusion and right and left lateral movements should be investigated for occlusal interferences. If these interferences are observed on the articulated diagnostic casts, they should be verified in the patient's mouth (see Chapters 18 and 19).

Evidence of interocclusal relationship of mandible to maxilla. The way in which the teeth of both jaws come together in the centric relation position will provide some indication of the degree of overbite and overjet relationship anteriorly and posteriorly and whether it lies within the normal range. Excessive overjet of the anterior maxillary dentition often contraindicates the selection of porcelain jacket crown restorations as contact with the maxillary teeth is often made in a location that would tend to fracture the delicate crowns. Buccal, labial, and lingual versions can be readily observed as well as anterior and posterior cross-bite relationships.

Evidence of alteration of midline location. Extraction of anterior teeth without immediate replacement is most commonly responsible for changes in the midline location. Deformities of the bony structure of either the mandible or the maxilla because of accident, surgical interference, or congenital defects can also produce noticeable changes in the midline location. Whatever the cause for the change, the esthetic considerations for an anterior bridge are often severely tested.

Evaluation of degree and direction of masticatory forces in a particular bridge area. Wherever possible functional masticatory forces should be directed parallel to the long axis of the supporting abutment teeth and to the opposing antagonist teeth. An assessment of the parallelism of all the teeth of both jaws involved in a particular bridge area must be made on the diagnostic casts together with an examination in the mouth to reassure the dentist that a fixed bridge is indeed indicated and will function satisfactorily in the environment it is placed.

Evaluation for need to establish a new occlusal plane. Estimation for the need to reduce certain overerupted teeth or rebuild other teeth that may be undererupted can be readily assessed on the diagnostic casts. Correction of a distorted

occlusal plane is a necessary prerequisite for satisfactory restoration of the posterior dentition.

Evaluation of "path of insertion" for proposed bridge. The path of insertion of a fixed prosthesis should be such that the completed restoration can be inserted and withdrawn without causing undue stress on the abutment and adjacent teeth. Although the degree of convergence or divergence of the abutment teeth may appear excessive when first assessed with the analyzing rod of the surveyor, it may be possible to modify the preparations or pontic design such that an acceptable path of insertion is achieved. Ideally this should be along the long axis of the abutment teeth and should be no greater than 25 degrees from parallelism. Additional factors such as pulp size, esthetics and malpositioned teeth may influence the choice of restoration and the path of insertion. The mechanical assessment of the latter then ceases to be the overriding factor in the bridge design (Fig. 1-8).

Evaluation of edentulous areas for selection and positioning of pontic facings and pontic forms. One can select manufactured pontic facings and forms from the manufacturer's mold charts by measuring the mesiodistal and either the occlusogingival or incisogingival height of the edentulous space and positioning the selected pontic in the area. When this type of pontic is to be used, one can often make a selection prior to preparation of the abutment teeth by positioning and stabilizing the pontic in the edentulous area and checking the relationship with the opposing arch and the alignment of contour with the approximating and opposing teeth.

LIMITATIONS OF DIAGNOSTIC CASTS AS A DIAGNOSTIC AID

It is generally agreed that semiadjustable articulators are an acceptable instrument on which study casts can be mounted. However, there are certain

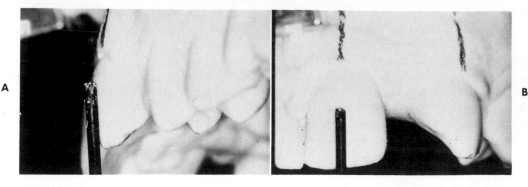

Fig. 1-8. A, Analyzing rod of surveyor is shown determining direction of proximal grooves for abutment tooth that is to receive a partial veneer crown. In this instance the rod simulates direction of incisal two thirds of labial surface of tooth. **B,** Analyzing rod of surveyor is shown determining long axis of tooth root of central incisor in which a pinledge abutment retainer is to be used. Direction of pinholes in central incisor must be parallel to long axis of tooth and to incisal two thirds of labial surface. They must also parallel the proximal grooves of cuspid tooth.

limitations in the articulator itself and the dentist would be wise to take into consideration the following precautions before arriving at a final diagnosis:

1. In cases where treatment other than minimal restorative dentistry is anticipated, an accurate assessment of the occlusal patterns is essential.
2. The diagnosis of occlusal abnormalities involves a thorough clinical examination of the occlusion in the mouth in addition to an examination of accurately mounted study casts.
3. One must relate the maxillary cast to the hinge axis and the horizontal member of the articulator to establish an anatomic relationship of the casts and the articulator.
4. An accurate centric relation record enables the clinician to check which teeth are involved with initial or premature contacts and the direction of the resultant compensatory mandibular movement necessary to achieve maximum intercuspation. The quality of the diagnosis is dependent on the accuracy of this record because it is from this starting point that subsequent border jaw movements are recorded and the articulator is set.
5. Mandibular border movements are

curved. With a semiadjustable articulator protrusive and lateral check bites only provide sufficient information to produce a straight-line record of these movements. Consequently, lateral check bites should be taken to the extent of expected lateral jaw movements. In this way the maximum degree of curvature is recorded over a minimal distance. A more accurate assessment of balancing side prematurities and of the existing anterior incisal guidance can then be made.

CLINICAL EXAMINATION OF MOUTH

Examination of the mouth will provide the clinician with the opportunity of reviewing the condition of the supporting tissues. The color, contour, and relationship to the cervical portions of the tooth crowns will provide an indication of general tissue health and may alert the clinician to complicating periodontal disease. The reaction of the tissue to previously placed restorations of all types including fixed bridges and partial dentures may be examined for tissue acceptability, and a measure of the patient's capability to maintain good oral hygiene may also be ascertained. Where bone loss has been demonstrated radiographically, the teeth may be tested by finger manipulation to determine the range of mobility. Visual examination of the tissues of the floor of the mouth and the hard and soft palate as well as the lateral borders of the tongue should be examined for suspicious lesions of any kind. Clinical examination of the mouth should be accompanied by dialog with the patient to establish the etiology of the conditions afflicting the hard and soft tissues that may present themselves. Mouth examination should be performed in a systematic manner with use of various types of mouth mirrors and explorers, water, air, dental floss, and a good light course. The procedure may be summarized in the following outline:

Clinical examination of mouth

1. Examination of all soft tissues associated with the oral cavity
2. Examination of tongue for lesions (note size and color)
3. Examination for any abnormal oral habits (horn players, pipe smokers, and so forth)
4. Examination of opening and closing movements in centric relation for the following:
   a. Deviation of the mandible
   b. Crepitus
   c. Cracking
   d. Range of movement of mandible in normal function
5. Examination of the integrity of all visible tooth-surface structure for the following:
   a. Carious lesions
   b. Color variations involving the enamel
   c. Areas of erosion
   d. Areas of abrasion
   e. Areas of occlusal wear
   f. Acceptability of present restorations including fixed bridges
   g. Recurring caries
   h. Sensitive areas of exposed dentin or cementum

Special tests may be required to augment the examination, such as transillumination, electrical examination of the pulp, and percussion tests.

6. *Examination of teeth* (clinical crowns and roots in conjunction with radiographic findings)
   a. Caries (new or recurring)
   b. Crown morphology (long, short)
   c. Relation of crown to crown roots
   d. Overall contour of crown type
   e. Rotations
   f. Axial changes in inclination
   g. Supraeruption and infraeruption of teeth
   h. Location of gingiva in relation to tooth crown
7. Examination of the occlusion (touch, sight, and sound) for the following:
   a. Premature and initial contacts
   b. Cuspal interferences in eccentric movements
   c. Presence of balancing side contacts

PERIODONTAL EXAMINATION OF MOUTH

A thorough periodontal examination of the mouth should be made to assess the patient's attitude and ability to practice rigid oral hygiene standards if they are to be required. Disclosing solutions may be used to demonstrate to the patient the degree and location of plaque accumulations.

Prior to an extensive periodontal examination, it is advisable that the patient receive a thorough prophylaxis together with deep quadrant scaling if deemed necessary to reduce the presence of infection. After an interval of time for healing, the periodontal examination can be subsequently performed more accurately and a preliminary judgment can be made on the patient's ability to carry out the necessary home care.

Periodontal treatment, if required, should ordinarily be completed prior to the preparation of the abutment teeth for a fixed bridge to provide an optimal state of health for the supporting tissues. If the periodontist anticipates that successful treatment may require extensive osseous surgery, which in his opinion may produce mobility of the teeth after surgery,

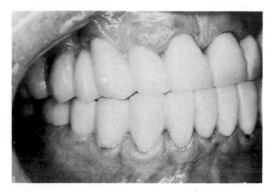

Fig. 1-9. Placement of provisional acrylic splints for both maxillary and mandibular arches prior to full mouth periodontal surgery. In this example bone loss about remaining teeth has been extensive and it is anticipated that corrective osseous surgery will leave the teeth in a mobile condition necessitating complete arch splinting for the completed reconstruction.

he may request the clinician to provide provisional acrylic splints before surgery is undertaken (Fig. 1-9).

The following steps need to be evaluated during the course of the periodontal examination:

1. Assessment of the patient's oral hygiene
2. Amount and location of residual plaque and calculus formation
3. Quality of investing tissues (tone, color, contour)
4. Measured crevice depths about all surfaces of all teeth
5. Recession of tissue because of pathologic or nonpathologic causes
6. Assessment of tooth mobility and its classification
7. Presence or absence of traumatic occlusion and its etiologic factors
8. Necessity to equilibrate the dentition concomitantly with periodontal treatment
9. Root bifurcation and trifurcation involvements and their classification
10. Presence or absence of mucogingival problems

Table 1-1. Dimensions of root surface areas

	1	2	3	4	5	6
Type of tooth	Average area (mm²)	Standard deviation	Coefficient of variation	Number of measurements	Relative sizes	Boyd (1958)
Maxilla						
Central	204	31.4	15.4	19	6	204.5
Lateral	179	24.9	13.9	25	7	177.3
Cuspid	273	43.9	16.1	26	3	266.5
First bicuspid	234	33.7	14.4	20	4	219.7
Second bicuspid	220	39.0	17.7	19	5	216.7
First molar	433	40.9	9.4	15	1	454.8
Second molar	431	62.5	14.5	10	2	416.9
Mandible						
Central	154	26.5	17.2	10	7	162.2
Lateral	168	21.5	12.8	10	6	174.8
Cuspid	268	42.2	15.7	18	3	272.2
First bicuspid	180	27.2	15.1	24	5	196.9
Second bicuspid	207	26.6	12.9	17	4	204.3
First molar	431	59.5	13.8	15	1	450.3
Second molar	426	69.7	16.4	10	2	399.7

From Jepsen, A.: Acta Odont. Scand. **21**:35, 1963.

SELECTION OF ABUTMENT TEETH

Dr. Irvin Ante in 1930 in discussing the suitability of abutment teeth pointed out that in fixed bridges the combined pericemental area of the abutment teeth should be equal to or greater in pericemental area than the tooth or teeth to be replaced. This statement has come to be known in the practice of fixed prosthodontics as Ante's law. A great deal of investigation has been carried out in relation to the measurement of root surface areas, and in 1963 Jepsen published the results of his research, which is summarized in Table 1-1. The results obtained by Boyd in 1958 are added for comparison.

Fig. 1-10 illustrates a healthy male patient 22 years of age with the mandibular second bicuspid and maxillary first bicuspid missing. Since the maxillary first bicuspid was extracted shortly after eruption, the remaining posterior maxillary teeth have moved mesially to restore the integrity of the arch and at the same time have maintained an acceptable axial relationship. Although a small diastema now presents between the maxillary left

cuspid and second bicuspid tooth, the situation could be regarded as stable and a satisfactory compromise for the loss of the first bicuspid. The opposing mandibular arch shows some mesial tipping of the first and second molars, but the difference in long-axis parallelism of the first bicuspid and first molar is not significant. Fig. 1-11, a radiograph of the area at the crown preparation stage, shows the crown-root ratio of the first bicuspid and first molar to be ideal for bridge construction. No periodontal disease exists and the morphologic characteristics of the abutment roots is more than satisfactory. By applying Ante's law, the two abutment teeth would account for over 600 mm² of pericemental area, more than sufficient to support the missing second bicuspid at approximately 200 mm². If, however, the mandibular first molar was also missing, the abutment teeth (i.e., the first bicuspid and second molar) would now have to support two missing teeth instead of one, a total of an approximately 630 mm² pericemental area if we accept Jepsen's measurements of tooth root surfaces. The second molar

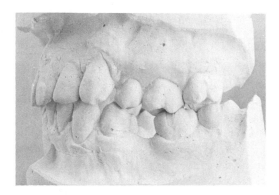

Fig. 1-10. Maxillary first bicuspid has been extracted shortly after eruption. Maxillary second bicuspid and first and second maxillary molars have moved mesially, maintaining a good axial relationship. A three-tooth bridge replacing mandibular second bicuspid will improve the occlusion and masticatory function of patient's left side.

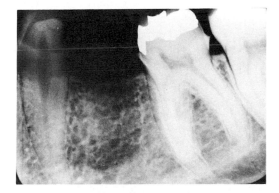

Fig. 1-11. Two prepared ideal abutment preparations for a three-tooth bridge. Although apex of first bicuspid root is not visible, combined pericemental area of both abutment teeth roots would account for over 600 mm², more than adequate to compensate for the missing second bicuspid at approximately 200 mm².

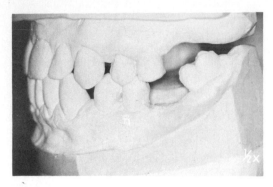

Fig. 1-12. Mandibular left posterior arch shows mesial tipping of second molar and posterior drifting of first and second bicuspids accompanied by partial rotation, after extraction of first molar. Some degree of overeruption of first bicuspid and second molar also exists. After osseous surgery for the correction of periodontal condition, combined pericemental area of cuspid, bicuspids, and second molar will approximate 480 mm², sufficient to compensate for missing first molar and to provide stability to mobile abutments.

and first bicuspid together account for only 606 mm² of pericemental support, an amount that falls short of the 630 mm² required to fulfill the principles of Ante's law. In this hypothetic case the selection of abutment teeth to support the proposed bridge should also include the mandibular left cuspid, which would then increase the pericemental support to approximately 870 mm². So far, the selection of abutment teeth has only been considered for the patient who presents with no serious etiologic factors, no periodontal disease, and therefore no concomitant loss of supporting bone. Fig. 1-12 illustrates an extreme case where bone loss from periodontal disease has been significantly complicated by tooth loss and subsequent tooth movement. In such a case the treatment by fixed bridgework is further compounded by the existence of occlusal interferences, supraeruption of the teeth, and mesial tipping of the mandibular second molar. These abnormal factors must be corrected prior to periodontal treatment and the subsequent construction of the mandibular bridge. To correct the reverse bony architecture resulting from the periodontal disease, the periodontist has indicated that osseous surgery involving the mandibular cuspid, first and second bicuspid, and second molar will reduce bone support about these teeth to less than one half the normal amount and will leave the teeth in a mobile condition. Therefore to replace the missing first molar tooth not only will the two bicuspids have to be utilized as abutment teeth but also the mandibular left cuspid, if Ante's law is to be satisfied. Obviously there are a number of other unfavorable conditions besides bone loss from periodontal disease, which may exist and contribute to modifications of Ante's law. These conditions may be summarized in Table 1-2.

It becomes increasingly obvious when dealing with the variety of patients that present for dental treatment that no fixed rules and regulations can apply to any one particular patient. In each case the abnormalities must be identified and their degree of seriousness assessed before the appliance to restore the lost teeth is designed.

MULTIPLE ABUTMENTS

In most bridges an abutment tooth is required at each end of the edentulous space to be restored. However, additional terminal abutment teeth are often required when the space to be restored replaces two or more contiguous teeth. Fig. 1-13 illustrates a case in which two posterior and an anterior edentulous space exists. The remaining teeth are periodontally involved when one can probe an average of 5 mm, which, when corrected with judicious osseous surgery will further reduce the overall bone support and may leave some of the teeth in a mobile condition. If the overall bone support after periodontal treatment is re-

Table 1-2. Factors modifying Ante's law

Condition existing	Probable modification in Ante's law
1. Bone loss from periodontal disease	Increase the number of abutments used for support
2. Mesial or distal tipping or changes in axial inclination	Increase the number of abutments used for support
3. Migration (bodily movement) of abutment teeth decreasing mesiodistal length of edentulous area	Decrease the number of abutments used (less pericemental support required)
4. Less than favorable opposing arch relationships producing increased occlusal load	Increase the number of abutments used for support
5. Endodontically restored abutment teeth with root resections	Increase the number of abutments used for support
6. Arch-form situations creating greater leverage factors	Increase the number of abutments used for support
7. Tooth mobility created after osseous surgery	Increase the number of abutments used for support (splinting procedure)

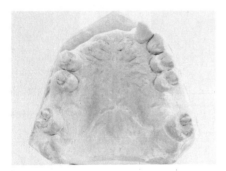

Fig. 1-13. Maxillary arch of patient with severe periodontal disease. After corrective periodontal surgery, bone support of remaining teeth will be reduced to less than one half the normal amount, rendering the teeth in a mobile condition. Since no complications of arch-to-arch relationships exist with occluding mandibular teeth, restoration of maxillary edentulous areas will be performed by splinting of all remaining abutment teeth together; thus a full-arch maxillary splint prosthesis is established.

duced to one half the normal amount, one will need to use all the remaining teeth as multiple abutments to restore the maxillary arch to integrity and function. The use of multiple abutments in such a case is referred to as a "splinting" procedure and implies the rigid connecting of two or more approximating teeth together. Splinting procedures are not only employed when the abutment teeth are

weakly supported or the edentulous space is long as in this example, but also when the occlusal plane is excessively curved or when the space includes a missing cuspid tooth. In all these situations additional abutment teeth are required to combat destructive forces that may arise as the result of unfavorable lever arms. Splinting of abutment teeth requires exact parallelism in preparation and placement and location of solder joints. Care must be exercised in preventing excessive contours of the casting, otherwise the natural embrasure space and form between the castings will be occluded. Solder joints must be properly placed to provide strength but should not be extended too far gingivally to cause food retention and subsequent tissue breakdown in the embrasure areas. Table 1-3, based on the conditions existing in a particular patient, will act as a guide in the selection of retainer types for a fixed bridge where the size of the space to be restored is arbitrarily designated as short, medium, or long.

DEVELOPING THE TREATMENT PLAN

At this stage of the patient's dental treatment a diagnosis of the patient's condition has been established, and the fact-finding leading up to the completion of

Table 1-3. Guide for selection of retainers according to varying spans

Length of span	Conditions existing	Selection of retainer type
Short span		
1. Cantilever (anterior maxilla replacing lateral incisor)	Good 1. Good crown-root ratio (no periodontal involvement) 2. No previous caries 3. No occlusal problems 4. Normal overbite, overjet relation	1. Pinledge retainer (V.I.P. system) 2. Intracoronal retainer 3. ¾ partial veneer crown
2. 3-T bridge	Good 1. Good crown-root ratio (no periodontal involvement) 2. No previous caries 3. No occlusal problems	1. Intracoronal retainers 2. Pin-ledge retainers (V.I.P.) 3. ¾ partial veneer crown
	Poor 1. Poor crown-root ratio 2. Some loss of bone 3. Occlusal factors need correcting 4. Previous caries experience	1. ¾ partial veneer crown 2. Complete veneer retainers 3. Splinting more than one abutment
Medium span		
3. 4-T bridge (2 pontics) (2 premolars) (1 premolar and 1 molar)	Good 1. Good crown-root ratio (no periodontal involvement) 2. No previous caries 3. No occlusal problems	1. ¾ partial veneer retainer 2. Extensive pinledge retainers 3. Complete veneer crowns
	Poor 1. Poor crown-root ratio 2. Some loss of bone 3. Some previous caries experience 4. Occlusal factors need correcting	1. Complete veneer crowns 2. Splinting more than one abutment
Long span		
4. Replacement of several teeth	Good 1. Good condition all around (no periodontal involvement)	1. Complete veneer crowns 2. Splinting more than one abutment 3. Lengthen crown surgically (increase incisogingival or occlusogingival length, or both)
	Poor 1. Periodontal involvement 2. Previous caries 3. Excessive bone loss 4. Tooth mobility	1. Complete veneer crowns (full arch splinting) 2. Partial denture (all types)

Student Name:

NORTHWESTERN UNIVERSITY
THE DENTAL SCHOOL

Student No.:

PLAN OF TREATMENT – FIXED AND REMOVABLE PROSTHODONTICS

Patient Name	Patient No.	Sex	Age	Marital Status	Date

Address — Phone No. — Occupation

SPECIAL POINTS OF DIAGNOSIS:

SUMMARY OF MOUTH PREPARATION:

RATIONALE FOR PROPOSED PLAN OF TREATMENT:

1

A

Fig. 1-14. A to **D,** Various pages of a special form designed for collection and integration of data necessary for treatment plan. *Continued.*

NUDS

SPECIAL ABUTMENT AND BRIDGE RETAINER PREPARATION

Tooth	Detailed Requirements

B

2

Fig. 1-14, cont'd

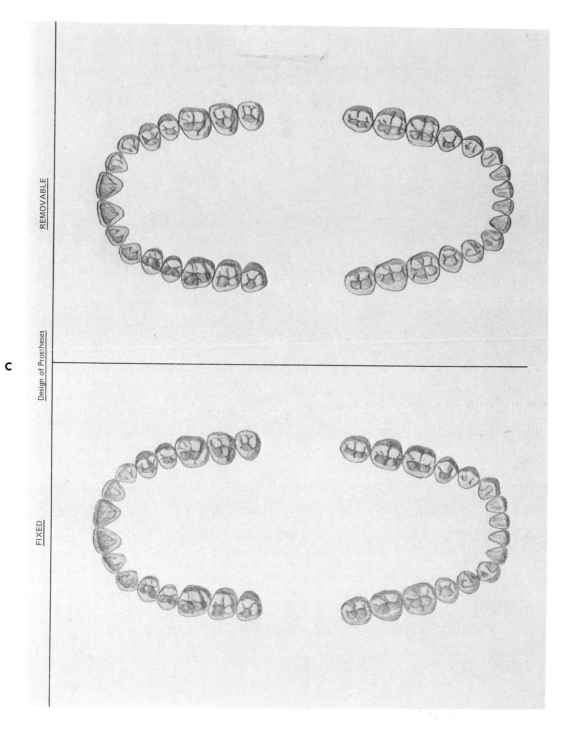

Fig. 1-14, cont'd

Continued.

NUDS

Details of prosthodontic treatment:

D

PROGNOSIS & ITS JUSTIFICATION:

PLAN OF TREATMENT APPROVED: Instructor

                                                                Instructor

Student Grade: . . . . Date

Fig. 1-14, cont'd

the patient's case history has been thoroughly investigated. Recognizing the fact that the patient's ultimate treatment will require fixed bridges or a combination of fixed and removable bridgework, it is advisable to use a special form for the collection and integration of data pertinent to these two clinical areas. Fig. 1-14, *A*, illustrates the first page of such a form requiring specific information in the areas of special points of diagnosis, summary of mouth preparation, and rationale for proposed plan of treatment. In a discussion of each of these areas in turn, the following information should be considered for each category:

Special points of diagnosis

The outstanding features of the case that make it different from routine dental care should be recorded. Consider the following areas:
1. General health, age, systemic disease (chronic or acute), types of medication, allergies, accident, and so forth
2. Clinical problems associated with analysis of the occlusion and articulation, assessment of occlusal vertical dimension, interocclusal clearance, and posterior path of closure
3. Presence of local clinical problems associated with severe bone loss, bruxism, attrition, unusual habit patterns, loss of vertical dimension, severe axial inclination, supraeruption and infraeruption, excessive fibrous tissue, and tooth mobility
4. Unusual and demanding esthetic requirements

Summary of mouth preparation

In this section an outline of the sequence of treatment required to restore the overall dental health of the patient should be recorded before one completes the treatment plan.
1. Overview of the treatment plan
   a. Evaluation of oral hygiene and occlusal analysis

b. Oral surgery
c. Periodontal treatment
d. Orthodontic treatment
e. Endodontic treatment
f. Operative dentistry
g. Fixed and removable prostheses
2. Clinical investigation and evaluation of all questionable teeth and their supporting tissue
3. Manner in which all phases of treatment will be coordinated

Rationale for proposed plan of treatment

This section requires a brief statement justifying the choice of a particular plan of treatment. Why has this particular plan of treatment been adopted? If the final choice of treatment is less than ideal, the reasons for the decision should be clearly stated. These reasons may be financial, the specific nature of the medical or dental condition, the time involved, the lack of dental appreciation, or the patient's availability for regularly scheduled appointments. Whatever the reason may be, it should be specifically recorded. It could have legal significance.

Special abutment preparation and selection of bridge retainers

Fig. 1-14, *B*, illustrates the second page of the form and is specifically directed to the recording of information for the individual teeth that have been selected as abutment teeth for fixed or removable bridgework.
1. List each tooth by number that is involved in either fixed or removable protheses that requires restoration.
2. Record the following information along with each abutment included in the prosthesis:
   a. Type of retainer and its design
   b. Modifications in preparation that may be required for supplemental retention, esthetics, and so forth
   c. Special requirements for splinting teeth that may be rendered

mobile after periodontal treatment

d. Special requirements for splinting teeth with a guarded periodontal prognosis

e. Modifications in preparation for partial denture abutments, that is, contour, guide planes, occlusal and cingulum rests, recessed reciprocating arms, location and amount of undercuts, and facings

f. Modifications of preparation required to receive intracoronal or extracoronal attachments—special attention should be paid to the alignment of preparations not necessarily in the same quadrant

Design of prostheses

Fig. 1-14, *C*, illustrates the third page of the combined fixed and removable treatment planning form and is specifically directed to the recording of the design of the prostheses. Two sets of the complete arch-form diagrams are presented, one to be used for the fixed prosthesis and the other for the removable prosthesis. The diagrams of the arch forms show the occlusal and incisal surface outlines, whereas the posterior teeth record a partial view of the buccal and lingual surfaces and the anterior teeth record most of the lingual surfaces but none of the labial.

The design of the prostheses should be indicated in both the fixed and removable sections, taking into account the following instructions:

1. Fixed prosthesis
   a. Indicate the outline of the abutment preparation in detail wherever possible. Make all drawings neatly and precisely.
   b. Use a color-coded system for abutment preparations, pontics, and so forth (for example, blue for abutment preparations and red for pontics).
   c. If splinting procedures are required within a single posterior

or a combination of both (cross-arch splinting), the solder joints should be indicated with an arrow located in the approximate embrasure space.

d. Horizontal nonparallel pin-retained abutment castings should be indicated by a short line running in a labiolingual or buccolingual direction. Vertical parallel pin–retained abutment castings or pinledge castings should be indicated by the placement of dots in the appropriate pin location.

e. If the category of bridge design is to be semifixed or cantilevered, it should be so stated in writing.

2. Removable prosthesis
   a. A precise diagram should indicate the location of saddle areas and retainers.
   b. Labels should indicate the type of retainer, amount of undercut, gage and type of wire if wrought, type of pontic including type of facing whether gum-set or not, details of acrylic anchorage, finish and seal lines, and guide planes.
   c. Any special feature that may be required and is not clear from an examination of the diagram on the cast model should be recorded on the diagram.
   d. Type of attachments and their location should be noted for partial or overlay dentures.

Details of treatment and prognosis

Fig. 1-14, *D*, illustrates the last page of the combined fixed and removable treatment planning form and is directed specifically to the details of prosthodontic treatment and the prognosis and its justification.

Details of prosthodontic treatment. In scheduling the details of treatment, the procedures that are to be achieved at each appointment should be listed on an appointment basis. All clinical and laboratory procedures should be included in this listing, with particular attention given to the following areas:

1. Preparation of tray for abutment teeth retainers; cases requiring precision attachments may require an impression of edentulous area (for example, 667).
2. Modifications in preparing abutment teeth (recessed areas and parallelism of axial walls on teeth on opposite sides of an arch may be required); adequate temporization.
3. Soldering procedure of precision attachments to castings and heat treatment.
4. Cement-fixed prostheses to protect precision attachments when necessary.
5. Prophylaxis, topical fluoride, and mouth preparation for removable ·prosthesis.
6. Fixed impression for removable prosthesis; incorporation of processing jigs into master cast (for example, 747, 604, 667).
7. Design of cast-metal partial framework with special notations if necessary (for example, gum-set teeth, retentive pins for precision attachments).
8. Try in the casting; index the precision attachment to framework, if necessary.
9. Take jaw relations (need for split-cast technique).
10. Trial insertion where necessary.
11. Insertion.
12. Postinsertion period—oral hygiene instruction, maintenance, prophylaxis, topical fluoride application.

All treatment procedures should be listed chronologically, particularly those involving both fixed and removable prostheses. The stages that need to be integrated should be clearly indicated. An estimated time for the completion of the case should be discussed with the patient. If all treatment procedures are properly listed in chronologic order, this should not be too difficult to assess.

Prognosis and its justification. A critical statement relating to the prognosis of the case should be recorded, not simply "good" or "poor." The evaluation of the prognosis should include an explanation of the reason, with attention to the patient's dental appreciation and cooperation, the supporting structures, occlusion, medical condition, and types of restorations. The prognosis should be related to the type of treatment performed, especially where less than optimal treatment has been carried out because of such limiting circumstances as personal, clinical, and financial problems.

SELECTED REFERENCES

1. Ante, I. H.: Abutments, J. Can. Dent. Assoc. **2:** 249-260, June 1936.
2. Beyron, H.: Occlusion: point of significance in planning restorative procedures, J. Prosthet. Dent. **30:**641-652, Oct. 1973.
3. Brehm, T. W.: Diagnosis and treatment planning for fixed prosthodontics, J. Prosthet. Dent. **30:**876-881, Dec. 1973.
4. Brown, M. H.: Causes and prevention of fixed prosthodontic failure, J. Prosthet. Dent. **30:**617-622, Oct. 1973.
5. Bull, A. W.: Diagnosis: a factor in the success of fixed partial dentures, J. Prosthet. Dent. **24:** 498-502, Nov. 1970.
6. Cavanagh, W. D.: Simplified crown and bridge treatment for the general practitioner, J. Can. Dent. Assoc. **25:**294-299, May 1959.
7. Coelho, D. H.: Present rationale of fixed restorations, J. Dent. Med. **7:**31-34, April 1952.
8. Coelho, D. H.: Criteria for the use of fixed prosthesis, Dent. Clin. North Am., pp. 299-311, March 1957.
9. Cohn, L. A.: Factors of dental occlusion pertinent to the restorative and prosthetic problem, J. Prosthet. Dent. **9:**256-277, March-April 1959.
10. Culpepper, W. D.: Concepts related to the preparation of teeth for fixed prosthodontics, J. Dent. Educ. **34:**258-262, Sept. 1970.
11. Dale, J. G.: Evaluation of proper procedures in oral diagnosis and their bearing on subsequent treatment planning, J. Can. Dent. Assoc. **24:** 511-527, Sept. 1958.
12. Davidson, G. B.: Diagnosis and treatment

planning in operative dentistry and in crown and bridge prosthesis, Dent. Clin. North Am., pp. 201-212, March 1963.

13. Douglas, G. D.: Principles of preparation design in fixed prosthodontics, J. Acad. Gen. Dent. **21**:25-29, March-April 1973.

14. Dykema, R. W.: Fixed prosthodontics, J. Tenn. Dent. Assoc. **42**:309-321, Oct. 1962.

15. Fridley, H. H., and Yurkstas, A.: Functional evaluation of fixed and removable bridgework, J. Dent. Res. **30**:475, Aug. 1951.

16. Greeley, J. H.: Planning for fixed prosthesis, J. Prosthet. Dent. **20**:412-416, Nov. 1968.

17. Herrick, P. W.: Classification of occlusal disharmony and restorations used pertinent to fixed bridge prosthesis, North-West Dent. **32**:92-102, April 1953.

18. Hursey, R. J., Jr.: Clinical survey of the failure of crown and bridge prosthesis, S. Carolina Dent. J. **16**:4-11, April 1958.

19. Kahn, A. E.: Considerations in the use of partial and full coverage in periodontal prosthesis, J. Prosthet. Dent. **15**:83-99, Jan.-Feb. 1965.

20. Ladenheim, R. N.: The temporary partial denture—its value and advantages in crown and bridge planning, J. Acad. Gen. Dent. **20**:13-16, May 1972.

21. Markley, M. R.: Broken-stress principle and design in fixed bridge prosthesis, J. Prosthet. Dent. **1**:416-423, July 1951.

22. Meadows, T. R.: Diagnosis and treatment: crown and bridge prosthodontics, J. Tenn. Dent. Assoc. **45**:425-30, Oct. 1965.

23. Mink, J. R.: Crown and bridge for the young adolescent, Dent. Clin. North Am., pp. 149-160, March 1966.

24. Moulton, G. H.: Functional demands of a posterior crown or bridge, J. Am. Dent. Assoc. **66**:534-536, Apr. 1963.

25. Moulton, G. H.: Importance of centric occlusion in diagnosis and treatment planning, J. Prosthet. Dent. **10**:921-926, Sept.-Oct. 1960.

26. Nuttall, E. B.: Diagnosis and correction of occlusal disharmonies in preparation for fixed restoration, J. Am. Dent. Assoc. **44**:399-408, April 1952.

27. Reed, O. M.: Why—fixed removable prosthesis, J. San Antonio Dent. Soc. **24**:10-11, March 1969.

28. Pugh, C. E.: Rationale for fixed prostheses in the management of advanced periodontal disease, Dent. Clin. North Am. **13**:243-262, Jan. 1969.

29. Ravinett, S.: Factors influencing fixed partial dentures for adolescents, J. Prosthet. Dent. **15**:880-888, Sept.-Oct. 1965.

30. Sauser, C. W.: Pretreatment evaluation of partially edentulous patients, J. Prosthet. Dent. **11**:886-893, Sept.-Oct. 1961.

31. Singer, F.: Co-report: indications for a fixed bridge, Int. Dent. J. **8**:352-353, disc. 359-60, 1958.

32. Shelby, D. S.: Tooth and tissue supported fixed partial dentures, J. Prosthet. Dent. **17**:590-595, June 1967.

33. Skurnik, H. R.: Treatment planning for occlusal rehabilitation, J. Prosthet. Dent. **9**:988-1000, Nov.-Dec. 1959.

34. Smith, G. P.: Factors affecting the choice of partial prosthesis—fixed or removable, Dent. Clin. North Am., pp. 3-12, March 1959.

35. Smyd, E. S.: Dental engineering as applied to inlay and bridge fabrication, N.Y. J. Dent. **21**:161-163, April 1951.

36. Tylman, S. D.: Crown and fixed bridge prosthesis: a phase of restorative dentistry, Int. Dent. J. **2**:457-467, June 1952.

37. Tylman, S. D.: Discussion of the biologic factors involved in the fixed partial denture, J. Can. Dent. Assoc. **23**:67-75, Feb. 1957.

38. Tylman, S. D.: Relationships of the structural design of dental bridges to their supporting tissues, Int. Dent. J. **13**:303-317, June 1963.

39. Tylman, S. D.: To what degree can the partially edentulous be rehabilitated by means of crowns and fixed bridges? J. Ontario Dent. Assoc. **30**:255-262, Aug.; 314-317, Oct. 1953.

40. Woodruff, H. S.: Construction of fixed bridges, N.Y. J. Dent. **21**:437-446, Dec. 1951.

41. Yurkstas, A., Fridley, H. H., and Manly, R. S.: Functional evaluation of fixed and removable bridgework, J. Prosthet. Dent. **1**:570-577, Sept. 1951.

GENERAL REFERENCES

Abramowsky, Z. L.: Splinting versus non-splinting of periodontally affected teeth, Anglo-Contin. Dent. Soc. **24**:12-17, April 1971.

Amsterdam, M., and Fox, L.: Provisional splinting—principles and techniques, Dent. Clin. North Am., pp. 73-99, March 1959.

Becker, R.: Semi-permanent periodontal splint. "A" splint, J. Mich. Dent. Assoc. **46**:306-309, Nov. 1964.

Ciancio, S., and Nisengard, R.: Resins in periodontal splinting, Dent. Clin. North Am. **19**:235-242, April 1975.

Chacker, F. M., and Serota, B. H.: Provisional periodontal prosthesis, Periodontics **4**:265-272, Sept.-Oct. 1966.

Cohn, L. A.: Integration of treatment procedures in occluso-rehabilitation, J. Prosthet. Dent. **7**:511, 1957.

Coppes, L.: Splinting, Acad. Rev. **13**:33-44, 1965.

Courant, P.: Use of removable acrylic splints in general practice, J. Can. Dent. Assoc. **33**:494-501, Sept. 1967.

Courtade, G. L.: Methods for pin splinting the lower anterior teeth, Dent. Clin. North Am. **14**:3-17, Jan. 1970.

Glickman, I., Stein, R. S., and Smulow, J. B.: Effect of increased functional forces upon the periodontium of splinted and non-splinted teeth, J. Periodontal. **32:**290-300, Oct. 1961.

Hileman, A. C.: Splinting and restorative dentistry in advanced periodontal disease, Caementum **23:**14-6, Jan. 1966.

Ivancie, G. P., and Fulkerson, R. D.: Periodontal splinting utilizing fixed prosthesis, J. Colorado Dent. Assoc. **43:**19-23, Dec. 1964.

Jantzen, J.: Definitive splinting, Quintessence Int. **1:**79-86, Feb. 1970.

Kallend, G. D.: Two-part posterior splintage, NACDL J. **15:**15, June 1968.

Larato, D. C.: Fixed splint for widely spaced mobile teeth, J. Prosthet. Dent. **20:**154-156, Aug. 1968.

Larato, D. C.: Immediate splint for stabilization of mobile teeth, Dent. Dig. **74:**11-3, Jan. 1968.

Levinson, E., and Gurr, R. H.: Splinting—a review and clinical investigation—preliminary report, J. Dent. Assoc. S. Africa **24:**284-288, Sept. 1969.

Linkow, L. I.: Abutments for full mouth splinting, J. Prosthet. Dent. **11:**920, Sept.-Oct. 1971.

Lytle, J. D.: Letter to the editor. Justification for splinting in periodontal therapy, J. Prosthet. Dent. **22:**704, Dec. 1969.

Meklas, J. F.: Splinting: a rationale, New Mex. Dent. J. **21:**13, 27-29, Feb. 1971.

Overby, G. E.: Esthetic splinting of mobile periodontally involved teeth by vertical pinning, J. Prosthet. Dent. **11:**112-118, 1961.

Overby, G. E.: Fixed-removable splinting technique in periodontics, Dent. Clin. North Am., pp. 197-211, March 1964.

Pound, E.: Cross arch splinting vs. premature extraction, J. Prosthet. Dent. **16:**1058-1068, Nov.-Dec. 1966.

Rateitschak, K. H.: The therapeutic effect of local treatment on periodontal disease assessed upon evaluation of different diagnostic criteria. 1. Changes in tooth mobility, J. Periodontol. **34:**540-544, 1963.

Rateitschak, K. H.: The therapeutic effect of local treatment on periodontal disease assessed upon evaluation of different diagnostic criteria. 2. Changes in gingival inflammation, J. Periodontol. **35:**155-159, 1964.

Rateitschak, K. H.: The therapeutic effect of local treatment on periodontal disease assessed upon evaluation of different diagnostic criteria. 3. Changes in appearance of bone, J. Periodontol. **35:**263-266, 1964.

Regan, J. E.: A simplified procedure for bilateral splinting of abutment teeth, J. Prosthet. Dent. **22:**544-554, Nov. 1969.

Rosen, H., and Gitnick, P. J.: Separation and splinting of the roots of multirooted teeth, J. Prosthet. Dent. **21:**34-38, Jan. 1969.

Renggli, H. H.: Splinting of teeth—an objective assessment, Helv. Odontol. Acta **15:**129-131, Oct. 1971.

Sayers, P.: A technique for splinting extremely mobile teeth, New Zeal. Dent. J. **62:**99-104, April 1966.

Waerhaug, J.: Letter to the editor. Justification for splinting in periodontal therapy, J. Prosthet. Dent. **22:**705, Dec. 1969.

Waerhaug, J.: Justification for splinting in periodontal therapy, J. Prosthet. Dent. **22:**201-208, Aug. 1969.

Weinberg, L. A.: Force distribution in splinted anterior teeth, Oral Surg. **10:**484, 1957.

Weiss, R. C.: A conservative and esthetic approach to intracoronal temporary splinting, J. Periodontol. **42:**590-591, Sept. 1971.

2

Biologic aspects of crown and bridge prosthodontics

Maury Massler

The purpose of this chapter is to bring into focus the fact that modern clinical prosthodontics demands of the clinician more than technical skill alone. The tooth is a living organ. The dentin contains cells whose nucleus protrudes into the pulp so that dentin and pulp are actually one connected tissue as are bones and bone marrow. Dentin is in fact a specialized bonelike tissue. It reacts to every insult imposed upon it from excessive attrition, abrasion, erosion, caries, and mode of cutting by either degenerative changes if the insult is severe, or by calcific repair if the damage is minor (Fig. 2-2). The periodontal ligament is also a vital and responsive tissue and the gingiva is a highly vascular modified mucosa frequently subjected to severe stresses, which would cause degeneration of most other soft tissues. Thus the prosthodontist must be concerned with the biologic aspects of his procedures as well as the technology if he seeks long-term success for his restorations or appliances as well as comfort for his patients (Fig. 2-1).

Another point that must be constantly kept in mind is that a single tooth does not stand alone. Each tooth is in dynamic balance with its neighbor at each side of it and with the opposing teeth. Each quadrant of teeth must mesh with the opposing quadrant and the whole must balance in a nontraumatic functional or "balanced occlusion."[1] Failure to analyze and take into account the occlusal forces acting upon a given tooth or quadrant of teeth when one plans a three-unit bridge, or even a single crown or onlay, invites unbalanced and destructive forces that shorten the life of the prosthesis.

The sophisticated prosthodontist goes even further. He recognizes that the physical forces acting upon the teeth must take into account the articulating mechanism of the jaws and the dental arches—the temporomandibular joint (TMJ) and musculature. An abnormal TMJ, whether tilted or unevenly articulated, causes unbalanced occlusal forces to strike upon the dental arches or individual teeth and shortens its functional life-span with great discomfort to the patient.[2] A good prosthodontist is therefore part orthodontist.[3] Both must pay attention to muscular balance (the lingual versus the buccal and labial muscle mass) as well as the strength of the patient's musculature.[4] Fixed or removable appliances constructed for a powerful male with massive masseter muscles must be designed differently for the delicate young woman who is sensitive to every slight defect in her natural or artificial dentition. Her tissues do not tolerate even expertly constructed prostheses. She tends to feel the appliance as a "foreign body."

As if all this were not complex enough, we must now add the influence of the oral

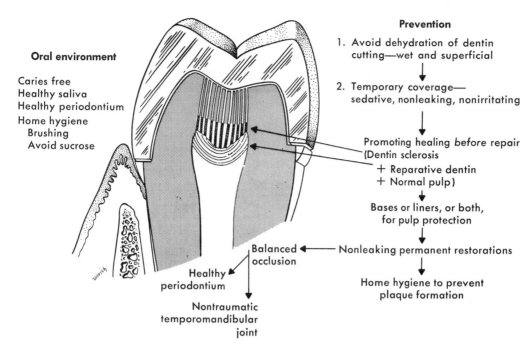

Prevention

1. Avoid dehydration of dentin cutting—wet and superficial

2. Temporary coverage— sedative, nonleaking, nonirritating

Promoting healing *before* repair (Dentin sclerosis + Reparative dentin + Normal pulp)

Bases or liners, or both, for pulp protection

Nonleaking permanent restorations

Home hygiene to prevent plaque formation

Oral environment

Caries free
Healthy saliva
Healthy periodontium
Home hygiene
  Brushing
  Avoid sucrose

Balanced occlusion

Healthy periodontium

Nontraumatic temporomandibular joint

Fig. 2-1. Diagram showing some biologic aspects that should be considered during crown and bridge construction. Oral environment must be made clean and free of cariogenic plaques and periodontal disease before restorations are delivered. Cavity preparation must not be injurious to pulp. Temporary and permanent coverage must not be injurious to tissues. Bases or liners should be used to protect the pulp and keep the tooth insulated from thermal and galvanic shock. Occlusion must be carefully balanced lest the temporomandibular joint becomes uncomfortable or injured.

environment, which bathes the teeth. The wet salivary environment contains hordes of living microorganisms, a variety of chemical compounds partly ionized but mostly bound to a variety of proteins. Saliva is a very complex and as yet poorly investigated fluid. Many foods in transit to the stomach cause temperature changes in the mouth that can destroy many new and old fillings by opening their margins. Since all restorations leak in the mouth, heat-insulating bases must be placed under all deep restorations, and cavity liners to seal the opened dentinal tubules should be placed under all shallow cavities.[5] This will effectively prevent salivary products from penetrating into the pulp.

If these complex biologic and physical variables were not enough to test the

acumen and abilities of even the most educated clinician, there is the human being attached to the teeth. Many patients present complex and variable behavior problems to the clinician seeking to restore a damaged and sometimes mutilated dentition. The fearful patient who refuses all attempts to educate her and the mercenary patient who rejects anything but cheap patchwork cause problems that modify treatment plans. Attempts to educate a fearful patient are at times frustrating, since the patient's anxiety blocks his logical thinking. He is afraid of any prolonged pain. Great patience on the part of the dentist is mandatory. Another patient may be concerned about the high cost of lengthy and careful treatment. For whatever reasons, he prefers the cheaper patchwork. The conscientious clinician must discuss these problems with his patient.

This chapter is directed toward the middle-aged and aging (geriatric) patients since they form the bulk of a prosthodontist's practice. He or she is different from the child and the young adult. The tissues have changed considerably and the response of the dentin, pulp, periodontal ligament, supporting bone, and gingivae to chemical and physical insults have become modified. These tissues change as much as the skin, eyes, hearing, and musculature and joints in other parts of the body. All this must be taken into consideration if the clinician dealing with a living biologic complex is to succeed above the level of the technician. Therefore, technical skill is not enough. The clinician must possess a

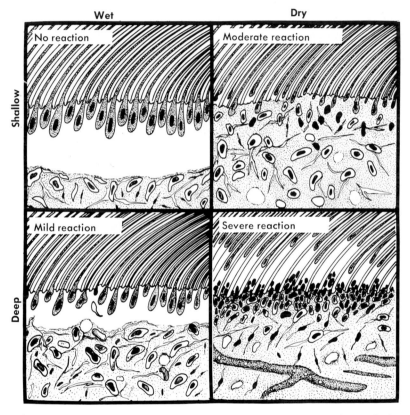

Fig. 2-2. Drawings illustrating pulpal reactions to operative procedures. *Left and right,* Compare cutting wet versus cutting dry. Upper compares shallow cuts (as for crowns) versus cutting deep (as for deep inlays). *Upper left,* Cutting shallow and wet shows no pulpal reaction. Note normal arrangement of odontoblastic layer and cell-free layer of Weil beneath. *Upper right,* Cutting dry results in dehydration even in a shallow preparation. Note aspiration of odontoblastic nuclei into dentinal tubules and invasion of cells into layer of Weil. Compare with *lower left* when a deep cavity preparation was made under a stream of water. The reaction is much milder and returned to normal in 30 days when cutting wet. *Lower right,* Severe reaction when a deep cavity preparation is made dry under a rubber dam. Note aspirated odontoblastic nuclei, invasion of cells and capillaries into cell-free layer of Weil, and engorged vessels deeper into the pulp. See also Tables 2-1 and 2-2 for further details. (From Weiss, M. B., Massler, M., and Spence, J. M.: Dent. Progr. **4:**6, 1963.)

strong biologic background and become a self-taught psychologist if he is to succeed in the field of prosthodontics. This chapter attempts to balance the many advances made in dental technology with some of the many advances made in oral biology toward implementing the broader concepts emerging from total patient care.

EFFECTS OF CAVITY AND CROWN PREPARATIONS
Effects of cavity depth

All cavity preparations produce some damage to the protoplasm within the tubules of the dentin and the nucleus of the odontoblasts. This damage can be very slight if the dentin is cut superficially

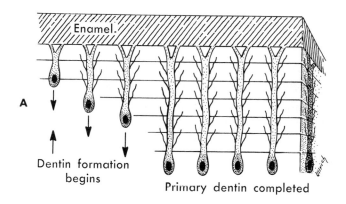

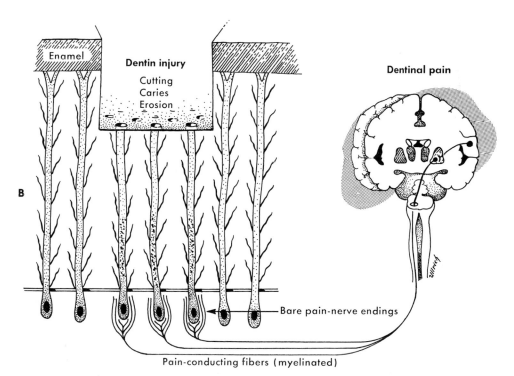

Fig. 2-3. A, Dentin formation. **B,** Pathways of pain from dentin. Note sclerosis under injured dentinal tubules.

wet, as for the usual full-crown preparation (Fig. 2-2). However the pain sensation is greatest when cutting is done at or just below the dentinoenamel junction (Fig. 2-3) because the protoplasmic branchings of the dentinal cell are greatest in this area, especially in young and previously uninjured dentin. Pain reaction becomes less as the cut is deepened, although damage to the odontoblast is increased. For example, superficial abrasion of the skin is more painful but less damaging than is a deep cut by a sharp razor.

Cutting to within 50 micrometers (μm) of the pulp produces as much damage as a bloodless pulp exposure so that indirect therapy to promote the formation of reparative dentin should be instituted before one attempts any further cavity preparation or even takes impressions.[7] Thus a deep preparation on the proximal surface for a large inlay is more destructive to the odontoblasts involved, than is

Table 2-1. Effects of operative procedures on the adult pulp

Operative procedure	Pulp reaction	Number specified	Burned dentin	Odonto-blastic layer	Subodonto-blastic zone of Weil	Body of pulp
Shallow wet	None	41	None	Normal	Normal	Normal
Deep wet	Mild	96	Small isolated areas usually in corners of cavity	1. Vacuoles or hemorrhage under areas of burned dentin 2. Disarrangement of odontoblasts 3. Reaction limited to cut tubules	Invasion by capillaries or inflammatory cells under areas of burned dentin; other areas essentially normal	Essentially normal
Shallow dry	Moderate	52	Larger area covering entire floor; does not penetrate deeply; dentin is a good thermal insulator	1. Aspirated nuclei of odontoblasts 2. Large vacuoles containing serum (edema) 3. Capillaries 4. Hemorrhage 5. Reduction in size and number of cells	Hemorrhage: invasion by capillaries and inflammatory cells into area under cavity	Engorgement of large vessels; thrombosis of some small vessels; increased numbers of inflammatory cells
Deep dry	Severe	36	Extensive; on walls as well as on floor; penetrates deeply into dentin	1. Cell body shrunken 2. Absence of odontoblasts 3. Large vacuoles filled with serum 4. Thrombosed capillaries	1. Large area of edema 2. Large and small blood vessels filled with coagulum 3. Many cells of inflammation	1. Coagulum in large vessels 2. Increase in density of ground substance
Total		225				

From Weiss, M. B., Massler, M., and Spence, J. M.: Dent. Progr. **4:**6, 1963.

the more extensive but more superficial crown preparation (Tables 2-1 to 2-3).

In this context, I should point out that ceramic-faced crowns, which require a deep labial shelf to accommodate the bulk of ceramic plus metal casting, also cut deeply toward the pulp and produce an effect upon the pulp similar to a deep proximal box. Since the gingival margin

Table 2-2. Reaction of dentin to operative procedures

	Acute injury
Mild reaction	a. Increased permeability of dentinal tubules
	b. Pulpodentinal membrane disrupted
	c. Odontoblastic layer disturbed
	c_1. Vacuolization between cells
	c_2. Beginning atrophy of cell body
	c_3. Nuclei migrate into tubules
	c_4. Complete atrophy of odontoblastic layer
	d. Subodontoblastic cell-free layer of Weil invaded by
	d_1. Small round cells
	d_2. Fibroblasts
	d_3. Capillaries
	e. Subodontoblastic body of pulp
Severe reaction	e_1. Cell infiltration
	e_2. Thrombosis of vessels
	e_3. Hemorrhage

Table 2-3. Clinical characteristics of dentinal and pulpal pains

Dentinal pain	Pulpal pain
Sharp lancinating pain	Dull throbbing ache
Easily located	Poorly localized
Stimuli: touch, cold, acid, dehydration	Responds slowly to heat or increased venous pressure during sleep
Origin: pain fibers around odontoblasts	Origin: pain fibers arising from pericytes around arterioles
Trigger: acetylcholine (?)	Trigger: inflammatory exudate or toxins
Conducted along small myelinated fibers in nerve trunk	Conducted along large unmyelinated fibers in nerve trunk

of all restorations is the most vulnerable to leakage and pulp damage, protection for this margin is especially necessary before, during, and after the restoration is completed. Under leaking temporary fillings or acid cement bases, recovery takes much longer or may not occur at all.

Effects of age

Cutting of dentinal tubules previously exposed by attrition or very slow caries is much less painful and less injurious to the pulp because the contents of the tubules have become modified (calcified or degenerated) and considerable reparative dentin has formed within the pulp.

Cutting wet versus cutting dry

The controversy of those who believe that physiologic considerations (that is, dentinal and pulpal protection) must be respected while one cuts through the living protoplasmic contents of the dentinal tubules versus those who believe that such damage is minimal when one cuts dry is now resolved through both experimental and clinical evidence.

Cutting dry causes the nucleus of the odontoblast to be drawn up (aspirated) into the tubule (Fig. 2-4). This produces a very painful response after the anesthetic wears off.[8] The postoperative sensitivity or pain does not disappear until the nucleus returns to its original position within the pulpal end of the odontoblastic process about 2 or 3 days later. The discomfort to the patient is not worth the increased visibility for the operator.

In addition to and concomitant with the aspiration of the nucleus into the dentinal tubule, excessive dehydration of the cut tubules produces a flow of liquid from the pulpal end into the dentinal floor. Whether this moisture is the "lymph" claimed by Bodecker or fluid from the pulp has not yet been determined.

In any case, physiologic cutting of either hard tissue (bone) or soft connective tissue should be done in a wet field to

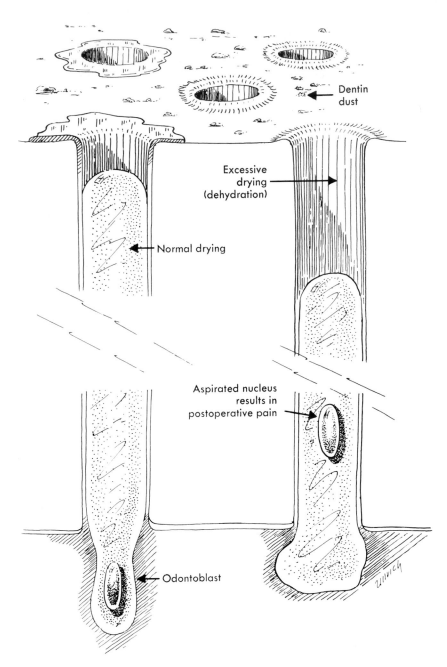

Fig. 2-4. Effects of dehydration of freshly cut dentin by cutting dry, using warm air for prolonged periods, and applying volatile chemicals such as chloroform, ether, or acetone. (From Brännström, M.: J. Prosthet. Dent. **20:**165-171, 1968.)

preserve the vitality of the protoplasm and the cells. Dentin is a living cellular calcified structure and its cellular contents should be protected.

Cleansing the cavity preparation

Cutting of enamel and dentin results in the production of debris (dust), which clings to the dentinal floor and interferes with proper cementation of the casting (Fig. 2-5).

Enamel crystals and shattered enamel rods are relatively large (5 to 20 μm) and are easily removed by thorough "flushing" of the preparation with a stream of warm water and wiping with moist cotton pellets. This removes most of the large particles. However, dentinal dust particles (2 to 5 μm) cling more tenaciously and the very small "dust" particles (0.5 to 2 μm) hang on to the cleanest floor as if by electrostatic attraction[9] (Fig. 2-5).

Acid cleansers have been used to remove these almost invisible dust particles. These remove the cavity dust, but at a high price (Fig. 2-6). The acids cause funneling of the opened ends of the dentinal tubules, dissolve also the outer ring of hypercalcified peritubular dentin (thus producing a softened cavity floor), and most importantly increase the permeability of the dentinal tubules so that penetration is greatly increased from the filling materials (tin and mercury from amalgam, monomer from plastics, and acids from cements) or from salivary ions if the margins leak (and *all* margins leak).

At present, the method of cleansing the cavity preparation, without damage to dentinal cells or pulp, is through the use

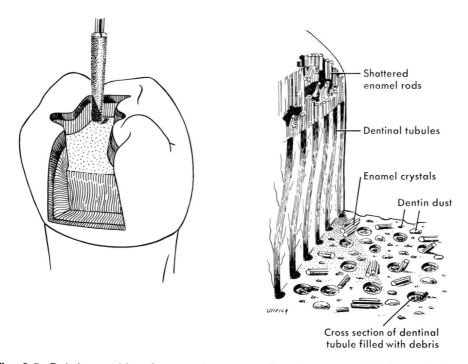

Shattered enamel rods

Dentinal tubules

Enamel crystals

Dentin dust

Cross section of dentinal tubule filled with debris

Fig. 2-5. Debris resulting from cavity preparation. Large crystals from shattered enamel rods can be removed by being flushed out with warm water. Larger particles of dentin dust can also be washed out. But very small particles adhere tightly to the cavity floor and fill the open dentinal tubules. These cannot be easily removed with water spray. Hydrogen peroxide is more effective. (From Brännström, M., and Johnson, G.: J. Prosthet. Dent. **31**(4):422-430, 1974.)

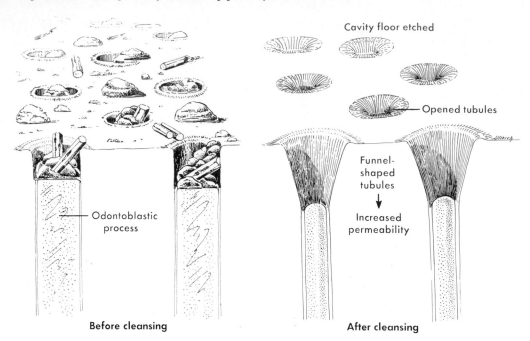

Fig. 2-6. Effects of acid cleansers upon freshly cut dentinal tubules. Although dentinal and enamel debris is removed, acid etches dentin floor and opens dentinal tubules. Acid then can penetrate into pulp and damages odontoblasts and causes engorgement of blood vessels in pulp. (From Brännström, M., and Johnson, G.: J. Prosthet. Dent. **31**(4):422-430, 1974.)

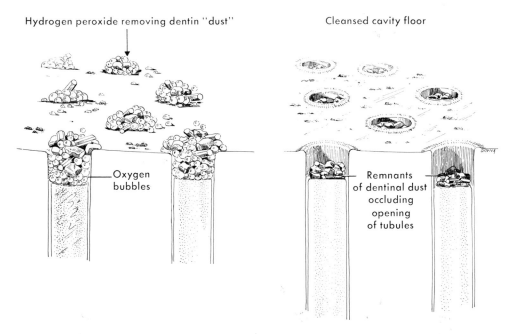

Fig. 2-7. Action of hydrogen peroxide (3%) as a cavity cleanser. This removes dentin dust effectively without damage to dentin or pulp. (From Brännström, M., and Johnson, G.: J. Prosthet. Dent. **31**(4):422-430, 1974.)

of 3% peroxide (Fig. 2-7). Peroxide is compatible with living tissues, as witness its use to debride soft-tissue wounds. The bubbling action of the oxygen (released by the peroxidase in the protoplasm) effectively removes even the smallest dust particles from the cavity floor.

It is not possible to cement a ceramic tile on a dusty concrete floor. Similarly, dust particles remaining under the cement of a crown or inlay will prevent adherence of the cement to the dentin.

Dentinal pain versus pulpal pain

It is important for the clinician to distinguish between dentinal pain and pulpal pain when dealing with a deep carious lesion or a very deep cavity preparation to determine whether the pulp has been injured beyond repair (necessitating endodontic therapy) or is still capable of recovery and healing. Many painful pulps can be saved by biologically sound, indirect pulp therapy and a period of rest to allow for repair; thus the vitality of both the pulp and the dentin are preserved.

Dentinal pain is characterized by a sharp lancinating quality and is initiated only after a specific stimulus such as cold, touch, acid, or sugar (Table 2-3). This pain sensorium is the result of injury to a living cell (the odontoblast), which releases a chemical substance (probably acetylcholine, according to Avery and Rapp, 1959) at the nuclear end of the dentinal cell that triggers off the pain impulse in the bare pain fibers from the pulp that surrounds the cell (Fig. 2-3).

In contrast, pulpal pain is recognized as a dull throbbing ache, a characteristic of all *deep* pain. This type of pain is a "vascular pain." The pulp is richly endowed with arterioles, which expand in response to inflammatory products, heat, physical trauma, and noxious substances. Nerve fibers (type A) originate from the contractile cells, which envelope all arterioles, and join the main nerve trunk.[10] These are

large unmyelinated fibers, in contrast to the small heavily myelinated and insulated nerve fibers that come from the odontoblasts.

Pulpal pain is a diffuse, not easily localized type of pain (coursing along unmyelinated fibers) that becomes worse when heat is applied to the tooth and when one lies down (which increases the venous pressure and causes a backup of blood in the arterioles). Cold relieves this "congested" pulpal pain, whereas cold elicits the dentinal pain (Table 2-3).

The patient should know that not all toothaches are reasons for extracting the tooth or the pulp. One can cause dentinal pain by cutting the protoplasmic ends of the odontoblasts. This pain is more severe if the cutting is dry. Cutting wet leaves the pulp less affected.

Effects of clamps and rubber dam applications

There is little doubt that cutting cavity and crown preparations under the rubber dam produces superior restorations, all other things being equal, including the operator's skill. However, placement of the rubber dam requires the use of a clamp. Proper and careful placement of the clamp requires practice and a modicum of skill to avoid damage to the cementum or the gingivae. The young tissue of the child and adolescent can quickly recover from such abuse. But this is not true in the middle-aged patient. The clamp must be applied with much greater caution and skill or damage to cementum (with subsequent painful exposed and injured dentin) and to the gingivae may be irreversible (Fig. 2-8).

SPLIT-TOOTH SYNDROME
Cracked enamel

Cracks in the enamel of anterior teeth occur very frequently and are more common as age advances. Incisal chippings are frequent in the older population. Cracked enamel can be very painful to

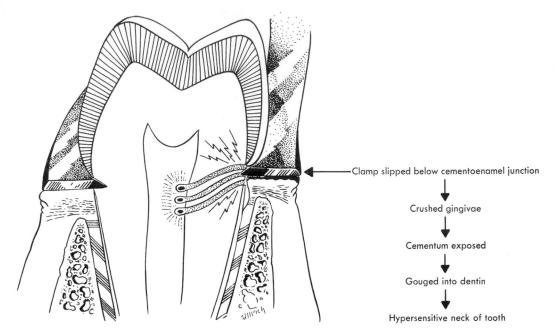

Fig. 2-8. Effect of clamps on gingivae and dentin. Cervical hypersensitivity after prolonged operative procedures under a rubber dam may be caused by clamp slipping below cementoenamel junction and gouging into cementum and dentin. This exposes dentinal tubules to oral environment (cold, touch, acid foods, and saliva) with postoperative pain resulting.

both old and young teeth if these cracks reach the dentinoenamel junction, and before the cracks are filled in with salivary debris (Fig. 2-9, *A*). In older teeth the cracks are filled in with a brown pellicle from the saliva similar to the brown pellicle that fills the occlusal pits and fissures in elderly people. One can visualize these cracks by applying a dye (such as toluidine blue 0.5% or erythrosine) to the enamel.

Cracks in the enamel may be caused by blows, biting on nuts, chicken bones, and perhaps extremes of temperature (ice cream after hot soup) since the enamel is a crystalline structure with very little flexibility. In the moist oral environment, cracked enamel adheres to the underlying dentin but separates easily after extraction and drying.

Filling in the painful cracks in young teeth can be hastened by topical application of stannous fluoride solution, 4% to 8%.

Cracked cusps

In posterior teeth, cusps adjacent to large, bulky metallic fillings may suddenly crack off during ordinary chewing. Cuspal fractures may be caused by overexpansion of the filling (usually an amalgam) because of excessive heat combined with marginal caries, which undermines the cusp (Fig. 2-9, *B*). Therefore, when very little dentin is left to support the cusp and the cusp stands alone as an island surrounded by amalgam, it is better to "shoe" the cusp and bind it to the tooth with a cast gold onlay.

Crazing of dentin

Dentin is much more flexible than the crystalline enamel because of its organic content (about 35%) and is therefore not

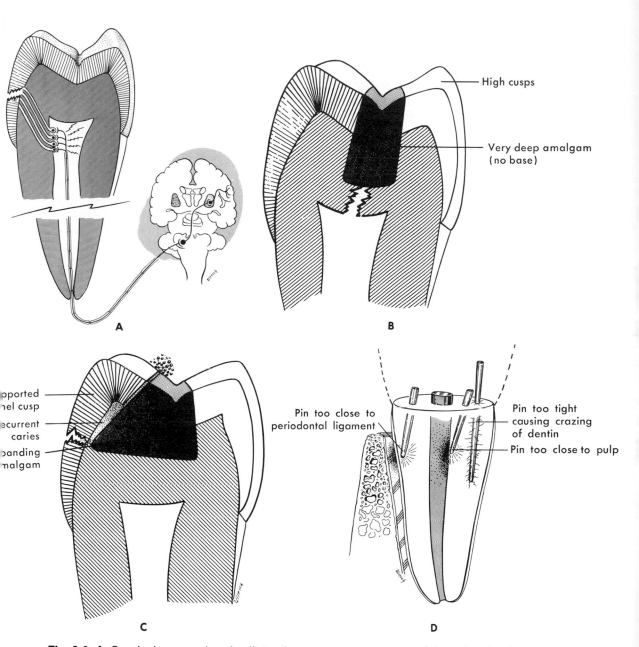

Fig. 2-9. A, Cracks in enamel and split teeth are a common cause of sharp lancinating pain during mastication. **B,** Split dentin. **C,** Cracked cusp. **D,** Biologic effects of pins. Pins placed under amalgams can be a source of discomfort when placed too close to pulp. Thermal changes from restoration to pulp through pin may produce pain. Pins placed too close to periodontal ligament may result in pain on biting. Pins placed too forcibly into dentin may cause crazing of dentin and dentinal pain. (**A** from Stanley, H.: In Clark, J. W., editor: Clinical dentistry, New York, 1976, Harper & Row, Inc.)

easily split but rather crazed, that is, fine hairlike multiple separations occur under excessive internal strains. The introduction of multiple pins to restore badly broken-down vital teeth and implanted post and core in endodontically treated teeth, has made possible the restoration of thousands of teeth otherwise doomed to extraction only a few years ago. However, excessive use of pins and excessive use of force in implanted posts can cause crazing of the dentin and even splitting of the tooth (Fig. 2-9, *C*).

Even properly placed pins in vital teeth can cause pain if placed very close to the pulp. Pins can transmit heat from the metallic restoration above almost directly into the pulp.

Split crown and root

Splitting of the crown or the root so that the pulp is breached but the tooth parts appear intact usually results when a very deep but narrow metallic filling is placed close to the pulp, without a base in premolar teeth with high cusps (Fig. 2-9, *D*). Excessive forces such as cracking a nut with the bicuspids can force the cusps apart and split the crown. A sharp lancinating pain is felt at the moment of cracking, but this pain disappears as the elastic dentin cusps return to close the crack. Thereafter, a sharp lancinating pain is felt intermittently and on biting. Most patients avoid biting on that tooth thereafter and seek relief from the dentist. However, since the crown or root fracture is not visible clinically nor in the x-ray film, the tooth is regarded as "normal" and the pain termed "of unknown origin" or "idiopathic." Positive diagnosis can be established by prying the cusps apart or having the patient bite cautiously on a wooden prop.[11]

Split roots are more difficult to detect than split crowns and are more often caused by large screw pins inserted with too much force. Diagnosis can be made by a history of intermittent sharp pain over a relatively long period of time. A sharp lancinating pain is elicited upon initiation or release of chewing pressure. When the pain is elicited upon release of biting pressure, the chances are that the fracture is incomplete and very difficult to demonstrate. Pulp testing gives a normal response. Hot gutta-percha or ice does *not* usually give a significant response or clue.

The split crown and root can be tied together with a carefully fitted crown, but preparation of the crown can cause further splitting of the tooth fragments. Root canal therapy is contraindicated, since such procedure forces the fragments farther apart. Most patients who suffer from the pain of undiagnosed split roots, with no relief over a long period of time, prefer extraction of the split tooth to further suffering.

EFFECTS OF VARIOUS RESTORATIONS
Silver amalgam

Advantages, limitations, and prevention. The following are biophysical effects of amalgam restorations.
Advantages
1. Plastic material, which can be manipulated readily
2. Cavity preparation less critical than for castings
3. Can be inserted into small preparations and into areas difficult to reach
4. Resists mastication fairly well
5. Relatively insoluble in oral fluids
Limitations
1. Oxidized readily (as silver sulfide and mercuric sulfide)
2. Corrodes much more rapidly than do previous metals (pitting)
3. Relatively high galvanic action
4. Darkens tooth substances by penetration of tin and mercury into dentinal tubules
5. Marginal leakage prominent immediately after insertion (marginal leakage tends to diminish after 3 to 6 months because of sealing of mar-

gins by corrosion products and salivary materials)

6. Percolation, facilitated by opening of and closing of margins because of expansion and contraction in hot and cold solutions

Prevention of deleterious effects

1. Use of nonacid cement base (reinforced with zinc oxide–eugenol cement preferred)
2. Use of copal resin varnish on walls and floor of cavity preparation to seal the space between tooth and amalgam (Fig. 2-8)

Disadvantages

Corrosion. Amalgam is a very useful, even essential, restorative material in dental practice. However, in the wet salivary environment, its metallic ions react with the high sulfide content of the saliva. The results are discoloration and corrosion of the filling with pitting and serious marginal defects (Fig. 2-10). Darkening of the dentin is caused by the penetration of tin and mercuric ions. This discoloration is prevented by the use of a proper insulating base or liner.

Marginal leakage. Because amalgam is

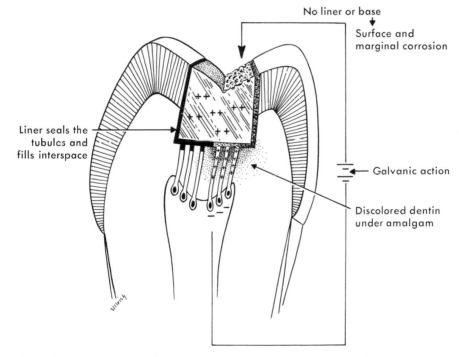

Fig. 2-10. Effects of oral environment on amalgam. Sulfides in saliva cause oxidation and corrosion of amalgam surfaces. Clinically, restoration becomes dark because of formation of metallic sulfides. Salivary sulfides and glycoproteins penetrate into marginal interspace and also cause corrosion products. These tend to reduce marginal leakage of amalgams. Amalgam is thus a self-sealing type of filling material in a non–caries active oral environment. If neither a liner nor a base is used under amalgam, metallic ions (mercury and tin) penetrate and discolor underlying dentin. Newly inserted amalgams have a strong galvanic action unless insulated from pulp.

A resin type of liner is used to seal freshly cut dentinal tubules and to fill marginal interspace. This prevents discoloration of underlying dentin and reduces surface corrosion. A nonacid base accomplishes the same results and also acts as a thermal insulator in a deep cavity close to the pulp. (From Massler, M.: In Clark, J. W., editor: Clinical dentistry, New York, 1976, Harper & Row, Inc.)

not adhesive to the walls of the cavity but merely abuts closely to them, a capillary space exists between the restoration and the cavity walls from 4 μm to approximately 20 μm in width at constant temperature (Fig. 2-10). These margins open and close as ingested hot and cold foods cause expansion or contraction of the metal. This is termed "marginal percolation." All fillings are therefore tested for marginal leakage in the laboratory by being cycled in hot and cold water.[5]

Marginal leakage decreases in vivo as corrosion products (metallic sulfides) and salivary materials fill into the marginal interspace (Fig. 2-10). Clinical impres-

sions suggest that this self-sealing of amalgam margins proceeds rapidly in the caries-free mouth, but slowly, if at all, in caries, active mouths. In the caries-active oral environment, penetration by cariogenic streptococci may cause marginal caries and prevent marginal sealing. This is a primary reason for eliminating *all* cariogenic plaques and *all* infected dentin from *all* precarious and carious lesions *before* one places any restorations or appliances in the mouth and institutes good home hygiene practices before beginning extensive restorative procedures.[12]

The deleterious effects of marginal leakage upon the underlying dentin and

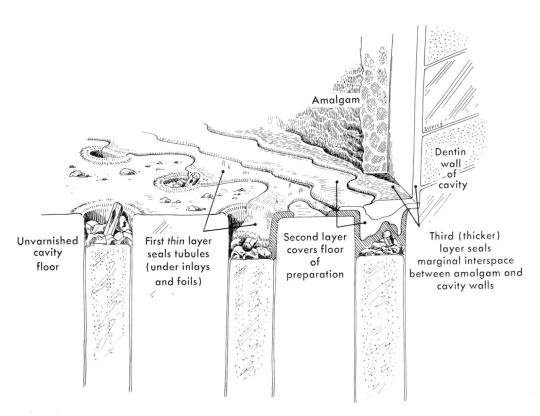

Fig. 2-11. Use of cavity varnish prior to placement of filling. First thin layer effectively seals opening of freshly cut dentinal tubules. Second layer covers floor of cavity preparation, and a third layer is used to fill interspace between amalgam and cavity walls. Only one layer of this varnish should be used under inlays, crowns, or foils to seal the dentinal tubules. Additional layers of varnish under inlays or foils could reduce retention of these filling materials.

pulp can be greatly reduced or prevented entirely by the use of a proper liner under shallow fillings or a proper base under deep restorations.

Bases and liners. Under a deep and large metallic restoration, the primary purpose of the base is to insulate the dentin and pulp against thermal shock. Direct contact of the metal on the protoplasm within freshly cut dentinal tubules results in a sharp lancinating pain when the metal is chilled. When the metal is close to the pulp, heat will cause a pulsating pain because of vascular engorgment. In addition, an insulating base or liner is a shield against galvanic shock and prevents the penetration of metallic ions and discoloration of the dentin.[13]

An acid phosphate cement should *not* be used under an amalgam restoration. The free acid increases galvanic action and may also undercut the restoration so that fractures are more frequent. Most experienced clinicians prefer to use one of the new modified zinc oxide–eugenol cements (increased hardness and accelerated set) as a base under deep and large amalgams for pulp protection and patient comfort.

In shallow cavities, a copal resin varnish or polystyrene liner is the material of choice. The varnish is applied in three successive layers. The first application seals the dentinal tubules against penetration of ions or molecules from the filling material itself and from organisms penetrating through the marginal interspace. The second layer seals the pores of the first layer produced during evaporation of the solvent (usually ether, chloroform, or acetone) and covers the floor of the cavity preparation. The third layer is applied just before the amalgam is inserted, to fill the marginal interspace (Fig. 2-11).

Fluorides. The presence of fluoride in silicate cements has been shown to increase the fluoride content of the adjacent enamel. This explains the resistance of silicate margins to carious attacks. The addition of fluoride salts to amalgam and to liners and bases to reduce the frequency of recurrent caries was therefore suggested. However, although the acid gel of a silicate allows the continuous release of fluoride ions, a similar release of fluoride from the set amalgam seems doubtful. Release of fluoride additives from liners and bases also seems questionable. A much more positive (and better documented) method of fluoridating the enamel and dentin of cavity preparations is to apply the fluoride solution to the cavity preparation before placing the temporary or permanent filling. The fluoride solution is conveniently prepared by placing one drop of Caulk's 30% stable solution of stannous fluoride (in water-free glycerin) into 10 drops of water. Topical application of stannous fluoride (about 3%) speeds up the remineralization of demineralized dentin.[14] This procedure is now used by many operators to reharden softened dentin. The assumption that fluoridizing the cavity preparation also retards secondary caries is probably valid but is not yet documented by *controlled* clinical studies.

Copper additives. Dispersion of small amounts of copper into the silver alloy has been shown to reduce corrosion and improve the marginal integrity of the restoration. (See more extensive descriptions and discussions in other restorative texts). The effect of the copper additive upon the dentin and the pulp is not yet known. Very little research has been conducted upon the biologic effects of copper amalgam since Manley demonstrated the deleterious effects of the old copper amalgams and copper cements in 1942 and 1944.

Composite resins

The composite resins have gained popular and extensive use because of their excellent esthetic qualities and ease of manipulation and because the silicate cements and unfilled methyl methacrylates are known to be injurious to young pulps. However, the speed of acceptance and use have outstripped the scientific tests and clinical evaluations so essential to modern practice. The effects of this material on the pulp are not yet thoroughly documented and the pulp protecting liners and bases not yet clearly established. Also the perfect finish of these materials has not yet been achieved.

The composite resins consist of about 70% glass spheres and rods coated with a water-repellent coupling agent bound together with modified acrylates that crosslink during polymerization. The material is completely water resistant and its translucent quality makes matching with the tooth color relatively easy. The filling is esthetically very pleasing.

Although originally intended for use in non–stress bearing areas (class III and class V restorations), it is now often used in class I cavities. The compressive strength is only three fourths that of amalgam so that at present it is not used in class II cavities. Excessive wear also restricts it from class II cavities. If further improvements are made, it may threaten to replace amalgam as a popular restorative material as it has already displaced the use of silicate cements in the anterior teeth, especially in young teeth.

Finishing and polishing the composite restoration has not yet been satisfactorily worked out. A surface glaze can be produced under a matrix band, but it is only fair. Polishing results in a rough surface so that plaque accumulation is high, as high as on unpolished enamel. Finishing burs and disks do not produce a smooth finish; in fact, the opposite occurs because the hard glass filler particles tear out from the much softer resin matrix. Marginal excess should be trimmed with a very sharp scalpel.

Marginal integrity is good when compared with amalgam, but microleakage and subsequent discoloration from salivary food products is high. Brännström and Nyborg (1972) found that this material is not bacteriostatic and that it shrinks excessively (2 to 20 μm), allowing bacteria (0.5 μm) and salivary debris to penetrate through the margins. They showed further that these bacteria can form a cariogenic bacterial plaque on the floor of the cavity and produce toxins to irritate the pulp. Chemical irritation to the pulp may also occur from the material itself, that is, the monomer or the polymerizing agents added to speed up the setting. Therefore a suitable liner should be used to protect the pulp under composite resins (as under silicates). Thus far, only Tubulitec (Buffalo Mfg. Co.), a polystyrene liner, has been tested. It gave considerable protection to the pulp when used under composite resin restorations.

Gold castings (inlays, onlays, and crowns)

Cast gold is ionically neutral and does not affect the dentin and pulp as does amalgam. As a metal it transmits heat and cold very quickly and efficiently. Chemically, the effect on the dentin and pulp can occur only through the cementing medium (or base). The cementing medium is usually one of the zinc phosphate cements. These luting agents seal the margins of these restorations adequately at first. But since they are soluble in saliva, they tend to wash out with time, leaving space for bacteria to establish bacterial plaques, especially within uncleansed proximal cervical margins. In caries-free mouths, these opened margins become filled with salivary debris. If the oral flora contains large numbers of cariogenic organisms, marginal decay may result.

Highly polished gold, like highly polished ceramics, does not irritate the gingivae as does amalgam and other rough surfaces. Plaque accumulation is also much less upon polished gold than upon unpolished amalgam surfaces or composites. A high polish is essential, especially on the proximal surfaces and all marginal areas in contact with the gingivae, to prevent plaque accumulation and gingivitis.

Porcelain

Gingival tissue is very tolerant of the highly polished surface of porcelain. Plaque accumulation is less than upon highly polished metallic restorations such as hard gold. However, the gingival margins of this nonductile material tend to be much more widely open than around ductile gold restorations where a fine knife-edge can be adapted in proximity to the tooth. Therefore, in-growth of connective tissue into open margins of porcelain jackets is fairly common. The nonadhesive cements available today wash out to leave the marginal openings subject to plaque formation and a bluish engorged gingivitis. Although the initial reaction of the gingivae around anterior jackets is excellent, the cervical gingivae soon become engorged. This defect has been greatly reduced in recent years by the use of metallic crowns with porcelain facings; thus the esthetic qualities of the porcelain are combined with the superior marginal adaptation of the metallic gingival collar.

Mechanical polishing of the porcelain after grinding is not enough. All porcelain materials must be reglazed by firing to achieve the highly polished surface layer that gives porcelain its unique tissue tolerance.

Gold foil

Gold-foil restorations are highly regarded by many practitioners because they can be placed into small cavity preparations and because the precious metal does not corrode and retians indefinitely its high polish in the salivary environment. Among all the restorations tested, gold foil showed the least marginal leakage. However, this has less significance than might appear at first glance.

The gold foil restoration did show some leakage after a relatively short test period. Furthermore, such leakage did *not* decrease with aging in the mouth. Finally, like all other restorations, marginal leakage was increased when subjected to temperature changes.

The pulp reacts strongly to the pounding force of the mallet on the dentin floor during insertion. The pulpal reaction is intense, with severe inflammation, but relatively brief. Since the insult is quickly withdrawn, the pulp soon recovers with the production of large amounts of reparative dentin. Newer materials that require much less malleting forces may be biologically more acceptable to the pulp. Electronic malleting devices, which employ much more rapid but less forceful condensing impacts, also reduce the pulpal and periodontal reactions. Dentin is a somewhat flexible material; so the dentin is able to absorb most of the forces produced by malleting modern materials with modern instruments except in very deep cavities where the dentin thickness is less than 0.1 mm.

Since metallic gold in direct contact with the freshly exposed protoplasmic contents of the dentinal tubules might transmit thermal shock to the odontoblasts, many gold-foil operators seal the cut tubules with a copal resin varnish prior to inserting the gold. This should not interfere with retention of the foil, which depends on gross undercuts to lock the condensed material within the cavity. However, I could not find documented studies on this subject; so the use of varnish under foils remains an empiric procedure that merits laboratory testing and clinical review.

EFFECTS OF TEMPORARY CROWNS AND BRIDGES

Temporary coverage of the crown preparation is essential to protect the freshly cut dentin and underlying pulp from thermal shock and from salivary con-

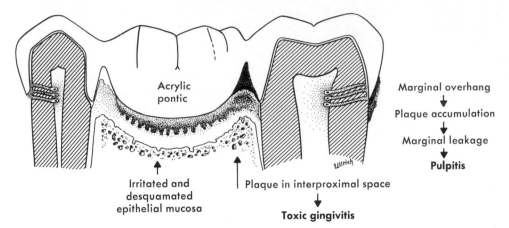

Fig. 2-12. Biologic effects of temporary acrylic crowns and pontic. Temporary crowns and bridges should help tissues to recover from operative procedures and should not injure them further. Avoid overhangs and grossly open margins. The patient must keep area free of plaque. Temporary acrylic crowns should be fabricated on models to avoid penetration of free monomer into dentin and pulp.

taminants such as bacteria, toxins, and debris from penetrating into the opened dentinal tubules (Fig. 2-12). These temporary crowns and bridges are now fabricated from fast-setting methyl methacrylate on plaster models. From the biologic point of view, this method of *indirect* fabrication is greatly superior to the direct fabrication of acrylic restorations practiced a decade ago. Pulpal damage by the free monomer and subsequent leakage because of excessive shrinkage occurred very frequently. Indirect fabrication of acrylic coverage avoids this damage.[15] However, leakage under these indirectly made acrylic crowns is still a major problem and one that has not yet been solved by the cementing medium. Zinc oxide–eugenol cements, even the new formulations, cannot be used under acrylic crowns because the free eugenol dissolves the adjacent acrylic. (NOTE: This may turn out not a bad feature since adhesion to the cement is increased). In addition, the volatile eugenol penetrates more deeply and discolors the acrylic.

Since the set acrylic is not a wettable material, zinc phosphate cement is not satisfactory because it cannot adhere nor

lute to the acrylic. Dycal has been used as a temporary cement. This material may adhere because of its resin content but does so poorly.

There is a real need to provide a cementing medium that (1) locks the acrylic to the dentin without damage to the latter and (2) prevents leakage into the margins of the crowns. These margins leak grossly so that the crown must not be expected to remain in place for more than short periods (2 weeks?). When these crowns become loose, the underlying dentin becomes very sensitive. At present, it is not known whether the sensitivity results from salivary products or the penetration of bacteria with formation of bacterial plaques over the freshly cut dentinal tubules. This suggests that even temporary crowns should not be placed into a caries-active oral environment. The mouth should be thoroughly cleansed and decontaminated, and the patient must practice good oral hygiene *before* restorative procedures are initiated.[16]

Sealing the freshly cut dentinal tubules with a copal varnish or a calcium hydroxide liner prior to cementation of the temporary or permanent crown greatly re-

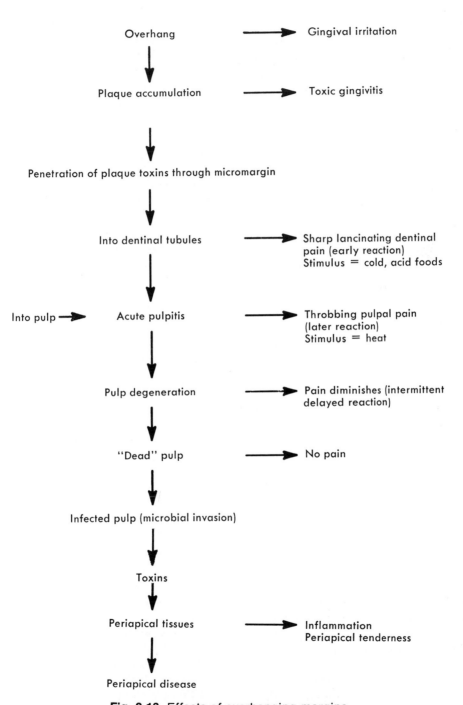

Fig. 2-13. Effects of overhanging margins.

duces the damage and the pain caused by leakage.

Gingival irritation

The effects of gross overhangs on the gingivae are usually quite severe and quickly reported by the patient (Fig. 2-12). It is not easy to finish the gingival margins of acrylic crowns to the knife-edge and close adaptations achieved with metallic crowns. Bacterial plaques quickly accumulate under these overhangs within 3 to 8 days so that bacterial irritants are added to the mechanical irritations. The gingivae soon become painful, swollen, and bleed easily (Fig. 2-13). The gingivitis disappears quickly after the temporary crown is removed.

Temporary pontics made of fast-curing acrylic should also be used for only a short period since the edentulous mucosa reacts to the acrylics as severely as do the marginal gingivae. No matter how smooth the finish of the acrylic in contact with the mucosa, the latter soon becomes irritated and red and the epithelium desquamates (Fig. 2-12). The latter may be attributable to the formation of bacterial plaque under the pontic.

Effects of various cements

Zinc phosphate cements. The chemical combination of zinc oxide with an acid to form a zinc cement has been in use by dentists for a long time. In the 1920s orthophosphoric acid was substituted for the highly injurious hydrochloric acid. Zinc phosphate (not oxyphosphate) cements contain free acids for approximately 6 to 12 hours after setting. The copper cements contain free acids for longer periods than do the ordinary zinc phosphate cements and produce greater damage to the pulp. In 1960, Smith substituted polyacrylic acid for the phosphoric acid and achieved a chelate type of cement that is not injurious to the pulp.[17]

The initial effect of the phosphoric acid on the pulp is similar to that seen under silicate cements. However, this damage does not continue, since the acid becomes gradually neutralized. The reparative process in the dentin then follows, particularly if the phosphate cement is used as a thin layer in a shallow cavity, as for cementation of a crown or inlay and especially in older teeth when placed over sclerotic dentin under which a good layer of reparative dentin has already been laid down. Experiments suggest that when a well-mixed thin layer of zinc phosphate cement is placed over old and sclerotic dentin, it may even act to stimulate new reparative dentin formation.

However, the placement of a thick base of zinc phosphate cement into a deep cavity over freshly opened and highly permeable dentinal tubules results in a severe shock of pain and acute pulpal damage, including some hemorrhage. This is particularly evident if the cement contains copper ions. For these reasons, it is biologically necessary to use a calcium hydroxide liner or a zinc oxide–eugenol cement rather than any of the phosphoric acid cements, in deep cavities, as a pulp-protective base. The zinc phosphate cements are useful as cementing media for metallic restorations and bands. It should not be used as a base. If used, an intermediary liner of copal varnish or calcium hydroxide should be used to protect the pulp, especially in young teeth or freshly cut tubules in older teeth.

Hydrophosphate cement. The powder of hydrophosphate cement contains zinc oxide and phosphoric acid and sets when mixed with water. However, the pH is the same as for the ordinary zinc phosphate cement and the pulpal reactions are very similar.

Silicophosphate cements. These mixtures are superior as luting agents, especially for permanent cementation of crowns and inlays. The pulpal reaction is somewhere between that caused by phosphate cement and silicate cement.[18]

Therefore a calcium hydroxide liner is necessary to protect the pulp in young teeth.

Zinc oxide–eugenol cements. The comparatively slow acceptance of zinc oxide–eugenol cement, biologically a more suitable temporary filling material than gutta-percha, and a biologically more desirable base under metallic restorations than zinc phosphate cement, is surprising in view of the extensive literature that documents the palliative action of zinc oxide–eugenol on the pulp. Berman (1958), James et al. (1959), Stanley (1961-1964), and others have demonstrated repeatedly that there is a reduction of inflammation and a distinctly palliative effect on the pulp after zinc oxide–eugenol is applied to cavity preparations even over severely inflamed pulps. In fact, most investigators now use zinc oxide–eugenol cement restorations as the standard against which to compare the biologic acceptability of other new and old filling materials.[19]

The palliative action of zinc oxide–eugenol cements may be attributable to (1) superior sealing qualities, (2) obtundent action of the eugenol, (3) bacteriostatic properties of the eugenol, or (4) a combination of these.

The extensive use of zinc oxide–eugenol cement and its modifications as a postsurgical periodontal pack, surgical pack in infected extraction sockets, temporary filling material, sealer in root-canal obturation, temporary (and permanent) cementing medium, impression paste in prosthetics, and so forth indicates a versatility of this material that is not yet fully appreciated. Dr. Jerome Brauer has published pioneering studies that show this material to have a chelate type of setting action. Further studies should be made of modifications to improve the physical properties of this material for specific uses. These include addition of polystyrene or acrylic resin (10% to 20% dissolved in the eugenol) for increasing

hardness of the cement, addition of alumina or ortho-benzoic acid (EBA), addition of Canada balsam (50%) for increased adhesiveness in root canal sealers and temporary cementation of crowns, addition of peanut oil or mineral oil to decrease adhesiveness of prosthetic impression pastes, addition of zinc acetate (up to 2%) to accelerate setting and use of finer and chemically purer zinc oxide and aluminum salts for increased rate of setting, lower solubility, and increased hardness. The action of these modifiers on the pulp is the same as zinc oxide–eugenol.

Polycarboxylate cement. The chemical and physical properties of this relatively new cement formed from the interaction between zinc oxide and polyacrylic acid are described elsewhere in this text. One of the first questions asked of this new cement was its effect upon the pulp when placed in bulk close to the pulp. A number of studies have now confirmed the fact that the pulpal response to this material is minimal and very similar to that observed under zinc oxide–eugenol preparations.[20] It is clear, therefore, that it can be used safely as a base under silicate and composite resin restorations and, probably, also under inlay and amalgam restorations.

No reactions were observed under old and sclerosed dentin. The reaction in very deep cavities under young and dehydrated dentin was mild and reversible.

GINGIVAL REACTIONS TO RESTORATIVE PROCEDURES
Gingival changes with age

The epithelial attachment shifts apically as age advances. In the partially erupted tooth of the child (with a deep but physiologic pocket the epithelium is "attached" to enamel. As the tooth slowly erupts, the epithelial attachment then migrates to the cementoenamel junction and the gingival pocket becomes a crevice. In the older person, the epithelial attachment continues to shift apically, often deepening the crevice until it may become a deeper but still "normal" or "physiologic" pocket. This area is kept clean by the exudate of gingival fluid, especially in slightly inflamed tissue. However, in the very deep pathologic pocket, this is not true, so that anaerobic bacteria may colonize and produce plaques within these non–self cleansing pathologic pockets. These plaques may be colonized by cariogenic organisms of *Odontomyces viscosus* and produce the cemental or root caries seen so often in patients past 50 years of age. Or these plaques may contain gram-negative toxin-producing organisms and produce a toxic gingivitis. These toxic plaques are seen most often in the young adult around full crowns with overhangs that foster the growth of bacterial plaques.

Termination of gingival floor

One of the problems that faced the clinician in the past and continues to plague him at present is just where to terminate the gingival floor of an inlay or crown. Should the gingival margin be placed just at the gingival crest for maximal cleansing (by gingival fluids or toothbrush)? Or just below the gingival crest and into the normal crevice as G. V. Black advocated on the basis that this area was self-cleansing and thus was considered "extension for prevention"? This may be true for the young adult. But suppose in the patient past 50 years of age, the crevice was deep (2 - 4 mm), or even considered as a pocket by the modern periodontist, where plaque may accumulate. Should the same generalization hold true? Or consider the geriatric patient, whose tissues are now ischemic and

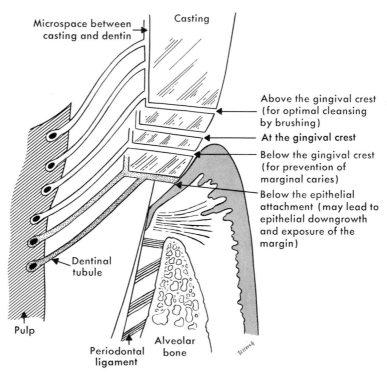

Fig. 2-14. Cervical margin of crown may be terminated at various levels. Most operators favor placement of cervical margin just below gingival crest, especially on proximal surfaces, for maximal protection against plaque accumulation and penetration of bacteria into margins of restoration.

whose gingivae shrink, and recession exposes the gingival margin so carefully placed inside the gingival crevice. What then?

Some clinicians are experimenting with terminating the gingival preparation 2 or even 3 mm *above* the gingival crest, on the buccal and lingual surfaces where the toothbrush can easily reach and keep the area clean of plaque (Fig. 2-14). Are they correct or to be condemned?

Unfortunately, there is no hard data, either clinical or experimental, to test these as hypotheses. But there are plenty of empiric observations and persons to defend each as a "fact."

Gingival retraction

Retraction of the gingivae to uncover the gingival margins of cavity and crown preparations in order to obtain a sharp impression of this area is essential to pre-

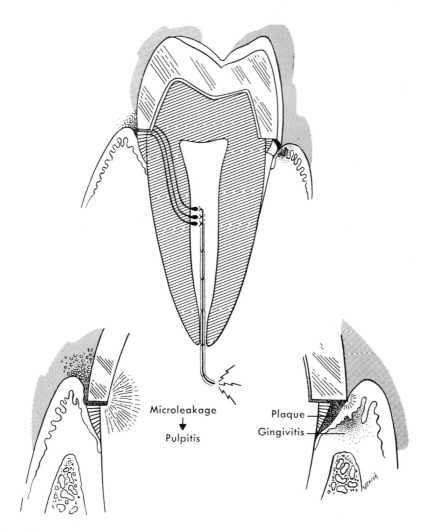

Fig. 2-15. Effects of microleakage and overhangs. All castings leave a microspace, which is filled by cement. When cement washes out, salivary products and bacteria can penetrate and affect dentinal tubules and pulp. The smaller the micromargin, the less likely that the cement will wash out.

cise crown and bridge construction. Retraction can be accomplished by mechanical pressure, astringents, gingivectomy or electrocautery. These measures are described and discussed elsewhere in this book.

The healthy gingivae of young patients quickly recover from such trauma to cover the gingival margin of the restoration properly. However, in the middle-aged patient the gingivae are likely to be ischemic and may not regenerate. Often the result of forceful retraction may be gingival atrophy, exposing the margin of the restoration rather than covering it, sometimes even exposing the cementum of the root. This leads to unesthetic elongation of the cllinical crown of the anterior teeth and cervical hypersensitivity of posterior teeth.

Desensitization of exposed sensitive necks by topical application of stannous fluoride solution (2% to 8%) is discussed elsewhere. This treatment is similar to that used by periodontists after gingivectomy for hypersensitive cementum and dentin.

Effects of restorative materials on gingivae

Very few precise investigations have been carried out on the effects of restorative materials on the gingival tissue that they contact, although there is no lack of speculative opinions based on the uncontrolled empiric observations. Waerhaug (1956), Zander (1957) and Newell (1964) studied the effects of zinc phosphate cement, silicate cement, and amalgam on the gingivae. These studies should be read in the original. More importantly, similar investigations should be repeated and extended. There is little doubt that different restorative materials have different biophysical effects on the gingival tissues, but these have not yet been studied in sufficient detail to permit generalizations or significant clinical applications at this time.

SUMMARY

Restorative materials must satisfy certain physical and chemical requirements before they can be certified for use in patients. They must also satisfy certain biologic requirements. Stated briefly, restorative procedures and restorative materials must not be injurious to the living tissues (dentin, pulp, bone or gingivae) by virtue of their chemical action or marginal leakage, since these may inhibit sclerosis of the dentinal tubules and reparative dentin formation (Fig. 2-15). Since few restorative materials now available can fully satisfy these requirements, properly selected liners and bases should be carefully considered for use under most, if not all, restorations. This is particularly true under amalgam restorations where a copal resin varnish tends to seal the margins, reduces galvanic action and corrosion, and prevents darkening of the underlying dentin by penetration of stannous and mercuric ions. A polystyrene liner should be used under composite resin restorations.

SELECTED REFERENCES

1. Fabrick, R. W.: Occlusal therapy in adolescents, Dent. Clin. North Am. **13**(2):451-456, April 1969.
2. Seltzer, S.: Classification of pulpal pathosis. Pages 331-349 in Siskin, M., editor: The biology of the human dental pulp, see General References at Siskin.
3. Rehak, J. R.: Corrective orthodontics, Dent. Clin. North Am. **13**(2):437-442, April 1969.
4. Kaleta, A. J., and Malone, W. F.: Masticatory muscle: a preview for the rationale of centric positions, Ill. State Dent. J. **43**(2):83-97, 1974.
5. Going, R. E.: Microleakage around dental restorations: a summarizing review, J.A.D.A. **84**:1349-1357, June 1972.
6. Weiss, M. B., Massler, M., and Spence, J. M.: Operative effects on adult dental pulp, Dent. Progr. **4**:6, 1963.
7. Marsland, E. A., and Shovelton, D. S.: Repair in the human dental pulp following cavity preparation, Arch. Oral Biol. **15**:411-423, 1970.
8. Brännström, M.: The effect of dentin desiccation and aspirated odontoblasts on the pulp, J. Prosthet. Dent. **20**:165-171, 1968.
9. Brännström, M., and Johnson, G.: Effects of various conditioners and cleaning agents on pre-

pared dentin surfaces: a scanning electron microscopic investigation, J. Prosthet. Dent. 31(4):422-430, April 1974.

10. Weine, F. S.: Endodontic therapy, St. Louis, 1972, The C. V. Mosby Co., pp. 68-102.

11. Silvestri, A.: The undiagnosed split-root syndrome, J.A.D.A. 92:930-935, May 1976.

12. Massler, M.: Restorative materials. In Clark, J. W.. editor: Clinical dentistry, New York, 1976, Harper & Row, Inc., vol. 4, ch. 15.

13. Going, R. E.: Status report on cement bases, cavity liners, varnishes, primers, and cleansers, J.A.D.A. 85(3):654-660, Sept. 1972.

14a. Wei, S. H. Y.: Remineralization of enamel and dentine; a review, J. Dent. Children 34(6):444-451, Nov. 1967.

14b. Wei, S. H. Y., Kaqueler, J. C., and Massler, M.: Remineralization of carious dentin, J. Dent. Res. 47(3):387-391, May-June 1968.

15. Sanjo, D.: Clinical studies on a cold-curing dental resin with a tri-*n*-butylborane catalyst, J. Dent. Res. 50:60, 1971.

16. Massler, M.: Therapy conducive to healing of the human pulp. Pages 308-316 in Siskin, M., editor: The biology of the human dental pulp, see General References at Siskin.

17. Smith, D. C.: A review of the zinc polycarboxylate cements, J. Can. Dent. Assoc. 37:22, Jan. 1971.

18. Phillips, R. W.: Report of the Committee on Scientific Investigation of the American Academy of Restorative Dentistry, J. Prosthet. Dent. 28(1):82-108, July 1972.

19. Stanley, H.: Preventive endodontics. In Clark, J. W., editor: Clinical dentistry, New York, 1976, Harper & Row, Inc., vol. 4, ch. 2.

20. Truelove, E. A., Mitchell, D. F., and Phillips, R. W.: Biological evaluation of a carboxylate cement, J. Dent. Res. 50:166, 1971.

GENERAL REFERENCES

Anderson, D. J., editor: Sensory mechanisms in dentine, London, 1963, Pergamon Press.

App, G. R.: Effect of silicate, amalgam and cast gold on the gingiva, J. Prosthet. Dent. 11:522, 1961.

Avery, J. K., and Rapp, R.: An investigation of the mechanism of neural impulse transmission in human teeth, Oral Surg. 12:190, 1959.

Barber, D., Lyell, J., and Massler, M.: Effectiveness of copal resin varnish under amalgam restorations, J. Prosthet. Dent. 14:533-536, 1964.

Barnes, D. S., and Turner, E. P.: Initial response of human pulp to zinc polycarboxylate cement, J. Can. Dent. Assoc. 37:265, 1971.

Baum, L.: Gold foil (filling golds) in dental practice, Dent. Clin. North Am., pp. 199-212, March 1965.

Baume, L. J. L., and Fiore-Donno, G.: Response of the human pulp to a new restorative material, J.A.D.A. 76:1016, 1968.

Berkman, M. D., Cucolo, F. A., Levin, M. P., et al.: Pulpal response to isobutyl cyanoacrylate in human teeth, J.A.D.A. 83:140-145, 1971.

Bernick, S.: Vascular and nerve changes associated with the healing of the human pulp. Pages 290-307 in Siskin, M., editor: The biology of the human dental pulp, see reference at Siskin.

Beust, T. B.: Demonstration of sclerosis of dentin in tooth maturation and caries, Dent. Cosmos 76:305-311, 1934.

Bhaskar, S. N., Cutright, D. E., Beasley, J. D., and Boyers, R. C.: Pulpal response to four restorative materials, Oral Surg. 28:126, 1969.

Bhaskar, S. N., and Lilly, G. E.: Intrapulpal temperature during cavity preparation, J. Dent. Res. 44:644-647, 1965.

Braden, M.: Heat conduction in teeth and the effect of lining materials, J. Dent. Res. 43:315-322, 1964.

Brännström, M.: The surface of sensitive dentine, Odontol. Revy 16:293, 1965.

Brännström, M.: Sensitivity of dentine, Oral Surg. 21:517, 1966.

Brännström, M.: The effect of dentin desiccation and aspirated odontoblasts on the pulp, J. Prosthet. Dent. 20:165-171, 1968.

Brännström, M., and Åström, A.: A study on the mechanism of pain elicited from the dentine, Arch. Oral Biol. 7:59, 1962.

Brännström, M., and Åström, A.: The hydrodynamics of the dentine; its possible relationship to dentinal pain, Int. J. Dent. 22:219, 1972.

Brännström, M., and Garberoglio, R.: The dentinal tubules and the odontoblastic processes—a scanning electron microscopic study, Acta Odontol. Scand. 30:291, 1972.

Brännström, M., and Johnson, G.: Movements of the dentine and pulp liquids on application of thermal stimuli, Acta Odontol. Scand. 28:59, 1970.

Brännström, M., and Johnson, G.: Effects of various conditioners and cleaning agents on prepared dentin surfaces: a scanning electron microscopic investigation, J. Prosthet. Dent. 31(4):422-430, April 1974.

Brännström, M., Linden, L. Å., and Johnson, G.: Movement of dentinal and pulpal fluid caused by clinical procedures, J. Dent. Res. 47:679, 1968.

Brännström, M., and Nyborg, H.: Pulp reactions to fluoride solutions applied to deep cavities: an experimental histological study, J. Dent. Res. 50:1548-1552, 1971.

Brännström, M., and Nyborg, H.: Pulpal reactions to composite resin restorations, J. Prosthet. Dent. 27(2):181-189, Feb. 1972.

Brännström, M., and Nyborg H.: Bacterial growth and pulpal changes under inlays cemented with zinc phosphate cement and Epoxylite CBA 9080, J. Prosthet. Dent. 31(5):556-565, May 1974.

Brännström, M., and Söremark, S.: The penetration of ^{22}Na ions around amalgam restorations with and without cavity varnish, Odontol. Revy **13**:331-336, 1962.

Carranza, F. A., and Romanelli, J. II.: The effects of fillings and prosthetic appliances on the marginal gingiva, Int. Dent. J. **23**(1):64-68, March 1973.

Dahl, B. L.: Some biological considerations in crown and bridge prosthetics, J. Oral Rehab. **1** (3):245-254, 1974.

Dahl, E., and Mjör, I.: The structure and distribution of nerves in the pulp-dentin organ, Acta Odontol. Scand. **31**:349-356, 1973.

Diamond, D. D., Stanley, H. R., and Swerdlow, H.: Reparative dentin formation resulting from cavity preparation, J. Prosthet. Dent. **16**:1127-1134, 1966.

Eccles, J. D.: The care of the gingival tissues near interproximal restorations, Dent. Practit. Dent. Rec. **14**:223, 1964.

Ehrlich, J., Hochman, N., Gedalia, I., and Tal, M.: Residual fluoride concentrations and scanning electron microscopic examination of roof surfaces of human teeth after topical application in vivo, J. Dent. Res. **54**(4):897-900, July-Aug. 1975.

Eich, J. D., Wilke, R. A., Anderson, C. H., and Sörensen, S. E.: Scanning electron microscopy of cut tooth surfaces and identification of debris by use of electron microprobe, J. Dent. Res. **49**:1359-1368, 1970.

Everett, F. G.: Desensitization of hypersensitive exposed root surfaces, Dent. Clin. North Am. **3**:221-230, 1964.

Fabrick, R. W.: Occlusal therapy in adolescents, Dent. Clin. North Am. **13**(2):451-456, April 1969.

Fesseler, A., Fetterroll, D., and Reiss, H.: Mechanische und histologische Untersuchungen über Durelon, Dtsch. Zahnaerztl. Z. **26**:241, 1971.

Frank, R. M.: Ultrastructural relationship between the odontoblast, its process and the nerve fibre. In Symons, N. B. B.: Dentine and pulp, London, 1968, E. & S. Livingstone Ltd., pp. 115-167.

Galan, J., Mondelli, J., and Coradazzi, J. L.: Marginal leakage of two composite restorative systems, J. Dent. Res. **55**(1):74-76, Jan.-Feb. 1976.

Gilson, T. D., and Myers, G. E.: Clinical studies of dental cements: IV. A preliminary study of a zinc oxide–eugenol cement for final cementation, J. Dent. Res. **49**:75, Jan.-Feb. 1970.

Going, R. E.: Microleakage around dental restorations: a summarizing review, J.A.D.A. **84**:1349-1357, June 1972.

Going, R. E.: Status report on cement bases, cavity liners, varnishes, primers, and cleansers, J.A.D.A. **85**(3):654-660, Sept. 1972.

Going, R. E.: Selection and use of intermediary materials. In Goldman, H. M., Gilmore, H. W., Irby, W. B., and Olsen, N. H., editors: Current therapy in dentistry, St. Louis, 1974, The C. V. Mosby Co., vol. 5.

Going, R. E., Massler, M., and Dute, H. L.: Marginal

penetration of dental restorations by dye and isotopes, J.A.D.A. **61**:285-300, 1960; J. Dent. Res. **39**:273-284, 1960.

Going, R. E., and Mitchem, J. C.: Cements for permanent luting: a summarizing review, J.A.D.A. **91**:107-117, July 1975.

Goto, G., and Jordan, R. E.: Pulpal response to composite-resin materials, J. Prosthet. Dent. **28**(6):601-606, 1972.

Grajower, R., Hirschfeld, Z., and Zalkind, M.: Compatibility of a composite resin with pulp insulating materials. A scanning electron microscopic study, J. Prosthet. Dent. **32**(1):70-77, July 1974.

Grajower, R., Kaufman, E., and Rajstein, J.: Temperature in the pulp chamber during polishing of amalgam restorations, J. Dent. Res. **53**(5):1189-1195, Oct. 1974.

Grajower, R., Kaufman, E., and Stern, N.: Temperature of the pulp chamber during impression taking of full crown preparations with modelling compound, J. Dent. Res. **54**(2):212-217, April 1975.

Horn, H. R.: The cementation of crowns and fixed partial dentures, Dent. Clin. North Am. **9**:65, March 1965.

James, V. E., and Schour, I.: Effect of cavity preparation alone on the human pulp, J. Dent. Res. **34**:758, 1955.

Jendresen, M. D., and Trowbridge, H. O.: Biologic and physical properties of a zinc polycarboxylate cement, J. Prosthet. Dent. **28**:264, Sept. 1972.

Johnson, G.: The hydrodynamics of the dentin and its clinical implications (doctoral thesis), Karolinska Institutet, Stockholm, Sweden, 1974.

Johnson, G., and Brännström, M.: Dehydration of dentin by some restorative materials, J. Prosthet. Dent. **26**:307-313, Sept. 1971.

Johnson, L. N., Jordan, R. E., and Lynn, J. A.: Effects of various finishing devices on resin surfaces, J.A.D.A. **83**:321-331, 1971.

Johnson, R. H., Christensen, G. J., Stigers, R. W., and Laswell, H. R.: Pulpal irritation due to the phosphoric acid component of silicate cement, Oral Surg. **29**:447, 1970.

Kanai, S., and Fusayama, T.: Effect of a cavity varnish on the retention of restorations, J. Dent. Res. **47**(3):403-406, May-June 1968.

Kaleta, A. J., and Malone, W. F.: Masticatory muscle: a preview for the rationale of centric position, Ill. State Dent. J. **43**(2):83-97, 1974.

Klotzer, W. T., and Langeland, K.: Tierexperimentelle Prüfung von Materialien und Methoden der Kronen-und Brückenprosthetick, Schweiz. Monatsschr. Zahnheilkd. **83**:163, 1973.

Kramer, I. R. H., and McLean, J.: The response of the human pulp to self-polymerizing acrylic restorations, Br. Dent. J. **92**:255-261, 281-287, 311-315, 1952.

Kurosaki, N., and Fusayama, T.: Penetration of elements from amalgam into dentin, J. Dent. Res. **52**(2):309-317, March-April 1973.

Landay, M. A., and Seltzer, S.: The effects of excessive occlusal force on the pulp. Pages 84-99 in Siskin, M., editor: The biology of the human dental pulp, see reference at Siskin.

Langeland, K.: Pulp reactions to cavity preparation and to burns in the dentin, Odontol. Tidskrift **68**: 463-470, 1960.

Langeland, K.: Prevention of pulpal damage, Dent. Clin. North Am. **16**(4):709-732, Oct. 1972.

Langeland, K., Dowden, W. E., Tronstad, L., and Langeland, L. K.: Human pulp changes of iatrogenic origin, Oral Surg. **32**:943, 1971.

Langeland, K., Dowden, W. E., Tronstad, L., and Langeland, L. K.: Human pulp changes of iatrogenic origin. Pages 122-159 in Siskin, M., editor: The biology of the human dental pulp, see reference at Siskin.

Langeland, K., and Langeland, L. K.: Pulp reactions to crown preparation, impression, temporary crown fixation and permanent cementation, J. Prosthet. Dent. **15**:129, 1965.

Lee, H., and Swartz, M. L.: Evaluation of a composite resin crown and bridge luting agent, J. Dent. Res. **51**:756, May-June 1972.

Liebman, F. M.: Pain and pressure in the human pulp. Pages 171-177 in Siskin, M. editor: The biology of the human dental pulp, see reference at Siskin.

Löe, H., and Rindom Schiøtt, C.: The effect of mouthrinses and topical application of chlorhexidine on the development of dental plaque and gingivitis in man, J. Periodont. Res. **5**:79, 1970.

Lyell, J., Barber, D., and Massler, M.: Effects of saliva and sulfide solutions on the marginal seal of amalgam restorations, J. Dent. Res. **43**:375-379, 1964.

Mandel, I. D.: Relationship of saliva and plaque to caries, J. Dent. Res. Part I. **53**(2):246-266, March-April 1974.

Marsland, E. A., and Shovelton, D. S.: Repair in the human dental pulp following cavity preparation, Arch. Oral Biol. **15**:411-423, 1970.

Massler, M.: Therapy conducive to healing of the human pulp. Pages 308-316 in Siskin, M., editor: The biology of the human dental pulp, see reference at Siskin.

Massler, M.: Restorative materials. In Clark, J. W., editor: Clinical dentistry, New York, 1976, Harper & Row, Inc., vol. 4, ch. 15.

Massler, M., and Barber, T. K.: Action of amalgam on dentin, J.A.D.A. **47**(4):415-422, Oct. 1953.

Matthews, B.: Cold-sensitive and heat-sensitive nerves in teeth, J. Dent. Res. **47**:974, 1968.

Messing, J. J.: A polystyrene-fortified zinc oxide–eugenol cement, Br. Dent. J. **110**:95, Feb. 1961.

Mitchell, D. F.: The irritational qualities of dental materials, J.A.D.A. **59**:955, 1959.

Moyers, R. E.: Some physiologic considerations of centric and other jaw relations, J. Prosthet. Dent. **6**:183-194, 1956.

Nelsen, R. J., Wolcott, R. B., and Paffenbarger, G. C.: Fluid exchange at the margins of dental restorations, J.A.D.A. **44**:228-295, 1952.

Newell, D. H.: Gingival reactions to restorative materials in rat molars, M.S. thesis, University of Illinois at the Medical Center, Chicago, 1964.

Parris, L., and Kapsimalis, P.: The effect of temperature change on the sealing properties of temporary filling materials, Oral Surg. **13**:982-989, 1960.

Peyton, F. A.: Effectiveness of water coolants with rotary cutting instruments, J.A.D.A. **56**:664-675, May 1958.

Phillips, R. W.: Cavity varnishes and bases, Dent. Clin. North Am., pp. 159-168, March 1965.

Phillips, R. W.: Report of the Committee on Scientific Investigation of the American Academy of Restorative Dentistry, J. Prosthet. Dent. **28**(1):82-108, July 1972.

Phillips, R. W.: Amalgam as a restorative material. In Clark, J. W., editor: Clinical dentistry, New York, 1976, Harper & Row, Inc., vol. 4, ch. 23.

Phillips., R. W., Avery, D. R., Mehra, R., Swartz, M. L., and McCune, R. J.: One-year observations on a composite resin for class II restorations, J. Prosthet. Dent. **26**:68-72, 1971.

Phillips, R. W., Gilmore, H. W., Swartz, M. L., and Schenker, S. I.: Adaptation of restorations in vivo as assessed by Ca[45], J.A.D.A. **62**:9-20, 1961.

Phillips, R. W., and Love, D. R.: The effect of certain additive agents on the physical properties of zinc oxide–eugenol mixtures, J. Dent. Res. **40**:294, 1961.

Phillips, R. W., Swartz, M. L., and Rhodes, B.: An evaluation of a carboxylate adhesive cement, J.A.D.A. **81**:1353, Dec. 1970.

Plant, C. G.: The effect of polycarboxylate cement on the dental pulp, Br. Dent. J. **129**:424, 1970.

Rao, S.: Pulp response in the rhesus monkey to "composite" dental restorative materials in unlined cavities, Oral Surg. **31**:676, 1971.

Rehak, J. R.: Corrective orthodontics, Dent. Clin. North Am. **13**(2):437-442, April 1969.

Sanjo, D.: Clinical studies on a cold-curing dental resin with a tri-*n*-butylborane catalyst, J. Dent. Res. **50**:60, 1971.

Schroeder, A.: Stand der Erfahrungen auf dem Gebiet der neuen Kunstoff-Kompositionsmaterialen auf Basis der Bowen-Formel, Schweiz. Monatsschr. Zahnheilkd. **81**:999, 1971.

Seltzer, S.: Classification of pulpal pathosis. Pages 331-349 in Siskin, M., editor: The biology of the human dental pulp, see reference at Siskin.

Seltzer, S., and Bender, I. B.: Modification of operative procedures to avoid post-operative pulp inflammation, J.A.D.A. **66**:503-512, 1963.

Seltzer, S., and Bender, I. B.: The dental pulp: biologic considerations in dental procedures, Philadelphia, 1965, J. B. Lippincott Co.

Silvestri, A.: The undiagnosed split-root syndrome, J.A.D.A. **92**:930-935, May 1976.

Silvey, R. G., and Myers, G. E.: Preliminary report of a three-year study of three luting cements, J. Dent. Res. (Abstr. 548) **53**:191, Feb. 1974.

Siskin, M., editor: The biology of the human dental pulp, St. Louis, 1973, The C. V. Mosby Co.; inquire only at American Association of Endodontists, P.O. Box 11728, Northside Station, Atlanta, Georgia 30305.

Shovelton, D.: Studies of dentin and pulp in deep caries, Int. Dent. J. **20**:283, 1970.

Shovelton, D. S.: The maintenance of pulp vitality, Br. Dent. J. **95**:95-101, 1972.

Smith, D. C.: A review of the zinc polycarboxylate cements, J. Can. Dent. Assoc. **37**:22, Jan. 1971.

Sotres, L. S., van Huysen, G., and Gilmore, H. W.: A histologic study of gingival tissue response to amalgam, silicate and resin preparations, J. Periodontol. **40**:543, 1969.

Sreebny, L. M., and Meyer, J., editors: Salivary glands and their secretions; proceedings of an international conference held at the University of Washington, Seattle, Aug. 1962, Oxford, 1964, Symposium Publications Division, Pergamon Press.

Stanley, H.: Dycal therapy for pulp exposures, Oral Surg. **34**(5):818, Nov. 1972.

Stanley, H.: Preventive endodontics. In Clark, J. W., editor: Clinical dentistry, New York, 1976, Harper & Row, Inc., vol. 4, ch. 2.

Stanley, H. R.: The cracked tooth syndrome, J. Am. Acad. Gold Foil Operators **11**(2):36-47, Sept. 1968.

Stanley, H. R., Going, R. E., and Chauncey, H. H.: Human pulp response to acid pretreatment of dentin and to composite restoration, J.A.D.A. **91**:817-825, Oct. 1975.

Suzuki, M., Goto, G., and Jordan, R. E.: Pulpal response to pin placement, J.A.D.A. **87**:636-640, Sept. 1973.

Symons, N. B. B., editor: Dentine and pulp, London, 1968, E. & S. Livingstone, Ltd.

Trivedi, S. C., and Talim, S. T.: The response of human gingiva to restorative materials, J. Prosthet. Dent. **29**:73, 1973.

Truelove, E. L., Mitchell, D. F., and Phillips, R. W.: Biologic evaluation of a carboxylate cement, J. Dent. Res. **50**:166, 1971.

von Fraunhofer, J. A., and Staheli, P. J.: The measurement of galvanic corrosion currents in dental amalgam, Corrosion Science **12**:767-773, 1972.

von Fraunhofer, J. A., and Staheli, P. J.: Gold-amalgam galvanic cells, Br. Dent. J. **132**:357, 1972.

Waerhaug, J.: Tissue reactions around artificial crowns, J. Periodontol. **24**:172, 1953.

Wei, S. H. Y.: Remineralization of enamel and dentine; a review, J. Dent. Children **34**(6):444-451, Nov. 1967.

Wei, S. H. Y., and Ingram, M. J.: Analysis of the amalgam-tooth interface using the electron microprobe, J. Dent. Res. **48**:317-320, March-April 1969.

Wei, S. H. Y., Kaqueler, J. C., and Massler, M.: Remineralization of carious dentin, J. Dent. Res. **47**(3)387-391, May-June 1968.

Wei, S. H. Y., and Wefel, J. S.: In vitro interactions between surfaces of enamel white spots and calcifying solutions, J. Dent. Res. **55**(1):135-141, Jan.-Feb. 1976.

Weine, F. S.: Endodontic therapy, St. Louis, 1972, The C. V. Mosby Co., pp. 68-102.

Weisenberg, M., editor: Pain (clinical and experimental perspectives), St. Louis, 1975, The C. V. Mosby Co.

Weiss, M. B., Massler, M., and Spence, J. M.: Operative effects on adult dental pulp, Dent. Progr. **4**:6, 1963.

Zach, L.: Pulp lability and repair; effect of restorative procedures, Oral Surg. **33**(1):111-121, Jan. 1972; also on pages 160-170 in Siskin, M., editor: The biology of the human dental pulp, see reference at Siskin.

3

Periodontal aspects of crown and bridge prosthodontics

Zigmund C. Porter and John K. Francis

The goal of every dentist is to maintain the dentition of his patients in health for as long as possible. If this truly is his responsibility, then it is necessary to understand the basic foundation of the mouth. With the strides that have been made in restorative dentistry, it is possible to rebuild almost the entire mouth when decayed to the root; however, it is very difficult to maintain the mouth after periodontal disease has removed most of the supporting structure. It is only through early recognition and then prevention that the dentist can serve his patients in the best possible way and for the longest period of time.

PERIODONTAL DISEASE
Attachment unit

To discuss the disease state, as with pathology, it is absolutely imperative that one understands the normal relationship of the tooth to the supporting structure, from both a histologic and an examination standpoint (Fig. 3-1). It is only by the deviation from normal that one is able to understand the extent of the disease. Fig. 3-2 shows a normal relationship of the gingival margin to the tooth, the epithelial attachment, and all the fibers that are attached from the cementum to the gingiva. One must understand what relationship the gingiva has to the tooth when it is being examined to evaluate whether it is normal or diseased. There are two

types of attachments, one the epithelial mucopolysaccharide type and the other the more tenacious fibrous connective tissue type.

The clinical gingival sulcus depth normally should measure 1 to 2 mm, whereas the epithelial attachment measures 1 mm and the connective tissue attachment 1 mm. Therefore the alveolar crest should be found approximately 2 mm apical to the base of the sulcus.[1] In the normal healthy patient there should not be a visible flow of sulcular fluid.[2] It is known that as the disease progresses the crevicular fluid flow increases.[3]

Periodontal ligament

The periodontal ligament is composed of collagen fibers arranged in bundles that are attached from the cementum of

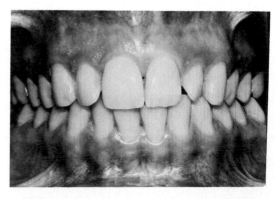

Fig. 3-1. Normal gingiva in young adult.

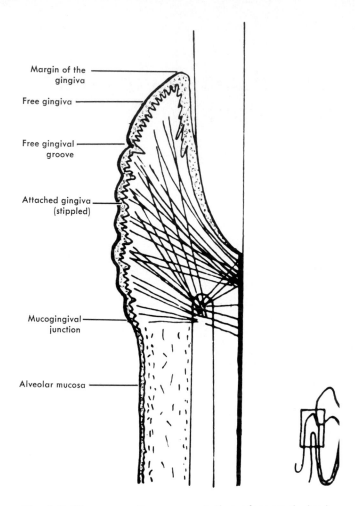

Margin of the
gingiva

Free gingiva

Free gingival
groove

Attached gingiva
(stippled)

Mucogingival
junction

Alveolar mucosa

Fig. 3-2. Diagrammatic representation of normal gingiva.

the tooth to the alveolar bone of the jaw. It is subject to the constant flux of change attributable to disease and masticatory forces. In health the periodontal ligament in functional occlusion is about 0.25 ± 0.1 mm wide. It is widest at the margin and apex and narrowest in the middle one third.

It is only after understanding the normal attachment of a tooth to the alveolar process that we can understand what the different measurements mean when we use a periodontal probe to establish the difference between health and disease. The two basic forms of periodontal disease are gingivitis and periodontitis.

Gingivitis

Gingivitis is defined as inflammation of the gingiva. Microscopically gingivitis may be characterized by the presence of an inflammatory cellular exudate and edema in the gingival lamina propria, destruction of gingival fibers, and both ulceration and proliferation of the sulcular epithelium.[4]

Periodontitis

Periodontitis is an inflammatory disease of the gingiva and the deeper tissues of the periodontium. It is characterized by pocket formation and bone destruction. Periodontitis is considered a direct

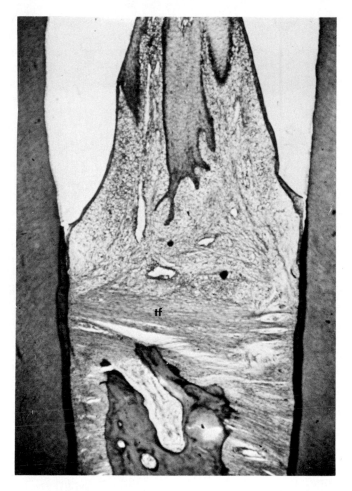

Fig. 3-3. Gingivitis. Beginning stages of the disease with local infiltration of inflammatory cells. Transseptal fibers, **tf,** are still intact and there is no apparent resorption of alveolar crest.

extension of neglected gingivitis. Periodontitis is caused primarily by extrinsic irritational factors and may be complicated by intrinsic disease, endocrine disturbances, nutritional deficiencies, periodontal traumatism, or other factors.[5]

Marginal lesion

The beginning stages of the disease can always be found histologically before any clinical manifestations are apparent, but it is not possible to take a biopsy of every papilla when one suspects a gingival problem (Fig. 3-3). Therefore one has to rely on clinical examination. Early recogni-

tion is the most important factor in preventing periodontal disease; therefore the dentist basically looks for any clinical change in the interdental papilla characterized by redness, swelling, tenderness, and bleeding. He must first be aware of it himself, and, second, make the patients aware of these subtle changes to enable them to bring the changes to the attention of the dentist when they first appear. A patient can be in a gingivally diseased state for many years and not be aware of such changes; however, when his mouth has been brought back to health by treatment and education, he is quickly alerted to an area becoming tender or to a very slight area of swelling and bleeding.

The disease is initiated with the formation of plaque. A tooth can appear to be clean and healthy, but a pellicle may have formed from the saliva[6] and bacteria will use this to hold on to the tooth. Plaque is invisible at this stage. When the plaque mineralizes, it becomes calculus. Bacterial substances that are attached to the tooth, through one form or another, will irritate the gingiva, therefore initiating inflammation. This is where the clinical signs of redness and swelling are visible. The inflammation then spreads from the lamina propria of the connective tissue to the alveolar bone. There is general agreement that there is a positive relationship between the presence of bacterial plaque and the existence of periodontal disease. One of the classic studies proving this point was performed by Löe[7] in 1965 and Theilade[8] in 1966. A group of dental students thoroughly cleaned their teeth before the study began and then stopped oral hygiene procedures. Gingivitis was noticeable in most of the subjects in a 10-day to 2-week period. They then initiated oral hygiene procedures and the gingivitis disappeared.

Löe then described the three phases of maturation of plaque. The first phase occurs within a 2-day period where there is a proliferation of gram-positive cocci and rods and a 30% gram-negative balance of cocci and rods. The second phase, which is between 1 and 4 days, shows the appearance of *Fusobacterium* and filamentous organisms. Phase three shows the appearance of spirilla and spirochetes within 9 days. It has been noted that at the time of infiltration by the polymorphonuclear leukocytes into the sulcular epithelium, the area begins to widen, encouraging the ingress of further antigens into the connective tissue area. If the retention of plaque around the tooth continues, the acute inflammatory lesion advances to a chronic inflammatory lesion by the ingress of mast cells, plasma cells, lymphocytes, and other mononuclear cells. It is through these cells that we begin to see the breakdown of the deeper connective tissue elements, either through immediate[9] or delayed hypersensitivities.[10]

Through the study of immunology dentists are beginning to understand the etiology of periodontal disease in its fullest form; however, there is still a lot of research to be done in order to elucidate the differences between all of our immunologic reactions.[11,11a] One factor that is clearly emerging is that the removal of plaque before the acute lesion starts seems to prevent periodontal disease. Once one allows the inflammatory lesion to form, all the other factors play the role of enhancing that lesion. Factors that seem to play the largest role are diabetes,[12] hormonal disturbances,[13] stress,[14] and altered nutrition.[15] In today's society, stress is playing more and more of an important role. The Selye studies[16] have proved the influence of stress on pathologic lesions.

Advanced lesions

Once the marginal lesion has developed to the point of chronic inflammation, the deeper layers of the connective tissues become involved with the ingress of the inflammatory cells, particularly the lymphocytes, which have been shown to be an enhancing factor to osteoclastic activity, resulting in the breakdown of the alveolar process[17] (Fig. 3-4). If, at the same time, the tooth is under trauma from the occlusion in the form of a prematurity or a bruxing habit, we know that this area is undergoing change. There can be a concomitant lesion of periodontal disease, with the occlusal traumatic lesion enhancing the loss of bone around the tooth. With further destruction the teeth will become mobile and eventually be lost. In consideration of the anatomic relationship, it is known that the tooth can

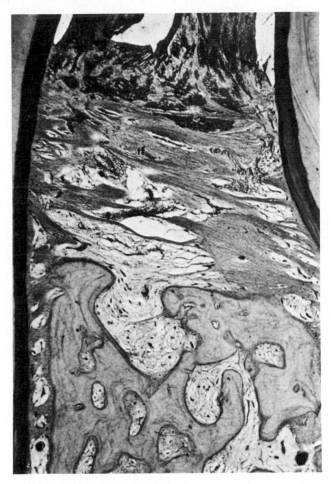

Fig. 3-4. Periodontitis. Local inflammatory cells have spread from gingiva into transseptal fiber area, **tf.** Note beginning stages of resorption of alveolar crest. (Courtesy Dr. Erwin Barrington, Chicago.)

withstand forces along the long axis because of the arrangement of its fibers better that way than in any other direction. Teeth only meet briefly during mastication and this is not enough force to create the problem of trauma to the supporting structure.[18] The trauma can only be instituted at times other than during mastication.

Occlusal traumatism

Occlusal traumatism is defined as a force that is created by the movement of the maxillary and mandibular teeth in such a way that it creates a pathologic lesion.

Primary occlusal trauma. Primary occlusal trauma is a pathologic lesion that has been created by a force that is strong enough to disturb a normal intact periodontium.

Secondary occlusal trauma. Secondary occlusal trauma is a lesion created by normal function on a weakened periodontium because of periodontal disease. The lesion caused by trauma is a noninflammatory type that comes in the form of pressure atrophy with the eventual death and necrosis of the affected area. Factors that enhance occlusal traumatism are clenching, grinding (bruxism), tongue thrusting, and nail biting. Of these, the one that appears to have the greatest effect is grinding. Again, there are discrepancies in the literature; one is that if an occlusal adjustment has been done correctly, a patient will stop his grinding habits; another is that grinding is entirely attributable to emotional distress and an individual will grind whether his teeth are in harmonious occlusion or not. The truth lies somewhere in between these two approaches.

Periodontal pocket

A periodontal pocket may be defined as a diseased periodontal attachment unit. It is the sign of a pathologic process that has involved the gingival unit. The pocket can result from the enlargement of the gingival tissue. In its customary form it is caused by the apical migration of the epithelial attachment with the loss of connective tissue attachment and eventually the loss of osseous support. The clinical significance of a pocket is that if an area has reached a level beyond 3 to 4 mm, compared to the normal level of 1 to 2 mm, the patient has increasing difficulty maintaining this area with his normal brushing and flossing techniques. As we already know, if an area cannot be maintained and the plaque is allowed to mature and stay adjacent to the epithelium, the disease process will continue. The ideal situation is for the total mouth to be free of pockets.

EXAMINATION
Visual examination

When one examines the patient, it is important to evaluate the color, consistency, texture, and shape of the gingival unit. It is important to be able to detect

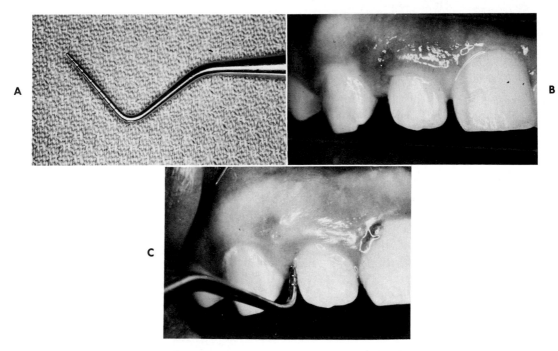

Fig. 3-5. A, Periodontal probe. Markings are in millimeters. **B,** Apparenty clinically healthy mouth of this 14-year-old boy. **C,** With probe in place, we have an 8 mm pocket on distal side of this lateral incisor.

the beginning stages of a marginal lesion through the change of color and consistency. The use of an adequate light source is essential to differentiate between normal and diseased tissue. Many times it is advisable to use a fiber-optic unit along with the mirror to be able to check lingual and distolingual areas in the mouth.

Probing

There are periodontal instruments designed to be used for probing (Fig. 3-5). One is advised to use the thinnest type of probe to enable traversal to the depth of a pocket without the patient being hurt and to allow for the greatest dexterity in differentiating the size and shape of the pocket. These probes are generally calibrated in millimeters. Probing can be one of the most difficult aspects of the examination, yet it is mistakenly taken for granted because it seems so easy to do. It is generally better for one to probe six areas around the tooth, paying specific attention to root anatomy. One should always evaluate bifurcation and trifurcation areas on the maxillary and mandibular molars and on the maxillary first bicuspids. To do this, it is mandatory to understand the anatomy of the root structure to be assured of what is being probed. Generally speaking, the mouth of a patient with poor oral hygiene habits will be very difficult to probe accurately. However, once good oral hygiene has been established, the patient may be probed to a greater degree of accuracy. During the probing procedure, one should also check for any bleeding or exudation that may be apparent, for these are also signs of periodontal disease. Clinically, the bleeding of the gingiva during probing is the symptom for the ulceration of the sulcular epithelium. One may also elect to use local anesthetic on the patient and probe for the bony contours to establish whether it is necessary to do surgery. This is generally done at the time of surgery before one decides the type of procedure that

will be performed. There are also special probes that can be used in the bifurcation or trifurcation areas. It is at the time of the probing procedure that one can determine whether it is necessary to place this patient on a prolonged scaling and curettage routine or whether one is dealing with a very fibrous pocket that might also necessitate osseous recontouring. There is much to be learned from probing and it is necessary to spend a great deal of time with this procedure during the examination.

Mobility

Mobility can be checked by using the handle end of the probe, along with the handle end of the mirror placed on the buccal and lingual surfaces of the tooth and applying pressure to the tooth with either the left or right hand. The extent of mobility of the tooth is then evaluated when pressure is applied. A classification of 1 to 3 is generally used, with 1 representing the early stage of mobility and 3 representing when a tooth is mobile in all directions and is depressible in its socket. Mobility is an indication of the loss of attachment of the tooth to the jaw. This can be seen radiographically in the form of a widened periodontal ligament space caused by occlusal trauma or orthodontic movement. It can also be caused by periodontal disease when the amount of the support has diminished sufficiently to loosen the tooth or it can be caused by overloading of the tooth with restorative work. Note that it is important to be able to determine the etiology for the mobility of this tooth or for an entire arch to be able to determine the prognosis for this tooth. I must emphasize that *because a tooth is mobile does not mean that the tooth will be lost.* Many times the whole mouth can exhibit a class I mobility and stay in this form for many years without the necessity of splinting any teeth together. If, however, the tooth is under secondary occlusal traumatism, one may

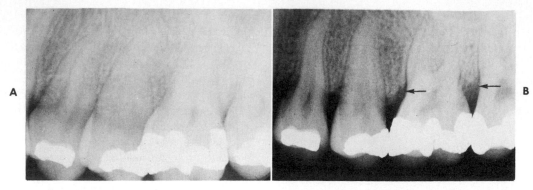

Fig. 3-6. A, Radiograph taken with short cone and poor technique. Note how alveolar crest appears to be at level of cementoenamel junction. This radiograph cannot be used for any diagnostic purposes. **B,** Radiograph taken by long-cone technique. Note alveolar crest defects that could not be seen previously in **A.** (Radiographs taken of same area on same day.)

need to splint a number of teeth together to obtain the required support for the teeth.

Radiographic examination

The normal radiographic relationship of the tooth to the bone has to be known before we can determine whether there has been any bone deterioration. The major consideration in examining radiographs is that the proper type of radiograph be taken. The one that best serves the purpose for evaluating the relationship of the tooth to bone is the long cone technique, as designed by Updegrave.[19] It is mandatory that a good amount of time be exercised in the taking of radiographs to ensure their use as a diagnostic aid (Fig. 3-6). The areas to be checked on the radiographs are the following:

1. Alveolar crest for signs of resorption (Fig. 3-7)
2. Integrity of thickness of the lamina dura
3. Evidence of generalized horizontal bone loss throughout the mouth
4. Evidence of vertical bone loss
5. Widened periodontal ligament space
6. Density of the trabeculae of both the maxillary and mandibular arches
7. Size and shape of the roots com-

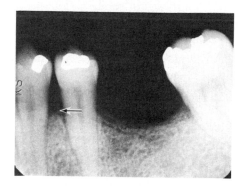

Fig. 3-7. Radiograph shows resorption of alveolar crest *(arrow).*

pared to the crown, so that the crown-to-root ratio can be determined according to the amount of bone available

The radiograph can determine the area of root that is still embedded in bone. This is important in our consideration for the prognosis of the total case. Often a case of short conical roots will have a minimal amount of bone loss but a maximum amount of mobility, and the prognosis for this case may be guarded to poor (Fig. 3-8). Some individuals can lose 50% of the bone throughout the mouth and yet have no mobility and the overall prognosis may be good because they have normal shaped roots.

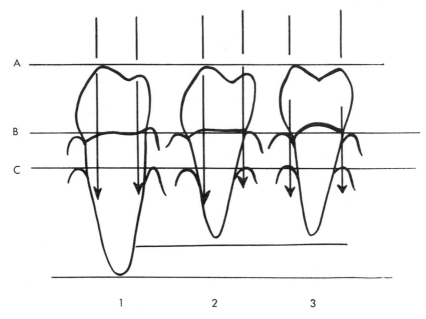

Fig. 3-8. Unfavorable distribution of functional forces associated with variations in crown-root relationship is accentuated in cases of reduced periodontal support. **1,** Normal premolar. Vertical forces of occlusion fall within confines of root when support is at cementoenamel junction, **B,** and also when height of periodontium is reduced, **C.** In the first instance the clinical crown is **A-B** and in the second instance **A-C. 2,** Premolar with normal crown and short root. Vertical forces of occlusion just barely fall within confines of root when periodontium is at cementoenamel line, **A.** However, when periodontium is reduced **(C),** vertical forces of occlusion fall outside root. **3,** Premolar with abnormally wide crown and short root. Vertical forces of occlusion are directed beyond periphery of root when periodontium is at cementoenamel line, **B,** and also when level of periodontium is reduced, **C.** (From Glickman, I.: Clinical periodontology, ed. 4, Philadelphia, 1972, W. B. Saunders Co.)

Habits

The major habit to consider is bruxism (Fig. 3-9). Visual examination of wear facct patterns and X-ray interpretation of thickened laminae durae and widened periodontal ligament spaces will many times determine if a patient grinds his teeth. It is important to discuss this with the patient to see if he is aware of this problem, but often an individual is not aware of the fact that he grinds his teeth during sleep. It is important to educate the patient to know what to look for and then reevaluate this factor at a later time.

One reason to suspect bruxism is a complete arch exhibiting mobility even where there appears to be good osseous

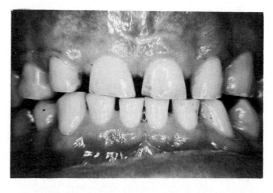

Fig. 3-9. Fifty-year-old male patient showing considerable wear in anterior portion of mouth.

support. Even though the tooth may not have been worn down because of the pressure of grinding, the whole tooth may have become mobile trying to give way to this force. You may also find wear facets on a tooth in areas where a person does not normally chew. Therefore, it is often difficult to diagnose a bruxism habit.

PREPARATION OF TISSUES

The most important aspect from a periodontal standpoint is for the patient to be totally informed of his problem and to educate him in the means and methods necessary to correct this problem. This should be done through a combination of audiovisual aids and reading material. After the patient has been examined and the proper diagnosis and prognosis have been established for the whole case, the final decision is discussed with the patient.

Treatment objectives as outlined by Goldman and Cohen should be followed:
1. Pocket elimination—obviation of the inflammatory lesion
2. Establishment of physiologic tissue contours necessary for self-cleansing and ease of physiotherapeutic management
   a. Thin, parabolically curved gingival margins
   b. Pyramidal interdental papillae that conform architecturally and adapt tightly to tooth contours while permitting the free egress of food and debris from the interproximal areas (Once surgical intervention is dictated because of existing disease, it is appropriate to eliminate the "col" form of gingiva interdentally and to substitute an occlusally convex tissue form shy of the contact areas between adjacent teeth.)
   c. Adequate width and rigidity of the zone of keratinizing attached gingiva (Rigidity implies density as well as firm attachment to tooth and bone.)
   d. Sufficient depth of the vestibular fornix to allow food to escape from the vestibular and gingival area (The musculature of the fornix, also the lips and cheeks, requires additionally the freedom of activity adequate to permit evulsion of food.)
3. Placement of teeth and the modification of their morphology in a manner to protect the periodontium from the effects of local environmental insults
4. Eradication of positive occlusal habits and control of their effects
5. Application of measures for tooth stabilization to protect the attaching tissues and to permit their full healing potential
6. The acquisition of patient cooperation and facility in the performance of preventive physiotherapeutic measures

It has been demonstrated that teeth can function and be stable despite the fact that they have lost a good deal of their investing and supporting tissues.[20]

Although these are all treatment objectives, it is mandatory that the dentist understands the objectives of the patient. It is important that time be spent with the patients to allow them to explain their objectives as a result of going through this therapy.

TREATMENT PLANNING
Initial preparation

Oral physiotherapy. The first stage of initial preparation is the teaching and demonstration of oral physiotherapeutic measure to enable the patient to maintain the mouth in a state of health for the rest of his or her life. The patient must have a complete understanding of what plaque is, how it is formed, and how to remove it. This is one area where we all too readily become discouraged. It's important to spend time with each and every patient by fully utilizing the auxiliaries. This will assure us that sufficient time can be spent

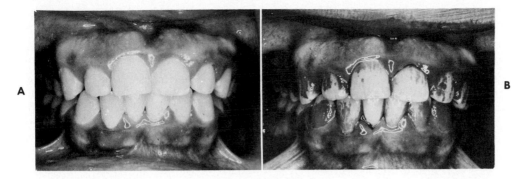

Fig. 3-10. A, Unstained dentition. Same patient as in Fig. 3-5, *B* and *C.* **B,** Teeth stained with disclosing solution. Comparison of views before and after shows how it was not possible to see the plaque before mouth was stained.

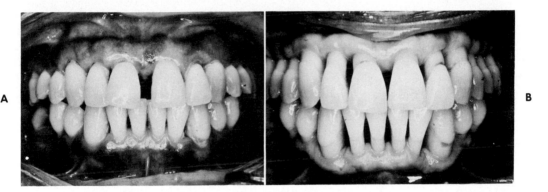

Fig. 3-11. A, Forty-five-year-old male patient before any periodontal therapy was initiated. **B,** Same patient 6 months later after initial preparation only. Surgery was not performed, only oral hygiene instructions and repeated scalings and curettage.

with each patient to educate him to maintain his mouth properly.

The plaque control record by O'Leary[21] is an excellent technique to demonstrate the efficiency of plaque removal on all four surfaces of the tooth. This allows the patient to visualize his progress in a percentage form (Fig. 3-10). The patient should reach a level of 20% to 10% efficiency before surgery is undertaken. The average periodontal patient starts at a level of 90% to 80%.

Preparation of oral tissues. The second most important aspect is to have the patient put his gingival tissues in condition to enable him to maintain these tissues properly once instructed. It is started by giving the patient a complete scaling and curettage of the root structures and the gingival tissues where indicated. The purpose of this is to accomplish the following:

1. Eliminate the irritant around the attachment area.
2. Smooth the root surfaces to make it easier for the patients to use their brushing and flossing technique.
3. Reduce swollen tissue to the stage where it is firmer and more manageable for surgery, if indicated; this may take one or more appointments, depending on the state of disease when the patient initiates periodontal therapy (Fig. 3-11).

At the same time we must follow up with:

1. Removal of all hopelessly involved teeth.

2. Excavation and temporization of all caries.
3. Evaluation of all teeth for possible endodontic involvement. This is an area in periodontal therapy that is overlooked much of the time. A necrotic pulp can be a hindrance in periodontal healing, especially when osseous transplants are done. A pulpal inflammation can be a serious problem with sensitivity, and the patient will not maintain his mouth properly.
4. Initiation of orthodontic tooth movement where indicated for selective cases.
5. Occlusal adjustment to eliminate a prematurity in centric occlusion and lateral and protrusive excursions.
6. Fabrication of a full acrylic occlusal night guard for the maxillary or mandibular arch to aid in cases of bruxism.
7. Reevaluation.

The entire mouth is now reevaluated with the periodontal probe to check for pocket depth and to determine whether it is necessary to go into the surgical phase of therapy. If the patient has not demonstrated his willingness to cooperate in proper oral physiotherapy, it is generally best to explain this to him and possibly stop therapy at this time and then to reconsider what the most conservative approach may be to keep this patient's teeth for as long as possible. When the patient is maintaining the mouth properly, by whatever index the dentist is using to determine plaque control, the dentist may proceed to surgical correction. Areas of 4 mm or more of pocket depth, or the lack of attached gingiva, necessitates the patient's undergoing a surgical technique to put his mouth in a healthier condition and enabling him to maintain this area in health.

Surgery

General principles. The rationale for surgery is found in the original objective as stated before. Pocket elimination and establishment of physiologic tissue contours are the prime goals. If scaling and curettage have not been able to produce these objectives, it is necessary to go into a surgical phase. To restore the integrity of the patient's mouth, it is important to differentiate between different surgical techniques, such as gingivectomy, mucogingival procedure, and mucoperiosteal flap entry with osseous recontouring. Ideally, we would like to rebuild all the lost osseous tissue along with all the attachment that has been lost because of periodontal disease. We are striving at this time through research and clinical evaluation to rebuild the mouth through different transplant techniques. It is a very predictable procedure for certain types of problems, but we still have a long way to go before it will work in every case. Therefore in most cases we are basically attempting to reestablish the physiologic architecture of the bone in the way nature originally had it before the disease but, of course, in a more apical location.

Advanced surgical techniques. Many times it is necessary to go into heroic periodontal procedures to save a part of a tooth for restorative commitments.

1. The mandibular molar can have one root removed in the form of a hemisection, a situation that enables the restoration of the tooth to function with a bridge.
2. On maxillary molars it is possible to remove either the distobuccal root or the mesiobuccal root and then to restore this tooth to function with the tooth's being splinted to its neighbor (Fig. 3-12).
3. Bone transplantation. Since 1960[22] dentists have been attempting to add bone to the osseous defects so that nature will regenerate the portion that has been lost because of the disease. The following are many ways of doing this:
   a. Swedge procedures[23]

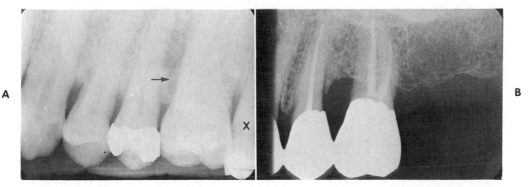

Fig. 3-12. A, Forty-two-year-old male patient with a class III furcation involvement around mesiobuccal root. *Arrow,* Radiolucency in this area. × marks tooth that was hopelessly involved and later extracted. **B,** Same areas but with mesiobuccal root removed and restoration in place 5 years later. (Courtesy Dr. Kenneth Molnar, Downers Grove, Ill.)

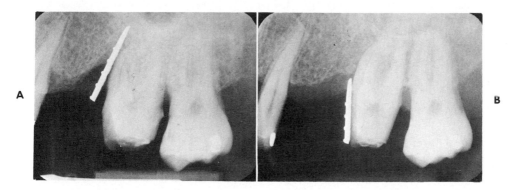

Fig. 3-13. A, Radiograph of infraosseous defect with a Hirschfeld point in place to show apical location of defect. **B,** Infraosseous three-wall defect was filled with an osseous coagulum, and radiograph shows the fill after 8 months. (Courtesy Dr. Nolan L. Levine, Oak Brook, Ill.)

b. Osseous coagulum procedures[24] (Fig. 3-13)

c. Bone from recent extraction sites[25] or trephine autografts

d. Bone from the posterior iliac crest[26] that has been removed by an orthopedic surgeon or hematologist

I must emphasize that these procedures are only done in selected cases where it is absolutely necessary to save this tooth for restorative commitments. However, many times it is better to sacrifice the tooth if the results are going to be questionable rather than to jeopardize the total restorative commitment.

Final preparation of tissues

1. A final scaling, curettage, and polishing of the total case to smooth the surfaces and allow the patient to maintain this area with plaque control.

2. A final occlusal adjustment to eliminate any interferences that may have developed after surgery.

3. Relieve patients of their tooth sensitivity. Root sensitivity is a problem for the periodontal patient. One must emphasize to the patient that more than 50% of his sensitivity is attributable to improper removal of

the bacterial products from the tooth. However, because of this severe sensitivity, he finds it very difficult to continue brushing at the same efficiency. The areas that should be checked are (1) caries, (2) traumatic occlusion, (3) bruxism, (4) plaque retention, and (5) degeneration of pulpal tissue. One of the best ways of correcting sensitivity (if the other areas have been checked) is by using an 8% fluoride solution with calcium phosphate burnished into the root. If this does not work, endodontic therapy may be indicated.

4. Reevaluation of the total case for restorative recommendations.
5. The improved condition of the patient's mouth necessitates a review of his oral physiotherapy techniques. The patient is now ready to go through the restorative treatment plan.

PERIODONTAL ASPECT OF FIXED OCCLUSION
Occlusion and its effect on periodontium

When there is increased functional demand upon the periodontium, it accommodates to a point to withstand these forces. This adaptive capacity varies in different persons and in the same person at different times and circumstances. The effect of occlusal forces upon the periodontium is influenced by their *severity, direction, duration,* and *frequency.*[27] When the severity is increased, the periodontal fibers thicken and increase and the alveolar bone increases in density. Changing the direction of the occlusal forces causes a change in the orientation of the periodontal ligament fibers.[20] These fibers are oriented so that they best withstand forces in the long axis of the tooth; thus, it is best, when one designs prosthetic appliances, to direct the forces into the long axis of the tooth. This will allow the greatest tolerances to work for the prosthetic appliance. Horizontal or lat-

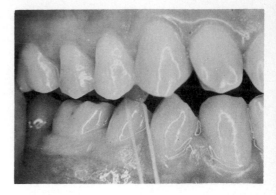

Fig. 3-14. Balancing side interference.

eral forces are usually found in balancing side interferences and they are injurious forces to the periodontium (Fig. 3-14). Lateral forces are marked by bone resorption in areas of pressure and by bone formation in areas of tension[28] (Fig. 3-15).

Rotational forces cause both tension and pressure on the periodontium and are the most injurious forces of all. The duration and frequency affect the response of the alveolar bone to occlusal forces because constant pressure on bone causes resorption but intermittent forces favor bone formation.[29,30] Recurrent forces over a short interval of time have essentially the same resorbing effect as constant pressure. When occlusal forces exceed the adaptive capacity of the periodontium, tissue injury results.[31-33]

Periodontal injury caused by occlusal forces is called trauma from occlusion. Occlusal traumatism does not affect the gingiva, nor does it cause bone formation. Inflammation will cause horizontal bone loss.[34] However, the inflammation in the presence of trauma from occlusion will change the pathway of this inflammation to allow it to enter into the periodontal ligament space and lead to intraosseous defects (infraosseous pockets).[31] Thus trauma from occlusion does not affect the marginal gingiva but affects the bone when there is inflammation present. This is called the zone of codestruction: trauma from occlusion in the

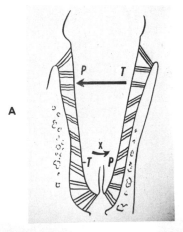

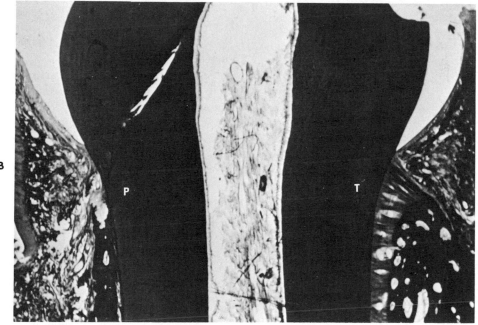

Fig. 3-15. A, Diagram showing center of rotation, ×. *P* is pressure and *T* is tension. **B,** histologic section through a tooth. *P* is pressure side; note tooth touching the bone. *T* is tension side; note widened periodontal ligament space at right of tooth on tension side and crushing of periodontal ligament fibers on pressure side.

presence of inflammation[27] (Fig. 3-16). Imagine, then, a poorly constructed partial denture that caused gingival irritation and at the same time was applying a twisting force to the abutment tooth. This would be a classic example of trauma from occlusion leading to bone destruction.

When there is increased functional demand upon the periodontium, it tries to accommodate to this demand. This adaptive capacity varies in different persons and in the same person at different times. The principal fibers of the periodontal ligament are arranged so that they best accommodate occlusal forces in the long axis of the tooth. When axial forces are increased, such as in restorative work,

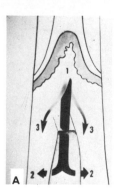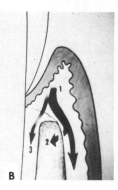

Fig. 3-16. Diagrams of pathways of inflammation. **A,** Interproximal view. *1,* Inflammation, which passes to bone, *2,* and then into periodontal ligament in inflammation, *3,* is pathway of inflammation with concomitant trauma from occlusion; inflammation goes directly into periodontal ligament space. **B,** Buccal view.

there is a distortion of the periodontal ligament and subsequent compression of the periodontal fibers and then resorption of the bone in the apical areas. The fibers in relation to the remainder of the root are placed under tension and new bone is formed. In designing dental restorations and prostheses, one should make every effort to direct occlusal forces in an axial direction to benefit from the greater tolerance of the periodontium to forces in this direction. Lateral or horizontal forces are ordinarily accommodated by bone resorption in areas of pressure and bone formation in areas of tension. A slightly more advantageous point of application of a lateral force is near the cervical line of the tooth. The reason is that as the distance from the center of rotation or the length of the lever arm is increased, and the force upon the periodontal ligament increases. Torque or rotational forces cause both tension and pressure, which, under physiologic conditions, result in bone formation and bone resorption, respectively. Torque is the type of force most likely to injure the periodontium.[34]

Trauma from occlusion occurs in three stages; the first is injury, the second is repair, and the third is a change in the morphology of the periodontium. Tissue injury is produced by excessive occlusal forces. Nature attempts to repair the injury and restore the periodontal tissues. This repair can occur if the force is diminished or the tooth, luckily, can drift away from it. Sometimes the moving away from the injurious force is called mobility. If the force is chronic, the periodontal tissues are remolded to cushion the traumatic force: the periodontal ligament is widened at the expense of the bone, angular (vertical) bone defects occur without pockets, and the tooth becomes mobile.[33]

Role of trauma from occlusion in etiology of gingivitis and periodontal disease. Everything in the periodontal tissues bears the touch of occlusion. Just as the occlusion is a critical environmental factor in the life of the healthy periodontium, its influence continues in periodontal disease. Inflammation in the periodontal ligament cannot be separated from the influence of occlusion. Because occlusion is the constant monitor of the condition of the health of the periodontium, it affects the response of the periodontium to inflammation and becomes a factor in most cases of periodontal disease. The role of trauma from occlusion in gingivitis and periodontitis is best understood if the periodontium is considered as having two zones, the zone of irritation and the zone of codestruction. The zone of irritation consists of the marginal and interdental gingiva, with its boundary formed by the gingival fibers. This is where gingivitis and periodontal pockets start.[35,36] They are caused by local irritation from plaque, bacteria, and calculus and by food impaction. With few exceptions, researchers agree that trauma from occlusion does not cause gingivitis or periodontal pockets.[37-39] In other words, such things as high restoration, orthodontic movement,

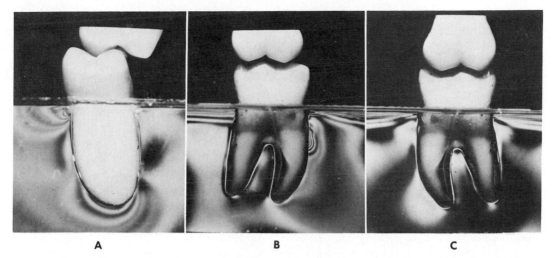

A   **B**   **C**

Fig. 3-17. A, Photoelastic model showing stress at apex when force is applied to cusp tip. **B,** Photoelastic model of forces at mesial aspect of molar such as that found when mesial neighbor is removed. **C,** Photoelastic model of forces at apex of root when force is in long axis of tooth. (Courtesy Dr. Irving Glickman, Boston.)

or the poorly designed rest of a partial denture that causes tooth trauma will *not* lead to a periodontal pocket. The reason is that the local irritants that start gingivitis and periodontal pockets affect the marginal gingiva, but trauma from occlusion affects only the supporting tissues. The marginal gingiva is not affected because its blood supply is sufficient to maintain it even when the vessels of the periodontal ligament are obliterated by excessive occlusal forces.[40] As long as the inflammation is confined to the gingiva, it is not affected by occlusal forces. When it extends from the gingiva to the supporting periodontal tissues, then inflammation does enter into the zone of codestruction. The zone of codestruction begins with the transeptal fibers and consists of supporting periodontal tissues: the bone, periodontal ligament, and cementum. When inflammation reaches the supporting periodontal tissues, its pathway and the destruction it causes come under the influence of the occlusion[43] (Fig. 3-17).

In ordinary inflammation without trauma, the inflammation follows the path

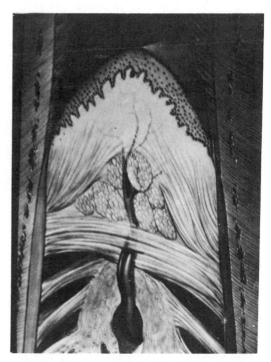

Fig. 3-18. Drawing of interdental area showing histologic features. Note blood vessel passing through transseptal fibers into crest of bone.

of least resistance. Its course is determined by the alignment of the transeptal fibers, and it goes into the crest of the bone by following a path along the circumvascular spaces[34] (Fig. 3-18). Trauma from occlusion changes the tissue environment around the inflammatory exudate in two ways: (1) it alters the alignment of the transeptal and alveolar crest fibers and thus changes the direction of the pathway of the inflammation so that it extends directly into the periodontal ligament, and (2) excessive occlusal forces produce periodontal ligament damage and bone resorption, which aggravate the tissue destruction caused by inflammation.[43] Combined with inflammation, trauma from occlusion leads to infraosseous pockets, angular (vertical), craterlike osseous defects, and excessive tooth mobility.

There is considerable variability in the response of the periodontium to the combination of inflammation and trauma from occlusion. The inflammation or the trauma may not be severe enough or the anatomy of the tooth or bone may not be conducive to pocket formation. In the absence of inflammation and local irritants, severe trauma from occlusion will cause excessive loosening of the teeth, widening of the periodontal ligament, and angular (vertical) defects in the alveolar bone *without pockets*.[41] Radiographic signs of trauma from occlusion are seen in Fig. 3-19. One will note the widening of the periodontal space, thickening of the lamina dura, and angular (vertical) bone loss, rather than that of horizontal bone loss. The furcation is the area most sensitive to trauma from occlusion.

Trauma from occlusion may be caused by (1) alterations in the occlusal forces, (2) reduced capacity of the periodontium to withstand occlusal forces, or a combination of both. The criterion that deter-

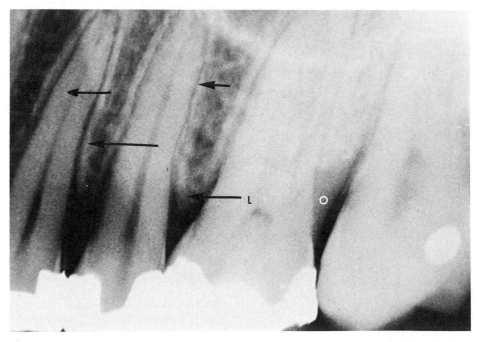

Fig. 3-19. Note widened lamina dura, *arrows;* trifurcation involvement, O; and loss of crestal lamina dura, *L.* These are classic signs of trauma from occlusion associated with inflammation.

mines whether an occlusion is traumatic is whether it causes an injury rather than how the teeth occlude with one another. A malocclusion is not necessary to produce trauma; it may be present when occlusion appears "normal."[42,43] Conversely, not all malocclusions are necessarily injurious to the periodontium.

Trauma from occlusion is either primary or secondary. In primary occlusal trauma the forces are excessive. It results from habits or compulsion such as clamping, clenching, or grinding the teeth. It is the parafunctional movements of bruxism that are significant in primary trauma from occlusion. Some other examples are "high" restorations, a prosthetic appliance that causes excessive forces on the abutment teeth or occluding teeth, orthodontic movement of teeth into functionally unacceptable positions, and the drifting or extrusion of teeth into spaces created by unreplaced missing teeth.[40]

Secondary periodontal traumatism occurs from normal forces such as mastication, but the support of the tooth is weakened by the loss of a portion of its attachment apparatus and it cannot withstand normal forces. Pressure from mastication is light and of only short duration, and it occupies only a small portion of the day. Swallowing occurs frequently but is also only a light contact. Bruxism and other parafunctional habits seem to be the major cause of excessive traumatic forces in a lateral or twisting manner,[44,45] along with poorly constructed bridges that violate good prosthetic rules and partial dentures that place too much stress upon abutment teeth.

Placement of margins of restorations

Except for decay going subgingivally, which would necessitate the subgingival preparation of the tooth in mouths susceptible to decay or for esthetic reasons, it would be best to end all preparations above the gingival margin. If periodontal therapy has been done and there is recession, one might best stop the preparations at the cementoenamel junction. Even if the tissue does not exhibit recession, again, it would be best to stop the preparations, if possible, away from the tissue margin.

Crown margins, when one needs to hide them subgingivally, should be located at the base of the gingival sulcus.[46,47] This is the level reached when one places a thin blunt probe without pressure into the gingival sulcus. In this position, the gingival fibers brace the gingiva against the tooth and the margin of the completed restoration.

The margin of the preparation should not be placed at the crest of the marginal gingiva, regardless of how perfect the margins of the restoration may be (Fig. 3-20). Microscopically, the margin is rough and a perfect place to harbor bacteria. Since the margin of the gingiva is

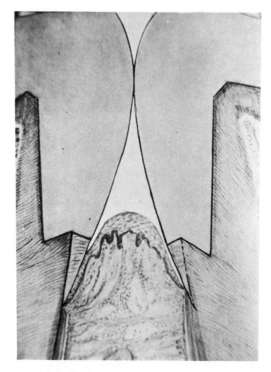

Fig. 3-20. Margins incorrectly placed, since they are in area where plaque forms. (Courtesy Dr. Max Perlitsh, Boston.)

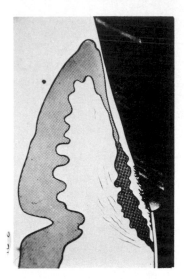

Fig. 3-21. Note restoration tearing epithelial attachment and deepening pocket. (Courtesy Dr. Irving Glickman, Boston.)

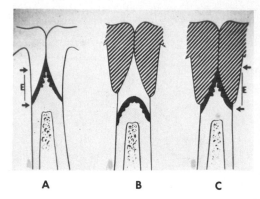

Fig. 3-22. A, Normal embrasure filled with tissue. **B,** Embrasure after periodontal surgery. **C,** Restructured crown shape restoring original embrasure. *E,* Height of free gingiva.

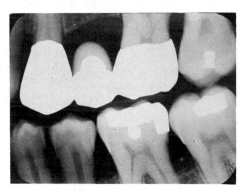

Fig. 3-23. Radiograph showing excellent margins and wide embrasures. (Courtesy Dr. Thomas K. Manolis, LaGrange Park, Ill.)

the place that plaque most frequently starts, this is the place that recurrent decay most frequently occurs.[27] If decay does not result, the plaque will cause periodontal involvement, which will always be at this most critical area. This is a non–self cleansing area.

On the other hand, restorations should not be forced subgingivally into the connective tissue beyond the epithelial attachment. This tearing of the epithelial attachment results in the epithelial attachment migrating apically and the sulcus deepening into a pocket (Fig. 3-21).

Embrasures

The teeth widen out into and touch in an area called a proximal contact. The spaces that widen out from the contact are known as embrasures. In health, the embrasures are usually filled with tissue (Fig. 3-22). Embrasures protect the gingiva from food impaction and deflect the food so as to massage the gingival surface. They provide spillways for food during mastication and relieve occlusal forces when resistant food is chewed. Embrasures are critical considerations in re-

storative dentistry. The proximal surfaces of dental restorations are important because they create the embrasures essential for gingival health. Restorations may be constructed so as to preserve the morphology of the crown and root relationship and thus retain the original morphology. In disease and periodontal therapy this tissue is reduced; the new restorations may create a new embrasure, which will locate the restorations close to the new level of the gingiva. The proximal surfaces of crowns should taper away from the contact areas on all surfaces (Fig. 3-23). Excessively broad proximal contact areas and inadequate contour in the cervical areas crowd out the facial and lingual gingival papillae. These prominent papillae trap food debris, which leads to gingival inflammation. Proximal contacts that are too narrow buccolingually create enlarged facial and lingual embrasures that do not provide sufficient protection against interdental food impaction.

Pontic design in fixed prosthesis

Pontic design and construction is a controversial subject complicated by an array of confusing terms and an abundance of empiric opinions and lack of extensive research. A pontic is important to a fixed prosthesis because a bridge alters the functional and environmental demands directed upon the teeth and the ridge. Any factor acting on any part of the fixed restoration affects the entire prosthesis. The pontic then, as it mechanically unifies the abutment teeth, covers a portion of the residual ridge, assumes a dynamic role as a component of this prosthesis, and cannot be considered as a lifeless insert of some material. In this role the pontic should restore the function of the tooth it replaces, insure adequate sanitation, be esthetic and comfortable, and be biologically acceptable to the oral tissues.

Questions relating to pontics concern two areas: material and design. From the material standpoint, there are many types, such as all gold, all porcelain, and combination pontics. The last group, combination pontics, includes gold-acrylic, porcelain fused to gold, and prefabricated porcelain-faced pontics. On the basis of design, pontics are variously described as saddle, modified saddle, ridge lap, modified ridge lap, sanitary contoured, bullet, spheroid, and modified spheroid. Disagreement arises as to the selection and success of these various pontic materials and designs.

Materials. The question of pontic materials has long been debated. The need for strength, rigidity, and durability has

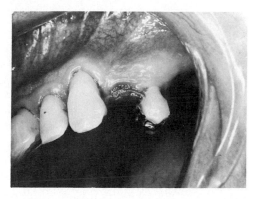

Fig. 3-24. Saddle area showing inflamed tissue under ridge lap pontic after removal of bridge.

been established.[48] Occlusal and incisal forces must be withstood, and yet optimal occlusion must be provided. The material must present or permit acceptable color and contour and must be kind to the adjacent and even contacting tissues. When examining the bioacceptability of materials, two factors must be considered: the effects of the material itself or the effects of the surface finish plus potential adherence, or both. Glazed porcelain has long been considered the most biologically acceptable material,[49-51] even to the claims that it has a stimulatory effect upon gingival tissue.[48,52] Investigators suggest glazed porcelain is, or at least appears to be, the most hygienic,[53] although it has been shown statistically to be the roughest of three pontic materials.[54] Gold has been blamed for an undesirable gingival response.[55] Attention has been drawn to a grayish mucinous accumulation under gold pontics as evidence of incomplete tolerance.[51] Gingival tissues under acrylic pontics have been found to be reddened and to be dramatically inflamed,[55] and acrylic has been widely condemned (Fig. 3-24). The water-inhibition potential of acrylic is unfavorable and attention has been drawn to the odor, noted when acrylic pontics are removed and examined.[56,57] The undesirability of a gold-porcelain or gold-acrylic junction in contact with gingival tissues is widely recognized.[58,59] Related to these various claims, it has been pointed out that although gold and acrylic are said to irritate the mucosa if they cover them it is generally agreed that the soft tissues of the lips, cheeks, and tongue are not affected by porcelain, gold, or resin.[60] There is increasing evidence that the surface finish is the significant factor in pontic materials. In histologic examinations of tissue from beneath pontics of glazed and unglazed porcelain, polished porcelain, polished gold, and polished acrylic, it has been found that though all materials produce some change, all were equally well tolerated.[61] A study of acrylic pontic tips placed deeply into extraction sockets did not demonstrate inflammatory changes except in the presence of plaque.[62] A 10-year study, though failing to find one material superior to another, did demonstrate that with altered pontic design, tissue health could be improved only if the pontic surfaces were carefully repolished or reglazed.[58] Studies comparing the relation of bacteria and plaque accumulation to surface roughness lend additional weight to the importance of surface smoothness. Porcelain, gold, and acrylic have all been found subject to plaque formation,[54] with unfinished pontic surfaces accumulating more debris and calculus than do polished or glazed materials. A study demonstrating the definite increase of bacterial numbers per unit of time on rough abraded surfaces emphasizes the problem.[63] The tissue irritation comes not from the rough materials themselves but from the bacterial plaque more readily accumulated on the rough surface.[64] It becomes apparent then that the finished and hygienic state in which it it is maintained are more important in tissue health than the material itself.

Design. Pontic design, with reference to form and contour, must be considered in relation to the gingival surface, the oc-

clusal surface, and the labial or buccal and lingual surfaces, and especially the proximal surfaces. In the anterior part of the mouth, design is compromised in favor of esthetics, whereas posteriorly, function and hygiene are the critical factors.

Gingival surface. The manner in which the pontic is related to the underlying gingival tissue has resulted in the multiplicity of descriptive names of various pontic shapes referred to above. The demands of esthetics often dictate tissue contact, whereas hygienic requirements favor tissue clearance. Techniques vary and include cast scraping and surgical insertion of a pontic tip into the gingival tissue,[65] major ridge coverage with a saddle pontic, minimal ridge contact as produced by the ridge lap pontic[47] and its modifications, and finally a definite separation between tissue and pontic exemplified by sanitary pontic designs.[66] The term "saddle pontic" refers to the pontic type sitting astride the alveolar ridge with greater tissue coverage than the ridge lap type (Fig. 3-25), which is fitted to the mucosa on the labial or buccal aspect and

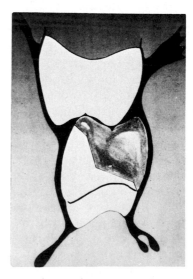

Fig. 3-25. Ridge lap pontic. (Courtesy Dr. Peter K. Thomas, Los Angeles, Calif.)

swings away from the crest of the ridge on the lingual side. The sanitary pontic, on the other hand, has the undersurface separated from the mucosa and is generally convex in all dimensions[67] (Fig. 3-26). Hygienic requirements are foremost in the arguments for and against the various designs. The ridge lap with minimum labial contact is said to retain plaque,[56] and the full saddle type of pontic is said also to be a food trap.[68]

It has been shown that inflammation under a saddle pontic can be progressively reduced by elimination of the tissue coverage lingual to the ridge crest and adjustment to a point contact.[46,58] The greater number of existing studies appear to rule against the use of the saddle pontic, however, the significance of oral hygiene must not be overlooked. With fastidious oral hygiene, it has been demonstrated that plaque formation can be controlled and gingival tissue maintained at a clinically normal level with saddle pontics, inserted both as an original design and as a subsequent modification.

There appears to be a general agree-ment that positive tissue pressure is an undesirable irritant.[56,58,61] Pressure on the tissue produced by scraping or relieving the cast is directly proportional to the tissue change.[51] Insertion of a pontic prosthesis did not prevent gingival tissues from returning to their original dimension, even after gingival excision, unless a permanent pathologic deformation of the ridge was created.[59]

The sanitary pontic is used in the absence of esthetic requirements, chiefly in the lower molar area.[58,67] The conventional design has its undersurface convex in all directions separated from the gingiva by at least 1 mm.[58] A recent modification suggests a concave tissue surface arching occlusally from one abutment to the other[66] (Fig. 3-27). Sanitary pontics are not indicated in the maxillary arch where a large resorption space between the pontic and ridge can interfere with tongue comfort and speech.[69]

Occlusal surface of a pontic. Three concepts exist relative to the occlusal surface of a pontic. One concept advocates the reduction of the occlusal table dimensions,[46,56,60] another maintains normal oc-

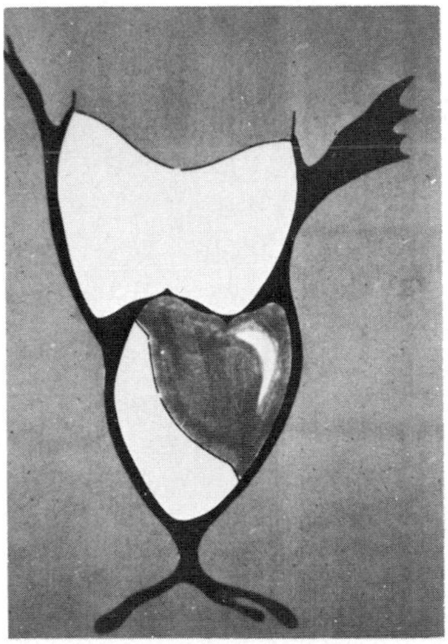

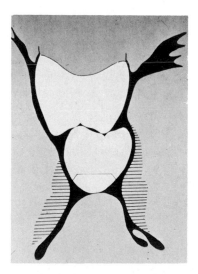

Fig. 3-26. Sanitary pontic. Note space between pontic and ridge. (Courtesy Dr. Peter K. Thomas, Los Angeles, Calif.)

Fig. 3-27. Stein or spheroid pontic. Note how it touches ridge at one point. (Courtesy Dr. Peter K. Thomas, Los Angeles, Calif.)

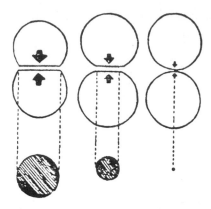

Fig. 3-28. Diagram showing various sizes of occlusal surfaces in same-shaped pontic. When shape is varied, amount of occlusal surface varies. However, amount of force carried by abutment teeth remains the same.

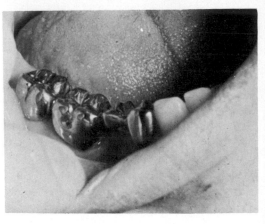

Fig. 3-29. Sanitary bridge replacing second bicuspid.

clusion width,[58] whereas the third approach tends to minimize the significance of occlusal dimension.[70,71]

The reduction of the occlusal width ranging from one fifth to one third the buccolingual dimension is specified to control the force on the abutment teeth (Fig. 3-28). Those who maintain occlusal width do so to provide a soft-tissue protective mechanism during mastication and to provide adequate occlusion with the opposing arch. Recent research points out the importance of the proprioceptive mechanism in regulating the occlusal force. It appears that such a mechanism can automatically control the occlusal forces, regardless of the dimension of the opposing food tables. Efficiency in mastication is achieved by well-developed occlusal ridges and sulci with adequate spillways to the buccal and lingual and into the proximal embrasures.[59,67]

Labial, buccal, and lingual surfaces. The labial aspects of anterior pontics are made to reproduce the natural teeth with their characteristic form and color. The greater accessibility of anterior pontics lessens the significance of the functional aspects of design.[67] Posterior pontic facial surfaces are varied from a natural tooth con-

tour to a nonanatomic gingival converging contour.[58,60] The differences reflect varying concerns over the functional importance of these axial contours. The protective function of the buccal and lingual surfaces is held by some to be important,[58] whereas others describe full contours as unnecessary on the basis of natural tooth form and position as exemplified by the lingual tilt of the lower molars.[72] Modifications include gingival conversion applied within the cervical one half of the buccal surface and cervical two thirds of the lingual surface. Nonanatomic designs, such as the bullet and modified sanitary pontics, place obvious emphasis on the hygiene aspects and disregard the functional theory of buccolingual contours (Fig. 3-29).

Proximal surface. Most clinicians agree that the embrasures in pontics should be designed so as to create conditions most favorable to the gingival and alveolar mucosa.[46] All clinicians concur with the contouring of the opening of the embrasures mesiodistally and buccolingually to facilitate proper oral hygiene. It has been shown that with poor oral hygiene the soft tissue within all types of embrasures develop inflammation, whereas with excellent oral hygiene the soft tissues remain clinically healthy, even when the embrasures were deliberately obliterated. A slight increase in the interdental gingival dimension after 1 year, even with optimum oral hygiene, has led to the suggestion that where oral hygiene is less than perfect, embrasures should be constructed to anticipate gingival enlargement.[46]

SPLINTING

Splinting is one of the most poorly understood and controversial areas of dentistry. One must remember that splinting is used for three purposes: (1) to protect loose teeth from injury while stabilizing them in a favorable occlusal relationship, (2) to distribute occlusal forces so that teeth weakened by loss of periodontal support do not become loose, and (3) to prevent a natural tooth from becoming loose and migrating. The number of teeth required to stabilize a loose tooth depends on the degree and direction of mobility, the amount of the remaining bone, the location of the mobile tooth in the arch, and whether it is to be used as an abutment tooth.

It is generally easier to reduce the mesiodistal component of mobility than the buccolingual component of mobility; this is so because of the approximating teeth in the arch, which aid in tooth support. For the reduction of buccolingual mobility, great reliance is placed on nonmobile teeth used in the splint. In general, it is much better to use more than one firm tooth to stabilize a mobile tooth. The more mobile the teeth, the greater the number of stable teeth are required to splint them. The exact number to splint the teeth varies, depending on the conditions present.

When a fixed bridge is used both to supply missing teeth and to stabilize natural teeth, the following should be noted: If the distal abutment of the bridge is the terminal tooth of the arch and it is mobile, multiple firm anterior abutments are required to stabilize this abutment. Remember, the splinting is the added mechanical factor used to prevent, reduce, or eliminate tooth movement. Alone, it is not always sufficient to accomplish the desired goal. To obtain maximum benefits, splinting should be combined with redesign of the crown surface and the tooth should be in functional harmony with the mandibular movements of the patient (Fig. 3-30).

Splinting refers to any joining together of two or more teeth for the purpose of stabilization. The benefits that can be derived from the effects of splinting are varied. Single or multiple mobile teeth with sufficient bone and evidence of parafunctional habits are *not* to be splinted but are to undergo occlusal correction and the construction of an appliance to prevent damage from the parafunctional habits. If the destructive forces can be reversed, the tooth or teeth with mobility should tighten up. If the mobile tooth is splinted to its neighbor without correction of the occlusal traumatism or parafunctional habit, *more* damage will occur because the tooth involved will not be able to avoid the trauma. In fact, the entire splint may become mobile. Splinting should not be used as an end approach to mobility or trauma from occlusion.

If, however, splinting is required, it will redirect the forces. This is probably the greatest benefit from splinting. Splinting "around the corner" expands the base in two directions and redirects both mesiodistal and buccolingual forces (Fig. 3-31). It is this principle of stress redirection that enables us to effectively save teeth with minimal remaining bone support. When teeth are joined together, any force on an individual tooth is redistributed to all of the splinted teeth. Root surfaces that may resist stresses poorly in one direction may provide good resistance in another. Thus the combined effect of splinting weak teeth together is

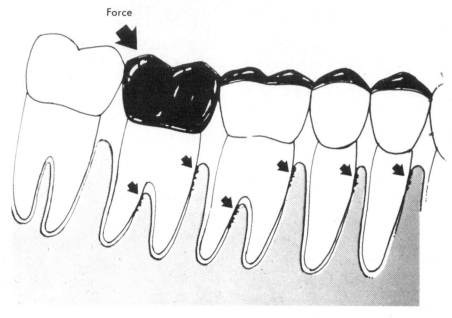

Fig. 3-30. Diagram showing how adverse force on splinted quadrant will transmit force to all the teeth.

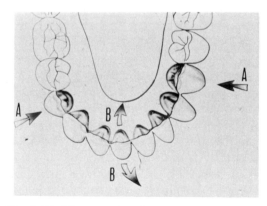

Fig. 3-31. Diagram showing cross-arch splinting that can withstand forces on all directions.

to capitalize on whatever strength any tooth can offer to the group. Splinting also prevents teeth from migrating and supererupting.

Methods used for splinting

Temporary or reversible splinting is used for a variety of purposes and may or may not be followed by permanent splint-ing. The stabilization that can be obtained by provisional splinting provides an environment that is conducive to periodontal healing or bone fill; it is also helpful after orthodontic movement. If after a period of time, usually 6 to 8 weeks, the teeth are stable, then it may not be necessary to continue to splint the teeth. On the other hand, it may be necessary to go on to more permanent stabilization. Some methods of reversible splinting are (1) ligature wire, (2) **A** splint or circumferential wiring, and (3) removable appliances, this last of which is divided into (a) Hawley appliance or retainer, (b) a continuous clasp type of denture, and (c) a swing-lock type of partial denture.

Splinting with ligature wire.[73] Stainless steel ligature wire can be used easily and quickly to stabilize anterior teeth. It is simple and reversible, but it really has no use in the posterior portion of the mouth because the wire has a tendency to slip into the narrower parts of the teeth. Dead soft 0.010 and 0.007 gage stainless steel

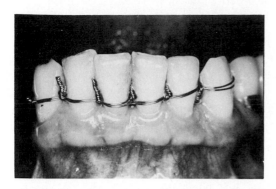

Fig. 3-32. Temporary double-wire splint with interproximal wires.

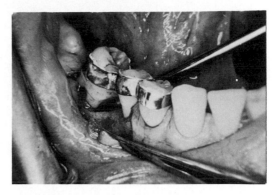

Fig. 3-33. Teeth splinted with orthodontic bands prior to surgery. Note intraosseous defect on mesial surface of molar.

ligature wire should satisfy all requirements. There are two techniques of applying the ligature wire: the inverted S tie and the interdental hairpin tie. In the inverted S tie, stainless steel ligature wire is wrapped around each tooth, through the contact, around the labial wire, and back through the contact. The procedure is repeated for each tooth and then it is twisted together with the labial wire at the distal of the last tooth to be splinted. Each loop is then twisted with pliers or an explorer until the wire is pulled tight around each tooth. The loops are then folded over the wire and they can be stabilized at the contact with autocuring acrylic applied with a brush. In the ligature wire splinting with interdental hairpin ties, the wire is wrapped around all teeth to be splinted and the wire is twisted at the end. A double wire may be used here if more strength is desired. Hairpin-shaped wires are placed at each contact and twisted tight. Contacts may be covered and stabilized with acrylic if desired (Fig. 3-32).

The A splint technique.[74] The A splint is an extracoronal splint and it is provisional. It is a fixed splint that involves minimal tooth reduction. It may be used anteriorly or posteriorly and provides good stability with acceptable esthetics. It can also be accomplished in one office visit. It is an economic way to provide

stabilization for fairly long periods of time, and it can be used to replace missing teeth provisionally. By use of an inverted cone bur or diamond stone, a channel is prepared on the lingual or occlusal surfaces of each tooth to be splinted. The anterior teeth should have the channel cut at the height of the contact. Braided multiple lengths of 0.010 stainless steel wire can be cut to size and adapted to the channel cuts. After a rubber dam is positioned, self-curing acrylic is placed in the channels.

Removable appliances. *Orthodontic retainers* may be used to splint teeth with a soldered lingual or buccal bar or even two soldered bands[75] (Fig. 3-33).

A *continuous clasp partial* is another way of splinting teeth. The advantage of this is that the appliance can be removed for easy cleaning of the appliance and the teeth.

Swing-lock partial dentures can be used in the stabilization of anterior teeth. This is accomplished quite effectively in combination with replacement of posterior teeth through a uniquely designed partial denture. The teeth are braced from the lingual by an extension of the palatal or lingual bar. A labial brace swings horizontally from a hinge on one side into labial contact with the anterior teeth and is locked into the partial denture on the other end of the brace.

Swing-lock partial dentures are effective, but one must remember that the saddle areas are rigidly connected to the anterior teeth and the partial is essentially a tooth-borne affair. Any settling of the saddle areas will cause damage to the anterior teeth.

Provisional splinting with full-coverage acrylic splints. This method is very commonly used with periodontally involved cases where the choice of fixed splints after periodontal therapy has already been selected. Before periodontal therapy the teeth are prepared, and temporary, processed acrylic splints are constructed and cemented in place with temporary cement. These splints can be removed, periodontal therapy performed, and the splints replaced. After healing of the periodontal surgery and allowance of time for the tissue to "mature," permanent splints can be placed.

Determination of abutments

There are many small factors in determination of which abutments are to be used. The first is the crown-to-root ratio; tooth stability is influenced by the leverage exerted upon the periodontium. The nature of this leverage depends on the amount of tooth that is retained in bone (clinical root) in relation to the portion of the crown out of the bone. Any increase in the length of the crown creates an unfavorable leverage upon the periodontium. The root may be short because of normal anatomy, too rapid orthodontic movement, bone loss, or even a combination of factors. There are two methods of modifying the tooth form to change the unfavorable crown-to-root ratio. One is the construction of a new crown in gold or porcelain to gold, and the other method is to change the occlusal surface of the tooth with an onlay. Lateral and tipping stresses arise during function when the cuspal inclines are too steep or the occlusal platform is too wide in relation to the root.[76] Ideally, forces applied to the teeth should fall within the peripheral contours of the root structure that is retained in alveolar bone. In the mandible, this force should be transmitted to the root by way of the buccal cusps. The location of the cusp in relation to the root in the buccolingual direction influences the direction of the transmitted force upon the periodontium.[1] If the direction of the functional forces falls within the lateral border of the clinical root, stress is directed vertically upon the periodontium.[77] If, on the other hand, the force is directed beyond the confines of the root, lateral or tipping stresses are induced. In most instances, the reduction of the length of the clinical crown, change of the cuspal position, and modification of the cuspal inclines can be accomplished simultaneously when one reconstructs the crown surface artificially. Narrowing the buccolingual width of the occlusal surfaces of the reconstructed crowns attains the correct location of the mandibular buccal and maxillary lingual cusps in relation to the root.[78]

Teeth normally have a certain range of mobility. One-rooted teeth are more mobile than multiple-rooted teeth. Mobility is usually in a horizontal direction, but it also occurs axially to a much lesser degree. Mobility beyond the physiologic range is termed "pathologic" and is attributable to one or both of the following factors: loss of alveolar bone and periodontal ligament support or severe trauma from occlusion. The amount of mobility depends on the severity and distribution of the tissue lost on various individual surfaces, the length and shape of the roots, and the root size compared with the crown. A tooth with short-tapered roots is more likely to be mobile than one with normal or bulbous roots with the same amount of bone loss. *The degree of mobility does not correspond with the amount of bone loss.* Trauma caused by excessive occlusal forces and abnormal occlusal forces, aggravated by emotional stress, is a common cause of tooth mobility. Mobility is also increased by hypofunction. Inflammation of an acute nature will also increase mobility greatly, as does periodontal surgery or pregnancy. Tooth mobility from loss of alveolar bone is not likely to be corrected. The likelihood of restoring tooth stability is inversely proportional to the extent of the loss of the alveolar bone.

Determination of prognosis

The alveolar bone should be examined radiographically. Three aspects of the alveolar bone should be considered: the amount of remaining bone, the distribution of remaining bone, and the pattern of bone loss. Obviously, the prognosis becomes less favorable as the amount of bone support decreases. Usually, if the bone loss extends to the apical third of the tooth, the prognosis is unfavorable. The prognosis varies as the distribution of the bone varies. If the bone is distributed unequally around the tooth, but if there is still at least one third of the bone remaining around the area of the greatest destruction, the prognosis is more favorable than if a similar amount of bone is distributed equally around the tooth. The pattern of bone loss is also important. If the bony defect is surrounded by bone and a surface of the tooth, as in a three-walled infraosseous defect, there is greater chance for filling in of bone than around a one-walled defect. Generally, the more bone that is around the defect, the better the prognosis. The clinician has to look at the number of remaining teeth, their size, the shape of the crown and the roots, and the relation of the amount of root in the bone to the amount of the tooth out of the bone (the crown-to-root ratio). The clinician also has to look at the distribution and arrangement of the remaining teeth. It is also important to look at the roots to see if they are within the bony housing. This last is important because a tooth may appear radiographically to have bone on all sides but a check of the position of the tooth in the arch might indicate that the tooth is in buccal version and that the bony housing does not extend over the buccal aspect of the root. Buccally, only gingiva may cover the root. This is called a dehiscence and is most commonly found in teeth that are prominent in the arch: cuspids, upper and lower first bicuspids, mesiobuccal roots of the upper first molars, and also any other tooth that is either pushed or moved (after orthodontics) into a buccal position.

CONCLUSION

The final success of fixed prosthetic work is measured by the longevity and durability of the prosthesis in function and in health. To achieve this success, the fixed prosthesis must be placed in the mouth in view of certain biologic principles that pertain to the relationship of the fixed appliance to the gingival tissues. These principles are broad and all encompassing: they have cleansability, allow for normal tissue shape and contour, do not exceed the adaptive capacity of the periodontium in matters of occlusion, follow the principles of occlusion in direction, duration, amount, and frequency of a force. One should make certain that the fixed appliance is placed into a healthy environment and should understand how to achieve this healthy environment and then how to maintain it. It is also important to diagnose a periodontal problem, subtle though it may be, through all of the subjective and objective signs that may be present. Only in this manner can one proceed to the next step—construction of a durable and healthy fixed prosthetic appliance.

We would like to thank Dr. Nolen Levine, Mrs. Joanne Pollack, and Ms. Jan Knauss for their help and understanding.

SELECTED REFERENCES

1. Gargiulo, A., Wentz, F. M., and Orban, B. J.: Dimensions and relations of the dento-gingival junction in humans, J. Periodontol. **32:**261, 1961.
2. Oliver, R. C., Holm-Pedersen, P., and Löe, H.: The correlation between clinical scoring, exudate measurements and microscopic evaluation of inflammation in the gingiva, J. Periodontol. **40:**201-209, April 1969.
3. Brill, N., and Krasse, B.: The passage of tissue fluid into the clinically healthy gingival pockets, Acta Odontol. Scand. **16:**233, 1958.
4. Grant, D., Stern, I., and Everett, P.: Orban's Periodontics, ed. 4, St. Louis, 1972, The C. V. Mosby Co., p. 206.
5. Ibid., p. 230.
6. Russell, A. L.: International nutrition surveys: a summary of preliminary dental findings, J. Dent. Res. **42:**233, 1963.
7. Löe, H., Theilade, E., and Jensen, S. P.: Experimental gingivitis in man, J. Periodontol. **36:**177, 1965.
8. Theilade, E., Wright, W. H., Jenson, S. B., and Löe, H.: Experimental gingivitis in man, II. A longitudinal, clinical and bacteriological investigation, J. Periodont. Res. **1:**1, 1966.
9. Nisengard, R.: Immediate hypersensitivity and periodontal disease, J. Periodontol. **45:**344, 1974.
10. Ivanyi, L., Wilton, J. M. A., and Lehner, T.: Cell mediated immunity in periodontal disease; cytotoxicity, migration inhibition and lymphocyte transformation studies, Immunology **22:** 141, 1972.
11. Brandtzaeg, P.: Local factors of resistance in the gingival area. J. Periodont. Res. **1:**19-42, 1966.
11a. Brandtzaeg, P.: Immunology of inflammatory periodontal lesions, Int. Dent. J. **23:**438, 1973.
12. MacKenzie, R. S., and Millard, H. D.: Interrelated effect of diabetes, arteriosclerosis and calculus on alveolar bone loss, J.A.D.A. **66:**191, 1963.
13. Wiener, R., Karshan, M., and Tenenbaum, B.: Ovarian function in periodontosis, J. Dent. Res. **35:**875, 1956.
14. Selye, H.: The general adaptation syndrome and the diseases of adaptation, J. Clin. Endo-1950.
15. Chawla, T. N., and Glickman, I.: Protein deprivation and the periodontal structures of the albino rat, Oral Surg. **4:**578, 1951.
16. See reference 14.
17. Horton, L.: Requirement for macrophage-lymphocyte interaction, J. Dent. Res. **53:**337, 1974.
18. Macapanpan, L. C., and Weinmann, J. P.: The influence of injury to the periodontal membrane on the spread of gingival inflammation, J. Dent. Res. **33:**263, 1954.

19. Updegrave, W. J.: Simplifying and improving intraoral dental roentgenography, Oral Surg. **12:**704, 1959.
20. Goldman, H., and Cohen, D. W.: Periodontal therapy, ed. 5, St. Louis, 1973, The C. V. Mosby Co.
21. O'Leary, T.: Plaque control record, J. Periodontol. **43:**38, 1972.
22. Pritchard, J.: A technique for treating infrabony pockets based on alveolar process morphology, Dent. Clin. North Am., p. 85, March 1960.
23. Ewen, S. J.: Bone swaging, J. Periodontol. **36:**57, 1956.
24. Robinson, R. E.: The osseous coagulum for bone induction technique, J. Calif. Dent. Assoc. **46:**18-27, Spring 1970.
25. Shellow, R. A., and Ratcliffe, P. A.: The problems of attaining new alveolar bone after periodontal surgery, J. West. Soc. Periodont. **15:**154, 1967.
26. Shallhorn, R. G.: Eradication of bifurcation defects utilizing frozen autogenous hip marrow implants, Periodontal Abstr. **15:**101, 1967.
27. Glickman, I.: Clinical periodontology, ed. 4, Philadelphia, 1972, W. B. Saunders Co., p. 329.
28. Glickman, I., Roeber, F., Brion, M., and Pameijers, J.: Photoclastic analysis of internal stresses in the periodontium created by occlusal forces, J. Periodontol. **41:**30-35, 1970.
29. Thurow, R. C.: The periodontal membrane in function, Angle Orthodont. **15:**18-29, 52-66, 1945.
30. Massoni, J., Gonzales, V., Haskel, E., and Sales, G.: Effect of traumatic forces applied on the molars of the rat, Odontológica Uruguaya **20:**5, 1964.
31. Glickman, I., and Weiss, L.: Role of trauma from occlusion in initiation of periodontal pocket formation in experimental animals, J. Periodontol. **26:**14, 1955.
32. Itoiz, M. E., Carranza, F. A., Jr., and Cabrini, R. L.: Histologic and histometric study of experimental occlusal trauma in rats, J. Periodontol. **34:**305, 1963.
33. See reference 18.
34. Orban, B.: Tissue changes in traumatic occlusion, J.A.D.A. **15:**2090, 1928.
35. Weinmann, J. P.: Progress of gingival inflammation into the supporting structures of the teeth, J. Periodontol. **12:**71, 1941.
36. Skillen, W. C., and Reitan, K.: Tissue changes following rotation of teeth in the dog, Angle Orthodont. **10:**149, 1940.
37. Bhaskar, S. N., and Orban, B. J.: Experimental occlusal trauma, J. Periodontol. **26:**270, 1955.
38. Stones, H. H.: An experimental investigation into the association of traumatic occlusion with periodontal disease, Proc. Roy. Soc. Med. **31:** 479, 1938.

39. Box, H. K.: Experimental traumatogenic occlusion in sheep, Oral Health **20**:642, 1930.
40. Glickman, I., Stein, R. S., and Smulow, J. B.: The effects of increased functional forces upon the periodontium of splinted and nonsplinted teeth, J. Periodontol. **32**:290, 1961.
41. Ramfjord, S. P., and Kohler, C. A.: Periodontal reaction to functional occlusal stress, J. Periodontol. **30**:95, 1959.
42. Goldman, H.: Gingival vascular supply in induced occlusal traumatism, Oral Surg. **9**:939, 1956.
43. Glickman, I., and Smulow, J. B.: Alterations in the pathway of gingival inflammation into the underlying tissues induced by excessive occlusal forces, J. Periodontol. **33**:7, 1962.
44. McCall, J. O.: Traumatic occlusion, J.A.D.A. **26**:519, 1939.
45. Robinson, J., Reding, G., Zepelin, H., Smith, V., and Zimmerman, S.: Nocturnal teeth-grinding: a reassessment for dentistry, J.A.D.A. **78**:1308, 1969.
46. Hirshberg, S. M.: Compatible temporary tooth health and gingival protection, J. Prosthet. Dent. **18**:151, 1967.
47. Waerhaug, J.: Tissue reactions around artificial crowns, J. Periodontol. **24**:172, 1953.
48. Boyd, H. R., Jr.: Pontics in fixed partial dentures, J. Prosthet. Dent. **5**:55, Jan. 1955.
49. Eissmann, H. F., Radke, R. A., and Noble, W. H.: Physiologic design criteria for fixed dental restorations, Dent. Clin. North Am. **15**:543, July 1971.
50. Harmon, C. B.: Pontic design, J. Prosthet. Dent. **8**:496, May 1958.
51. Hobo, S., and Shillingburg, H. T., Jr.: Porcelain fused to metal: tooth preparation and coping design, J. Prosthet. Dent. **30**:28, July 1973.
52. Allison, J. R., and Bliatia, H. L.: Tissue changes under acrylic and porcelain pontics, J. Dent. Res. Abstr. **37**:66, Feb. 1958.
53. Cavazos, E., Jr.: Tissue response to fixed partial denture pontics J. Prosthet. Dent. **20**:143, Aug. 1968.
54. Coelho, D. H.: Pontic construction and assemblage, J. 2nd Dist. Dent. Soc. (N.Y.) **32**:162-168, April 1946.
55. Podshadley, A. G.: Gingival response to pontics, J. Prosthet. Dent. **19**:51-57, Jan. 1968.
56. Clayton, J. A., and Green, E.: Roughness of pontic materials and dental plaque, J. Prosthet. Dent. **23**:407, April 1970.
57. Adams, J. D.: Planning posterior bridges, J.A.D.A. **53**:647, Dec. 1956.
58. Gade, E.: Hygienic problems of fixed restorations, Int. Dent. J. **13**:318, June 1963.
59. Pine, B.: Pontics for gold-acrylic resin fixed partial dentures, J. Prosthet. Dent. **12**:347, March-April 1962.
60. Stein, R. S.: Pontic residual ridge relationship: a research report, J. Prosthet. Dent. **16**:251, March-April 1966.
61. Wing, G.: Pontic design and construction in fixed bridgework, Dent. Pract. Dent. Rec. **12**:390, July 1962.
62. Masterson, J. B.: Recent trends in the design of pontics and retainers, Dent. Pract. Dent. Rec. **15**:131, Dec. 1964.
63. Swartz, M., and Philips, R. W.: Comparison of bacterial accumulations on rough and smooth enamel surfaces, J. Periodontol. **28**:304, Oct. 1957.
64. Waerhaug, J.: Effect of rough surfaces upon gingival tissues, J. Dent. Res. **35**:323, April 1956.
65. Kayser, A. F.: The gingival design of the pontic, Oral Res. Abstr. **5**:162, Feb. 1970.
66. Perel, M. L.: A modified sanitary pontic, J. Prosthet. Dent. **28**:589, Dec. 1972.
67. Meyers, G. E.: Textbook of crown and bridge prosthodontics, St. Louis, 1969, The C. V. Mosby Co.
68. Krajicek, D. D.: Periodontal consideration for prosthetic patients, J. Prosthet. Dent. **30**:15, July 1973.
69. Klaffenbach, A. O.: Biomechanical restoration and maintenance of the permanent first molar space, J.A.D.A. **45**:633, Dec. 1952.
70. Anderson, D. J., and Picton, D. C.: Masticatory stresses in normal and modified occlusion, J. Dent. Res. **37**:312, April 1958.
71. Ramfjord, S. P., and Ash, M. M.: Occlusion, ed. 2, Philadelphia, 1971, W. B. Saunders Co.
72. Morris, M. L.: Artificial crown contours and gingival health, J. Prosthet. Dent. **12**:1146, Nov.-Dec. 1962.
73. Hirschfeld, L.: The use of wire and silk ligatures, J.A.D.A. **41**:647, 1950.
74. Obin, J. N., and Arvens, A. N.: The use of self-curing resin splints for the temporary stabilization of mobile teeth due to periodontal involvement, J.A.D.A. **42**:320, 1951.
75. Block, P.: A wire band splint for immobilizing loose posterior teeth, J. Periodontol. **39**:17, 1968.
76. Pugh, C. E., and Smerke, J. W.: Rationale for fixed prosthesis in the management of advanced periodontal disease, Dent. Clin. North Am. **13**:243, 1969.
77. Glickman, I.: Role of occlusion in the etiology and treatment of periodontal disease, J. Dent. Res. **50**:199, 1971.
78. Burch, J. G.: Ten rules for developing crown contours in restorations, Dent. Clin. North Am. **15**:611, 1971.

4

Distribution of abutments, crowns, and fixed partial dentures relative to patient's sex and age

As long as the dental arches are complete, we may expect them to function in a normal way, both mechanically and physiologically. However, when one or more of the natural teeth are lost or missing either through caries, accident, or some other cause, an immediate impairment of their functions takes place in proportion to the number of teeth missing and their relative importance in the arch. Although the loss of a tooth is harmful to the continued welfare of the masticatory mechanism, the dangers of such a condition may be mitigated or prevented to a large degree by replacing the tooth with a prosthetic appliance at the earliest possible time.

Because a patient continues to take food and apparently leads a normal, natural, and healthy existence does not alter the fact that the efficency of his chewing mechanism has been disturbed and that additional strains have been placed upon the remaining natural teeth. Since unnatural conditions develop from the loss of teeth, it is logical to expect a new environment and the development of new stresses. Nature cannot always accommodate herself to a new arrangement, and, unless rehabilitated by means of prosthethetic appliances, the entire arch may eventually be destroyed.

LOSS OF ONE TOOTH

It is, therefore, the duty of every dentist to appraise in the patient not only the mechanical deficiencies which result from the loss of a single tooth, but also the biologic changes that follow such a loss and that extend their destructive local influences to involve the entire upper and lower arches. Such disturbances in the dental structure and the resulting malpositions of teeth may be found in every mouth in which an edentulous area has been permitted to exist for any length of time without being reconstructed.

It has been estimated that the loss of one tooth, particularly the lower first molar, results in a 10% decrease in the function of the dental arch. This instant decrease in function may be increased to 30% if immediate steps are not taken to replace the lost tooth and thus to maintain normal functions and relationships.

Fig. 4-1 presents a condition that has resulted from the extraction of a lower molar. Because the lost tooth was not immediately replaced, we find a mesial drifting and tilting of the posterior teeth; this results in the loss of most of their chewing efficiency since they contact the opposing arch only in the area of the distal marginal ridges. Such an occlusal relationship is traumatic in its possibilities, creating a predisposition toward periodontal disease and pulp involvement. Because the contact areas on the distal surfaces are also lost, we find a tendency for food impaction and the development of pockets.

With the continued forward inclination

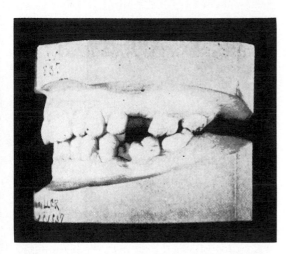

Fig. 4-1. Shifting and tilting of teeth caused by extraction of first molars in upper and lower arches.

of the tooth, the alveolar process on the mesial surface, together with the periodontal membrane in this area, is destroyed, leaving the cementum of the tooth exposed; such a condition makes this area vulnerable to sensitiveness and caries. Eventually a deep pocket develops, necessitating the removal of the tooth.

Because the lower first molar is the most frequently lost tooth in the arch, it is usually found that the second molar moves forward and is subject to the symptoms and changes just described. It is also noticed that the bicuspids sometimes move distally into the edentulous space. There are times when the distal movement of the second bicuspid equals the full width of the tooth. Because a tendency also exists for lower molars to incline lingually, excessive destruction of the periodontal membrane and alveolar process on this surface is frequent. If the lingual inclination of the tooth becomes excessive, it may not only prove a handicap to speech but may also result in an inflammation of the soft tissues of the tongue.

That the deleterious changes are not limited to the individual or adjacent teeth

is shown by the fact that teeth in the opposing arch also become directly involved. The removal of a lower tooth causes the loss of occlusal function with an opposing upper tooth; hence the upper tooth gravitates beyond its normal occlusal plane. In so doing, it changes or loses its contact with its proximating teeth, and the resultant unusual egression promotes pathologic possibilities, since it produces an unusually rapid and extensive epithelial detachment and cementum exposure. Moreover, such egressed teeth later prove to be serious obstacles when the restoration of the edentulous condition is undertaken.

Because patients are less prone to chew their food on a partially edentulous side, the disuse of these teeth will assist in the development of an unhygienic condition. Such a habit frequently is a predisposing cause of caries and excessive calculus formation with its accompanying gingivitis. As previously indicated, teeth not used habitually or used only to a minor degree induce definite tissue changes. Not only is the structural form of the alveolar process changed or modified, but also the lack of functional stimulation results in an area of lowered resistance, making the periodontal membrane and the gingival tissues easy prey for infective organisms.

LOSS OF SEVERAL TEETH

Noticeable changes in the facial contour of patients frequently may be traced to the loss of several teeth and to the edentulous space that was permitted to remain for a long time. Such unnatural oral conditions are very often reflected unfavorably in temporomandibular joint disturbances. Several investigators[1-5] have indicated an apparent relationship between the two conditions.

The majority of reports dealing with the loss of permanent teeth invariably indicate that the first molar is the tooth most frequently lost; this is especially true of the lower first molar. This view is also substantiated by data that have been compiled from clinical records of several thousand crown and bridge clinic patients extending for a period of over 40 years.

The following discussion concerns itself with, first, those teeth restored with crowns, and, second, those missing teeth that were restored with bridges during the first 17 years of the research. A recent recapitulation shows no appreciable deviation in the sex and age distribution of patients or in the teeth or types of restorations involved. Our clinical data and observations cover 12,000 crowns and 6,000 fixed structures made by students. An analysis of the first 17 years of clinical data presents the following findings.

CROWNS AND FIXED PARTIAL DENTURES

There were 1,075 crowns for teeth having vital pulps. These were placed for 378 men and 574 women patients.

Tables 4-1 and 4-2 indicate the distribution and location of the teeth restored. It is significant that for upper teeth with

vital pulps the greatest number of crown restorations are placed on the central and lateral incisors. This is attributable largely to the use of complete porcelain veneer crowns subsequent to operative restorations. In the lower arch the first and second bicuspids, also the first molar, are the teeth most frequently crowned. This is attributable largely to the fact that biscuspids with vital pulps are very frequently retained and crowned in order that they may be used as direct retainers for removable partial dentures. In studying this group of patients, the investigators found that all except 126 patients had normal occlusion; 60% were in good health; 39%, in fair health; and 1%, in poor health. These patients were divided almost equally between those who were and those who were not susceptible to caries.

Table 4-3 shows the sex and age distribution of patients requiring crowns on teeth with vital pulps.

It is interesting to note that although the quantity of the work was done for pa-

Table 4-1. Crowns for teeth with vital pulps—distribution of restored teeth

	Upper																	
Times restored	3	17	26	32	21	31	51	62	81	59	22	19	23	28	21	9		
Tooth	8	7	6	5	4	3	2	1	1	2	3	4	5	6	7	8		
R		Lower																L
Tooth	8	7	6	5	4	3	2	1	1	2	3	4	5	6	7	8		
Times restored	3	26	45	45	56	22	4	5	6	3	27	65	54	40	23	8		

Table 4-2. Crowns for teeth with vital pulps—location of restored teeth

Upper teeth		Total	Order	Lower teeth		Total	Order
Central	(1)	143	1	Central	(1)	11	5
Lateral	(2)	110	2	Lateral	(2)	7	6
Cuspid	(3)	53	5	Cuspid	(3)	49	4
First bicuspid	(4)	40	6	First bicuspid	(4)	121	1
Second bicuspid	(5)	55	3	Second bicuspid	(5)	99	2
First molar	(6)	54	4	First molar	(6)	85	3
Second molar	(7)	38	7	Second molar	(7)	49	4
Third molar	(8)	12	8	Third molar	(8)	11	5

tients between the ages of 20 and 40 years, the maximum for women occurred in the 30- to 39-year period, whereas for men it was in the 20- to 29-year group.

There were placed 1,350 crowns on teeth without pulps, 707 for women and 506 for men patients.

In studying Tables 4-4 and 4-5, note that the majority of crowned pulpless teeth are also in the upper arch. Again, the two upper incisors predominate in the frequency of their restoration, whereas in the lower arch the first molar is the tooth most frequently restored; the cuspid and the two bicuspids follow next in order. The occlusion of these patients is normal in all but 220 patients. Approximately 70% of the patients were susceptible to caries, whereas 75% were in good health, 24% in fair health, and 1% in poor health. It is significant that here again the largest percentage of restorations was placed for patients between 20 and 40 years of age.

Table 4-3. Crowns for teeth with vital pulps—sex and age distribution of patients

	Age of patient				
	17-19 years	**20-29 years**	**30-39 years**	**40-49 years**	**50 years and over**
Male	51	89	76	41	33
Female	78	92	157	93	41

Table 4-4. Crowns for pulpless teeth—distribution of restored teeth

Upper																		
Times restored			40	55	42	54	56	88	100	104	120	55	65	50	47	37		
Tooth	8	7	6	5	4	3	2	1	1	2	3	4	5	6	7	8		
R					**Lower**													L
Tooth	8	7	6	5	4	3	2	1	1	2	3	4	5	6	7	8		
Times restored	4	30	58	38	43	42	15	3	3	10	42	38	40	65	33	2		

Table 4-5. Crowns for pulpless teeth—location of restored teeth

Upper teeth		Total	Order	Lower teeth		Total	Order
Central	(1)	204	2	Central	(1)	6	7
Lateral	(2)	208	1	Lateral	(2)	25	6
Cuspid	(3)	111	4	Cuspid	(3)	84	2
First bicuspid	(4)	119	3	First bicuspid	(4)	81	3
Second bicuspid	(5)	92	6	Second bicuspid	(5)	78	4
First molar	(6)	102	5	First molar	(6)	123	1
Second molar	(7)	79	7	Second molar	(7)	63	5
Third molar	(8)			Third molar	(8)	6	7

Table 4-6. Crowns for pulpless teeth—sex and age distribution of patients

	Age of patient				
	17-19 years	**20-29 years**	**30-39 years**	**40-49 years**	**50 years and over**
Male	114	154	122	61	55
Female	170	202	193	107	37

Table 4-7. Fixed partial dentures—distribution of restored teeth

	Upper																
Times restored	7	88	65	64	60	190	42	59	49	37	162	66	91	58	98	13	
Tooth	8	7	6	5	4	3	2	1	1	2	3	4	5	6	7	8	
R	Lower																L
Tooth	8	7	6	5	4	3	2	1	1	2	3	4	5	6	7	8	
Times restored	43	113	18	109	60	30	8	3	49	37	30	44	80	14	91	37	

Table 4-8. Fixed partial dentures—location of restored teeth

Upper teeth		Total	Order	Lower teeth		Total	Order
Central	(1)	108	6	Central	(1)	52	6
Lateral	(2)	79	7	Lateral	(2)	45	7
Cuspid	(3)	352	1	Cuspid	(3)	60	5
First bicuspid	(4)	126	4	First bicuspid	(4)	104	3
Second bicuspid	(5)	155	3	Second bicuspid	(5)	189	2
First molar	(6)	123	5	First molar	(6)	32	8
Second molar	(7)	186	2	Second molar	(7)	204	1
Third molar	(8)	20	8	Third molar	(8)	80	4

Table 4-6 shows that the highest percentage of restorations for men is between 20 and 29 years of age, whereas for women the requirements are almost equally divided between the 20- and 30-year groups.

Tables 4-7 and 4-8 are concerned with 853 fixed partial dentures constructed for 462 female and 391 male patients. Here again we observe the distribution of women requiring dental service; it is evident that upper teeth are more frequently restored than the lower teeth. Since the upper cuspid is common to the anterior, median, and posterior bridge components, it is the tooth most frequently employed as an abutment. Because of the frequent loss of the first molars, we find that the second bicuspids and the second molars are next in the frequency of their use as abutments. As expected, the lateral incisors and third molars are the teeth least used as abutments.

A study of the lower arch presents a slightly different situation, for the second molars and the second bicuspids are the teeth most frequently used as abutments; the first bicuspid is next in order. That the third molar is used as often as it is may at first seem incredible. Yet, it is recalled that the lower first molar is the tooth most frequently lost and that the second molar has a high mortality because of mesial tilting; as a result there frequently is no alternative left except to use the lower third molar for the bridge abutment. The significant fact is that the lower first molar is used the least number of times as a bridge abutment.

Of the total number of abutments used for fixed bridges, 1,439 were teeth with vital pulps, whereas 300 were pulpless. Although the ratio of vital to pulpless teeth is nearly 5:1, periodic examinations, both clinical and roentgenographic, have shown that the pulpless tooth may be used satisfactorily as a bridge abutment, provided; first, that the prognosis for treatment is favorable; second that the treatment and filling of the root canal are carried out under aseptic and controlled conditions; and third, that the treated tooth is kept under periodic surveillance.

The 1,739 abutment teeth supported 1,559 pontics. This gives a ratio of 1.7:1.5 of abutment tooth to pontic. A further

Table 4-9. Fixed partial dentures—sex and age distribution of patients

	Age of patient				
	17-19 years	**20-29 years**	**30-39 years**	**40-49 years**	**50 years and over**
Male	24	153	104	54	33
Female	35	120	153	81	22

Table 4-10. Semifixed partial dentures—distribution of restored teeth

		Upper																
Times restored		44	21	75	32	68	12	38	35	15	68	26	74	23	40	3		
Tooth	8	7	6	5	4	3	2	1	1	2	3	4	5	6	7	8		
R							Lower											L
Tooth	8	7	6	5	4	3	2	1	1	2	3	4	5	6	7	8		
Times restored	9	105	22	98	29	7	1	—	2	—	4	22	96	15	100	10		

Table 4-11. Semifixed partial dentures—location of restored teeth

Upper teeth		Total	Order	Lower teeth		Total	Order
Central	(1)	73	4	Central	(1)	2	7
Lateral	(2)	28	7	Lateral	(2)	1	8
Cuspid	(3)	136	2	Cuspid	(3)	11	6
First bicuspid	(4)	58	5	First bicuspid	(4)	51	3
Second bicuspid	(5)	149	1	Second bicuspid	(5)	194	2
First molar	(6)	44	6	First molar	(6)	37	4
Second molar	(7)	84	3	Second molar	(7)	205	1
Third molar	(8)	3	8	Third molar	(8)	19	5

analysis discloses 706 four-tooth bridges and 147 three-tooth restorations. Although the ideal bridge has two abutment teeth for every restored tooth, clinical evidence indicates that the four-tooth restoration is a biologically acceptable restoration.

The occlusion was normal in 35% of the patients; 80% kept their mouths habitually clean, whereas slightly more than 50% were susceptible to caries. Moreover, 75% of these were in good health, 24%, in fair health, and 1%, in poor health.

Table 4-9 again emphasizes that crown and bridge prosthesis is primarily a service for the 20- to 40-year age group. Again note that the maximum requirement for men is in the 20- to 29-year period; for women it lies within the 30- to 39-year span.

In the semifixed bridges, employing a flexible or nonrigid connector at one terminal, we find that of 683 restorations of this type 355 were constructed for women, whereas 287 were made for men.

A study of the data in Tables 4-10 and 4-11 indicates that this type of bridge is used most frequently to restore an upper first bicuspid and upper lateral incisor, for we find that the second bicuspids, cuspids, and central incisors are used most frequently as abutments. We also find evidence here of the frequent restoration of the upper first molar, since the second molar is used 84 times as an abutment. The tabulation likewise emphasizes the infrequent use of the upper lateral incisors and third molars as bridge abutments.

In the lower teeth we find that the first molar is most frequently restored by

Table 4-12. Semifixed partial dentures—sex and age distribution of patients

	Age of patient				
	17-19 years	**20-29 years**	**30-39 years**	**40-49 years**	**50 years and over**
Male	34	128	57	26	8
Female	30	100	125	48	10

means of a bridge. The second molars and second bicuspids are most frequently used, whereas the central and lateral incisors are employed the least number of times as abutments.

Of the abutments used, 1,070 had vital pulps, whereas 221 were pulpless. These teeth supported 944 pontics, with a ratio of 2 abutment teeth to 1.5 of pontics. In this instance it is found that of the total number of bridges constructed, 66% are the three-unit type, that is, two teeth supporting one pontic. Of these patients, 80% had normal occlusion and 75% of them kept their mouths habitually clean. The records disclose that fully half of the patients were susceptible to caries, whereas 75% were in good health, 15% in fair health, and 10% in poor health.

Table 4-12 again emphasizes the 20- to 40-year bracket for this type of service; likewise, the fact that the male requirement has its optimum in the 20- to 29-year group, whereas the women find their greatest need in the 30- to 39-year period.

The foregoing data are factual; what, if any, biologic significance is attached to these findings remains for future investigators to determine.

Since the ratio of teeth with vital pulps to pulpless teeth is approximately 5:1, it is frequently necessary to decide whether a pulpless tooth should be retained or extracted, and, if retained, what the possibilities are of its giving satisfactory service. Although it is unquestionably true that a tooth with a vital pulp is better than one without it, one should make the decision by ascertaining what the response has been and what service the patient has obtained from his or her previously treated teeth. If radiographic evidence indicates an unfavorable biologic reaction to treated teeth, then it is unwise to employ such teeth for additional bridge abutments.

SELECTED REFERENCES

1. Hildebrand, G. Y.: Studies in mandibular kinematics, Dent. Cosmos **68**:449, 1936.
2. Hildebrand, G. Y.: Studies in the masticatory movements of the human lower jaw, Berlin, 1931, Walter De Gruyter & Co.
3. Hildebrand, G. Y.: Studies in dental prosthetics, Stockholm, 1937, Swedish Dental Association, A. B. Fahlcrantz Boktryckeri.
4. Brodie, A. G.: The temporo-mandibular joint, Illinois Dent. J. **8**:2, 1939.
5. Maves, T. W.: Radiology of the temporo-mandibular articulation with correct registration of vertical dimension for reconstruction, J.A.D.A. **25**:585, 1938.

GENERAL REFERENCES

Anderson, D. J.: Measurement of stress in mastication, J. Dent. Res. **35**:664, 1956.

Brekhus, J. J.: Dental disease and its relation to the loss of human teeth, J.A.D.A. **16**:2237, 1929.

Cheyne, V. D., and Drain, C. L.: Dental caries and permanent tooth extraction: a study of age, sex and location of the incidence of first permanent molar extraction in 8,677 school children, J. Dent. Res. **19**:570-584, 1960.

Finn, S. B.: Prevalence of dental caries, Publ. 225, National Academy of Sciences, Washington, D. C., 1952, National Research Council.

Grewe, J. M., and Meskin, L. H.: Loss of teeth, Northwest. Dent. **46**(3):156-158, 1967.

Kishi, Y., Uchida, T., and Kasai, A.: [Statistical observation on artificial crowns and fixed partial dentures], Aichi Gakuin J. Dent. Sci. **9**(3):116-125, Dec. 1971.

Knutson, J. W., and Klein, H.: Studies on dental caries, IV: tooth mortality in elementary school children, U. S. Public Health Rep. **53**:1021, 1938.

Lundquist, C.: Tooth mortality in Sweden: a statistical survey of tooth loss in the Swedish population, Acta Odont. Scand. **25:**289-322, 1967.

McCollum, B. B.: Is it necessary to replace missing teeth? J.A.D.A. **24:**442, 1937.

Salzmann, J. A.: A study of orthodontic and facial changes, and effects on dentition attending the loss of first molars in five hundred adolescents, J.A.D.A. **25:**892, 1938.

Silness, J.: Distribution of crowns and bridges, Bergen, Norway, 1968, University of Bergen.

Weinberg, L. A.: Force distribution in mastication, clenching and bruxism, Dent. Dig. **63:**58, 72, 1957.

Weiner, S.: Evaluation of success of prosthetic treatment using fixed partial dentures, Prosthet. Stomatol. **21**(5):337-342, 1971.

Westin, G., and Wold, H.: 1942 års tandmönstring av inskrivningsskyldiga, Odontol. Tidskrift **51:** 487-616, 1943.

5

Biomechanical considerations of tooth preparation for fixed prosthodontics

William F. P. Malone, Boleslaw Mazur, Stanley D. Tylman, and Hosea F. Sawyer

Perceptive diagnosis by the dentist and the quality of the tooth preparation predetermine the longevity of the majority of fixed prostheses. Biologically tolerant fixed prosthodontic procedures are initiated by prudent tooth preparation. Tooth preparation is referred to as the mechanical treatment of dental diseases or injury to hard tissues that will restore a tooth or teeth to original form and prevent future destruction. Tooth preparation in fixed prosthodontics has the additional responsibility of maintaining the support of the prosthesis that is placed over the edentulous areas.

The advent of high-velocity instrumentation has transformed extremely arduous tooth preparation into ordinary dental treatment. Conversely, high-speed tooth preparation proceeded initially without concomitant longitudinal studies in the science of occlusion. This is also true of the development of optimal morphologic contours for restorative units.

TOOTH PREPARATION

A great percentage of failure of cast restorations are justifiably attributed to the violation of basic preparation design. Tooth preparations that remove an inordinate amount of tooth structure should be considered prohibitive. Oversimplification or omission of the principles of cavity preparation established by G. B. Black[1] and crown and preparation emphasized by S. D. Tylman[2] commonly result in clinical failure. A premise that must be conveyed to the patient, understood by the technician, and realized by the dentist is the fact that crown preparations or restorations are seldom performed on healthy teeth. However, the ideal design for a preparation must be visualized by the dentist so that modifications of classic treatment can be employed. Satisfactory tooth preparation remains the primary premise for all fixed prosthodontics.

Objectives of tooth preparation in fixed prosthodontics

Objectives of restorative preparation procedures must be clearly defined. All fixed prosthodontic procedures are potentially a failure if any of the following objectives are not considered:

1. Removal of caries and the clinical evaluation of existing restorations
2. Acceptable structural design of the fixed restorations to withstand functional forces
3. Strengthening of remaining tooth

structure by uniform tooth reduction to provide sufficient support for the retainers

4. Preservation of existing healthy tooth structure to provide resistance against displacement of the retainer

5. Satisfactory gingival marginal design for an acceptable seal of the restoration

6. Conservative but pragmatic tooth reduction to encourage a clinically acceptable supportive tissue response[3]

CARIES-CONTROL PROGRAM

A more sagacious approach to comprehensive patient care would be the initiation of a caries-control program, which would reduce the infectious process as a disease entity prior to any prosthodontic procedures. The severity of the carious involvement and the age of the patient will determine the merit of an individual's caries-control program. Caries-control programs will also allow a programmed sequence of treatment so that fixed prosthodontics can be performed over a period of time, with priority for patient esthetics, comfort, or functional needs. Further benefits are the following:

1. The time lapse created by use of the caries-control concept will result in more biologically tolerant restorations by allowing an accommodation period for the patients.

2. The caries control will also provide the patient with time to ease financial stress for professional services rendered. This will make more refined procedures available to a greater percentage of the populace.

3. The dentist, in turn, can evaluate the success of oral hygiene methods instituted. A realistic preventive program should be routinely instituted prior to insertion of cast restorations.

It is only reasonable to expect that the caries-control program instituted for a patient should be followed up by a more refined treatment plan within an acceptable length of time. Failure to accomplish a proper subsequence of definitive treatment defeats the entire rationale of comprehensive health care delivery. If this crucial procedure is not instituted, ultimately a "bad name" results from worthwhile clinical therapy.

Removal of caries

The amount of caries removed and how, is an alternative exercised by the dentist based upon existing clinical conditions. The removal of caries during actual tooth preparation is possible when there is limited loss of the original tooth structure. Carious tooth structure and existing restorations are methodically removed after establishing the traditional form of the intended preparation. This procedure is performed to preserve the vitality of the teeth involved. Capricious removal of caries or existing restorations without a preconceived concept of the final form of the tooth preparation commonly renders the tooth inoperable. Conversely, the most common error associated with caries removal is incomplete excavation of active caries in the dentinoenamel junction under the cusps.

The coronal portion of the tooth preparation must provide adequate retention for the casting. Therefore the removal of caries during tooth preparation is possible only if there is limited loss of the original tooth structure.

A common practice is to remove caries and existing restorations during preparation and to "base out" these defects on the working dies. One drawback is the effect of severe undercuts, which may compromise the elastic properties of the impression materials. Another consideration is the disorientation of the dentist to the position of the pulp while he removes large portions of tooth structure during tooth preparation. Teeth with nonvital pulps and loss of retention can result from this direction of therapy.

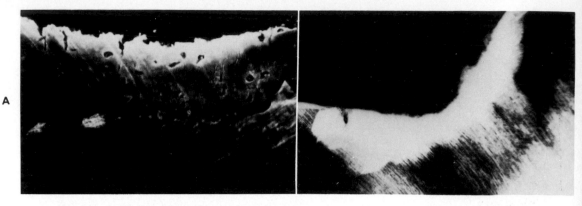

Fig. 5-1. A, Penetration of caries into dentin, which threatens vitality of pulp. Tooth preparations place additional stress upon recovery mechanism of tooth. **B,** Sclerotic dentin resulting from host response to irritants.

Extensive caries involvement or the presence of large restorations require a caries-control program. Caries-control procedures are initiated in the form of traditional-quadrant cavity preparations with high-velocity instruments. Rubber-dam utilization is a preemptive measure during caries removal and quadrant placement of amalgam restorations.[4]

There are three classic steps involved in caries-control programs.

1. Quadrant removal of all infected carious tooth structure
2. Protection and maintenance of tooth vitality or initiation of endodontic therapy, or both (Fig. 5-1)
3. Restoration of destroyed tooth structure with amalgam restorations prior to the preparation of teeth for cast restorations

Carious tooth structure is removed by meticulous use of a slowly revolving large round bur, that is, no. 6 or no. 8. Undue pressure on pulpal tissue should be avoided. Ultrasharp spoon excavators have limited use in deep caries removal.

Sequence of caries control

Complete dentistry for all patients in short time intervals is usually a ludicrous approach that must not be confused with comprehensive patient care. The caries control is usually accomplished by plac-ing amalgam restorations in quadrants with the use of a rubber dam. Endodontic therapy and periodontal treatment are initiated concomitantly. Canines and terminal molars are given priority provided that the dentist has already addressed his attention to patient discomfort, such as emergency esthetics or pain-relieving therapy. The first molars, because of their crucial arch position, would be the next teeth to treat after the canines and terminal molars.

In summary:

1. Caries control is a practical procedure designed to eliminate the infectious process of dental caries as a disease entity.
2. Caries control enables a logical sequence of complex treatment plans.
3. A programmed evacuation of caries with quadrant amalgam restorations is presently the most effective approach for a predictive caries control (Fig. 5-2).
4. The age group that will benefit most in this type of procedure is the 12- to 18-year-old individuals who are in an active growth and development period.[5]
5. Whenever the complexity of a given case exceeds normal treatment direction, a caries-control program instituted to restore the teeth with

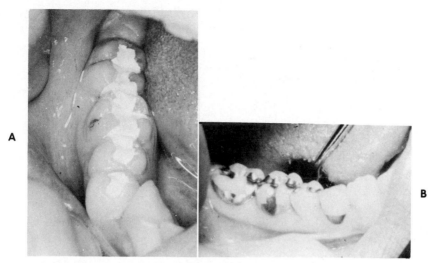

Fig. 5-2. A, Caries is removed and sedative treatment restorations are placed to eliminate the disease entity prior to fixed prosthodontics. Sedative treatment restorations have only limited clinical value because of their inability to withstand forces of mastication. **B,** Quadrant amalgam restorations provided a realistic approach to oral treatment. (From Malone, W. F., and Sarlas, C. H.: Dent. Clin. North Am. **13**(2):461, April 1969.)

high priority in the arch by concomitant periodontal therapy, is the most sensible approach.

UNIFORM TOOTH REDUCTION

One factor merits thoughtful consideration in preparing teeth for all types of retainers; it is the insatiable desire of the air rotor for tooth structure. The removal of mineralized tooth structure is swift and irreversible. Previously, preparations were performed by a combination of cleavage, planing, and abrasion. Small amounts of tooth structure were tediously cut away.

Uniformity of tooth reduction should prevail in high-velocity instrumentation. As a general rule teeth that are in an undesirable or poor arch position warrant a more perceptive diagnosis and treatment plan sequence than do teeth in a normal arch position. Diagnostic wax-ups of secondary "study" casts assist the development of a workable occlusal plane and set the stage for more conservative crown preparations (Fig. 5-3, *A*). The dentist can then program the reduction of tooth surfaces to provide parallelism and improve arch position with selective tooth reduction. Deviations from normal or uniform reduction become more apparent in gross skeletal disparities in the maxillomandibular relationship, for example, class III relationship and crossbites.

Sequence of uniform tooth reduction

A common fault during preparation is insufficient or excessive reduction during tooth reduction (Fig. 5-3, *B*). Diagnostic casts are indicated as the complexity of the preparation increases. The casts are a mandate when multiple maxillary or mandibular preparations are anticipated (Fig. 5-4). Perceptive diagnosis reduces the untoward results of multiple or single preparations.

The following are the most common steps of tooth preparation:
1. Occlusal or incisal reduction
2. Axial reduction: proximal, buccal (labial), and lingual reduction

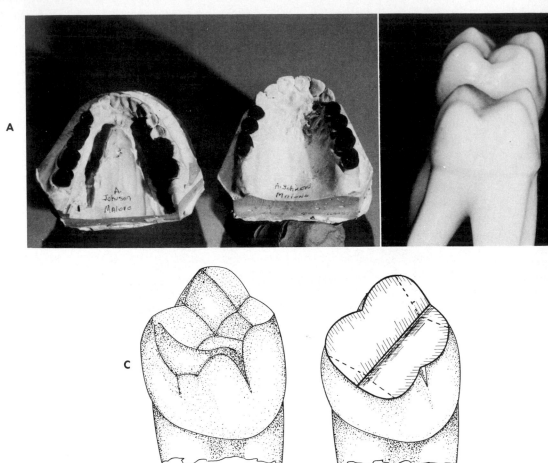

Fig. 5-3. A, Diagnostic wax-ups on casts prior to tooth preparation assist the dentist in determining occlusal relationship, establishing esthetics, and providing satisfactory treatment restorations for interim coverage. **B,** Complete crown preparation for an upper molar. Uniform tooth reduction from original tooth morphology is desirable. Occlusal topography serves as a prescription during laboratory fabrication. **C,** Uniform reduction is started with occlusal (central groove) reduction to maintain satisfactory arch position and adequate occlusal clearance. (**A,** Courtesy Dr. Albert Johnson, Riverside, Ill.)

3. Resistance and retention form established
4. Refinement and smoothing after gross axial and occlusal reduction
5. Establishment of gingival termination

Occlusal reduction

Occlusal of incisal reduction is performed *first* to provide adequate clearance between the prepared surface and the teeth in the opposing arch. Approximately 2 mm is considered adequate. Variations will depend upon the maxillomandibular relationship, the arch position of potential abutment, and the age of the patient. The dentist must have a working knowledge of border movements and stamp cusp performances so that a comprehensive reduction in the areas of maximum occlusal load will result. Minimal load sections of the preparation can

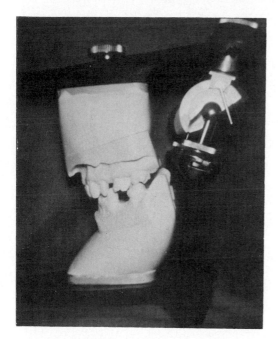

Fig. 5-4. Diagnostic casts mounted on an arcon articulator to establish diagnosis and coordinate sequence of treatment. Degree of refinement of articulator is usually dictated by difficulty associated with treatment phases for patient. (From Malone, W. F., and Sarlas, C. H.: Dent. Clin. North Am. **13**(2):461, April 1969.)

be conservatively prepared to provide resistance and retention.

The occlusal reduction will dictate the necessity for additional forms of retention when the axial walls are reduced vertically to the point of barely acceptable length. Patients whose interocclusal clearance is minimal present a variety of problems. A template designed from diagnostic casts is an aid to establishing a satisfactory occlusal reduction. The use of a registration medium such as a wax index in centric and eccentric positions during preparation will act as a gage for the determination of the amount of restorable interocclusal space. Occlusal reduction also allows an assessment for retaining the existing restorations when a caries-control program was deemed unnecessary. Initiating tooth preparations

with the more accessible occlusal reduction is also easier for the patient.

The occlusal reduction usually is accomplished in one of three ways:
1. Uniform reduction of cusps and fossa to resemble the original occlusal topography
2. Height reduction in two planes, that is, buccolingually in posteriors, or labiolingually in the upper anterior area
3. Onlay-inlay type, for example, mesial one-half crowns, pin-ledge preparations

A uniform reduction permits sufficient thickness of gold to resist normal stresses and withstand forces during function. The "corrugated" topography type of occlusal reduction also helps to maintain the orientation of the operator during preparation, and reduces the frequency of inadvertent pulpal involvement.

Flat plane reduction is associated with teeth that have a nonvital pulp and with aged patients whose interocclusal relationship is minimal (Fig. 5-5, *A* and *B*). The onlay-inlay combination preparation eliminates the occlusal grooves of the tooth and is prepared to the traditional outline form. Proximal slice preparations are common with onlay-inlay preparations. Cavosurface margins of this type of occlusal reduction may involve two or more cusps. Perceptive occlusal reduction will assist in establishing a harmonious or at least an innocuous maxillomandibular relationship.

Most failures caused by inept occlusal or incisal reduction will be realized during fabrication of interim restorations or at the time of insertion of the restoration or prosthesis. However, a more insidious failure can result belatedly in the form of occlusal discrepancies with eventual vertical bone loss.

Narrowed occlusal table. Narrowing the occlusal table of a restorative unit is possible only if the dentist was perceptive enough to narrow the buccolingual width

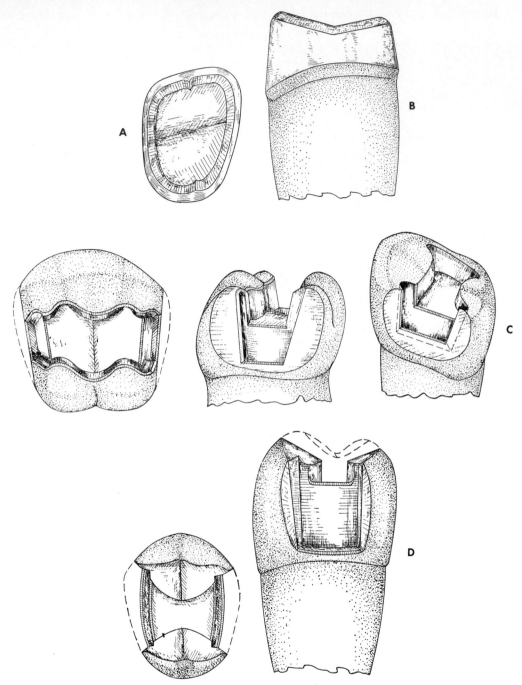

Fig. 5-5. A and **B,** Type 2 occlusal surface reduction having buccal and lingual plane reduction. Type 1 is shown in Fig. 5-3, *B.* **C,** Traditional boxing with slice preparations. Two-plane reduction of buccal and lingual cusps would result in onlay restoration. **D,** Three-surface intracoronal preparation without proximal slice in upper bicuspid, with both cusps restored. **E,** Occlusal onlay restoration also illustrating broad proximal slice preparation. **F,** Tooth preparation for a terminal abutment with a narrowed buccolingual width after prior pin amalgam reinforcement. **G,** Model that illustrates type 1 occlusogingival axial reduction to enhance optimal resistance and retention form. **H,** Note parallelism of proximal walls. (**F** from Malone, W. F., and Balaty, J.: Ill. Dent. J. **37**(2):138, 1968.)

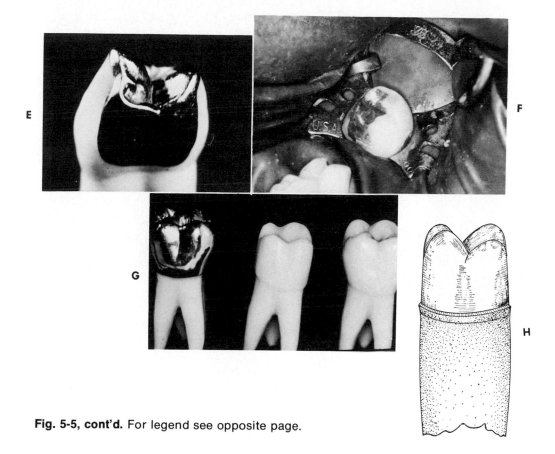

Fig. 5-5, cont'd. For legend see opposite page.

on the preparation (Fig. 5-5). The resultant buccolingual width of the retainer
tends to place:

1. The functional stresses toward the
   long axis of the tooth.
2. It also reduces the incidences of
   deleterious working-side and balancing-side prematurities during
   lateral excursions of the mandible.

Conservatism can be well served by a
knowledgeable assessment of the existing biomechanical requirements for a
routine fixed prosthesis.

Guidelines merely outline traditional
preparations to allow incorporation of
modifications that will serve the clinical
needs of the patient. Patients with class
III malocclusions and crossbites will necessitate alterations of, and dictate modifications of, the amount of buccolingual
axial tooth reduction.

Axial reduction

Axial reduction represents the restorable space for a proximal contact area
(that is, mesiodistal to two teeth) and the
first step to narrow the buccolingual
width of an occlusal table. The vertical
height of axial reduction occlusogingivally represents the degree of resistance and
retention that a given restoration possesses (Fig. 5-5, *G*). Axial reduction may
or may not encompass the entire circumference of the tooth. Preparation of
the proximal axial walls infers a 2- to 5-
degree taper occlusogingivally from the
long axis of the preparation.[6] The finish of
the axial reduction may involve a combination of all four types of gingival margins.

Failure to provide sufficient separation
between teeth during preparation of the
proximal axial walls results in improper

contact areas with the predictable periodontal implications. Conversely, excessive reduction in the proximal axial walls undermines the entire concept of resistance and retention form, which provide sufficient tooth structure to resist functional forces. Splinted multiple preparations decrease the need for 2- to 5-degree maximum taper mesiodistally. However, preservation and restoration of the dentition should have a sound biomechanical basis. Involvement of additional teeth to rectify a diagnostic problem should be rare. Axial reduction buccolingually will

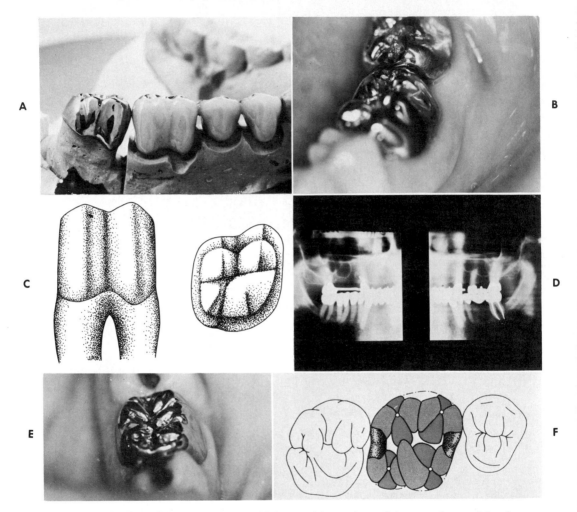

Fig. 5-6. A, Fluted lower molars, which provide a cleansible area for oral hygiene. Periodontally treated patients are more likely to require this type of axial reduction. **B,** Conventional gingival bulge for a complete gold crown. Design of buccal axial reduction is dictated by clinical conditions, that is, crossbite occlusal relationships. **C,** Diagram of fluted upper molar. Note gingival finish follows radicular surface of buccal cusps. A narrowed occlusal table is also enhanced by this type of preparation. **D,** Radiographic panoramic survey of 5-year-old oral rehabilitation showing supportive tissue response to fluted lower molars. **E,** Lower molar whose restoration has a flattened buccal contour. **F,** Programmed appositional wax technique to assist occlusal therapy for a narrowed occlusal table for a complete crown. Note triangular formation of cuspal inclines. (**A** courtesy Dr. Francis W. Summers, Maywood, Ill.)

provide the opportunity of developing an occlusal table that is congruent with harmonious occlusal dictates of the patient.

Cervical areas of the proximal surfaces of restorations are somewhat inaccessible to routine oral hygiene measures. Perceptive preparation by the dentist will allow the opportunity to maintain a *relatively* plaque-free state for these vulnerable areas. Prosthodontically designed morphologic contours of the clinical crown should enhance the degree of accessibility for practical oral hygiene, for example, fluted molars. The buccal and lingual contours of the retainer starts with a tooth preparation in which axial reduction was perceptively accomplished.

Contour

According to Yuodelis et al.,[7] the final retainer or restoration should not mimic the original anatomic crown but recreate the contour of the root portion. Tooth preparation for periodontally treated patients should be fluted just short of the furcation areas eliminating the triangular region formed by the cervical bulge and the roots. The flattened restoration will enable a more cleansible area for home care (Fig. 5-6). Supervised technical construction is necessary to ensure that this procedure is performed consistent with the preparation. Laboratory procedures that ignore the fluted areas of the preparation are worthless. Explicit instructions by the dentist will reduce these improprieties. The slopes and contour of the crown or retainer should reflect the fluted preparation, which enhances gingival health. Section E of Chapter 6 provides a more detailed discussion of crown contour.

Conclusion of the discussion on axial reduction

1. Occlusogingival length of the axial walls should provide retention.
2. Proximal walls should be nearly equal in length occlusogingivally because the retention of the retainer will be only as effective as its shortest wall.
3. Mesial and distal walls must possess a 2- to 5-degree taper and be consistent with the path of insertion.
4. Facial and lingual walls must be more convergent from the occlusal one third to provide an opportunity for cusp warpage, that is, narrowed occlusal table.
5. The short axial walls indicate the need for accessory methods of retention, such as boxing, grooves, and pins.

Gingival termination cannot be divorced from the subject of contour, but it is discussed separately.

Applied physical forces

Basic principles of resistance and retention form are commonly compromised in the majority of preparations for a fixed prosthesis because of the condition of the abutment teeth. For example, it is customary to have an edentulous area in a patient with a carious or periodontally involved abutment. However, if the dentist blatantly violates the basic principles of resistance form, a failure results. The concepts of retention are usually related to friction and surface area covered by the restorations. Modifications from traditional preparation design to satisfy the needs of individual and multiple tooth preparations, esthetics, and excursive occlusal demands *cannot* be oversimplified. Forces are placed on teeth from a myriad of angles. A force placed upon a retainer can result from mastication, bruxism, biting habits, a demanding dietary intake, and a host of intangible, unpredictable stresses (Fig. 5-7).

Retention

Retention may be either extracoronal or intracoronal, but a combination is possible (Fig. 5-8). The blending of both types of retention makes the seating of a casting arduous. Intracoronal retention is synon-

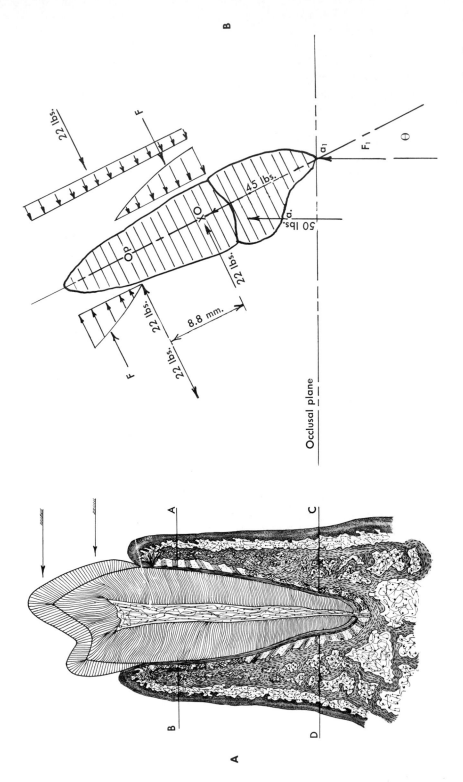

Fig. 5-7. A, Areas of tension, *A* and *D*, and those of compression, *B* and *C*, in periodontal membrane; center of rotation lies between apical one third and occlusal two thirds of root. **B,** Analysis of effects of incisal force on upper central incisor.

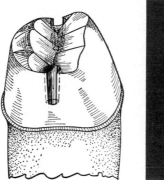
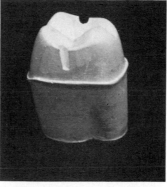

Fig. 5-8. Shoulder type of preparation for a complete crown modified by preparing two proximal keyways for additional resistance to displacement.

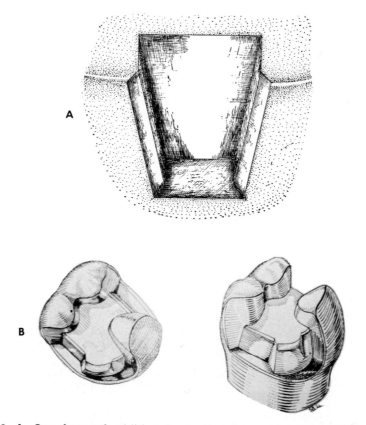

Fig. 5-9. A, One form of additional retention for crown preparation in teeth with extensive proximal carious involvement. **B,** Modified three-surface intracoronal preparation. (**B** from McElroy, D. L., and Malone, W. F.: Handbook of oral diagnosis and treatment planning, Huntington, N.Y., 1974, R. E. Krieger Publishing Co.)

ymous with friction exemplified in a tapered, wedged plug. Extracoronal retention is circumferential by nature and is associated with type one occlusal tooth reduction and axial reduction that does not exceed 2 to 5 degrees occlusogingivally on the mesial and distal aspects of the preparation. The greater the surface area, the more retention usually attained by the dentist.

Intracoronal designs

Intracoronal abutment designs have decreased in popularity since the advent of high-velocity tooth reduction. However, principles of intracoronal resistance and retention form are still employed for crowns that house precision attachments for reception of fixed-removable prosthodontics. Wedge-shaped retention boxes are also utilized to augment retention for full coverage when there is a lack of healthy tooth structure (Fig. 5-9).

The advantage of intracoronal preparations is the undisturbed gingival attachments buccolingually with reduced disturbance of occlusal relationships. An obvious disadvantage of these restora-

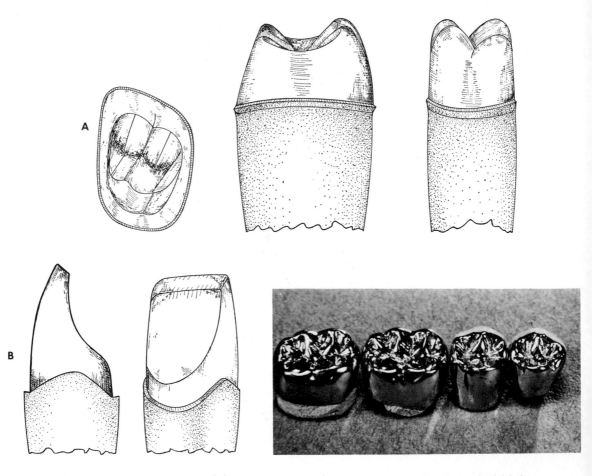

Fig. 5-10. A, Near-parallel proximal axial walls and narrowed buccolingual width from the occlusal one third is desirable. **B,** Complete crown preparation for an anterior porcelain jacket. **C,** Complete metal crowns possess maximum retention form, but present formidable occlusal restorative problem. Programmed recall system to monitor extensive restorative therapy is a mandate.

tions is the wedgelike effect that drives the cusps of the tooth apart when it is used as a bridge abutment. Onlays have minimized this problem. Deleterious pulpal responses are common with extensive intracoronal preparations. Perfection of marginal seal with intracoronal retainers has been an elusive aim for the most fastidious dentists. Intracoronal tooth preparations are contraindicated for patients with a high DMF, malpositioned teeth, and a reduced interocclusal clearance.

Full coverage

Complete crowns have the distinct advantage of allowing warpage of cusps during wax-ups to a beneficial arch position. Complete crowns also provide strength to teeth that otherwise would be incapable of withstanding the forces of mastication. Increased esthetic demands have made complete veneer crowns the standard-bearer for fixed prosthodontics. The increased surface areas also have an obvious retentive feature (Fig. 5-10).

The main disadvantage of using full coverage is the replacement of occlusal topography so that it is in harmony with its approximating and opposing teeth.

Optimal gingival termination design for full-coverage restorations also does not enjoy the consensus of discerning clinicians. In addition, anterior esthetics have always been and will continue to be a problem for both intracoronal and extracoronal preparations.

In summary, the retention of any restoration is directly proportional to the surface area. Increasing the surface area will increase the retention. However, if one axial surface is increased disproportionately in relation to an opposing axial surface of the same tooth, the retentive and resistant properties of the preparation are appreciably reduced.

Additional retention

One method of increasing resistance and retention without lengthening axial surfaces is to use grooves that are V-shaped or miniature box forms. However, rounded grooves have a distinct advantage when evaluated in light of the resistance form and ease of preparation. A seven-eighth or three-quarter crown preparation is an example of how these retentive grooves can be effectively used (Fig. 5-11). The groove design for a preparation may also be paramount to the

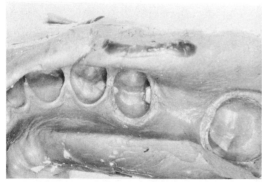
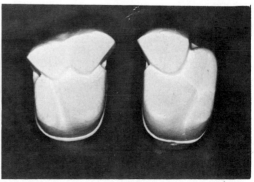

A

B

Fig. 5-11. A, Mercaptan rubber-base impression showing V-shaped groove on mesial surface of the premolar and traditional "box" form on distal aspect of same abutment. **B,** Traditional three-quarter crown on *left* and seven-eighth crown on *right* illustrate V-shaped groove. Boxlike proximal and rounded V grooves are common modifications of the preparations. (**A** from Malone, W. F., and Manning, J. L.: J. Prosthet. Dent. **20**(5):417, 1968.)

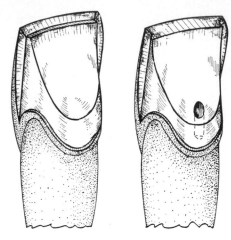

Fig. 5-12. Lingual pin placement to increase retention on traditional anterior three-quarter crown preparation.

success of full-coverage restorations that are placed in patients with minimal interocclusal clearance. It is generally accepted that the V-shaped, Tinker's, groove is used only in teeth that are more round in cross section. The boxlike proximal modification is used in teeth that have a parallelogram shape.

Pin retention

Pins are also used to increase retention in cases where axial retentive surfaces are insufficient to withstand displacement forces. Pins theoretically improve retention by establishing cylindric pinholes, which increase surface area (Fig. 5-12). There is insufficient comprehension of the exact manner in which pins add to retention of cast restorations. Nevertheless, the accuracy of the pin casting contacting the tooth preparation, the diameter and length of the pin itself, and the number of pins to augment the retention are important. Cast restorations should also have the pinhole placed parallel to the long axis of the main tooth preparation. There are two types of pins commonly used. The tapered wedge provides a strong form of additional retention. The second type, parallel-walled pins, have

failed to illustrate the stability when tested experimentally. A comprehensive review of pin-and-box configuration for retention and resistant form has been reported by Guyer.[8] In conclusion, the following are five ways to resist displacing forces:

1. Conservative preparation of the axial wall maintaining 2 to 5 degrees from parallelism
2. Perceptive preparation of the gingival finish
3. Prudently contoured and placed contact areas
4. Occlusal locks, such as dovetail, boxes, and grooves
5. Tapered and paralleled pins.

A more comprehensive review of the mechanical principles of tooth preparation with an accompanying bibliography, is available in Chapter 13 of Tylman's sixth edition.

CONSERVATION OF TOOTH STRUCTURE

One of the objectives of tooth preparation is the preservation of the existing healthy tooth structure. All preparation designs should enhance the resistance and retention forms of the classic preparations. Parallelism provides the most effective means of opposition to displacement. Parallelism is synomous with conservatism in most cases. The taper of the proximal walls of a preparation can exceed 8% only if the axial length of the tooth is excessive. Additional retentive means should be utilized to compensate for excessive taper or lack of tooth surface area, for example, teeth that have been severely weakened by caries. Pin-retained amalgam restorations are another means of coronal radicular stabilization for teeth with vital and nonvital pulps.

However, pin-reinforced teeth restored with amalgam prior to placement of cast restoration have been shown to succumb to induced stresses that could result in additional fractures (Fig. 5-13). The extension of the gingival margin of the res-

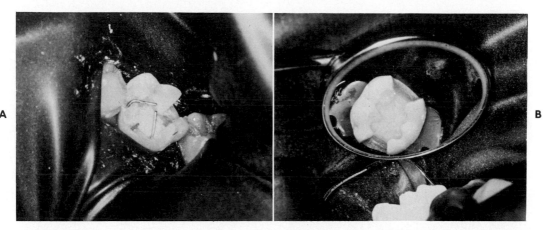

Fig. 5-13. A, Pin-retained amalgam preparation that will be restored with a complete crown. **B,** Caries-control procedure in amalgam prior to construction of a complete crown abutment. Complete metal crown retainer should be extended beyond gingival termination of amalgam restoration if possible. (**A** from Malone, W. F., and Manning, J. L.: Ill. Dent. J. **36**(11):724, 1967. **B** from Malone, W. F., and Balaty, J.: Ill. Dent. J. **37**(2):138, 1968.)

toration beyond the termination of the amalgam buildup would act as a collar to strengthen and protect the integrity of a given abutment. Termination of the gingival margin of the cast restoration short of the amalgam buildup gingivally is not desirable but may be a necessity in elderly patients. Periodontal treatment prior to placement of a fixed prosthesis is usually a mandate in cases of this nature.

PULPAL RESPONSE

From the standpoint of pulpal response, the most conservative preparation is the three-quarter crown, because the three-quarter crown may have its sole dentinal contact in the retentive grooves. This preparation was the standard-bearer for fixed prosthodontics until the advent of the air rotor. A three-quarter crown has limited use in a patient with a high DMF rate and where esthetics is a priority. Intracoronal preparations present an antithesis. Inlay type of retainers are not conservative if one considers the number of dentinal tubules involved during preparation. They are only conservative if re-

viewed with the total amount of enamel left exposed and the minimal soft-tissue involvement. In addition, the stress factor in intracoronal retention tends to spread or eventually split the abutment. Conventional inlays superficially appear more conservative but are considered a poor retainer when evaluated in light of stress concentration, microleakage, and pulpal involvement. Some dentists prefer onlays. The occlusal implications are obvious, but onlays are superior when gingival response is a major restorative problem (Fig. 5-14).

STRESS

Extensive stress concentration studies have been performed to inform clinicians of the optimal preparation designs to reduce the resulting strain factors.[9] these studies are superb. Fortunately, the role of the periodontal ligament provides the dentist with additional latitude, which reduces strain values. The magnitude of stress concentration occurs during function (Fig. 5-15). This implies that the occlusal aspects of preparation design can-

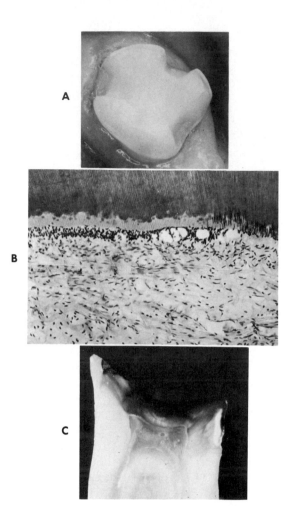

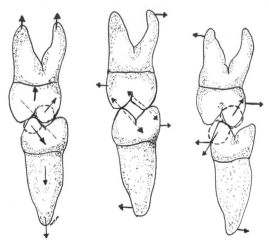

Fig. 5-15. Functional cusp height showing horizontal component of three-dimensional mandibular motion in relation to differentials of motions. Obviously establishment of cusp height and occlusal table are of notable significance.

Fig. 5-14. A, Modified onlay preparation with hooded buccal and lingual cusps. There is an inordinate number of dentinal tubular involvements with these types of preparations. However, gingival tissue response will be superior to a complete crown retainer. **B,** Histological section of tooth illustrating the common odontoblastic response of irritation from deep intracoronal preparations. **C,** This specimen of arrested caries illustrates the incomplete formation of secondary dentin just superior to the pulpal chamber. Prudent preparation and selection of bases will create a climate for favorable pulpal response. (**A** from Malone, W. F., and Manning, J. L.: J. Prosthet. Dent. **20**(5):417, 1968. **C** from Malone, W. F., and Manning, J. L.: Ill. Dent. J. **36**(11):724, 1967.)

not be overemphasized. Concepts of occlusal therapy are discussed in Chapters 6, 18, and 19 by Reynolds and Henneman. However, guidelines for an innocuous occlusion are initiated with appropriate tooth preparation. These guidelines are congruent with conservative tooth reduction:

1. Maintain a near parallelism of 2 to 5 degrees at the proximal walls.
2. Narrow the buccolingual width of the tooth from the occlusal one third.
3. Design the gingival termination for a satisfactory circumferencial seal.

GINGIVAL TERMINATION
Types of margins

Basically there are four types of marginal design. They are the shoulder or butt joint, bevel or shoulder with bevel, chamfer or hefty knife-edge, and shoulderless or featheredge. Restorative dentistry stipulates four basic criteria for successful marginal design, as follows:

1. Acceptable marginal adaptation

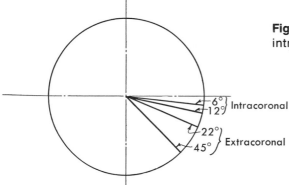

Fig. 5-16. Different angles of gingival bevels of intracoronal and extracoronal retainers.

2. Surfaces that are reasonably tissue-tolerant
3. Adequate contour to support tissue
4. Sufficient strength to resist deformity during function

Angles or bevels will be influenced by the classification of retainers (Fig. 5-16).

Shoulder preparations

The shoulder gingival margin is usually associated with complete porcelain crowns or at times with porcelain fused to metal crown. It is one of the most arduous to prepare, difficult to obtain an accurate fit, and the least conservative when evaluated in light of dentinal tubular involvement. Bulk removal and pulpal insult are paramount considerations during preparation. It is also improbable, because of caries and other reasons, that the dentist can routinely prepare a shoulder with an even width around the entire circumference of the tooth (Fig. 5-17). Carious attacks of the tooth and periodontal conditions rarely provide tissue attachments that are within normal limits for ideal preparations. Caution must be exercised to follow the crest of the gingival tissue to provide adequate tissue support after placement of a restoration. Full shoulders for posterior teeth are extremely difficult. Routine employment of such clinical practices are difficult to justify in light of microleakage, stress analysis, and pulpal response research.

Modification of the full shoulder in posterior teeth with a bevel might be a more acceptable direction of treatment.

Conversely, the increased tooth reduction performed during shoulder preparation permits more latitude when one establishes the gingival contour of the retainer of single restoration. In addition, the narrowed buccolingual width of the restoration is enhanced.

Shearing stresses were found to be concentrated more on the buccal than the lingual surfaces of cusp-fossa type of occlusions. If the occlusion is within normal loading limits, marginal configuration is not a major factor.[9] A full-shoulder gingival termination becomes more important in cases of concentrated point loading, for example, long span bridges and cases of malocclusion in general.

Beveled shoulders

The beveled margin has a diverse connotation because of the angle of the finish line. If the angle from the tooth is perpendicular to the long axis, it is called a shoulder. Currently, veneer crowns use a modified shoulder in conjunction with a gingival bevel. The angle of this bevel approaches the path of insertion of the restoration. The "bevel" with a rounded axial angle on the shoulder portion is a more popular preparation for porcelain-fused-to-metal crowns. This particular preparation, although subject to modi-

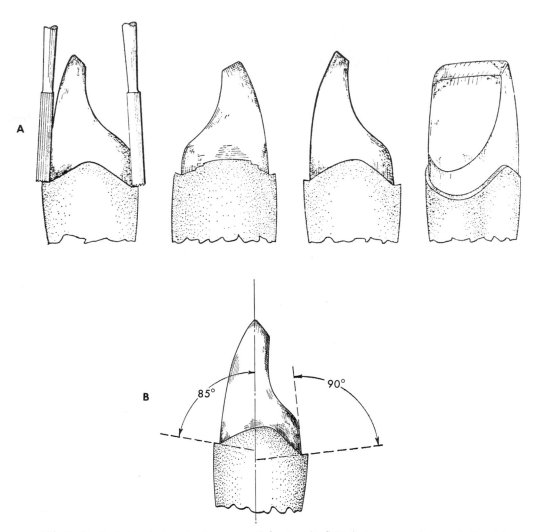

Fig. 5-17. A: *1,* Use of plain fissure, *left,* and end-cutting burs, *right,* to cut shoulder. *2,* Irregularly prepared shoulder having steps instead of continuous plane. *3* and *4,* Sharp-line angles where axial surfaces meet incisal and lingual surfaces are rounded and polished with discs. **B,** Plane of shoulder made at right angle to axial surface of tooth. **C,** Full-shoulder preparations for various classifications of teeth. Note proximal contour of shoulder support on underlying structures. **D,** Full-shoulder tooth preparation for a molar illustrating development of narrow occlusal table. Conversely, most fastidiously prepared tooth will not reflect the perceptive thinking of dentist if crown is overwaxed during construction. **E,** Complete metal-veneer crown with a two-plane reduction of buccal surface. This provides additional space for a veneered crown.

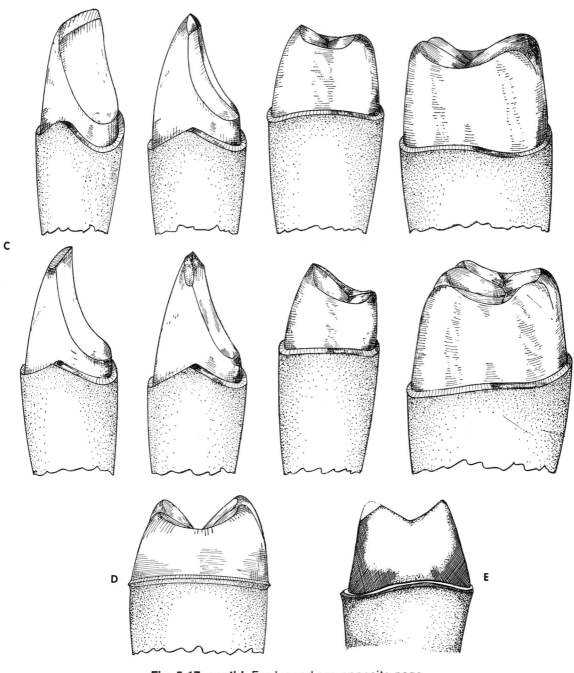

Fig. 5-17, cont'd. For legend see opposite page.

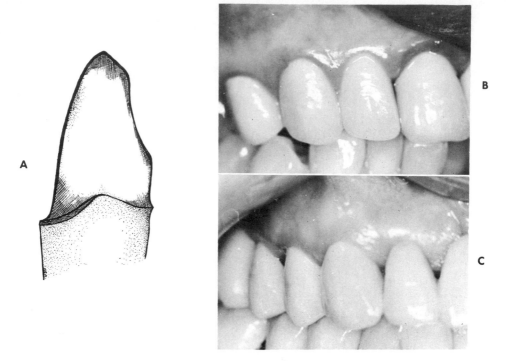

Fig. 5-18. A, Veneer crown preparation for a porcelain-fused-to-metal crown. Beveled shoulder extends facially from proximal to proximal surface with a chamfer or knife-edge finish lingually. **B,** Anterior porcelain-fused-to-metal crowns showing a fair-to-poor tissue response. Oral hygiene procedures of patient play an important role in maintenance of extensive restorative procedures. **C,** Maxillary porcelain-fused-to-metal splint showing a more favorable soft-tissue response. The canine-premolar splinted-abutment area is particularly vulnerable to adverse tissue reaction.

fication, also has a smooth evenly distributed chamfer from proximal to proximal on the lingual surface (Fig. 5-18, *A*). The gingival margin is developed by rotary burs or hand instruments with ample vision. A rounded shoulder supplies the internal bulk of metal to resist functional distortion, and the bevel provides an improved marginal adaptation. Esthetics will be determined by the tissue response of the patient to preparation, retraction, treatment restorations, and inherent patient adaptation (Figs. 5-18, *B* and *C*).

A variation of the beveled shoulder is the utilization of a short, heavy type placed on a posterior full-crown prepara-tion with a flame-shaped diamond. This is commonly referred to as a chamfered shoulder.

Chamfer

A chamfer is an obtuse-angled gingival termination. There is usually a misconception as to the angle and size of the actual chamfer. A chamfer is a definite concave extracoronal gingival marginal finish line that possesses a greater angulation than does a knife-edge but one that has less width than a shoulder (Fig. 5-19). Accurate gaging of a predetermined, equal width around the entire circumference of the tooth is difficult but considered desirable. Variations of depth and

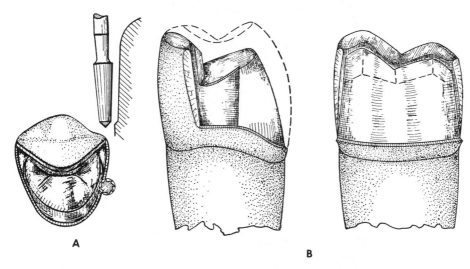

Fig. 5-19. A, Posterior partial veneer crown with a chamfer as a gingival margin. Instrumentation usually is a matter of dentist's preference. **B,** Proximal and lingual view of gingival finish molar partial veneer crown.

angulation of the gingival one third of the tooth preparation will vary the instrumental approach of the dentist while he develops the chamfer.

It is the prime purpose of definite gingival margins to supply sufficient thickness of the metal casting for an adequate gingival seal. The more a clinical preparation approaches ideal traditional guidelines, the more easily the restoration can be fabricated. According to el-Ebrashi et al.,[10] chamfered margins provide a gingival area with an optimal stress distribution and an adequate seal and require only minimal uniform tooth reduction. This latter fact enables competent "die dissection" for technical fabrication of all restorations.

Shoulderless gingival margins

Shoulderless margins are commonly called knife-edge or featheredge (Fig. 5-20). The shoulderless gingival margin is the easiest to prepare with rotary instruments but the most difficult to fabricate. This latter fact is true because of the fragile nature of the finish and one's inability to determine the finish line during laboratory procedures. Waxing and pol-

ishing features of construction become crucial. Casting the featheredge restoration accurately also becomes difficult. There are clinical situations where knife-edge margins are an advantage, such as in younger patients and barely accessible areas of the oral cavity. Knife-edge preparations are also employed for areas other than gingival termination. Slice preparations, pinledge preparations and the outline form for partial veneer crowns are also an indication for knife-edge termination. The difference between a knife-edge and the featheredge is the thickness. Featheredge margins are thin, whereas knife-edge margins are thicker. Earlier prepared designs used the featheredge retainer because of the malleability of the metal used for posterior complete crowns and poor cutting instruments.

In summary, the chamfer edge possesses internal bulk and better marginal adaptation extracoronally. It presently represents the optimal gingival termination for posterior crowns placed on molars. Full-shoulder crowns are the classic preparation for complete porcelain crowns, whereas beveled shoulders are

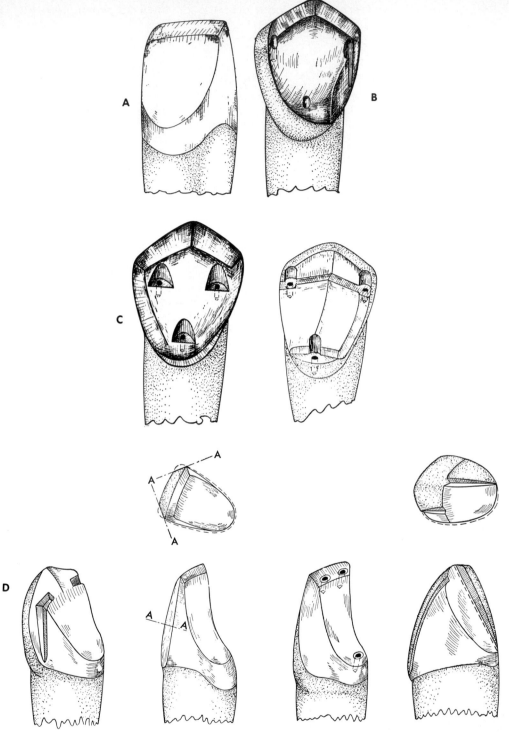

Fig. 5-20. A, Shoulderless preparation for complete veneer crown. This type of gingival margin may be a necessity for a younger patient because of trauma and mineralization distrubances. A small collar of metal is commonly employed to provide sufficient bulk for veneer. **B,** Pinledge shoulderless anterior preparations. **C,** Types of pinledge restorations with various forms of stabilization. **D,** Various types of shoulderless preparation that are infrequently used.

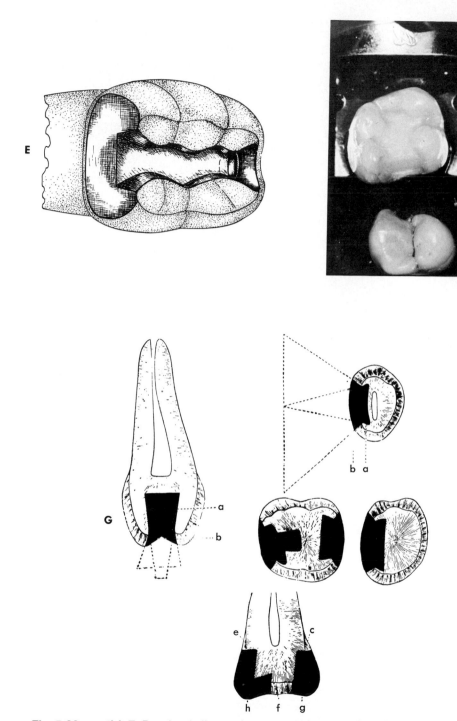

Fig. 5-20, cont'd. E, Proximal slice on intracoronal restoration. Additional grooves and occlusal coverage is a common variation. **F** Tooth preparation for intracoronal retainer on posterior abutment. Note lingual extension for additional retention. Inlays are used infrequently as retainer for fixed prosthesis. **G,** Principles of slice-and-channel retentions, illustrated in 1894 by Weeks. *Continued.*

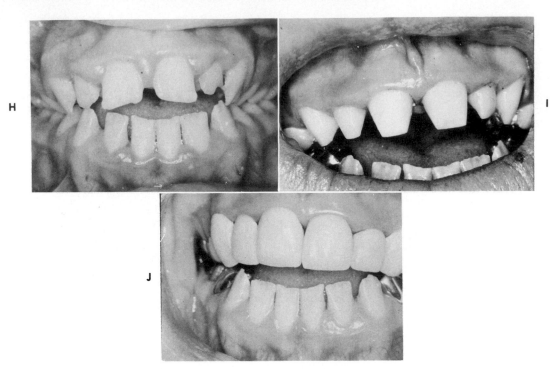

Fig. 5-20, cont'd. H, This picture illustrates an indication for the shoulderless anterior preparation. The patient had amelogenesis imperfecta with classic manifestations of large pulp, little or no enamel, and poor soft-tissue profile. **I,** Shoulderless preparations used in conjunction with the anterior teeth. **J,** Resin type of veneer placed after removal of treatment restorations. (**H** to **J** from Malone, W. F., and Sarlas, C. H.: Dent. Clin. North Am. **13:**(2):461, April 1969.)

used for teeth with veneers. Knife-edge and featheredge preparations are used posteriorly for younger patients and inaccessible areas of the oral cavity. These generalizations are obviously tempered by clinical conditions, technical logistics, and the dentist's preferences.

TERMINATION OF TOOTH PREPARATION IN RELATION TO THE GINGIVA

All tooth preparations terminate in a margin. Some margins end on the occlusal and axial surfaces and are commonly referred to as a cavosurface angle. The margin that evokes the most controversy is the gingival margin.[11] Increased use of full-coverage restorations, current oral research, and belated, but justifiable, emphasis on periodontal support are responsible for repudiation of the traditional extension of crown margins into the gingival crevice. It has been previously recommended to extend margins in most clinical circumstances into the gingival crevice. The gingival crevice was purported to be immune to caries. Deviation from this established norm was viewed as irresponsible despite the fact that there is strong evidence to support keeping the margins above the gingival tissue. Abnormal plaque formation and inflammatory changes associated with the inherent limitations of restorative work are ample evidence for employment of supragingival margins.

However, subgingival margins are considered necessary in the following clinical conditions:

1. Esthetics in the anterior portions of dental arches

2. Patients with a high incidence of caries with actual loss of tooth structure, such as teenagers

3. Patients whose interocclusal clearance is insufficient, such as those whose mechanical retention is a necessity by axial extension of the preparation[12]

There is one precept that is commonly omitted in the discussion of gingival margins; it is that the soft tissue approximating the tooth to be prepared is usually unhealthy prior to preparation.[13] The reason is that the original contours that preserve or protect the soft tissue have been eliminated by caries or modified by existing intracoronal restorations. The elimination of this tissue with questionable architecture and regrowth of protected tissue is a rational direction of treatment. Perhaps interceptive periodontics should be initiated by early recognition of symptoms.[14]

Obviously, the all-or-none laws are not valid. Glittering generalities of where the margins should be placed for an optimal contour requires well-designed research. The subgingival area is not an immune area. If there is any credence to the theory of passive eruption, the subgingival margin could be supragingival in a surprisingly short period of time. The latter point should be noted by clinicians who verbally condemn a prosthesis without inquiry into the longevity of the existing crown or fixed prosthesis.

Supragingival versus subgingival

Ideally, the most innocuous position of the margin for soft-tissue health is above the gingival crest. The more esthetic position for anterior restorations would be a midpoint subgingivally between the epithelial attachment and the crest of the gingiva. Gentle air pressure from a syringe would reveal the condition of the margin in the latter. It is notable that the area immediately above the gingival crest could be far more susceptible to caries.

Serious thought should precede a supragingival approach with a younger patient who is caries prone or a patient who exhibits decalcification in the gingival third of a potential abutment.

Overcontoured restorations in the gingival third, regardless of types of gingival termination, are objectionable.[15] Supragingival margins are usually advocated for restorations placed subsequent to periodontal surgery and elderly patients who exhibit a normal recession without bone loss (Fig. 5-21). The exception to these latter guidelines are usually esthetic demands by the patients.

IDEAL ABUTMENT

Primarily, the ideal abutment tooth possesses a vital pulp. The foremost consideration while one prepares vital teeth for fixed prosthodontics is tooth conservation. This is accomplished by uniform tooth reduction. All procedures that could ultimately result in pulpal degeneration should be minimized. One must not infer that an abutment tooth with a nonvital pulp is undesirable. For years, endodontically treated teeth have performed an invaluable service. Usually they require some form of additional coronal-radicular stabilization, which is difficult but general guidelines exist.[16]

A second qualification for an ideal abutment is substantial alveolar bone support with a healthy soft-tissue profile. The amount of alveolar bone is clinically determined by the examination of periodontal attachment. Radiographic surveys obviously serve as the ultimate method of alveolar bone appraisal. The type of bone present ordinarily reflects the degree of function of the abutment. Abutment teeth sustain forces of a type and magnitude that an individual tooth is not commonly required to bear. The type and the profile of the supporting structures are of paramount importance. Ideally an abutment tooth should have sufficient bone to withstand the forces to which it will be sub-

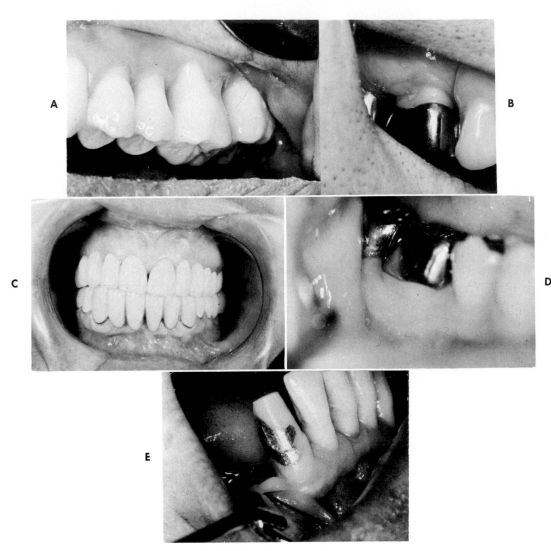

Fig. 5-21. A, Periodontally treated patient who is caries free. If restorations were to be placed, gingival margins should be supragingival. **B,** Supragingival margins of partial denture retainer in periodontally treated patient. Note plaque accumulation in area of trifurcation; nevertheless, area remains accessible for oral hygiene techniques available to patient. **C,** Patient showing restoration after periodontal surgery with a full maxillary splint with subgingival margins for esthetics. Mandibular arch has supragingival margins. Strictly enforced oral hygiene programs are essential for continued gingival health. **D,** Complete metal crown preparation with a supragingival termination. **E,** Complete metal-veneer crown preparation to be used for removable partial denture abutment.

jected susequent to placement of a fixed prosthesis.

If a tooth has lost more than one third of its supporting structure, it becomes questionable whether the tooth should be retained as an abutment. Splinting of teeth with poor periodontal support, unless it is a terminal clinical approach for a fixed prosthesis, is usually a heroic therapeutic approach.[17]

The third qualification for an ideal abutment is an optimal arch position for resistance to occlusal forces. Ideal arch position would permit near-parallel walls for retention and minimize tooth reduction to allow seating of the prosthesis. Optimal arch position also enhances a desirable esthetic result.

Tissue-compatible morphologic axial contours and harmonious occlusal topographic surfaces would encourage the maintenance of an acceptable level of supportive tissue health. One must understand that the presence of any restoration in contact with soft tissue elicits a histologically unfavorable response, but usually allows a clinically tolerable tissue profile.[18-20] Gingival marginal termination above the tissue is the most biologically acceptable but is not always possible or indicated.[21-23]

Deflective gingival morphologic design is obviously unfavorable for good gingival health.[24] In summary, the arch position of the tooth and the patient's innate tissue adaptation may render all prosthodontic contour designs less effective.

The fourth qualification for an ideal abutment is that the existence of a proportional relationship exists between the lengths of crown and root.[25-27] If the root is excessively short, it is incapable of furnishing the necessary resistance to the forces of mastication developed during various functional movements of the mandible. Additional biologic and mechanical forces directed toward a fixed prosthesis will cause short-rooted or

bone-deficient teeth to fail as abutments. Radiographic surveys and periodontal-ligament instrument examinations are the most objective methods of determining the acceptable crown-root ratios.

Additional qualifications of abutment teeth

In addition to the four qualifications of an ideal abutment, the clinically acceptable abutment must be prepared by the dentist so that it:

1. Is capable of supporting the additional forces to which it will be subjected.
2. Possesses retentive characteristics congruent with the span of prosthesis.
3. Maintains and safeguards the normality of the pulp.
4. Provides continued integrity of the tooth structure against fracture or caries.

Underlying principles of any technique must be comprehended; so a reasonable expectation of performance is predictable. The dentist is often overwhelmed with varying, if not diametrically opposed, directions of treatment.[28,29] Basic principles of the traditional tooth preparation designs must be comprehended before valid modification can be instituted by any dentist.

COMMON ERRORS IN TOOTH PREPARATION

1. Insufficient occlusal or incisal reduction
2. Nonuniform reduction of a labial or buccal surface preventing maximal achievement of esthetics
3. Minimal axial reduction on the buccal and lingual sides of posterior crowns that increases the incidence of balancing-side prematurities
4. Insufficient proximal reduction to ensure a cleansable embrasure space
5. Overreduction of teeth in the more accessible areas of the mouth

6. Insufficient gingival reduction to accommodate a definite finish line
7. Presence of undercut areas on the distolingual portion of the preparation
8. Inadequate parallelism of the proximal walls to ensure retention

SELECTION OF TYPES OF RETAINERS

The selection of the types of retainers is merely the coronal extension of the preparation of the abutment teeth of a fixed prosthesis. A lack of perception during preparation is magnified during the construction of the retainer. All factors concerned with a given case must be weighed in a regimented differential diagnosis. The oral-hygiene habits or the DMF rate of the patient, or both, may preclude the use of intracoronal types of retainers. Complete crowns, which are not so vulnerable marginally, are sometimes preferable under such conditions. There is a considerable amount of latitude in the selection of retainers when the patient is nearly immune to caries or has a belated low DMF rate as age becomes a factor. This latter remark is predicated upon the existence of a healthy periodontium.

Exposure to a variety of patients with knowledge of the limitations of clinical treatment ultimately results in practical abutment selection.

Although the periodontal ligament of the abutment teeth determines the limit of force that a bridge can endure, the length of the bridge span and the type of bridge used also determines the type of retainer selected. Retainer selection for terminal abutments is constantly a crucial determination. Retainer selection is usually dictated by the following:

1. Age
2. DMF rate
3. Edentulous span
4. Periodontal support
5. Arch position of the teeth
6. Skeletal relationships
7. Interocclusal and intraocclusal conditions, such as crown length
8. Existing and projected oral hygiene of the patient
9. Vitality of the potential abutment

A step-by-step discussion of the most frequently used preparations is illustrated in Chapter 6.

IDEAL RETAINERS

The prime mechanical function of a retainer is to support and connect the body of the bridge with the abutment. It may also restore the form, function, and esthetics of the abutment. The retainer should also forestall any future harm to both the tooth and its adjacent tissues.

The first attribute of an ideal retainer should be that it can be constructed for the mouth without injury to pulp and supporting structures. Secondly, the retainer should protect and maintain the pulp against thermal and galvanic shock. A third attribute is the ability of the retainer to provide safety for the tooth during the lifetime of the restoration. The fourth ideal property is the establishment of the self-cleaning property of the retainer. It should be at least readily cleansable. This implies that the retainer is resistant to corrosion and tarnish. The last and necessary condition is that fabrication of the ideal retainer is within the realm of all dentists.

Lastly, the retainer that involves the least amount of tooth reduction and alteration of tooth contour is more desirable than those that dictate excessive tooth loss. Conservation and uniformity of reduction of the abutment tooth are prerequisites for ideal retainers. The stress of function should be dispersed to the more receptive areas of the abutment. The greater the surface contact between the abutment and a retainer, the less the strain subjected to any one part of the abutment. Selection of an adequate luting agent becomes important.

CLASSIFICATION OF INDIVIDUAL RESTORATIONS AND RETAINERS FOR TOOTH PREPARATION

Class I—extracoronal restorations

The preparation of the tooth and its cast retainer lies externally to the body of the coronal portion of the prepared tooth and restores a tissue-compatible contour for the crown. The retention and resistance to displacement is developed between the inner walls of the casting and the external walls of the prepared tooth, such as in complete gold and porcelain crowns.

Complete crowns

1. Complete gold crown
2. Complete porcelain crown
3. Complete porcelain-fused-to-metal crown
4. Complete gold crown with acrylic resin facing

Partial crowns

The preparation of the tooth lies largely external to the coronal portion of the prepared tooth and complements the morphology of the axial portion of the tooth, such as in three-quarter and seven-eighth crowns. The retention and resistance to displacement depend on the internal surfaces and the auxiliary retentive means such as grooves, boxing, and pins.

Division 1—anterior
1. Three-quarter crown
2. Variations of three-quarter crown, such as the Selberg crown

Division 2—posterior
1. Mesial one-half crown
2. Three-quarter crown
3. Seven-eighth crown

Class II—intracoronal restorations

The prepared cavity and its cast retainer lie within the body of the coronal portion of the tooth. It is within the body of the coronal portion of the tooth and also within the contour of the crown. Retention and resistance are developed between the casting and the internal walls of the prepared cavity. However, cuspal coverage might lend additional surface for retention and resistance to normal forces.

1. Inlays
2. Onlays
3. Pin ledge
4. Combinations

Class III—radicular retainers

The dowel type of retention is confined to the root portion. Retention and resistance to displacement is developed by the extension of an attached metal dowel into the radicular portion of the tooth. Most teeth with nonvital pulps have a crown placed on them with a cervical apron on the crown to reduce the chance of fracture. Additional techniques may be used in combination with each other to improve the quality of coronal-radicular stabilization. Longitudinal studies are needed to substantiate the empirical statement that with nonvital pulps, teeth are more brittle. Do they fracture because of their weakened condition prior to pulp removal or does the access procedure render these teeth more susceptible to functional fracture? Incisors and premolars fracture more frequently after treatment. Molars are notable exceptions to

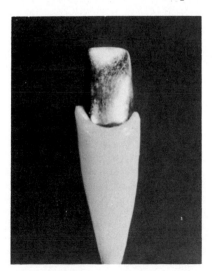

Fig. 5-22. Core and dowel for maxillary incisor. Preformed coronal forms will eventually facilitate coronal-radicular stabilization.

the empirical fracture theories. Resected teeth are obviously in dire need for coronal-radicular stabilization. Selection of one technique depends largely on the remaining percentage of healthy tooth structure (Fig. 5-22).

1. Cast core
2. Blue Island posts
3. Parapost techniques
4. Kürer technique

SELECTED REFERENCES

1. Black, G. V.: Operative dentistry, ed. 7, Chicago, 1956, Medico-Dental Publishing Co., vol. 2.
2. Tylman, S.: Theory on practice of crown and fixed partial prosthodontics, ed. 6, St. Louis, 1970, The C. V. Mosby Co.
3. Douglass, G. D.: Principles of preparation design in fixed prosthodontics, J. Acad. Gen. Dent. **21:**25-29, March-April 1973.
4. Malone, W. F., and Balaty, J.: The rubber dam dilemma, Ill. Dent. J. **37:**138-143, March 1968.
5. Malone, W. F., and Manning, J. L.: Caries control, Ill. Dent. J. **36**(11):724-729, Nov. 1967.
6. Gilbar, D. B., and Teteruck, W. R.: Fundamental of extracoronal tooth preparation. Part I. Retention on resistance form, J. Prosthet. Dent. **32:**651-656, 1974.
7. Yuodelis, R. A., Weaver, J. D., and Sapkos, S.: Facial and lingual contours of artificial complete crown restorations and their effects on the periodontium, J. Prosthet. Dent. **27:**61-65, 1973.
8. Guyer, S. E.: Multiple preparations for fixed prosthodontics, J. Prosthet. Dent. **23:**529-553, 1970.
9. Farah, J. W., and Craig, R. G.: Stress analysis of three marginal configuration of full posterior crowns by three-dimensional photoelasticity, J. Dent. Res. **53**(5):1219, Sept.-Oct. 1974.
10. el-Ebrashi, M. K., Craig, R. C., and Peyton, F. A.: Experimental stress analysis of dental restorations, J. Prosthet. Dent. parts I-IX, 1967-1970.
11. Löe, H., Reactions to marginal periodontal tissues to restorative procedures, Int. Dent. J. **18:**4, 759-778, Dec. 1968.
12. McElroy, D. L., and Malone, W. F.: Handbook of oral diagnosis and treatment planning, Springfield, Ill., 1969, Charles C Thomas, Publisher.
13. Malone, W. F.: Electrosurgery in dentistry, Springfield, Ill., 1975, Charles C Thomas, Publisher, Chapter 6.
14. Eisenmann, D., Malone, W. F., and Kusek, J.: Interceptive periodontics with electrosurgery, J. Prosthet. Dent. **22:**135, Nov. 1969.
15. Mahajan, M.: Tissue responses to dental rehabilitative procedures (Postdoctoral master's thesis), Loyola Medical Center, Loyola University, Chicago, 1976.
16. Malone, W. F., Dinga, P. and Smulson, M.: Clinical guidelines for coronal-radicular stabilization, Loyola University Clinical Manual, Maywood, Ill., Feb. 1975, Loyola University Press.
17. Glickman, I., Stein, R. S., and Smulow, J. B.: The effect of increased function forces upon the periodontium of splinted and non-splinted teeth, J. Periodontol. **32:**290, 1961.
18. Morris, M. L.: Artificial crown contours and gingival health, J. Prosthet. Dent. **12:**1146-1156, 1962.
19. Perel, M. L.: Axial crown contours, J. Prosthet. Dent. **25:**642-649, 1971.
20. Marcum, J. S.: The effect of crown marginal depth upon gingival tissue, J. Prosthet. Dent. **17:**479-487, 1967.
21. Waerhaug, J.: Histologic considerations which govern where the margins of restorations should be located in relation to the gingiva, Dent. Clin. North Am., pp. 161-176, March 1960.
22. Volchansky, A., Cleaton, J. P., and Retuf, D. H.: Study of surface characteristics of natural teeth and restoration adjacent to gingivae, J. Prosthet. Dent. **31:**411-421, April 1974.
23. Heilando, R. E., Lucca, J. J., and Morris, J. L.: Forms, contours and extension of full coverage restorations in occlusal reconstruction, Dent. Clin. North Am. **6:**147-162, 1962.
24. Larato, D.: Effect of cervical margins on gingiva, J. Calif. Dentists Assoc. **45:**19-22, 1969.
25. Hood, J. A., Farah, J. W., and Craig, R. G.: Modification of stresses in alveolar bone induced by a tilted molar, J. Prosthet. Dent. **34**(4):415, 1975.
26. Gordon, T.: Where to avoid pitfalls in periodontal prosthetics, Bull. Acad. Gen. Dent., Issue 11, p. 24, June 1965.
27. Brewer, A. A., and Morrow, R. M.: Overdentures, St. Louis, 1975, The C. V. Mosby Co.
28. Dawson, P. E.: Evaluation, diagnosis, and treatment of occlusal problems, St. Louis, 1974, The C. V. Mosby Co.
29. Brecher, S. C.: Conservative occlusal rehabilitation, J. Prosthet. Dent. **9**(6):1001-1016, 1959.

GENERAL REFERENCES

Berman, H., and Lustig, L. P.: Primary substructures and removable telescopic superstructures in dental reconstruction, J. Prosthet. Dent. **10:**724-732, 1960.

Brill, N.: Adaptation and the hybrid prostheses, J. Prosthet. Dent. **5:**811, 1955.

Contino, R. M., and Stallard, H.: Instruments essential for obtaining data needed in making a functional diagnosis of the human mouth, J. Prosthet. Dent. **7**:66, 1957.

Dolder, E. J.: The bar joint mandibular denture, J. Prosthet. Dent. **11**:689, 1961.

Gordon, T.: Telescope reconstruction: an approach to oral rehabilitation, J.A.D.A. **72**:97-105, 1966.

Hollenback, G. M.: A plea for a more conservative approach in certain dental procedures, J. Alabama Dent. Assoc. **46**:16, 1962.

Malone, W. F., Gerhard, R. J., Ensing, H., and Morganelli, J.: Imaginative prosthodontics, J. Acad. Gen. Dent. **18**:21-25, June 1970.

Maruyama, T., Simoosa, T., and Ojima, H.: Morphology of gingival capillaries adjacent to complete crowns, **35**:179-184, 1976.

McAllister, H. H.: The tilted molar abutment, Dent. Clin. North Am., pp. 25-32, March 1965.

Miller, P. A.: Complete dentures supported by natural teeth, J. Prosthet. Dent. **8**:924-928, 1958.

Morrow, R. M., Feldman, E. E., Rudd, K. D., and Trovillion, H. M.: Tooth supported complete dentures: an approach to preventive prosthodontics, J. Prosthet. Dent. **21**:513-521, 1969.

Nuttall, E. B.: Abutment preparations using high speed instruments, J. Kentucky Dent. Assoc. **13**:161, 1961.

Prichard, J. F., and Feder, M.: Modern adaptation of the telescopic principle in periodontal prosthesis, J. Periodontol. **33**:360-364, 1962.

Pugh, C. E., and Smerke, J. W.: Rationale for fixed prostheses in the management of advanced periodontal disease, Dent. Clin. North Am., pp. 243-262, January 1969.

Schweitzer, J. M., Schweitzer, R. D., and Schweitzer, J.: The telescoped complete denture: a research report at the clinical level, J. Prosthet. Dent. **10**:724-732, 1960.

Smith, D. E.: Fixed bridge with tilted mandibular second or third molar as an abutment, J. South. Calif. Dent. Assoc. **6**:131, 1939.

Seltzer, S., and Bender, I. B.: The dental pulp: biological considerations in dental procedures, ed. 2, Philadelphia, 1965, J. B. Lippincott.

6

Individual tooth preparation for fixed prosthodontics

William F. P. Malone, Boleslaw Mazur, Hosea F. Sawyer, Stanley D. Tylman, Raymond Henneman, and Lee M. Jameson

---

Complete cast crown

DEFINITIONS

anatomic crown Portion of a natural tooth that extends from its cementoenamel junction to the occlusal surface or incisal edge.

clinical crown Portion of a natural tooth that extends from the bottom of the sulcus (epithelial attachment) to the occlusal surface or incisal edge.

artificial crown Fixed restoration of the major part or of the entire coronal part of a natural tooth, restoring its anatomy, function, and esthetics; usually of metal, porcelain, synthetic resin, or their combination.

HISTORY

The complete metal crown employed today has undergone considerable change since its introduction by W. N. Morrison in 1869. Originally the Morrison crown consisted of two pieces of gold plate, an axial band, and a swaged occlusal cap soldered together. Because the finished crown reproduced the tooth form by means of a thin shell, it was also known as the "gold shell" crown. The accepted procedure during the latter part of the nineteenth century was to devitalize the teeth requiring crowns. Because a certain percentage of treated teeth ultimately failed, the loss of crowned treated teeth was not attributed to a poor root-filling technique, but to the fact that the tooth was crowned. Unfortunately, this mistaken idea has convinced the medical profession as well as the laity that a crown constructed of a metal is dangerous to the health of a patient and that it should not be used in good dental health service. It took organized dentistry a long time to educate people that, where indicated and when adequately prepared, a complete metal crown is a safe and useful type of restoration.

INDICATIONS

The complete metal crown may be used as an individual restoration or it may serve as a bridge retainer. The gold crown is used whenever a tooth cannot be more conservatively restored. Any complete crown is the last resort in the reclamation of a carious or fractured tooth. On the other hand, there are indications for the placement of a complete gold crown even when the tooth could be repaired with other restorations. For example, there are teeth so weakened and undermined by caries that the placement of a complete crown affords the best protection against possible fracture of the remaining tooth structure. Complete gold crowns usually have shorter marginal lines than do the intracoronal restorations. In a mouth in which caries is very active or oral hygiene is rather poor, it frequently serves more of a preventive purpose to place a complete crown instead of extensive intracoronal restorations with multiple cavosurface margins. High DMF rates are also an indication for complete coverage.

Where it is impossible to correct the alignment or occlusion in malpositioned teeth with ordinary restorations, the complete gold crown may be employed. When it is necessary to use a noncarious tooth for a bridge abutment, ordinarily some type of intracoronal or partial extracoronal retainer is preferred. If, however, the gingivo-occlusal height of the tooth is relatively short, there may be considerable difficulty in getting sufficient retention with an onlay or the partial veneer retainers, in which event the complete crown is indicated.

A gold crown may be constructed on both vital and pulpless anterior or posterior teeth. When used anteriorly to the second bicuspid, the esthetic requirements are fulfilled by placement of a porcelain or acrylic resin veneer on the buccal or labial surface of the crown. Unless modified, the complete metal crown is rarely, if ever, used in the anterior teeth.

REQUIREMENTS
Pulp conservation

Every precaution will be taken during the preparation of the tooth and after the crown has been completed and cemented, so as not to jeopardize the vitality of the pulp. The indiscriminate or deep cutting of a tooth usually results in the degeneration or death of the pulp.

Restoring function and anatomy

The complete metal crown, as Orton[1] so ably expressed it over five decades ago,

"must be one that will exactly reproduce in all its essential details that particular tooth which it is intended to replace, bearing in mind the age of the patient and the variation from the normal which it may be necessary to reproduce in order to have the crown in harmony with its environment."

Not only the axial and occlusal contours of the individual tooth, but also those relationships that exist between the other restored teeth and its adjacent or opposing teeth; that is, correct contact areas, proximal embrasures, occlusal wear, and proper functional coordination with the other teeth must be replaced.

Protection of investing tissues

An acceptable gold crown requires that its gingival margin must be correctly adapted to the tooth as prepared and placed in its proper relationship to the gingival tissues. The gingival termination of the crown should never be extended so far rootwise that it will cause a recession of the gingival tissues or result in detrimental effects to the periodontium. In younger patients the gingival margin of the crown can terminate at or slightly above the crest, or barely into the gingival crevice.

An adequate fit and above all satisfactory contour of the crown will enhance the health of the investing tissue.

Uniformity of tooth reduction

Original occlusal anatomy should be maintained after the tooth is prepared. Cusps and grooves are always in the same relative position but at a lower level. Normal occlusal anatomy of prepared teeth will have been reduced to a configuration that increases the strength, stability, and retention of the metal crown. On axial surfaces enough tooth structure is removed to eliminate undercuts and provide room for the type of veneer diagnosed.

The advantages of the complete metal

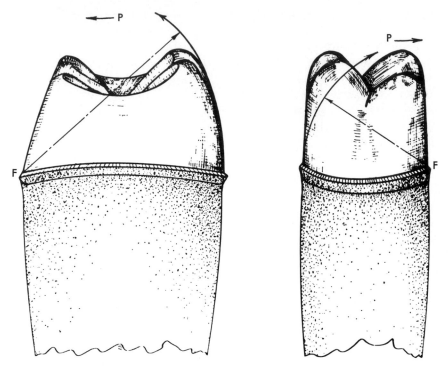

Fig. 6-1. Complete crown preparation with exaggerated gingival chamfer on vital tooth for cast gold crown.

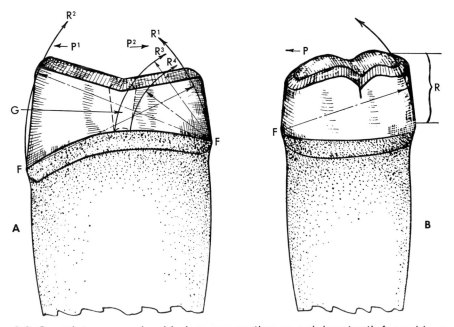

Fig. 6-2. Complete crown shoulderless preparation on pulpless tooth for gold crown.

crown are that it is inherently strong and it may be so constructed that it possesses superlative retentive powers, being dislodged with difficulty. This is accomplished by satisfactory preparation of the occlusal and axial surfaces of the tooth, as explained, and because it follows the strongest principle of engineering design, that of a circle.

Proper alloy

The requirements of an acceptable metal crown also demand that the materials used in its construction be intrinsically strong enough to withstand the forces and wear of mastication to which the crown will be submitted. Therefore, the alloy must be carefully selected for the purpose it is intended to serve. This presupposes that the nobility of the alloy will be such as to prevent tarnish or corrosion from oral fluids.

Retention and resistance form

It is observed in Fig. 6-1 that the mesial and distoaxial walls are most favorable for developing parallelisms essential to displacement resistance. The buccal and lingual surfaces, because of their natural contour, do not afford the same opportunity for paralleling walls. Where possible, the occlusal planes are reproduced at a lower level; these planes help considerably to assist stability or displacement. Where it is impossible to reproduce the normal occlusal anatomy, or if the tooth is pulpless, a buccal and a lingual occlusal plane are developed as shown in Fig. 6-2. These offer resistance to lingual or buccal forces. When necessary and where indicated, additional resistance may be obtained by placing pins, grooves, or boxes in any available surface where the length of this surface is adequate.

In Fig. 6-2, A, one may see that, if an occlusal force p_1 is directed buccally, the lingual portion of the crown tends to be dislodged occlusally and buccally with the point of rotation situated at F; this

displacement is resisted by the lingual surface when it lies outside the arc R_1.

On the other hand, an occlusal force p_2 directed lingually is likely to dislodge the crown lingually, since the buccal wall of the preparation lies within the tipping path of the arc R_2. When such a condition prevails either in the buccal or lingual wall, resistance to displacement can be developed by placement of two proximal grooves at G in the mesial and distal surfaces shown in Fig. 6-2, A. In Fig. 6-2, B, it is evident that an occlusal force P directed mesially will not dislodge the crown, since the distal wall of the preparation lies outside the tipping path of arc R.

DISADVANTAGES
Lack of esthetics

One of the chief disadvantages of the gold crown is that it lacks ordinary esthetic requirements. When the crown is made entirely of metal, it is limited to the posterior teeth. The preparation of a tooth for the reception of a gold crown, today, is generally regarded as a mundane task. Even with the advent of the high-speed cutting techniques, it should be one of the most meticulous operations that the dentist is called upon to perform. An ill-fitting crown placed on a hastily prepared tooth can stay in place for many years before the resultant serious injury to other dental morphologic tissues is discovered.

Possibility of gingival irritation

Although the complete gold crown should be placed where indicated, promiscuous usage should be discouraged because of the difficulty of reestablishing the acceptable axial contours and satisfactory gingival continuity of the axial surfaces once they have been removed or altered.

Danger of incipient caries

Incipient caries at the gingival margin of the full metal crown is often difficult to detect and should be one of the primary objects of a recall examination. Caries sometimes penetrates the seal of the crown and remains undiscovered. The damage done can be irreparable, because of difficulty in radiographic detection.

TYPES OF COMPLETE METAL CROWNS

The complete metal crown may be one of the following categories: (1) cast, (2) swaged, (3) swaged-cast combination, and (4) the metal pins plus fired porcelain to metal or the acrylic resin combination. Each of these may be further subdivided into the shoulder and shoulderless types and may be used on either the posterior or the anterior teeth.

With the introduction of improved impression materials and casting techniques "swaged" or "swaged-cast" categories of crowns have become almost obsolete, leaving only the cast type of crown.

ADVANTAGES OF CAST CROWN

Dressel enumerated the merits of the all-cast type of complete crown as compared to the all-swaged plate crown, by stating that (1) the former is a stronger and sturdier crown, (2) proper contact areas may be established, (3) adequate embrasures and interproximal spaces may be established, (4) satisfactory buccal and lingual anatomic form may be obtained, and (6) it achieves a more acceptable occlusion.

As previously stated, the complete metal crown, though primarily being a restoration for posterior teeth, is used in anterior teeth as veneer crowns.

COMPLETE METAL CROWN AS A SINGLE RESTORATION

Before preparation of a metal crown is started assay the condition of the tooth. Remove all carious lesions of the tooth *by use of the traditional outline forms.* Keep in mind the age of the patient, type and depth of decay, and proximity of the pulp. Also remove any other restorative material placed in the tooth.

While removing decay, as a suggestion, use a large round bur, rotating at a low speed. This method seems to afford less danger of exposure of the pulp than the one with use of sharp hand instruments for excavation.

The hardness of the dentin and not discoloration is used as a guideline in removing decay. After removal of decay and the removal of old restoration materials, evaluate the remaining tooth structure. Often it is substantial enough to provide retention for a complete gold crown, but if not the tooth requires a restorative buildup prior to completion of the tooth preparation.

The tooth is now ready for preparation. The suggested step-by-step procedures will help to achieve this goal.

STEP 1—OCCLUSAL REDUCTION

A review of the literature will disclose many different ways of occlusal reduction, resulting in a varied occlusal topography.

The principle of "uniform tooth reduction and preserving vitality of the pulp" indicates that the tooth is reduced in such a way as to maintain the primary occlusal grooves and cusps. The primary anatomy is maintained, but 1.5 to 2 mm away from the existing plane of occlusion. One should pay attention that the position of the cusps of the prepared tooth is not changed.

Gross reduction is accomplished by diamond wheels and burs. The resulting preparation will be rather coarse, with rounded grooves and indefinite cusps. The anatomic features are sharpened with a cylindric diamond (the larger being 770-7P, 1 mm in diameter, and the smaller 769-7P, 0.5 mm in diameter). The cusps are sharpened and the primary grooves are deepened (buccal, lingual, as well as central). The cusps are developed with smooth lines. The position of the cusps in relationship to the opposite tooth is not usually changed and centric occlusal clearance is checked and maintained.

There may be difficulty in checking visually, as well as with the explorer, the amount of reduction of the lingual cusps. In such a case, the dentist can take a piece of base-plate wax (which is 2 mm thick), soften it, place it over the prepared tooth, and ask the patient to close (in centric occlusion). When the wax hardens, he can remove it and examine against the light. If the reduction is uniform and of proper depth, the wax will be bent, conforming to the preparation.

If the cusps are cutting into the wax (wax looks thinner in this area), this is an indication that a particular cusp has not been reduced enough. Further reduction is required.

The occlusal clearance of preparation should be checked also in lateral excursion. Sometimes there is an edentulous space opposite the tooth to be prepared. In such a case, the dentist cannot use an antagonist to check adequate occlusal reduction. The dentist can use the occlusal surfaces and marginal ridges of the adjacent teeth as guides for reduction. If there are no adjacent teeth, the dentist should resort to other techniques. One method is to construct bite rims, establishing an acceptable plane of occlusion.

Finally, if there is no other way of guiding the operator to the correct amount of occlusal reduction, one can, before any occlusion reduction is started, place 2 mm control grooves on the tips of the cusps and in the grooves (see Fig. 6-3). If the tooth is reduced to the deepest parts of these notches, the result will be uniform and will be an acceptable occlusal reduction.

STEP 2—PROXIMAL REDUCTION

The next step in the complete gold crown preparation is proximal reduction. All precautions are instituted not to injure the adjacent teeth. Proximal reduction can be accomplished by any of the following methods:

1. The first method involves a stainless steel matrix that can be placed on the teeth adjacent to the one to be prepared. This stainless steel matrix will provide some protection, but the bur may still cut the band and injure the adjacent teeth.

2. The second and most common method of making the proximal cuts is the use of a very thin, tapered diamond point or bur. If this diamond or bur point is placed directly in the contact area, the tooth to be prepared and the adjacent tooth will be inadvertently cut.

Place the diamond point or bur some distance (that is, slightly more than the diameter of the diamond point) from the contact area on the buccal or lingual surface and direct the thin tapered diamond or bur as in buccolingual preparation. Direct the diamond point or bur so that it will cut through the contact point slightly above the interdental papilla (see Fig. 6-4).

The retention and resistance form in complete gold crown preparation depend

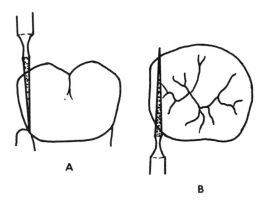

A

B

Fig. 6-4. Proximal reduction by long, thin diamond points or burs. **A,** Buccal view of diamond placement for proximal reduction. **B,** Occlusal view.

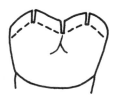

Fig. 6-3. Uniform occlusal reduction (note control grooves).

on the parallelism of the sides of the prepared tooth. The walls should be close to parallelism (2 to 5 degrees) on the mesial and distal surfaces.

Buccal and lingual walls are naturally tapering occlusally; so when the tooth is reduced, excessive tapering will be increased as the tooth is reduced more at the occlusal surface than at the gingival finishing line.

STEP 3—BUCCAL AND LINGUAL AXIAL REDUCTION

After occlusal and proximal reductions, the next step is to reduce buccal and lingual surfaces. For bulk reduction the dentist can use a large, coarse, tapered diamond cylinder (770-7P) or burs. The operator should initially carry the preparation to the gingival crest. The gross-reduction diamonds or burs are not designed to be placed into the sulcus.

Note that the gingival portion of buccal surface is close to paralleling the lingual surface rather than the occlusal one third of the tooth. To increase perfect parallelism (retention and resistance form), the dentist would have to make rather wide gingival shoulder. This axial wall increases retention; however it would not necessarily increase resistance to lingual displacement (see Fig. 6-5).

Unless a tooth has a class V restoration, where part of the shoulder is already prepared, placing shoulders for the purpose of making part of the buccal surface parallel to the lingual axial surface is a questionable approach.

The lingual portion of the tooth is reduced in a similar way. The resulting surface will be rather straight, occlusogingivally curving in its occlusal one third toward the central groove to narrow the occlusal table.

During this step of preparation, care is exercised to reduce buccal and lingual surfaces enough to place cusp tips for satisfactory occlusal relationship. Otherwise, the occlusal table of the prepared

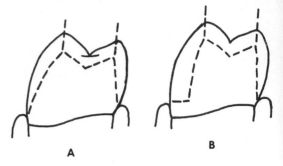

Fig. 6-5. A, Correct preparation. **B,** Attempt to make buccal and lingual walls perfectly parallel to each other would necessitate making wide buccal shoulder.

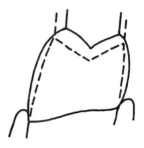

Fig. 6-6. Tips of cusps of prepared tooth are farther apart than they originally were.

tooth would be larger than the buccolingual width of the unprepared tooth (see Fig. 6-6). The most common error of preparing the buccal and lingual walls is an attempt to make them parallel. This results in having the tips of the cusps of the prepared tooth farther apart than they were originally. The crown does not have the necessary amount of metal in the occlusal third on the buccal and lingual, or the crown will be too wide buccolingually and will increase the width of the occlusal table.

STEP 4—PROXIMAL LINE ANGLE

A small tapered cylindric diamond or bur is moved from the proximal surfaces to the buccal surfaces, with the sharp corners being rounded off. Elimination of undercuts is concomitantly accom-

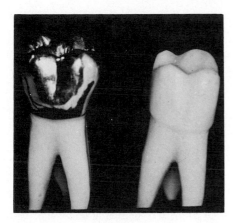

Fig. 6-7. Restored tooth (complete prepared tooth with gold crown).

plished. The same procedure is repeated on the lingual of the tooth, so that the buccal, lingual, and proximal surfaces blend without any sharp angles and are devoid of gross undercuts.

With a thin, fine diamond or bur, one smooths the entire preparation (eliminating the markings of the coarse diamond or bur) and carries the finishing line barely below the crest of the gingivae. If the rubber dam was not used to retract the gingival tissue, a fine diamond or bur will reduce the possibility of injuring the gingivae (see Fig. 6-7).

SELECTED REFERENCES

1. Orton, F. H.: Absence of standards in crown work, Dent. Items Int. **39**:345, 1917.
2. Ante, I. H.: The gold crown as you make it, Aust. Dent. J. **10**:1, 1938.
3. Dressel, R. P.: Principles of fixed bridge construction, Dent. Cosmos **72**:565, 730, 853, 941, 1173, 1272, 1930; **73**:130, 253, 342, 1931.
4. Selberg, A.: Cast gold crowns, J. Tenn. Dent. Assoc. **29**:21, 1949.
5. Woolson, A. H.: Restorations made of porcelain baked on gold, J. Prosthet. Dent. **5**:65, 1955.

GENERAL REFERENCES

Asgar, K., and Peyton, F. A.: Pits on inner surfaces of cast gold crowns, J. Prosthet. Dent. **9**:448, 1959.
Asgar, K., and Peyton, F. A.: Effect of the investment material and mold temperature on the quality of the union achieved during gold casting to embedded attachment metals, Int. Assoc. Dent. Res. **40**:93, 1962.
Baker, C. R.: Banded-cast metal crowns, J.A.D.A. **56**:522, 1958.
Barishman, H.: Impression making for complete crown restorations, J.A.D.A. **61**:161, 1960.
Beeson, P. E.: The use of acrylic resins as an aid in the development of patterns for two types of crowns, J. Prosthet. Dent. **13**:493, 1963.
Carter, R.: Electrolytic action in the presence of gold crowns placed over amalgam restorations: case report, Aust. Dent. J. **10**:317-319, 1965.
Craig, R. G., el-Ebrashi, M. K., and Peyton, F. A.: Experimental stress analysis of dental restoration, I: Two-dimensional photoelastic stress analysis of crowns, J. Prosthet. Dent. **17**(3):292-302, 1967.
Ewing, J. E.: Construction of accurate full crown restorations for an existing clasp by using a direct metal pattern technique, J. Prosthet. Dent. **15**:889, 1965.
Ewing, J. E.: Direct metal pattern technique for full crown restorations, J.A.D.A. **63**:822, 1963.
Ewing, J. E., and Bentman, D.: Porcelain-veneered full-crown restorations made with cadmium patterns, J. Prosthet. Dent. **18**(2):140-150, 1967.
Hausman, M.: Occlusal reconstruction using transitional crowns, J. Prosthet. Dent. **11**:278, 1961.
Henschel, C. J.: Double cast crowns, Oral Hyg. **52**:37, 1962.
Herlands, R. E., Lucca, J. J., and Morris, M. L.: Forms, contours, and extensions of full coverage restorations in occlusal reconstruction, Dent. Clin. North Am., pp. 147-162, March 1962.
Herrick, P. W., Shell, J., Timmermans, J., and Turpin, D.: Investigation of hygroscopic investment (control water added) for casting multi-unit bridges, J. Dent. Res. **40**:774, 1961.
Herrick, P. W., Shell, J. S., Timmermans, J. J., and Turpin, D. L.: One-piece casting of multi-unit bridges, Dent. Progr. **2**:93, 1962.
Hirshberg, S. M.: Compatible temporary tooth health and gingival protection, J. Prosthet. Dent. **18**:151, 1967.
Killebrew, R. H.: Crown construction for broken down partial denture abutments, J. Prosthet. Dent. **11**:93, 1961.
Kuratli, J.: Restoration of broken down vital teeth for fixed partial denture abutments, J. Prosthet. Dent. **8**:504, 1958.
Lavine, S.: Construction of cast-gold crowns and fixed partial dentures by use of gold bands, J. Prosthet. Dent. **10**:959, 1960.
Leff, A.: Evaluation of high speed in full-coverage preparations, J. Prosthet. Dent. **10**:314, 1960.
Lewis, R. M., and Owen, M. M.: Mathematical solution of a problem in full crown construction, J.A.D.A. **59**:943, 1959.
McCabe, D. J., and Rinne, V. W.: Treatment of carious teeth: disadvantage of full coverage, Dent. Clin. North Am., p. 639, Nov. 1960.

Malson, T. S.: Anatomic cast crown reproduction, J. Prosthet. Dent. **9:**106, 1959.

Marcum, J. S.: The effect of crown marginal depth upon gingival tissue, J. Prosthet. Dent. **17:**479, 1967.

Miller, I. F., and Feinberg, E.: Full coverage restorations, J. Prosthet. Dent. **12:**317-325, 1962.

Miller, I. F., and Belsky, M. W.: The full shoulder preparation for periodontal health, Dent. Clin. North Am., pp. 83-102, March 1963.

Modjeski, P. J.: Cavity preparation pertaining to fixed partial dentures, Ill. Dent. J. **16:**408, 1947.

Raucher, F.: Systematic approach to full crown preparations using high speed instruments, N.Y. Dent. J. **27:**284, 1961.

Schweitzer, J. M.: Gold copings for problematic teeth, J. Prosthet. Dent. **10:**163, 1960.

Segat, L.: Restoration of non-vital teeth, J. Michigan Dent. Assoc. **44:**254, 1962.

Selberg, A.: Full cast crown technique, J. Prosthet. Dent. **7:**102, 1957.

Strickland, W. D., and Sturdevant, C. M.: Porosity in the full cast crown, J.A.D.A. **58:**69, 1959.

Swartz, M. L., and Phillips, R. W.: Study of adaptations of veneers to cast gold crowns, J. Prosthet. Dent. **7:**817, 1957.

Tylman, S. D.: Ultrasonic techniques for crown and bridge retainers, J. Prosthet. Dent. **8:**167, 1958.

Wagman, S. S.: Tissue management for full cast veneer crowns, J. Prosthet. Dent. **15:**106-117, 1965.

Weinberg, L. A.: Double casting of metal to metal in full coverage, J.A.D.A. **63:**821, 1961.

Wheeler, R. C.: Restoration of gingival or cervical margins in full crowns, Dent. Cosmos **73:**238, 1931.

SECTION B

Complete porcelain crown

The complete porcelain crown, more commonly referred to as the porcelain jacket crown, has been utilized for nearly three fourths of a century. Land (as reported by Clark[1]) and Schneider[2] combined their efforts to develop an esthetic restoration that has undergone only slight modification since its technical development. Porcelain jacket crowns have been successfully employed over the years by the practicing profession, which is a tribute in itself to the ingenuity of the perceptive clinicians who conceived and developed the restoration. Porcelain crowns are capable of meeting the most exacting esthetic requirements, and many of the characteristics (Fig. 6-8) and peculiarities of an individual tooth within a given dentition can be reproduced.

Clinical evidence indicates that a satisfactorily fabricated and contoured porcelain crown is one of the most acceptable restorations to the supporting soft tissue. One possible reason for the favorable soft-tissue response is the labial contour of porcelain jacket crowns, which is similar to the morphology of the original tooth. When the tooth is adequately

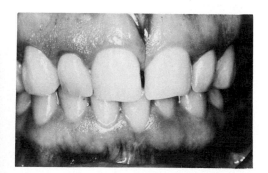

Fig. 6-8. Porcelain crown placed on maxillary incisors. Variation of morphology and color are possible with this type of restoration.

prepared and the porcelain crown satisfactorily fabricated, the soft tissue is not so distended in the cervical area as other anterior complete crowns.

When combined with the appropriate luting media, porcelain jackets protect the pulp of the tooth against thermal shock.

INDICATIONS

The primary reason for using porcelain jackets is to achieve optimum esthetics. Indications for the use of this type of crown on anterior teeth include the following:

1. When incisal angles have been fractured beyond a point where a conservative restoration can serve equally well in terms of function and esthetics
2. When proximal decay is excessive or has caused multiple restorations to be placed in the past
3. When incisors are discolored because of mineralization disturbances during formation, or with excessive amounts of tetracycline and fluoride
4. When malformation occurred because of nutritional deficiencies
5. When the anterior teeth are rotated or laterally displaced and orthodontic treatment is not feasible
6. When tooth discoloration after endodontic treatment cannot be corrected with simple bleaching procedures
7. Where maximum esthetics is required for professional reasons related to show business, politics, and so forth

The preparation for a complete porcelain crown is one of the most demanding of all complete crowns. The uniformity of

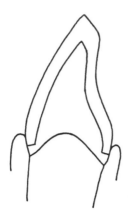

Fig. 6-9. Complete porcelain crown preparation for upper central incisor. Uniform reduction of tooth is object of preparation.

tooth reduction, the angle of the shoulder, and the design of the proximal contours to support the investing soft tissue are crucial to the longevity of this restoration. Fig. 6-9 diagrammatically illustrates the tooth reduction needed for a successful esthetic result.

Porcelain jacket crown preparations are more difficult for the upper lateral incisors because of their size and restriction at the cervical portion of these teeth. Porcelain veneer crowns have replaced the porcelain jacket as an individual restoration on the lower anteriors for the same reasons. Since the porcelain crown is primarily indicated for individual maxillary incisor teeth, the porcelain-fused-to-metal veneer crown with its superior

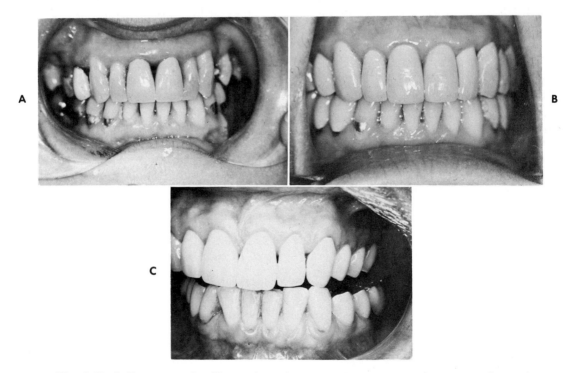

Fig. 6-10. A, Prerestorative illustration of patient who has undergone extensive periodontal surgery. **B,** Postoperative illustration of same patient in **A** 6 months after placement of porcelain-veneer crowns. Length of coronal aspect of periodontally treated teeth and the constricted cervical portion of these teeth prohibit placement of porcelain jackets. **C,** Porcelain jackets placed on four maxillary incisors with porcelain-fused-to-metal crowns on canines provide maximum esthetics with superior strength during lateral excursions of mandible.

strength has also replaced the porcelain jacket for restoration of the canines and premolars.

Aluminous porcelain, introduced by McLean, improved the strength of porcelain jackets and in some cases enhanced their esthetics. However, this contribution was minimized by the versatility of porcelain-fused-to-metal crowns. McLean discusses the manipulation of aluminous porcelain in detail in Chapter 25.

CONTRAINDICATIONS

1. Younger patients with large vital pulps
2. Individuals engaged in contact sports and rigorous occupations where the incidence of fracture is high
3. Patients who have a reduced interocclusal relationship or edge-to-edge occlusion, that is, accompanying heavy masticatory musculature
4. Patients who have had periodontal surgery (Fig. 6-10) or cervical erosion making tooth preparation impossible or impractical
5. Anterior teeth with a constricted cervical circumference
6. Patients with a high DMF rate
7. Patients who have a short clinical crown either naturally or because of abrasion or attrition

If the patient is made aware of the risk of fracture or the possibility of belated endodontic therapy attributable to the cutting away of enamel and dentin with close pulpal tissue, the needs and demands of the patient may subjugate the known difficulties associated with this restoration.

The dentist may elect to place the porcelain jacket crowns despite their shortcomings. The technical advancements made with porcelain-fused-to-metal crowns in recent years related to color and strength should make this type of decision less frequent.

DISADVANTAGES

There are also several disadvantages associated with the porcelain jacket that are worthy of mention:

1. They are prone to fracture because of an inherent weakness of the material.
2. They are arduous to prepare since the reduction of sufficient tooth structure is necessary to accommodate the restoration and for the establishment of a uniform shoulder.
3. Reproduction of the color of some natural teeth can be problematic.
4. Time expenditure in mastering the technical aspects of fabrication is lengthy.
5. Securing an accurate impression with minimal tissue trauma is also difficult.

REQUIREMENTS AND PULPAL CONSIDERATIONS

It is essential that a sufficient amount of the tooth structure remain after preparation to withstand the functional forces of occlusion and protect and maintain the normality of the pulp. The preparation of the tooth in ideal arch alignment should also be designed to mimic the morphology of the tooth prepared. If the tooth is in malalignment, the pulpal integrity is of paramount consideration. Belated pulpal degeneration and undercut preparations are not uncommon when malalignment exists. Preparations on healthy teeth in good alignment are infrequent; consequently a certain percentage of belated pulpal and support tissue problems are indigenous to crown preparations. The added insult of extensive tooth preparation can exceed the ability of the tooth to recover. In the cases of younger adults, where arch alignment is not a problem, not all of the enamel covering the anatomic crown need be removed.

Sedative bases with pin buildups of the coronal portion of the involved teeth prior to preparation is one method of treatment to combat these problems. The advent of polycarboxylate cements has also reduced the incidence of belated, deleterious pulpal manifestations. However, extirpation of the pulp becomes a necessity in many cases. The use of a core and dowel or some type of acceptable coronal-radicular stabilization becomes necessary.

CLASSIFICATION

Oppice[3] has classified the types of preparations for complete porcelain crowns as follows:

1. Teeth possessing vital pulps
   a. With the gingival tissue attached to the enamel as well as the cementum
   b. With the gingival tissues attached to the cementum only
2. Teeth without a vital pulp
   a. Requiring a full core
   b. Requiring a partial core

In addition, Tylman[4] gives the following:

3. Special preparation for shoulderless crowns with some form of reinforcement
4. Teeth that serve as abutments, that is, complete porcelain crowns for thimble bridges

Restoring function and anatomy

The anatomic features of the complete porcelain crown are sometimes difficult to implement. Horizontal and vertical labial surface anatomy, which renders the restoration its natural appearance, requires sufficient tooth removal to allow manipulation of the porcelain. Ceramic manipulation is a refined art and science. The greater the labial bulk of porcelain, the more latitude the ceramist can exercise during laboratory fabrication. Conversely, the more labial the reduction, the greater the pulpal involvement. One answer to this problem is uniform tooth reduction to place a crown in harmony with its environment.

Functional occlusal relationships may determine the validity of placing porcelain jackets. Although esthetics are the prime consideration for a complete porcelain crown, the anticipated forces placed on the restoration cannot be taken lightly. Reduced interocclusal clearance might prohibit this placement. Porcelain jackets are adequate to withstand normal functional relationships (Fig. 6-11) when prepared with a uniform shoulder preparation.

Protection of investing tissue

One advantage mentioned previously is the labial and lingual gingival contour of the complete porcelain crown. The full shoulder type of preparation should permit a gingival contour that mimics the natural tooth. If a satisfactorily designed preparation has been realized and care has been exercised in the placement of the treatment restorations and final cementation, the response of the tissue is usually acceptable.

In younger patients, a certain amount of gingival recession over a period of years is predictable. This is true also with patients who have additional systemic complications where tissue response is a problem, such as in diabetes. Conservative preparation initially will allow the crown to be remade after a period of time with the usual preparation modifications if the tissue recession becomes objectionable after a period of years.

Uniformity of tooth reduction

This requirement is possible only if the proper diagnostic aids are utilized prior to preparation. Radiographs are preemptive measures for all restorative procedures. Diagnostic casts should be mounted on an articulator if multiple tooth preparation is involved.

Radiographic surveys will assist the dentist in determining the status of the supportive structures, periapical condition of the pulp, and possibly the pres-

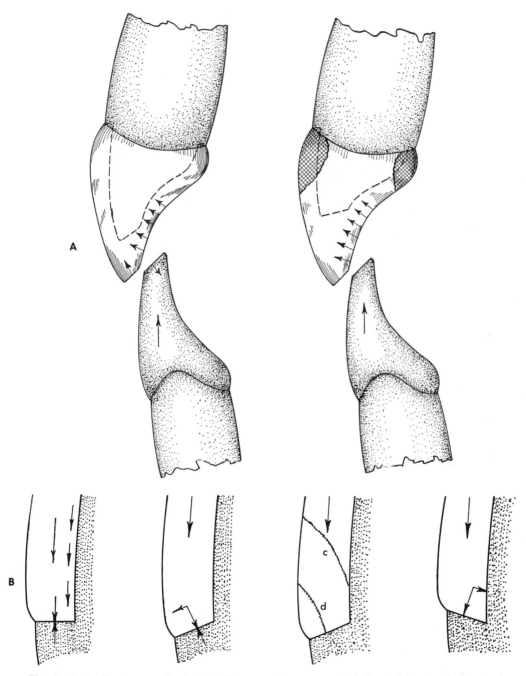

Fig. 6-11. A, Forces applied to tooth properly prepared, *left,* and to one improperly prepared, *right,* causing fractures of crown. **B,** Acute or right angle is preferred to obtuse angle of shoulder in relation to axial surface of preparation.

ence and position of pulpal horn extensions. Accessibility and visibility can hamper the operator during preparations; so chair position is also important.

PREPARATION

The preparation for a complete porcelain crown prior to the 1950s was very time consuming. High velocity instrumentation has reduced the preparation time, depending on the dentist, by as much as two thirds. However, the uniform reduction of the tooth and establishment of a full shoulder that will adequately support the investing tissue still demands concentration and a disciplined sequence of procedures. The sole objective of tooth preparation is not speed per se, but the biologic objectives and principles of procedure in preparing the tooth still remain the same, that is, (1) that the operator remove the least amount of tooth tissue consistent with necessary mechanical retention, (2) that he do this with the least harm to the periodontal tissues and the pulp, (3) that it be done with the least discomfort to the patient, and finally (4) that no pathologic reactions be initiated in the pulp.

SEQUENCE OF PREPARATION AND INSTRUMENTATION

Ultrahigh speeds of cutting instruments have modified the traditional method of full crown preparation. The air turbine has changed the method, but not the sequence or the steps of preparation. Diamond stones and carbide burs are constantly being improved. Hence we will not attempt to describe the various burs or diamond stones but merely provide guidelines with the illustrations.

Over 95% of the patients receive local anesthesia during preparation or for soft-tissue manipulation. Routine use of local anesthesia has alleviated the task of the dentist and rendered these refined dental procedures more acceptable to a greater number of patients.

Step 1—incisal reduction

Although the literature will disclose a variety of methods or steps of tooth reduction, there is usually general agreement that incisal reduction is first. A minimum of 1.5 to 2 mm is usually removed with a donut-shaped diamond stone bathed in water spray (Fig. 6-12, *A*). Removal of more than 2.5 mm of tooth structure incisally usually reduces vertical retention and encourages fractures of the porcelain at the gingival margin.

Incisal reduction also affects the esthetics if it is not uniform. Inadequate reduction will jeopardize the restoration during function, causing its fracture, that is, during protrusive movements of the mandible. Clearance should be checked visually in all excursions of the mandible to ensure sufficient tooth removal. Proper reduction can be checked by placement of a piece of wax interocclusally to make sure the wax immediately adjacent to the preparation is not penetrated (or too thin) during static positions and functional movements.

In keeping with the rule that planes are placed at right angles to applied forces, the incisal edge of the upper anterior teeth slopes lingually (Fig. 6-12, *C* to *E*), whereas that of the lower teeth slopes labially. This latter comment, concerning the slope of the incisal edge of the lower toward the labial, generally applies only to complete crown preparations.

The fundamental physical laws that govern or determine the traditional preparation design for the complete porcelain crown are elaborated in Chapter 24 of the sixth edition of this book.

In summary:

1. The incisal edge of this tooth preparation should be as close to the incisal edge of the porcelain crown as possible to be consistent with esthetics and still withstand functional forces.
2. The incisal edge will assist in absorbing the gingival forces during function by helping form a properly,

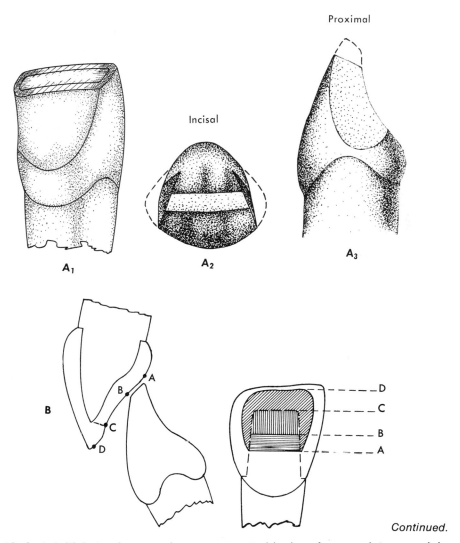

Proximal

Incisal

A₁

A₂

A₃

B

Continued.

Fig. 6-12. A, *1,* Initial step in preparing upper central incisor for complete porcelain crown; *2,* incisal view of incisal reduction for maxillary anterior teeth; *3,* proximal view. **B,** In area *A* to *C,* porcelain is supported by underlying tooth tissue; in area *C* to *D* it is not. **C,** Central incisors prepared for complete porcelain crowns: *1,* maxillary with lingual slope of the incisal edge; *2,* mandibular with labial slope of the incisal edge. **D,** Incisal reduction of maxillary central incisor as viewed from lingual surface. **E,** Incisal reduction of a maxillary central incisor as viewed from labial surface.

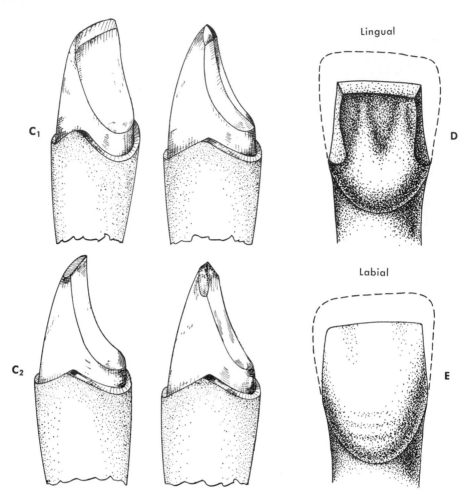

Fig. 6-12, cont'd. For legend see p. 143.

Step 2—proximal reduction

prepared angle between the shoulder and the labial wall.

All precautions are taken not to injure the adjacent teeth. Proximal reduction is accomplished by use of a very thin, tapered diamond stone (approximate size, 669L bur). The diamond stone is placed about 1 mm from the contact area (Fig. 6-13) and employed similarly to a slice preparation. Tapered diamond stones have replaced the diamond discs, which were cumbersome and dangerous to the soft tissue if the patient inadvertently moved.

The proximal slice is initiated from the labial surface and directed to almost one half the labiolingual width of the tooth. The next step is to join the labial slice with a slice started from the lingual proximal surface. The tip of the diamond point is directed to connect the labial and lingual slice slightly above the interdental papilla. Parallelism of 2 to 5 degrees is the desired result in the mesial and distal surfaces. The depth of the proximal reduction depends on the depth of the gingival crevice. Ordinarily, an effort is made to locate it midway between the crest of the gingiva and the bottom of the crevice.

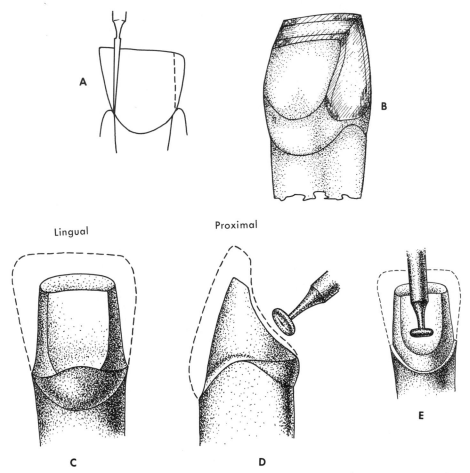

Fig. 6-13. A, Position of a diamond stone for mesial slice reduction of tooth. *Dotted line,* Distal cut to be made. **B,** Starting point, direction, and termination of proximal cuts; note no shoulder at gingival portion of cut. **C,** Proximal and incisal reduction of maxillary central incisor as shown from lingual surface. **D,** Proximal, lingual, and labial reduction as viewed from proximal surface. **E,** Lingual view of maxillary incisor showing a donut-shaped diamond stone used to develop lingual concavity.

The proximal preparations *do not* include the early development of the gingival shoulder. Since the depth of the gingival crevice varies not only in different areas of the oral cavity but also in different regions of the same tooth, a flat, thin periodontal membrane explorer is used to determine the depth of the crevice on both proximal surfaces.

One must keep in mind that the proximal gingival tissue must be supported by a gentle proximal elevation of the shoulder. The height of the elevation should be similar to the proximal tissue height.

Step 3—removal of labial enamel and establishment of vertical lingual retention

The removal of the labial enamel is accomplished by a tapered, cylindric diamond stone that is moved in sweeping motions across the water-bathed surface. After the removal of the enamel (Fig. 6-14) so that the labial gingival termina-

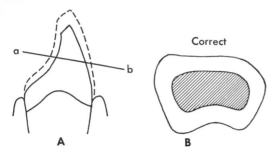

Fig. 6-14. Axial gross tooth reduction. **A,** Proximal view. **B,** Cross-cut view of **A** at *a-b* level.

tion is made at or just above the crest of the labial gingival face, the vertical retention area immediately below the cingulum is then prepared. This area represents an additional area of retention and resistance to displacement.

Step 4—preparation of lingual surface and proximal line angles

The lingual tooth structure is removed uniformly in sweeping motions with a donut-shaped diamond stone (Fig. 6-13, *D* and *E*) bathed in an air-water spray. In the case of maxillary tooth preparation, special attention should be given to providing sufficient clearance during function. If any tooth of the opposing arches appear supraerupted, they should be adjusted to provide smooth excursions of the mandible in lateral and protrusive movements.

The proximolabial and the proximolingual line angles of the tooth are removed with a medium-length, tapering, cylindric diamond stone. The grade of the diamond stone should decrease in coarseness as the preparation nears completion. Step 4 finishes the gross reduction of tooth structure (Fig. 6-14) and leaves the tooth without undercuts *prior to* the establishment of the gingival termination.

One of the common errors of dentists is to start the shoulder preparation initially, prior to gross reduction. Soft-tissue and

pulpal integrity will be better served by completion of step 4 before initiation of the shoulder preparation. Obviously, more experienced operators are capable of modifications of this sequence of preparation for full shoulder preparations. Concomitant preliminary shoulder preparation with labial and lingual reduction is acceptable, but full shoulder preparation prior to labial reduction presents a myriad of problems. Pulpal exposures are commonly involved in an effort to eliminate undercuts from an inordinately large shoulder preparation.

Step 5—preparation of gingival margin

The next step is cutting and refining the gingival margin. Complete porcelain crowns terminate, whenever possible, in a full shoulder that lies slightly below the level of the gingival crest. Gingival margins for this crown are prepared to terminate midway between the crest of the soft tissue and the bottom of the gingival crest. Age, variations in tissue height, caries, and the arch position of the individual teeth will determine the need to modify these guidelines.

The shoulder rarely exceeds a width of 0.5 to 0.75 mm. Ideally, the plane of the shoulder is cut at right angles to the axial surface of the preparation. Cylindric diamond stones and gingival finishing carbide burs are the most common cutting instruments used to complete the accessibility and visibility. In carrying this cut from labial to lingual, one should exercise caution that the plane of the shoulder is paralleled to the *level of the crest* of the gingival tissue. If the shoulder is cut in a straight line labiolingually, the gingival tissue is left unsupported and the fibers of the periodontal membrane can be severed.

To minimize this occurrence, the cutting stone, hand instrument, or bur (Fig. 6-15, *A* and *B*) is not sunk initially to its full diameter. The end of the cutting stone is moved back and forth at the crest

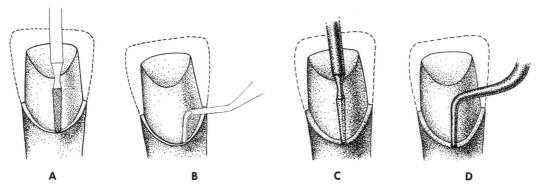

A   **B**   **C**   **D**

Fig. 6-15. A, Labial view of shoulder preparation of maxillary central incisor. Tapered diamond stone or fissure bur, or both, are commonly used for this procedure. **B,** Labial view of maxillary central incisor showing use of hand instrument used for development of labial shoulder. **C,** Labial view of maxillary incisor showing increased labial shoulder width after further refinement with tapered diamond stone. **D,** Labial view of maxillary incisor showing hand-instrument refinement for finishing of labial shoulder. Line running mesiodistally and superior to the hand instrument illustrates the direction of rotary or hand instrument by dentist.

of the labial tissue, with gentle planing of the tooth in smooth strokes. Gradually the full diameter of the cutting instrument (Fig. 6-15, *C* and *D*) has established the shoulder. Cautiously, the shoulder is extended from the labial to the lingual, following the curvature of the free soft tissue.

The same procedure is duplicated in cutting the shoulder on the lingual surface (Fig. 6-16). Ordinarily, the lingual shoulder is extended around the lingual and proximal line angles uniting with the labial and proximal cuts. Visibility during the proximal shoulder preparation is absolutely necessary. The patient should be positioned in the chair to permit easy access.

Formerly, with lower cutting speeds, the shoulder was completed supragingivally and then the shoulder was lowered to the desired level. With the air turbine, the establishment of the full shoulder is brought to its desired subgingival depth after gross reduction. Care must be taken to avoid soft-tissue damage and excessive reduction of the tooth. While the shoulder is being prepared, the air rotor is not

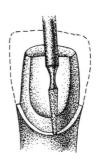

Fig. 6-16. Lingual view of maxillary incisor showing tapered diamond stone used to develop lingual shoulder.

usually run at full speed. End-cutting burs and smooth diamonds are later used to finish the full shoulder preparation (Fig. 6-17). There are usually a series of steps at different levels, instead of a smooth, continous plane. With the end-cutting burs or diamond stones, there is less chance of undercutting the axial walls of the coronal portion of the preparation. The angulation of the shoulder can be smoothed and checked as shown in Fig. 6-15, by use of a chisel, hoe, or special files softly across the shoulder in a sweeping motion. Sandpaper discs are used to finish the coronal portion of the

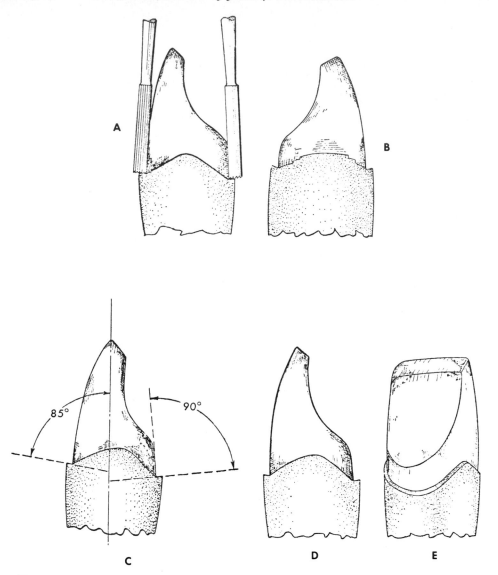

Fig. 6-17. A, Use of plain-fissure, *left,* and end-cutting burs, *right,* to cut shoulder. **B,** Improperly prepared shoulder having steps instead of continuous plane. **C,** Plane of shoulder made at right angle to axial surface of tooth. **D** and **E,** Sharp-line angles where axial surfaces meet incisal and lingual surfaces are founded and polished with discs.

preparation and eliminate subtle undercuts (Fig. 6-15).

FINISHED PREPARATION

The finished preparation should be a miniature reproduction of the original teeth with certain modifications:

1. An incisal plane placed at a 45 degree angle to meet the forces of mastication at right angles
2. All axial surfaces converging slightly toward the axis of the preparation
3. A labial surface that is convex mesiodistally and gingivoincisally

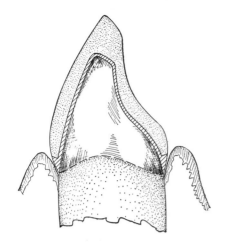

Fig. 6-18. Shoulder type of porcelain-veneer crown used with shoulderless metal casting.

4. A lingual surface on the central and lateral incisors slightly concave mesiodistally and gingivoincisally and extending from the incisal plane to the crest of the cingulum
5. Adequate clearance linguoincisally to allow for a sufficient amount of porcelain between the preparation and the opposing tooth
6. The gingival third region of the lingual surface is prepared from a convexity to an axial wall converging incisally
7. A gingival shoulder located at or below the crest of the investing tissue

MODIFICATION OF COMPLETE PORCELAIN CROWN PREPARATION— SHOULDERLESS TYPE

Both,[5] in 1937, stated that the shoulderless preparation (Fig. 6-18) is indicated for a tooth when it is so narrow at its cervical diameter that the vitality of the pulp would be endangered by cutting a shoulder. Both listed the teeth more likely to need preparation modification because of possible pulpal involvement, such as the following:
1. Lower incisors
2. Maxillary lateral incisors

3. Teeth from which the gingival tissue has receded beyond the enamel matrix

Both[5] and Wheeler,[6] in 1931, had different viewpoints. Wheeler believed that a porcelain gingival margin must be shouldered to be a successful restoration.

Ewing,[7] in 1952, pointed out that the dentist must compromise between shoulder and shoulderless types of preparations. Biologic and mechanical reasons were enumerated. Trauma is naturally reduced by the elimination of the full shoulder preparation.

Ewing's description of the "atypical" porcelain jacket crown preparation was perceptive and his modifications are now commonly employed for the porcelain-fused-to-metal crowns. The advent and refinement of porcelain-fused-to-metal techniques has made this clinical problem obsolete.

CONCLUSIONS

The greatest advantage of the complete porcelain crown is its superior esthetics. An obvious disadvantage is the amount of tooth reduction necessary for proper support of the porcelain. In addition to the initial and belated pulpal response, the preparation for a complete porcelain crown is arduous and demands a regimented approach where the dentist has very little latitude for preparation modifications. Currently, complete porcelain crowns are used more frequently as individual restorations on the maxillary central and lateral incisors where superior esthetics are demanded.

The flexibility in preparation design to control biomechanical problems is more available to the dentist in complete porcelain-fused-to-metal crowns. A complete porcelain-fused-to-metal crown has the added advantage of being a versatile bridge retainer.

The technical aspects for fabrication of porcelain crowns is discussed in Chapter 25.

SELECTED REFERENCES

1. Clark, B. E.: Requirements of the jacket crown. J.A.D.A. **26**:355, 1939.
2. Schneider, A. E.: The preparation of a tooth for a porcelain veneer crown, Chicago, 1916.
3. Oppice, H. W.: A résumé of ideas on porcelain jacket crown preparations, J.A.D.A. **21**:1030, 1934.
4. Tylman, S. D.: Theory and practice of crown and fixed partial prosthodontics (bridge), ed. 6, **24**:505, 1970, The C. V. Mosby Co.
5. Both, H. S.: Newer methods in preparing vital teeth for porcelain jacket crowns, Dent. Dig. **43**:481, 1937.
6. Wheeler, R. C.: Restoration of the gingival or cervical margins in full crowns, Dent. Cosmos **73**:238, 1931.
7. Ewing, J. E.: Atypical porcelain jacket crown preparations, J. Prosthet. Dent. **2**:865, 1952.

SECTION C

Veneer crown preparation: porcelain-fused-to-metal acrylic veneer crowns

Although the complete metal crown fulfills all the biomechanical requirements, its use in the past was confined to the posterior quadrants of the oral cavity. Currently, the complete metal crowns are modified for the anterior quadrants of the patient by use of a porcelain or acrylic veneer. This modification is commonplace with the anterior ten maxillary teeth and eight mandibular teeth but occasional with the maxillary first molar.

When the porcelain or acrylic facing is used, the tooth preparation is modified by establishment of a shoulder on the labial or buccal surfaces. This modification is made to allow additional space for the thickness of porcelain and acrylic. There are some dentists who consider the use of acrylic veneer crowns as a disservice;

however, there are indications for use of acrylic veneer. They are economics, establishment of a posterior occlusal relationship, and full arch splints or transitional crowns, or both, for adolescents. Acrylic veneers are therefore included in the discussion. Improvements and research in the chemistry of plastics will eventually render acrylic more acceptable for routine usage.

The use of porcelain as a veneer was formerly designated as a Hollenbach crown. The porcelain veneer facing was a customized porcelain denture tooth that was adapted to fit a given preparation. After the facings were adapted with lateral recesses, it was waxed (Fig. 6-19) into a prepared crown. The facing was removed from the wax-up and luted with

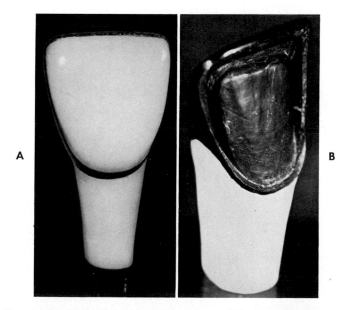

A   **B**

Fig. 6-19. A, Porcelain denture facing waxed to model of prepared crown. **B,** Facing removed to show recesses in wax into which lateral extensions of porcelain facing extend. Hollenbach and Richmond crowns, now classified as obsolete, were harbingers of current veneer crowns.

cement after the casting was finished and polished. The assembled two-part crown was then cemented to the patient's tooth. Variations of the Hollenbach crown were introduced.

Acrylic denture teeth were substituted for porcelain facings. The advantage to this modification was the durability of the acrylic and the ease of fabrication. Currently, acrylic veneer crowns have their facings processed to the cast metal. Although used extensively, the resin veneer crown did not possess the natural tooth shades. The earliest resins were porous and were easily stained. It was also common to see abrasion or washing out of the processed resin despite the fastidious attention to the laboratory fabrication processes. Porcelain-fused-to-metal crowns were the next logical advancement.

PORCELAIN-FUSED-TO-METAL VENEER CROWNS

Woolson[1] presented an early effort to overcome the difficulty that arises when porcelain is fired to metal. Porcelain fired directly to gold alloys developed cracks after firing because of the different coefficients of contraction and expansion of the two materials. The problem was temporarily resolved when he interposed a slip plane so that each material could manifest its own physical laws of contraction and expansion. Metallurgic research has provided many advancements, such as vacuum firing and superior ceramic mixtures, to enhance the use of complete porcelain-fused-to-metal crowns since the early 1940s. Porcelain-fused-to-metal crowns till the late 1950s lacked natural color and vitality when used as a restoration for the maxillary four incisors.

Improvements in the bonding of the porcelain to the metal and the properties of the porcelain itself have also made this restoration more acceptable. Porcelain-fused-to-metal complete crowns are used extensively both as an individual restoration and as a bridge retainer.[23] Fig. 6-20 shows the labial view of the tooth preparation for a porcelain-fused-to-metal crown for a maxillary central incisor. Fig. 6-21 diagrammatically shows the proximal view of a porcelain-fused-to-metal crown preparation.

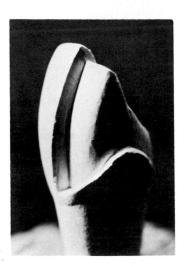

Fig. 6-20. Amount of labial reduction needed for veneer crown.

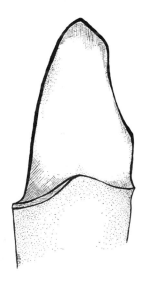

Fig. 6-21. Proximal view of porcelain-fused-to-metal veneer crown preparation.

INDICATIONS

The primary reason for using complete porcelain-fused-to-metal crowns is similar to indications for the complete porcelain crown on p. 137. However, the veneer crown is more versatile because of its common employment as a bridge retainer. It is also used as a single restoration in the posterior quadrants of the oral cavity where esthetics is a consideration.[4,5] In addition to the indications for the complete porcelain crown, the porcelain-fused-to-metal veneer crown is also indicated for the following:

1. Single and multiple restorations for both anterior and posterior teeth
2. Retainers for a removable partial denture prosthesis
3. Fixed prosthodontic units of veneer crowns, both anterior and posterior, will add strength to the teeth and still maintain esthetics
4. Superstructures for splinted periodontal prosthesis
5. Mandibular anteriors where full shoulder preparations are prohibitive
6. Peg-shaped laterals or teeth with similar morphologic deviations
7. Patients with a reduced interocclusal clearance or those who exhibit a strong masticatory musculature

A satisfactory preparation is a primary premise to all crowns. The porcelain-fused-to-metal crown is no exception. Although this crown is similar to the preparation for a porcelain jacket, there are major points of difference between the two preparations, as follows:

1. The labial shoulder is usually slightly wider and has a rounded gingival shoulder at the gingival axial line angle.
2. More of the labial axial wall of the tooth would be removed consistent with the larger labial shoulder.
3. The lingual and linguoproximal margins that extend to half the distance labially on each proximal

surface are prepared as a chamfer instead of a shoulder.

4. Less of the lingual surface of the tooth is removed.
5. The use of a beveled labial or buccal margin that extends gingivally beyond the rounded shoulder from proximal to proximal mesiodistally. This modification (Fig. 6-21) is left to the discretion of the dentist.

Actually with the refinements in metals and ceramics,[6] the porcelain-fused-to-metal tooth preparation can be more conservative than the complete porcelain crown. Additional strength is added to the tooth by the coronal-radicular stabilization[7,8] gained by use a labial or buccal beveled shoulder. Crown preparations for resin veneers do not differ basically with the porcelain-fused-to-metal veneer. However, the resin veneer crown preparation is modified in the following aspects:

1. The resin veneer preparation requires slightly less width to the labial shoulder.
2. The labial gingival shoulder is not rounded but is a point angle similar to the complete porcelain jacket preparations.
3. The proximal wall where the labial

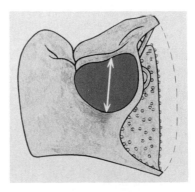

Fig. 6-22. Acrylic-veneer crown illustrating position of proximal contact area. Note retentive devices used on buccal surface to secure processed facing. (Courtesy The J. M. Ney Co., Bloomfield, Conn.)

shoulder and the lingual chamfer join can be more abrupt in the resin veneer crown preparation.

The beveled labial or buccal shoulder is again up to the discretion of the dentist and the clinical conditions presented by the patient. The buccal or labial surface of a resin veneer must be protected by metal (Fig. 6-22). This is particularly true on the buccal of mandibular teeth because of their stamp cusp function.

DISADVANTAGES

Although the application of veneer crowns is diverse, there are some disadvantages and difficulties incident to their use, as follows:

1. The porcelain-fused-to-metal veneer is susceptible to fracture whereas the resin veneer is vulnerable to color instability upon aging.
2. Creation of the labial shoulder for all complete veneer crowns subjects the pulp and investing tissue to trauma.
3. Development of esthetics that is tissue tolerant is more difficult because of the overcontour of the veneer crowns regardless of type.
4. The longevity of these restorations is diretly related to the durability of their veneers.

Along with the disadvantages, there are clinical conditions that limit the use of complete veneer crowns:

1. Younger patients with larger pulps dictate modification of the labial shoulder preparation.
2. Establishment of satisfactory occlusal relationships is demanding, particularly with complete porcelain-fused-to-metal crowns.
3. Patients with poor hygiene restrict the latitude of the dentist in the placement of the gingival margin.

As with other crowns, the limitations of any restoration are placed in the relative order of importance. The dentist, with the permission of the patient, may elect to place complete veneer crowns despite the difficult clinical implementation. Belated periodontal complications are not uncommon. The rough areas of overcontoured margins of complete veneer crowns within the gingival sulcus cause inflammation. Whenever the gingival sulcus is involved, the material selected, and the preparation phase completed, all must be performed with minimal trauma to restore a tooth to its former form and function.[9,10] However, recent research seems to show that some inflammation of the periodontal tissue is indigenous to all crowns whose margins are subgingival.

REQUIREMENTS
Pulpal considerations

The labial shoulder is usually the area responsible for pulpal involvement. However, there are few individual crowns placed on healthy teeth. The prepared teeth have previously received a carious, periodontal, or traumatic insult. Belated pulpal responses after preparation and crown placement is a definite reality in all fixed prosthodontics. Preparation of a healthy tooth as an abutment for a fixed prosthesis is one exception. The opportunity of cutting an ideal preparation, without the usual modifications that are associated with fixed prosthodontics, is a rare occurrence for a dentist; nevertheless near-ideal preparations are also possible if a regimented caries-control program with amalgam restorations or composites is performed prior to placement of cast restorations.

Restoration of function and anatomy

The complete metal veneer crown can meet nearly all the requirements of a successful dental restoration if it is placed where indicated and if the tooth is satisfactorily prepared. It is possible not only to simulate the natural tooth but also to restore esthetics and function. In addition, the complete metal veneer crown allows the dentist more latitude in developing or restoring a tooth to normal occlusal relationships.

The use of porcelain-fused-to-metal veneer crowns with total occlusal coverage of porcelain for an entire quadrant presents a problem. One of the reasons gold was used as a restorative material, in addition to its noble-metal attributes, was that its attrition rate is similar to that of tooth structure. When porcelain is placed on opposing teeth or on maxillary to mandibular molars or is used in key occlusal relationships, a bisque-baked try-in is necessary. The use of full porcelain coverage on posterior teeth demands more longitudinal studies to warrant this direction of therapy as a routine clinical approach. Patients with an immediate canine disocclusion who require maximum esthetics may permit the use of full porcelain occlusal coverage posteriorly. Patients with a group-function occlusion with maximum intercuspal articulation during lateral excursions of the mandible may present overwhelming complications. Some of the problems noted by the dentist may be immediate in the form of porcelain fractures, whereas the belated problems may be exhibited as supportive bone loss. The crown that uses a resin as the veneer presents the same problems, but the occlusal adjustment of gold occlusal surfaces is much easier for the dentist. Many gnathologists prefer using gold occlusal surfaces with processed resin or Pyroplast as the veneer. They believe it is arduous enough to obtain a satisfactory gold-to-gold interocclusal relationship that is amendable at chairside.

Porcelain-to-porcelain surfaces are near impossible to adust without additional porcelain firing. Fig. 6-4 illustrates an ideal contact area on a posterior acrylic veneer crown. Contact areas on porcelain-fused-to-metal crowns are usually more bulky unless technical implementation is precisely exercised.

Investing tissues

Complete metal veneer crowns, whether porcelain-fused-to-metal or resin type, restore the entire coronal portion of the tooth. Optimum contours for labial and buccal surfaces of these crowns are still being closely reviewed by clinicians and scrutinized by researchers.[11] Overcontoured crowns, misplaced proximal contacts, and poorly designed occlusal relationships sponsor adverse supportive tissue responses. The concept of splinting crowns to obtain a more favorable supportive tissue response is also still a matter of discretion. Splinting may add support to a tooth or teeth, but limits the patient's approach to certain aspects of oral hygiene procedures. Additional studies are needed to determine when a given case should be splinted.[12] To date, it would appear the disadvantages outweigh the advantages unless the restorative measures are a terminal attempt to avoid placement of a removable prosthesis. Single units are more conducive to supportive tissue health.

Uniformity of tooth reduction

Diagnostic aids in the form of radiographs and diagnostic casts will enhance this objective. Crowns placed on the posterior teeth present a formidable problem from the standpoint of access and visibility. Modifications of traditional preparation designs are made for a myriad of reasons, but mainly because of extensive caries, which is not an unusual occurrence during preparation for complete metal veneer crowns. Periodontally involved teeth will also require fluting and possibly supragingival margins.

INSTRUMENTATION

Ultrahigh speed cutting instruments have made extremely arduous procedures simple. The selection of diamond stones and carbide burs become a matter of preference to the dentist. Four-handed dentistry, versus the solo operator ap-

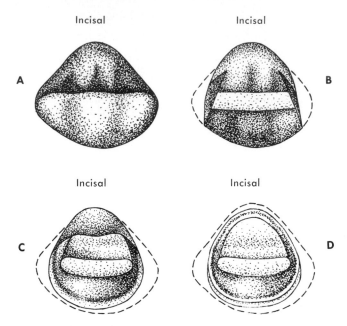

Fig. 6-23. A, Incisal view of maxillary incisor prior to preparation. **B,** Incisal and proximal surface reduction of a maxillary incisor for veneer crown preparation. **C,** Partial coronal preparation of a porcelain-faced metal preparation as shown from incisal surface. **D,** Porcelain-fused-to-metal veneer crown preparation on a maxillary incisor as viewed from incisal surface.

proach, also plays a role in the manipulation of the instrumentation. However, guidelines will be presented during the discussion of the steps in preparation for a complete metal veneer crown.

SEQUENCE OF PREPARATION
Step 1—incisal reduction

The incisal plane is reduced from 1.5 to 2 mm (Fig. 6-23) so that there is suitable thickness of gold or porcelain. Incisal reduction should be adequate to ensure clearance in protrusive movements of the mandible, permit satisfactory esthetics, and enhance optimal function.

The occlusal reduction for a posterior veneer crown is similar to that of the complete metal crown. The occlusal reduction of 2 mm is accomplished with a donut-shaped diamond stone. Clearance is checked by the dentist during the various excursions of the mandible with an interocclusal wax wafer.

Step 2—proximal reduction

Proximal reduction is accomplished with a long, thin, tapered diamond stone or crosscut carbide burs, such as no. 700 and no. 669. The cut is started on the incisal or buccal plane 1 to 1.5 mm from the proximal surface. A diamond stone is directed gingivally so that when the cut is made through the body of the tooth the proximal plane will emerge at or slightly above the crest of the gingiva (Fig. 6-24) without the creation of a gingival ledge. The other proximal is treated similarly. Gross reduction is identical for both types of veneer crowns. A frequent problem arises when insufficient space is created for establishment of a contact area with adequate interproximal embrasures (Fig. 6-24).

Step 3—removal of labial enamel

The removal of enamel from the labial and buccal surface is performed in the

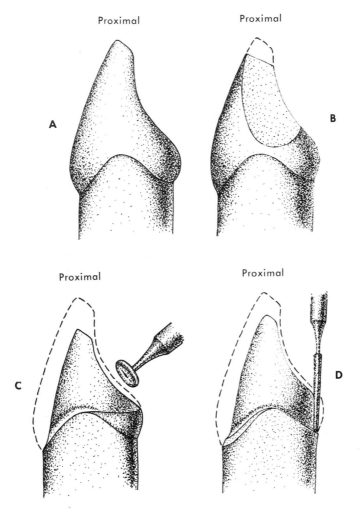

Fig. 6-24. A, Proximal view of maxillary incisor prior to preparation for a veneer crown. **B,** Proximal view of maxillary incisor illustrating incisal reduction and proximal slice. **C,** Proximal view of gingivoincisal and lingual reduction of a veneer crown preparation. Lingual reduction is commonly performed with donut-shaped diamond stone. **D,** Proximal view of veneer crown preparation showing labial shoulder with bevels. Proximal line angles are finished with long medium-grit diamond stone.

same manner (Fig. 6-25) as it is in the complete porcelain crown, that is, in a smooth controlled motion from mesial to distal. Depth orientation channels or control grooves are indicated for the difficult preparations. The most common problem in labial reduction is to ensure that the labial axial surface is convex mesiodistally and gingivoincisally. Failure to observe this operative procedure results in a

more protrusive veneer (Fig. 6-26) than desired because of lack of space at the incisal plane. This is called "biomechanical reduction."

Step 4—reduction of lingual surface

All the enamel need not be removed from the lingual surface of complete metal veneer crowns. Adequate reduction for strength to withstand the forces of oc-

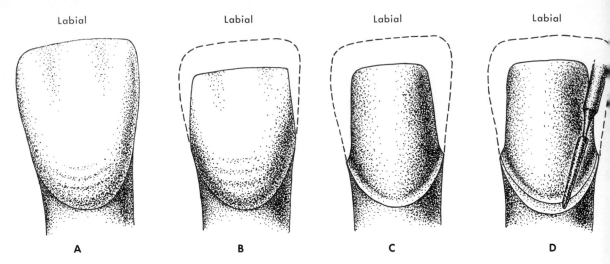

Labial   Labial   Labial   Labial

A   B   C   D

Fig. 6-25. A, Labial view of maxillary incisor prior to preparation. **B,** Labial view of maxillary incisor showing amount of incisal reduction necessary. **C,** Labial view of a maxillary incisor showing usual amount of proximal and incisal surface for veneer crown preparation. **D,** Placement of bevel on labial shoulder of maxillary incisor for veneer crown.

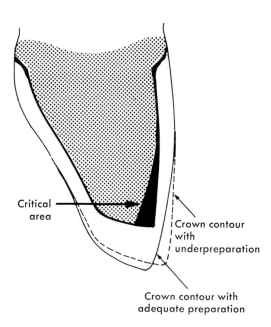

Critical area

Crown contour with underpreparation

Crown contour with adequate preparation

Fig. 6-26. The most common problem with veneer crown preparation is insufficient labial reduction. (From Fischer, W. F., editor: Hospital Dental Service Bulletin, R.D.A., Oct. 1969, Walter Reed Army Hospital.)

clusion is the routine guideline. The porcelain-fused-to-metal veneer requires more reduction than does the resin type of veneer. Step four is accomplished with a donut-shaped diamond stone in the anterior quadrants, whereas the lingual vertical reduction would be performed with a medium-sized cylindric diamond stone. The proximal line angles can be prepared both anteriorly and posteriorly (Fig. 6-27) with the same-shaped diamond cutting instrument.

The gingival margin is usually a chamfer, or possibly a knife-edge for resin crowns. A lingual chamfer is preferable for definite marginal termination.

Step 5—preparation of gingival margins

The labial shoulder preparation is 0.5 to 0.75 mm in width for complete metal veneer crowns. However, the labial shoulder meets and is continuous with the chamfer midway on the proximal surfaces. This differs from the complete porcelain crown in which the shoulder con-

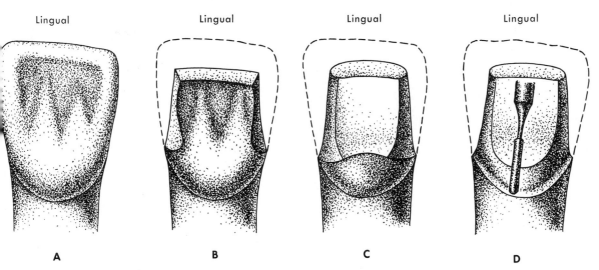

Fig. 6-27. A, Lingual view of maxillary incisor prior to preparation. **B,** Lingual view of maxillary incisor showing lingual and initial proximal reduction for veneer crown preparation. **C,** Reduction of lingual surface in preparation for veneer crown. **D,** Lingual axial reduction is performed with medium-length diamond whose rounded end assists in making a lingual gingival chamfer.

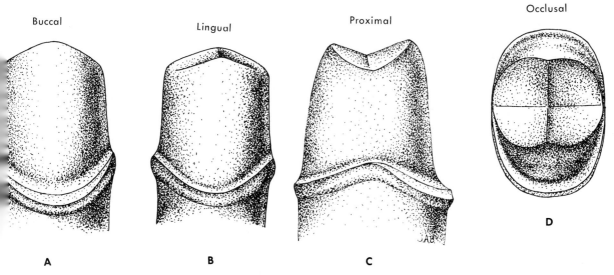

Fig. 6-28. A, Buccal view of completed porcelain-fused-to-metal veneer crown preparation on a premolar. Note buccal bevel and the gradual modification of buccal shoulder as it proceeds lingually. **B,** Lingual view of lingual chamfer of porcelain-fused-to-metal crown preparation on maxillary premolar. **C,** Proximal view of porcelain-fused-to-metal veneer crown preparation on maxillary premolar. Note gradual "fade-away" of beveled buccal shoulder. **D,** Occlusal view of maxillary premolar showing modified buccal shoulder and lingual chamfer.

Buccal Lingual

Proximal Occlusal

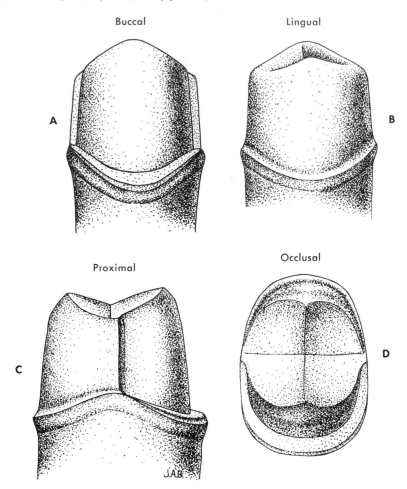

Fig. 6-29. A, Buccal view of maxillary premolar for acrylic-veneer crown preparation. Note abrupt proximal preparation in contrast to gradual lingual "fade-away." **B,** Lingual view of acrylic-veneer crown preparation. Note lingual chamfer. **C,** Proximal view of acrylic-veneer crown preparation. Note more rigid proximal preparation. **D,** Occlusal view of acrylic-veneer crown preparation on maxillary premolar. Note difference in proximal preparation, between porcelain-fused-to-metal and acrylic-veneer preparations.

tinues around the entire lingual surface. However, the establishment of a labial shoulder has a similar instrumentation to that of the tooth preparation for a porcelain jacket.

Differences between the porcelain-fused-to-metal (Fig. 6-28) and acrylic veneer crown preparations (Fig. 6-29) have been discussed; that is, the line angle at the labial shoulder can be more rounded for the porcelain and the proximal junction of the labial shoulder, and the lingual finish line at the proximals can be more abrupt for the resin type of veneer crown.

Development of a labial or buccal bevel is usually associated with the porcelain veneer, but it can be used for the acrylic veneer as well. The use of a bevel, long or short, is at the discretion of the dentist. Labial shoulders with bevels are accomplished by the combined use of a long, smooth cylindric diamond cutting instrument and hand instruments. Visibility is necessary for an adequate subgingival margin.

Tissue management to secure gingival margins is reviewed in Chapter 7. Cords and electrosurgical techniques are both advocated.

The cervical margin is normally placed slightly below the crest of the soft tissue labially. More latitude can be built in by the dentist during preparation of the lingeral surface. Placement of the labial margin subgingivally usually enhances esthetics. If the smile lip line of the patient terminates below the gingival crest or below the cervical third of the clinical crown, this procedure is less critical. Posteriorly, the buccal margin on the premolars is subject to the same rules as the incisiors, but the gingival margins on the molar can terminate at a position more supragingivally to promote the health of the soft tissue. This last statement is particularly true in the case of periodontally treated patients.

CONCLUSION

The finished preparation should be a miniature reproduction of the original teeth with shoulder modification.

There seems to be few contraindications for the use of porcelain veneer crowns. Porcelain-fused-to-metal crowns presently enjoy unparalleled popularity among restorative dentists. However, one must remember that the longevity of a veneer crown is directly proportional to the durability of its veneer. Veneers placed on molar teeth should be a rare occurrence, such as in exceptionally demanding esthetics.

Improvements in both porcelain-fused-to-metal and acrylic veneer crowns will be welcomed by the entire profession.

SELECTED REFERENCES

1. Woolson, A. H.: Restorations, made of porcelain baked on gold, J. Prosthet. Dent. **5**:65, 1955.
2. Dawson, P. E.: Evaluation, diagnosis and treatment of occlusal problems, St. Louis, 1974, The C. V. Mosby Co.
3. Guyer, S. E.: Multiple preparations for fixed prosthodontics, J. Prosthet. Dent. **23**:529-553, 1970.
4. Brecker, S. C.: Porcelain fused to gold, J. Calif. Dent. Assoc. and Nevada Dent. Soc. **36**:425-429, 1960.
5. Johnston, J. F., Mumford, G., and Dykema, R. W.: Porcelain veneers bonded to metal castings, Practical Dent. Monogr., pp. 3-32, March 1963.
6. Shell, J. S., and Nielsen, J. P.: Study of bond between gold alloys and porcelain, J. Dent. Res. **41**:1427-1437, 1962.
7. Shillingburg, H. T., Hobo, S., and Fisher, D. W.: Preparation design and margin distortion in porcelain fused to metal restorations, J. Prosthet. Dent. **30**:28-36, 1973.
8. Hobo, S., Shillingburg, H. T.: Porcelain fused to metal: tooth preparation and coping design, J. Prosthet. Dent. **30**:28-36, 1973.
9. Myers, G. E.: Textbook of crown and bridge prosthodontics, St. Louis, 1969, The C. V. Mosby Co., pp. 68-92.
10. Weinberg, L. A.: Esthetics and the gingiva in full coverage, J. Prosthet. Dent. **10**:737, 1960.
11. Kahn, A. E.: Partial vs. full coverage, J. Prosthet. Dent. **10**:167, 1960.
12. Lorey, R. E., and Myers, G. E.: The retentive qulities of bridge retainers, J.A.D.A. **76**:568, 1968.

GENERAL REFERENCES

Baker, C. R.: Banded-cast metal crowns, J.A.D.A. **56**:522, 1958.

Craig, R. C., el-Ebrashi, M. K., and Peyton, F. A.: Experimental stress analysis of dental restorations. I. two-dimensional photoelastic stress analysis of crowns, J. Prosthet. Dent. **17**(3):292-302, 1967.

Ewing, J. E., and Bentman, D.: Porcelain veneered full crown restorations made with cadmium patterns, J. Prosthet. Dent. **18**(2):140-150, 1967.

Gordon, T.: Telescopic reconstruction: an approach to rehabilitation, J.A.D.A. **72**:97-105, 1966.

Herrick, P. W., Shell, J., Timmermans, J., and Turpin, D.: Investigation of hydrogroscopic investment (control water added) for casting multiunit bridges, J. Dent. Res. **40**:744, 1961.

Isaacson, G. O.: Telescopic crown retainers for removable partial dentures, J. Prosthet. Dent. **21**:458-465, 1969.

Jameson, L. M.: Comparison of crevicular fluid volumes between restored and non-restored teeth (master's thesis), Loyola University Dental School, Chicago, 1976.

Leff, A.: Evaluation of high speed in full coverage preparations, J. Prosthet. Dent. **10**:314, 1960.

Lyon, D. M., Cowger, G. T., Woycheshin, F. F., and Miller, C. B.: Porcelain fused to gold—evaluation and esthetics, J. Prosthet. Dent. **10**:319, 1960.

Marcum, J. S.: The effect of crown marginal depth upon gingival tissue, J. Prosthet. Dent. **17**:479, 1967.

Miller, I. F., and Feinberg, E.: Full coverage restorations, J. Prosthet. Dent. **12**:317-325, 1962.

Schweitzer, J. M.: Gold copings for problematic teeth, J. Prosthet. Dent. **10**:163, 1960.

Swartz, M. L., and Phillips, R. W.: Study of adaptation of veneers to cast gold crowns, J. Prosthet. Dent. **7**:817, 1957.

Wagman, S. S.: Tissue management for full cast veneer crowns, J. Prosthet. Dent. **15**:106-117, 1965.

Weinberg, L. A.: Double casting of metal to metal in full coverage, J.A.D.A. **63**:821, 1961.

SECTION D1

Partial veneer crowns

Prior to constructing a fixed partial denture, the dentist must make a comprehensive examination of the existing oral condition as well as the general condition of the patient. Complete clinical and roentgenographic records and a set of mounted diagnostic casts are prime requirements for a meaningful diagnosis and for determining sound biologic and mechanical plans of treatment before, during, and after oral treatment. Not only is the preparation of the teeth for crowns of bridge retainers important and likewise an evaluation of the type of the existing arch position of the teeth and dynamics of tooth articulation, but also the treatment of pathologic conditions of the supporting and contiguous soft tissues is needed.

Diagnostic study casts mounted in centric relation on an articulator are extremely helpful in determining the design and method of preparing a tooth for a crown or bridge retainer.

After the biologic tolerance of the abutment teeth, the periodontal membrane, and the bone support have been appraised clinically and radiographically, the physical and mechanical engineering aspects of the prosthesis require equal consideration. First is the total structure itself: (1) the number, size, position, and anatomic integrity of each abutment tooth; (2) the length, dimensions, and curvature of the bridge span and the forces that may be placed upon the structure; (3) the materials and their manipulation, of which the appliance is to be made; (4) the design of the supporting retainers to tolerate the anticipated displacing forces of occlusion; (5) instrumentation and steps of procedure; (6) construction of pontics; (7) methods of connecting the component units of the bridge (connectors); and finally (8) the

methods of fixation and postoperative procedures.

Bridge retainers are classified into two general groups, the intracoronal and the extracoronal. The intracoronal retainers may be placed in the anterior and the posterior teeth and involve three or more surfaces: the distolingual (DL), mesiolingual (ML), mesio-occlusal (MO), disto-occlusal (DO), and MOD, as well as the MODL and similar types are examples of this class.

PARTIAL CROWNS

According to Boucher's *Current Clinical Dental Terminology,* a partial crown is a restoration that covers two or three or more surfaces but not all surfaces of a tooth. The surfaces involved are usually the lingual, proximal, and occlusal (or incisal). A partial crown is an extracoronal restoration. As a basis, one can differentiate the following types of partial crowns:

1. Three-quarter crown
2. Seven-eighth crown
3. Mesial-half crown

Three-quarter crown

The three-quarter crown covers three fourths of the gingival circumference of the tooth, leaving one, usually the buccal or labial, intact. It can be placed on anterior as well as posterior teeth.

General considerations. The cast partial veneer retainer is universal in its application. It may be used on most of the anterior or posterior teeth of the upper or lower arches. Its virtue lies in the fact that the maximum retention may be obtained with the least danger to the normal pulp and a minimum sacrifice of tooth structure. Its esthetic values permit its use in the anterior as well as the posterior regions, whereas from a mechanical or retentive standpoint, it greatly approximates the values of a complete veneer crown if properly constructed.

Indications. Although the three-quarter crown is primarily indicated on sound normal teeth, it may be employed on teeth having small carious lesions on the proximal or lingual surfaces. It should be used for patients with a low DMF rate and where sufficient tooth structure is available. The general acceptance of this type of retainer is largely attributable to the following facts:

1. The preparation conserves most of the tooth structure.
2. The clamplike locking effect of the three-quarter design minimizes the possibility of a tooth fracturing from the forces of mastication.

A three-quarter crown can be used as a bridge retainer as well as a single restoration. It has been found that the square type of anterior teeth, relatively thick labiolingually, are more suitable for this type of restoration than the ovoid type of teeth, which are not so thick in their incisal third.

To be successful, the three-quarter crown requires, in addition to the correct placement of the proximal grooves and walls, that at least a type 3 gold be used.

Anterior three-quarter crown

Outline form. Before any tooth preparation is begun, the outline form, especially that of the labial and proximal surfaces, should be accurately determined. This is extended into an area that is cleansable, but at the same time there should be no unnecessary display of metal. To avoid this undesirable display of metal, the exact locations of the labioproximal and the incisal margins should be determined from the labial aspect. The incisal margin should not be carried onto the labial surface so that it is visible. It should terminate at the line where the labial and incisal surfaces meet. Although it is es-

sential that the proximal margins be carried labially into cleansable or immune areas, this can be accomplished without an excessive display of gold.[1] The gingival margin is placed slightly beneath the crest of the gingival tissue, following its curvature.[2] In instances of gingival recession where the cementoenamel junction is exposed, no attempt is made to carry the margin below this line. When cementum is exposed, the gingival margin is placed in a cleansable area above the cementoenamel junction in the enamel parallel to the gingival curvature.

Principles of retention. Vertical occlusal forces acting on the anterior three-quarter crown have horizontal resultants. Consequently, the displacing forces tip or rotate a restoration out of the preparation. The tipping is in a lingual direction and the rotation occurs mesiolingually or distolingually. The retention form of the partial veneer crown is more readily understood if the method used to resist both the lingual tipping and the torsional displacement or rotation is analyzed.[3]

In Fig. 6-30, *A*, observe the proximal groove *ab*. If a force *P*, directed lingually, is applied at the incisal edge, it will have a tendency to tip the casting out of the cavity, turning on the center of rotation often designated as the fulcrum point. The resistance to this displacement is furnished by the rib of gold that lies in the axial groove *ab*, also by that part of the axial wall lying lingually to the axial groove, and encompasses arcs *c* and *f*.

It will be observed that the lingual wall of the incisal groove does not furnish any resistance to lingual displacement, since the plane of this wall lies in the tipping path of arc *c*. For this reason the incisal portion of the preparation is usually prepared with one plane instead of a two-plane groove.

Fig. 6-30, *B*, discloses an incisal view of the same three-quarter crown preparation and a bevel at the cervical margin. When force *P* is applied mesiolingually to the

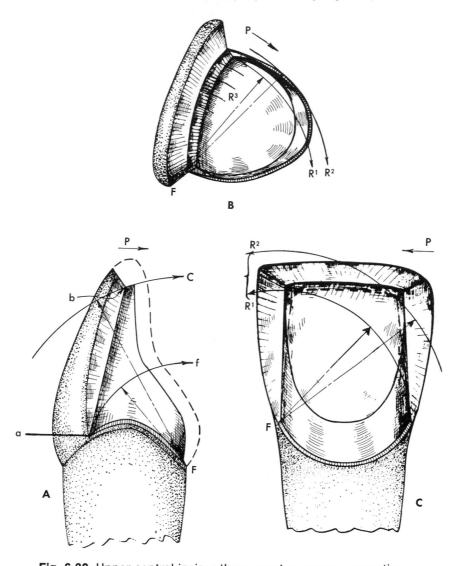

Fig. 6-30. Upper central incisor three-quarter crown preparation.

margin ridge of the upper central, the tendency is to rotate the restoration out of the mesiolabial wall of the cavity, point F acting as the center of rotation. Obviously then the resistance to this rotational displacement is furnished by the distoproximal groove and that portion of the proximal surface lying within the arcs R^1 and R^2.

Analogous resisting forces are present when acting forces are in a distolingual direction; then the distolabial wall acts as

the point of rotation and the mesioproximal groove and wall furnish the resistance to displacement.

The incisal groove is indicated when its lingual wall is needed to resist lingual displacement under torsional forces and when the tooth is relatively thick labiolingually. The incisal groove is especially contraindicated in those teeth that are thin labiolingually. In such a case, the incisal plane or bevel is used.

In Fig. 6-30, *C*, there is a horizontal

force P applied mesially to the incisal area. This has a tendency to tip the casting mesially, rotating on point F. This displacing force is resisted by the proximodistal groove and that portion of the proximodistal surface lying between the arcs R^1 and R^2.

Proximal grooves. The direction of insertion and position of the proximal grooves can be determined on the diagnostic study casts. In order that the proximal grooves in anterior teeth exert their maximum resistance to displacement, it is necessary for them to be placed as follows[5]:

1. They parallel the incisal two thirds of the labial surface.
2. These grooves, in their gingivoincisal relationship to each other, are nearly parallel.
3. Their convergence incisally does not exceed 5 degrees from parallelism.

Placing the proximal grooves parallel to the incisal two thirds of the labial surface results in the following[6]:

1. There is formed a retainer that automatically enables its labial margins to be extended into a cleansable area.
2. It makes a retainer that encompasses three fourths of the circumference of the tooth.
3. It furnishes proximal grooves that are comparatively longer and hence stronger than grooves placed parallel to the long axis of the crown.

Axial walls. Every effort should be made to prepare the opposing proximal walls as close to parallelism as possible. At any rate, the convergence should be between 2 and 5 degrees. Such near parallelism will add greatly to the retention qualities of the preparation.

Steps and instrumentation of preparation. The first step in the preparation of the proximal surfaces is comparatively simple. In making this procedure, one should not injure the adjacent tooth. This must

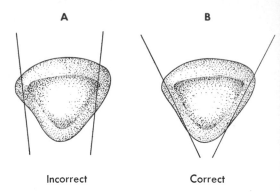

Fig. 6-31. Initial steps in preparation of upper central incisor for partial veneer extracoronal retainer. Long thin tapered diamond stone is used to break proximal contact areas. Incorrect and correct initial proximal-cut angulation.

be accomplished by one of the following methods:

1. Mechanically separate the teeth.
2. Place a steel matrix band on the adjacent tooth for its protection.
3. Use a thin, pointed diamond stone or bur.

The simplest, most convenient way to make the proximal cuts (Fig. 6-31, *B*) is to use a very thin tapering diamond point or bur. Place the thin, tapering diamond point or bur lingually to the contact point on the tooth at least the thickness of the diamond point away from the contact area. Direct this point labially, cutting the tooth. Keep in mind that the purpose of the first cut is to remove the contact area. Careful proximal cuts (Fig. 6-32) will maintain the normal labial contour of the tooth without displaying an unnecessary amount of metal.

Incisal reenforcing grooves. A bevel or a plane is prepared labiolingually (Fig. 6-33) and is carried mesiodistally uniting the two proximally relieved areas. The labial margin of this bevel is positioned in such a way that the metal will not be visible from the labial aspect through the enamel. The angle of the plane labiolingually is approximately 45 degrees to the long axis of the tooth. The purpose of the inclined plane is to give the incisal portion of the tooth a sufficient bulk of alloy to be approximately 1 mm thick. Diamond wheels or inverted cone burs can be used to make this cut.

Lingual preparation. The reduction of the lingual surface is usually accomplished in two phases. The first involves the removal (Fig. 6-34) of enamel on the lingual surface to a minimum depth of 0.5 mm, extending from the crest of the cingulum (Fig. 6-35) to the lingual margin of

the incisal plane (Fig. 6-34, A). During the lingual reduction one will find that on an upper central incisor the surface is concave incisogingivally and mesiodistally, whereas in a cuspid the lingual surface (Fig. 6-36) will consist of two planes that rise and meet in a central lingual ridge.

The preparation of the lingual surface may be accomplished by the use of barrel-shaped or wheel-shaped (with round edge) diamond stones. The second phase of the lingual preparation consists of the reduction of the lingual enamel lying between the crest of the cingulum and the crest of the gingiva.[4] This phase of the preparation could be postponed until after the proximal grooves have been prepared. The wall between the crest of the cingulum and the gingivae should be parallel to the proximal grooves in order to produce another retentive plane. The instrument used is the small straight or tapered diamond stone.

Incisal groove. The incisal groove is formed by two very definite planes—a labial and a lingual—which meet at a

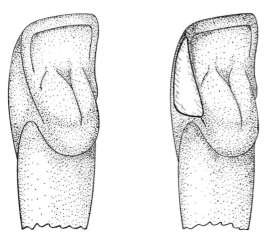

Fig. 6-32. Amount of enamel removed in initial proximal cut that will maintain normal labial contour after step 1.

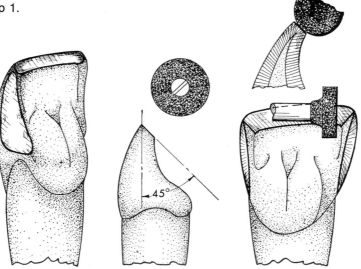

Fig. 6-33. Incisal reduction at the expense of lingual surface in step 2.

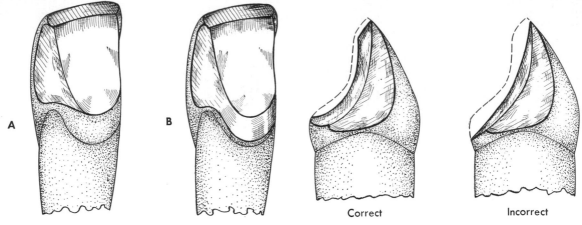

Fig. 6-34. Step 3 involves preparation of lingual surface. **A,** Reduction is made from incisal edge to cingulum. **B,** Reduction is shown from cingulum to level of crest of gingival side.

Fig. 6-35. Correct and incorrect amount of enamel removal on lingual surface.

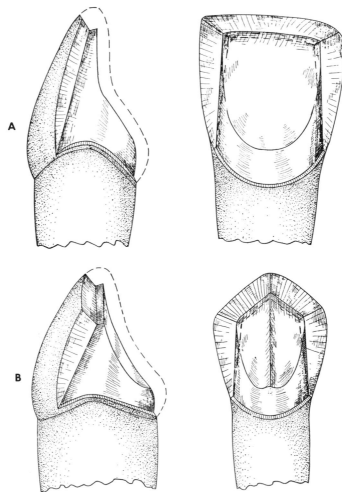

Fig. 6-36. Lingual view of upper teeth, prepared for three-quarter crown. **A,** Upper central incisor. **B,** Upper cuspid.

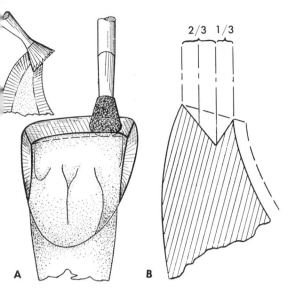

Fig. 6-37. A, Placing the incisal groove. **B,** Shape of incisal groove.

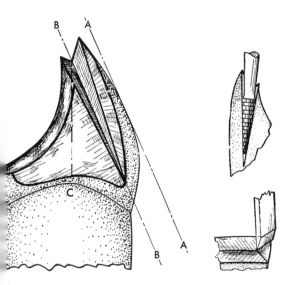

Fig. 6-38. Correct shape, direction, and relative parallelism of axial grooves are important in obtaining maximum retention in retainer.

and lateral incisors, the incisal groove extends in a continuous curve mesiodistally. In the cuspid the grooves rise from the mesial and distal and merge at the cusp. In starting the incisal groove, a small inverted-cone diamond stone or bur is placed in the center of the incisal plane in such a position that the base of the cone of the stone or bur faces lingually and the sides of the cone of the stone or bur face toward the labial plate of enamel. The revolving stone is moved from the mesial to the distoproximal cuts, gradually cutting a V-shaped groove (Fig. 6-37). The labial plane is twice as high as the lingual. After the cut has been carried to the desired depth with the cutting instrument, the labial and lingual planes must be finished with fine sandpaper or garnet discs.

Axial proximal grooves. Since the proximal grooves furnish the major retention of a partial veneer restoration, it is essential that they be prepared adequately and be placed satisfactorily in relation to the axis of the preparation (Fig. 6-38). The partial veneer retainer is prepared so that it sheds from the tooth gingival area in an incisal direction. Such a path of insertion eliminates the necessity of including any of the labial surface of the enamel. Best results are obtained when the proximal grooves are parallel to the incisal two thirds of the labial surface of the tooth. The depth of the groove must lie in dentin. Proximal grooves so located enable the completed retainer to encircle three fourths of the circumference of the tooth. When the grooves are parallel to the incisal two thirds of the labial surface, they must be also parallel to each other. Their convergence toward the incisal should not exceed 5 degrees.

The proximal groove starts at the bottom of the incisal groove, or on a thin tooth midway labiolingually to the incisal plane. It is directed labiogingivally so that it terminates at or slightly below the crest of the gingival tissue. The groove is

right or at a slightly acute angle. The bottom of the groove lies in dentin just lingual to the labial plate of enamel. The labial wall of the incisal groove is twice the length of the lingual plane. The incisal groove parallels the general contour of the labial incisal edge. In the central

started with a thin, tapered diamond stone or bur placed midway along its length and brought into the tooth structure to its full diameter for depth. Check the position and direction of the started groove. If satisfactory, the groove is extended gingivally, becoming shallower as it nears the gingival tissue without forming any definite step. The labial walls (Fig. 6-39) are made smooth either by the use of straight chisels no. 15 and no. 20 or with very fine tapering polishing stones or sandpaper discs. Krause[7] files are sometimes used to accentuate the triangular shape of the grooves. During planing of the labial wall of enamel, care must be exercised not to overextend the labial cavosurface margins.

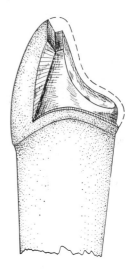

Fig. 6-39. Axial grooves shown with cingulum and its same path of "seat."

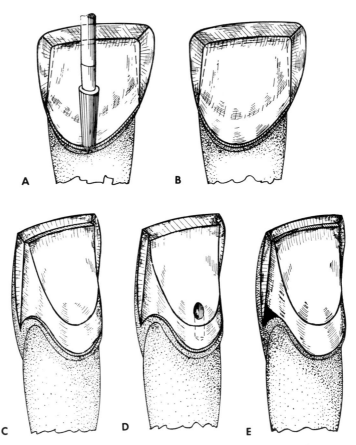

Fig. 6-40. A to **D,** Preparation and finished chamfer at cervical plane of upper central incisor. **E,** Triangular area of enamel is removed with tapering stone or bur.

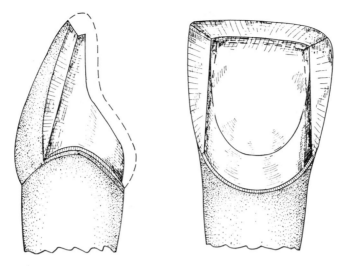

Fig. 6-41. Completed three-quarter crown preparation on maxillary central incisor.

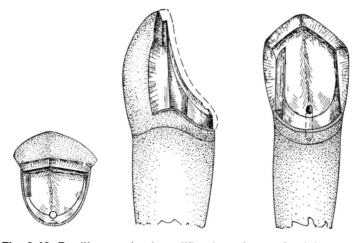

Fig. 6-42. Boxlike proximal modification of one of axial grooves.

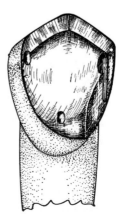

Fig. 6-43. Pin and groove placement employed in principles of retention of a partial veneer. (From Kabnick, H. H.: Dent. Items Interest **53**:376, 1931.)

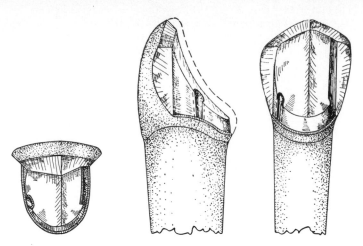

Fig. 6-44. Supplementary grooves and keyways for additional retention.

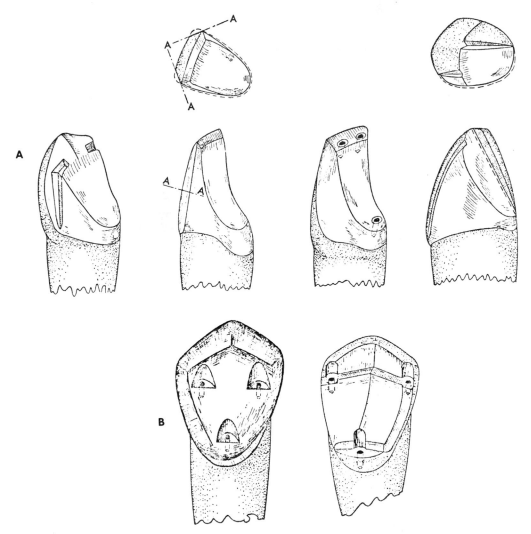

Fig. 6-45. A, Designs of extracoronal preparations designed by MacBoyle. *A-A,* Linguolabial convergence of planes. **B,** Frequently used pinledge retainer.

Some clinicians prefer to end the groove in a definite step at the gingival margin, thereby getting a stronger rib of gold in the finished cast retainer. This mechanical advantage is offset, however, by the resulting closeness of the gold casting to the pulp and the necessity of cutting away a greater amount of tooth structure. The diagnosis of the type of groove that is to be prepared is influenced by the following:

1. Labiolingual size of the tooth
2. Presence and extent of proximal caries
3. Presence and extent of old restoration
4. Necessity to provide room in the retainer for a stress-breaker (precision or nonprecision) if the three-quarter crown is part of a bridge

Cervical margin preparation. The preparation of a partial veneer crown ends slightly below the crest of the gingiva in a chamfer or bevel. In the preparation of this chamfer, care should be exercised not to injure the gingival tissue.

Use a small tapered diamond point (with round tip) and place it in a proximal groove, moving it slowly back and forth (Fig. 6-40) from one proximal groove to the other, till a chamfer is prepared. This diamond point should be kept parallel to the proximal grooves while the chamfer is being cut.

The advantage of using an even narrow chamfer lies in the fact that it affords a definite finishing margin for the wax pattern and the casting and yet at the same time eliminates excessive cutting of tooth structure (Fig. 6-41).

Fig. 6-42 to 6-45 illustrate some modifications used with anterior partial veneer crowns. These modifications are dictated by retentive, esthetic, and functional needs.

SELECTED REFERENCES

1. Thompson, M. J.: Exposing the cavity margin for hydrocolloid impression, J. South. Calif. Dent. Assoc. **19**:17, 1951.
2. Pagenkopf, A. A.: Hydrocolloid method: if not, why not? Northwest Dent. **34**:93, 1955.
3. Selberg, A.: Cast gold crowns, J. Tenn. Dent. Assoc. **29**:21, 1949.
4. Malone, W., Eisenmann, D., and Kusek, J.: Interceptive periodontics through electrosurgery, J. Prosthet. Dent. **22**:555, 1969.
5. Tinker, E. T.: Some of the fundamentals in the construction and application of crown and bridge restorations, J.A.D.A. **12**:1347, 1935.
6. Tinker, H. A.: Three-quarter crown in fixed bridgework, J. Can. Dent. Assoc. **16**:125, 1950.
7. Krause, O. G.: Cast attachments for bridgework, with special reference to vital teeth, J.A.D.A. **21**:4, 1934.

SECTION D2

Posterior three-quarter crowns

POSTERIOR PARTIAL CROWN

Fig. 6-46 shows that the same general displacing forces are present in the posterior partial crown as in the anterior partial crown, but the ability of this retainer to resist displacement is more favorable than in the anterior teeth. In Fig. 6-46, *A*, the occlusal forces may be occlusal, horizontal, or any one of the other component forces as indicated by letter *P*. Minimal problems exists when the force is vertical, for the reaction is

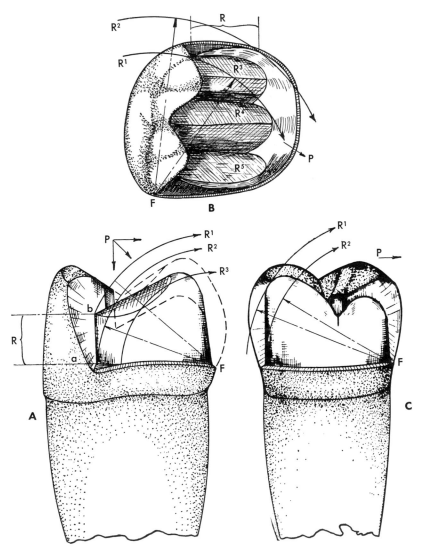

Fig. 6-46. Upper molar partial veneer preparation that illustrates principles of retention.

equal and opposite. When the force tends to displace the casting lingually, it does so along the paths R^1, R^2, and R^3, with its rotation center at point F. Resistance to this displacing force is furnished by the ribs of gold lying within the axial groove *ab* and by that portion of the proximal surface extending lingually from the proximal groove and lying within the arcs R^1, R^2, and R^3. In addition to this, the occlusal surface lying on the plane R^2-R^3 offers resistance.

Fig. 6-46, *B*, shows horizontal and occlusal views of the same preparation. When force P is applied in a mesiolingual direction, the tendency is to rotate the casting mesiodistally, with the rotation center being point F, the mesiobuccal wall. The resistance to this displacing force is developed by the rib of gold lying in the distoproximal groove and by the portion of the casting coming in contact with the proximal surface lying between the arcs R^1 and R^2. Additional resistance to displacement is offered by the occlusal inclined planes R^3, R^4, and R^5.

Fig. 6-46, *C*, illustrates occlusal force P being directed in the distal direction. The tendency is to rotate the casting occlusally, with its dislodgment along the arcs R^1 and R^2, with F serving as the point of rotation. The resistance to this displacing force is furnished by the rib of gold lying in the mesioproximal groove and also by the buccal and mesioproximal walls lying within the areas R^1 and R^2.

The displacement of a bridge retainer to a direction opposite to its line of insertion is resisted by (1) the cement holding the retainer in position, (2) an acceptable fit of the casting, and (3) axial walls prepared as nearly parallel as possible (2- to 5-degree convergence).

The mechanical retention in posterior partial and complete veneer. crowns is obtained mainly by internal stresses developed between the external axial walls in the dentin of the preparation and the internal surfaces of the metal retainer when the restoration is cemented.

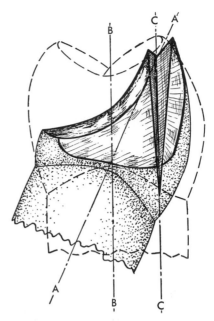

Fig. 6-47. Directions of axial grooves in anterior and posterior teeth prepared for partial veneer retainers. *A-A*, Long axis of cuspid. *B-B*, Long axis of molar. *C-C*, Direction of axial groove with reference to labial or buccal surfaces of cuspid or of molar.

The posterior partial veneer retainer does not differ fundamentally from the anterior, since the principles of its retention and preparation are similar to those of anterior teeth. In the anterior retainers the proximal grooves are placed parallel to the incisal two thirds of the labial surface, but in the posterior teeth, the axial grooves are made parallel with the long axis of the tooth (Fig. 6-47). In posterior retainers, the two proximal, the occlusal, and the lingual surfaces are involved on all teeth with the exception of the lower molars. In the lower molars, the natural inclination of these teeth would necessitate a great deal of tooth cutting if the lingual surfaces were to be included.

In preparing a posterior tooth to receive a partial retainer, place the proximal grooves at the junction of the buccal and middle thirds. By placement of the grooves in this position, the following will be true:

1. Three fourths of the circumference

of the tooth will be encompassed within the casting.

2. The proximal outline of the preparation will be extended sufficiently to the buccal vestibule and the margins will lie in a cleansable area.
3. The grooves will be buccally to the highest point of interdental papilla, permitting advantageous length.

The V-shaped groove is used in those teeth that are round in cross section, whereas the boxlike proximal modifications are used in those teeth that are of a parallelogram shape.

The boxlike modification is indicated for the following conditions:

1. If caries is present in the proximal surfaces of the abutment tooth
2. If the retainer is to receive an interlocking key used with the semirigid principle
3. If the restoration such as an inlay or amalgam had to be removed
4. If the teeth are of medium or short length

INDICATIONS

Although the partial veneer retainer may be used on most posterior teeth having a sufficient amount of tooth structure, their use is indicated primarily on teeth having vital pulps.

The advantages of partial crowns are as follows:

1. The preparation is conservative.
2. It can be confined mostly to enamel.
3. The retentive grooves are usually distant from the pulp.
4. The restoration possesses sufficient mechanical retention.

Where caries is present, it is advisable for the dentist to first remove the decay to determine its extent and enable him to decide what deviation from the normal must be made.

OUTLINE FORM

Since all but one surface of the crown are involved in the preparation, the normal outline form for upper posterior teeth brings the buccal margins onto the buccal surface. The gingival margin is normally carried slightly below the crest of the soft tissue into the gingival crevice. The location of the occlusal margin varies with the type of preparation made. In a maxillary bicuspid or molar that is noncarious and contains a vital pulp and the partial crown is not a bridge retainer (individual restoration), the buccal cusps do not need to be included. The occlusal buccal margin extends from one proximal groove to the other in a curved line that leaves intact as much of the buccal cusps as possible. If the partial crown serves as a retainer for a bridge, the buccal cusp is commonly included in the preparation.

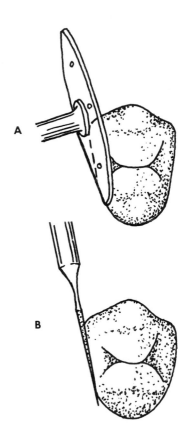

Fig. 6-48. Proximal reduction for posterior three-quarter crowns can be ably performed with a safe-sided disc, **A,** or a long thin diamond stone, **B.**

STEPS OF PREPARATION (UPPER POSTERIOR TEETH)

There is little difference in the preparation of an upper premolar and molar. For simplicity, the preparation of an upper premolar will be described.

Proximal cuts

The same precautions as described in an anterior tooth preparation should be exercised here. The cuts can be made either with a safe-sided disc (Fig. 6-48, *A*) or a thin, long, tapering diamond point or bur. This diamond point can be placed on the lingual surface of the premolar away from the contact point by the thickness of the diamond point. With a high-speed diamond point, the slice is made from the lingual toward the buccal. The same cut is performed on the opposite surface. Note the taper of the cuts to each other.

Looking from the buccal, note the slight gingival taper of these cuts (Fig. 6-49, *A*). The cuts end at or slightly below the interdental papilla. If the proximal cuts are made parallel to the long axis of the tooth, the buccal anatomy of the prepared tooth will be altered and an unnecessary amount of metal will be displayed.

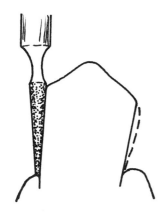

Fig. 6-49. Care must be exercised during proximal reduction in order not to display an inordinate amount of metal.

Occlusal reduction

If the tooth being prepared is pulpless or will serve as an abutment for a bridge, the entire occlusal surface is involved in the preparation. Using a tapered diamond stone or tapered fissure bur (no. 701), make a cut from one proximal (Fig. 6-50) to the other, to a depth of 1.5 to 2 mm, preserving the buccal cusp.

In the maxillary molar, the occlusal groove is cut following the central groove, (Fig. 6-50, *B*) in a manner similar to MOD inlay preparation. With diamond stone no. 770-7P the entire occlusal surface is reduced but the general anatomic form is maintained. The tooth is reduced uniformly and the slopes of the buccal and lingual cusps are retained.

In a maxillary molar, the distobuccal direction of the lingual groove and the direction and size of the oblique ridge must be maintained in the prepared tooth. The inclined slopes of the cusps assist in the development of resistance form (Fig. 6-50, *C*).

Proximal grooves

The proximal retention grooves are placed parallel to the long axis of the tooth. These grooves, one on the mesial and one on the distal surface, are placed buccally at the junction of the buccal and middle thirds of the tooth. Every effort should be made to keep the grooves as nearly parallel to each other as possible (Fig. 6-51). The proximal groove in the bicuspids and molars have a definite gingival wall.

During placement of the grooves toward the buccal third, the greatest amount of tooth structure is encompassed within the grip of the retainer, resisting any tendency toward lingual displacement.

To prepare the groove, place a no. 700 crosscut tapering fissure bur or tapered diamond stone parallel to the long axis of the tooth between the buccal and middle thirds of the tooth and carry it gingivally

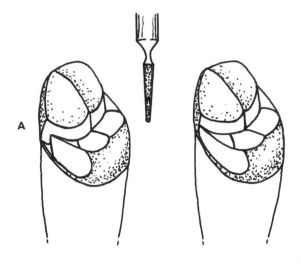

Upper posterior three-quarter crown molar

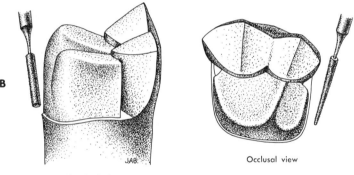

Proximal view

Occlusal view

JAB

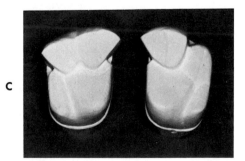

Fig. 6-50. A, Every effort is made to preserve the buccal cusp of tooth during preparation. **B,** Three-quarter crown preparation for maxillary molar is a conservative preparation with more than ample retention for use as a bridge abutment. This preparation is commonly placed in patients with a low DMF rate. Proximal modification of traditional Tinker's groove is possible. **C,** Occlusal view of posterior three-quarter crown, *left,* and seven-eighth crown, *right,* on a maxillary molar. Seven-eighth crowns can surpass the retention and resistance form of the three-quarter crowns without an inordinate display of metal.

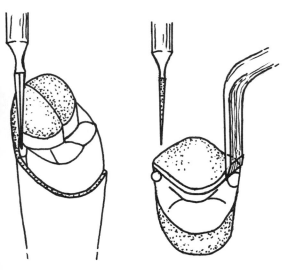

Fig. 6-51. Grooves appearing as nearly parallel to each other as possible.

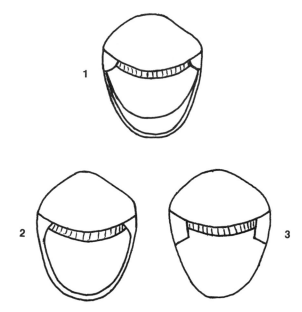

Fig. 6-52. Lingual wall of groove can be finished in any of three ways.

so that it terminates in a flat gingival plane slightly beneath the crest of the gingival tissue. The groove at the occlusal end may be in the dentin.

After the initial cut with the bur or stone, the buccal surface of the groove is moved from the inner angle of the groove buccally so that the buccal margins are extended into cleansable or self-cleansing areas. This is done with no. 15 and no. 20 chisels, or with a superfine taper diamond stone.

These walls must be finished with fine sandpaper discs. Care must be taken not to undercut the walls. The lingual wall of the groove can be finished in any of three ways (Fig. 6-52):

1. Leave it concave.
2. Round it proximolingually, removing the sharp angle; the groove will be triangular in shape; the triangular shape of the groove can be accentuated with chisel no. 15 or with Krause files.
3. It can be moved lingually to change the V-shaped groove into a boxlike form; this modification increases the bulk of the metal, and the lingual

wall of the box increases the retentive qualities of the preparation.

It is desirable to bevel the cavosurface margin of the gingival wall of enamel approximately 6 degrees from the horizontal plane. This step is carried out with the gingival margin trimmer. This bevel removes any unsupported enamel rods at the gingival wall margin and is continuous with and blends into the gingival chamfer or bevel, which is subsequently established around the lingual wall.

Lingual reduction

The lingual surface may best be reduced by use of a small tapering diamond stone or bur. No effort is made to remove all the enamel. Only enough of the enamel is removed to make the preparation slightly convergent gingivo-occlusally. No effort is made at this time to lower the axial preparation below the crest of the gingival tissue.

Gingival chamfer

It is well at this point in the preparation of the tooth to examine all axial surfaces

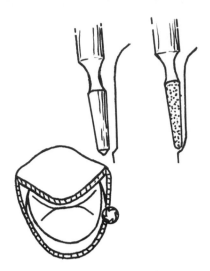

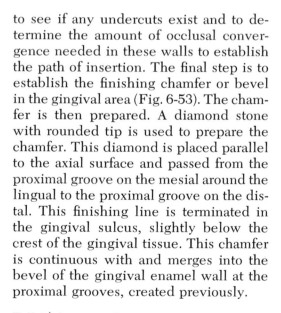

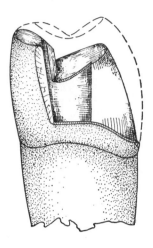

Fig. 6-53. Instrumentation for preparation of gingival margin can vary, but chamfer type is preferable.

Fig. 6-54. Lower molar partial crown preparation, with lingual cusps protected.

to see if any undercuts exist and to determine the amount of occlusal convergence needed in these walls to establish the path of insertion. The final step is to establish the finishing chamfer or bevel in the gingival area (Fig. 6-53). The chamfer is then prepared. A diamond stone with rounded tip is used to prepare the chamfer. This diamond is placed parallel to the axial surface and passed from the proximal groove on the mesial around the lingual to the proximal groove on the distal. This finishing line is terminated in the gingival sulcus, slightly below the crest of the gingival tissue. This chamfer is continuous with and merges into the bevel of the gingival enamel wall at the proximal grooves, created previously.

Toilet of preparation

The final step in the preparation consists of finishing all the axial and occlusal walls to remove any sharp angles or undercuts. Any scratches created by burs or coarse diamond stones are smoothed and eliminated with a pointed superfine diamond. A smooth paper disc can be used for this purpose.

MODIFICATIONS OF POSTERIOR PARTIAL CROWNS
Lower crowns

As previously stated, in the mandibular molar the buccal surface is included in the preparation instead of the lingual (Fig. 6-54). This is attributable to the anatomy as well as to the position of the tooth in the arch. The natural inclination of the lower molar is such that one would need a great deal of tooth removal if the lingual surface were to be included in the preparation.

The steps of preparation of mandibular molars are the same as those of the maxillary. When proximal cuts are made on the lower molar, the planes are cut buccolingually so that they have a slight convergence buccally instead of lingually, as is done in the upper teeth. The proximal grooves in the lower molars are placed at the junction of the lingual and middle thirds of the tooth. The lingual cusps can be left intact if the restoration is not a retainer for a bridge. If it is a bridge retainer, the lingual cusps of lower molars should be protected in the same way as the buccal cusps of the upper molars are prepared for partial gold crown.

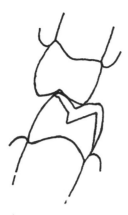

Fig. 6-55. Buccal cusp of restored tooth is protected with metal coverage.

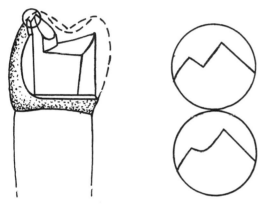

Fig. 6-56. Buccal preparation increases resistance and retention form.

Lower premolars

In the preparation of lower premolars for partial crowns, some modification is necessary. The basic principles of retention and resistance as well as the steps of preparation and instrumentation are the same as those for upper posterior teeth. Importantly, however, the buccal cusp of the lower premolars is the stamp cusp of prime importance.

If the buccal cusp of the lower premolar were prepared in the same manner as that of the upper premolar, the buccal cusp of the upper premolar would be hitting the junction of the metal and tooth (in centric occlusion) (Fig. 6-55). To avoid this, the buccal cusp of lower premolars are "hooded." "Hooding" means that there is an additional step in preparation—the reduction of the bucco-occlusal part of the buccal cusp. The extent to which this buccal step is carried gingivally depends on the type of occlusal pattern, size of cusps, and depth of grooves (vertical overjet) as well as the size of the lower premolar. This "hood" (Fig. 6-56) also increases retention and resistance to displacement of the restoration.

GENERAL REFERENCES

Alpert, C. C.: Anterior pin-ledge abutment, J. Dist. Columbia Dent. Soc. **34:**11, 1959.

Arbo, M. A.: A simple technic for castings with pin retention, Dent. Clin. North Am., pp. 19-29, 1970.

Baker, C. R.: Replacement of lost mandibular incisor or incisors: 1. fixed; 2. removable appliances, Int. Dent. J. **5:**287, 1955.

Baum, L.: New cast gold restorations for anterior teeth, J.A.D.A. **61:**1, 1960.

Baum, L., and Contino, R. M.: Ten years of experience with cast pin restorations, Dent. Clin. North Am., pp. 18-41, 1970.

Beck, P. B.: Parallel pins in fixed prosthodontics, J. South. Calif. Dent. Hyg. Assoc. **34:**237-240, 1966.

Brigadier, L. R.: The anterior one-half pin-lay, Dent. Dig. **45:**448, 1939.

Burgess, J. K.: The pinledge attachment, Dent. Items Int. Q. Rev. **4:**33, 1920.

Burgess, J. K.: The preparation of abutments and construction of pinlay and pinledge attachments for bridge work, Pacific Dent. Gaz. **24:**559, 1916.

Burns, B. B.: Pin retention of cast gold restorations, J. Prosthet. Dent. **15:**1101-1108, 1965.

Carlson, N. C.: Selection of proper abutments for anterior bridges, J. Kansas City Dist. Dent. Soc. **30:**12, 1954.

Carpenter, E. E.: Pinledge attachments for anterior bridgework, Dent. Items Int. **72:**132, 1950; Indiana Dent. Rev. **20:**67, 1951.

Chechik, M. M.: Retention simplified: employing prefabricated tapered gold pins, Dent. Dig. **61:** 386, 441, 1955.

Courtade, G. L.: Pin pointers, III: self-threading pins, J. Prosthet. Dent. **20:**335, 1968.

Courtade, G. L.: Methods for pin splinting the lower anterior teeth, Dent. Clin. North Am., pp. 3-17, 1970.

Courtade, G. L., Sanell, C., and Mann, A. W.: The use of pins in restorative dentistry, part I: parallel pin retention obtained without using paralleling devices; part II: paralleling instruments, J. Prosthet. Dent. **15:**502-516, 691-703, 1965.

Cowger, G. T.: Retention, resistance and esthetics of the anterior three-quarter crown, J.A.D.A. **62**: 167, 1961.

Doxtater, L. W.: Procedures in modern crown and bridgework, New York, 1931, Dental Items of Interest Publishing Co.

el-Ebrashi, M. K., Craig, R. G., and Peyton, F. A.: Experimental stress analysis of dental restorations, part V, the concept of occlusal reduction and pins, J. Prosthet. Dent. **22**:565-577, 1969.

Falkner, P. L.: Anterior bridges—full or partial coverage? Roy. Can. Dent. Corps Q. **2**:7, 1961.

Fisch, G. M.: The three-quarter crown as a filling for anterior teeth, J.A.D.A. **18**:2393, 1931.

Fridge, D. S.: Forming pin-ledge holes and paralleling grooves, Denver, 1966, Densco Mfg. Co.

Fusayama, T., Hosoda, H., and Wakumoto, S.: A one-piece cast permanent splint, J. Prosthet. Dent. **16**:572-582, 1966.

Gade, E.: Function and aesthetics of anterior bridges, Int. Dent. J. **12**:18, 1962.

Gamer, S., Klein, E., and Zusman, S. H.: Position finder: an improved design for paralleling preparations, J. South. Calif. Dent. Assoc. **33**:566-567, 1965.

Gamer, S., and Zusman, S.: Position finder for parallelism, J. Prosthet. Dent. **65**:717, 1965.

Gillett, H. W., and Irving, A. J.: Gold inlays by the indirect system, New York, 1932, Dental Items of Interest Publishing Co.

Hoelzel, S. H.: Dowel pin locators for hydrocolloid impressions, North-West Dent. **41**:100, 1962.

Iwanson, R.: The pinledge attachment and its use for fixed bridges, Dent. Items Interest **46**:207, 1934.

Kabnick, H. H.: The "pinledge" as a cast bridge attachment, Dent. Items Interest **53**:376, 1931.

Kaloyiannides, T.: A method for the attainment of parallel grooves on three-quarter crown construction, Acta Stomatol. Hellen. **2**(1):3-13, 1967.

Karlstrom, G.: Parallel pins and fixed partial dentures, J. Prosthet. Dent. **19**:615, 1968.

LaForgia, A.: Tissue retraction for fixed prosthesis, J. Prosthet. Dent. **11**:480, 1961.

Lamb, R. T.: Varied applications of direct pin inlays, J. Can. Dent. Assoc. **22**:282, 1956.

Le Huche, R.: Molded key inlay lock for bridges, Rev. Stomatol. **41**:533, 1939.

Le Huche, R.: Inlays and onlays, bridges on living teeth, Paris, 1951, Julien Prélat; J.A.D.A. **45**:619, Nov. 1952.

Linkow, L. I.: Reconstruction of anterior teeth with an extreme vertical and horizontal overlap, J. Prosthet. Dent. **12**:947, 1962.

Lorey, R. E., Embrell, K. A., and Myers, G. E.: Retentive factors in pin-retained castings, J. Prosthet. Dent. **17**(3):271, 1967.

McAdam, D. B.: Maxillary cuspid three-quarter crown preparation of increased retentive form, J.

Can. Dent. Assoc. **28**:291, 1962; Dent. Dig. **68**: 522, 1962.

MacBoyle, R. E.: Crown and fixed bridgework, from the point of view of our present knowledge, J. Natl. Dent. Assoc. **8**:635, 1921.

Manes, R. J.: Pinledges as bridge anchorages, pins and inlays combined, Dent. Abstr. **2**:81, 1957.

Mann, A. W., Courtade, G. L., and Sanell, C.: The use of pins in restorative dentistry, part 1: parallel pin retention obtained without using paralleling devices, J. Prosthet. Dent. **15**:502-516, 1965.

Mittleman, G.: Use of pins in difficult cases, J.A.D.A. **49**:163, 1954.

Moffa, J. P., and Phillips, R. W.: Retentive properties of parallel pin restorations, J. Prosthet. Dent. **17**:387-400, 1967.

Moffa, J. P., Razzano, M. R., and Doyle, M. G.: Pins —a comparison of their retentive properties, J.A.D.A. **78**:529-535, 1969.

Mollersten, L.: An impression technique for teeth prepared for parallel pins, J. Prosthet. Dent. **18**: 579, 1967.

Mosteller, J. H.: Parallel pin gold castings, Practical Dent. Monogr., pp. 5-29, Nov. 1963.

Mosteller, J. H.: Pin castings by a paralleling device and hydrocolloid technique, Dent. Clin. North Am., pp. 53-61, 1970.

Nally, J. N.: Fixed bridge for anterior teeth, Int. Dent. J. **12**:1, 1962; Chir. Dent. Fr. **22**:57, 1962 (French).

Nealon, F. H.: A new approach to parallel pin restorations, Ney Technical Bulletin, Bloomfield, Conn., 1964, The J. M. Ney Co.

Nealon, F. H., and Sheakey, H. G.: An extra-oral pin technique, J. Prosthet. Dent. **22**:638-646, 1969.

Overby, G. E.: Esthetic splinting of mobile periodontally involved teeth by vertical pinning, J. Prosthet. Dent. **11**:112-118, 1961.

Parmlid, A.: A new intraoral parallelometer, J. Prosthet. Dent. **18**:469-475, 1967.

Peterka, C. A.: A modern three-quarter veneer crown, J.A.D.A. **27**:1175, 1940.

Pruden, K. C.: A hydrocolloid technique for pinledge bridge abutments, J. Prosthet. Dent. **6**:65, 1956.

Pruden, K. C.: A hydrocolloid technic for pinledge bridge abutments, J. Prosthet Dent. **6**:65, 1956

Rosen, H.: The incisal insertion pin inlay, J. Prosthet. Dent. **19**:263, 1968.

Rudin, B. M.: Conservative abutment restoration for anterior fixed partial dentures, J. Prosthet. Dent. **11**:272, 1961.

Sanell, C.: Vertical parallel pins in occlusal rehabilitation, Dent. Clin. North Am., pp. 755-778, 1963.

Sanell, C., Mann, A. W., and Courtade, G. L.: The use of pins in restorative dentistry, part III: the use of paralleling instruments, J. Prosthet. Dent. **16:**286-296, 1966.

Shapiro, F. M., and Rosen, B. S.: Fixed splint for lower anterior teeth, J. New Jersey Dent. Soc. **33:** 95, 1961.

Shooshan, E. D.: A pinledge casting technique—its application in periodontal splinting, Dent. Clin. North Am., pp. 189-206, March 1960.

Smith, C. L.: Prefabricated parallel pin castings, Dent. Clin. North Am., pp. 31-41, 1970.

Sobel, S. L.: A technique for using parallel pins, J. Prosthet. Dent. **20:**526, 1968.

Steen, P. M.: Positive pin retention for bridge work and inlays, Dent. Survey **30:**757, 1954.

Timmermans, J. J., and Courtade, G. L.: Nonparallel threaded pin retention of fixed prosthesis, J. Prosthet. Dent. **19**(4):381-392, 1968.

Wagner, A. W.: Pin retention for extensive posterior gold onlays, J. Prosthet. Dent. **15:**719-721, 1965.

Willmott, J. T.: Pin retention for indirect inlays utilizing rubber-base impression material, Br. Dent. J. **102:**359, 1957.

SECTION E

Questionable abutments

A common dilemma faced by dentists is the use of a questionable tooth as an abutment. This experience is often associated when a patient prefers a fixed rather than a removable prosthesis. Any abutment may be periodontally involved, partially fractured, polycarious, or in poor arch position.

The continued success of the fixed prosthesis can also be related to the dental I.Q. of the patient and the coordinated interspecialty treatment preceding tooth preparation and impression techniques. A frequent professional omission in cases of this nature is not to fully inform the patient of the obvious limitations associated with treating questionable abutments.

CLASSIFICATION OF QUESTIONABLE ABUTMENTS IN FIXED PROSTHODONTICS

There are problematic teeth that are recognizable. These teeth consistently require perceptive decisions during diagnosis and formulation of a treatment plan of difficult clinical conditions. Because of the diversity of existing clinical conditions, only guidelines to treatment and several approaches to problems will be suggested. The following outline is presented as a guideline for identification of teeth that are difficult to use as abutments for fixed prosthodontics:

1. General disorders
   a. Mineralization
      (1) Amelogenesis imperfecta
      (2) Dentinogenesis imperfecta
      (3) Hypocalcification
      (4) Ectodermal dysplasia
      (5) Discolorization because of drugs, such as tetracycline (Fig. 6-57)
      (6) Fluoridosis
      (7) Internal resorption
   b. Congenital and growth deformities
      (1) Malformed dentition
      (2) Malposed teeth
      (3) Skeletal disparities of maxillomandibular relationships
      (4) Oligodontia, that is, congenitally missing teeth
2. Local problems commonly associated with questionable abutments
   a. Polycarious teeth
   b. Periodontally involved teeth
   c. Occlusal plane correction
   d. Endodontically treated teeth
      (1) Previously treated
      (2) Currently treated
   e. Tilted teeth
   f. Attrition, abrasion, or erosion

The questionable abutment teeth that have generalized mineral disturbances are usually restored with full-coverage restorations. Esthetic desires and functional needs are more adequately met by this direction of treatment. Although the mineralization disturbances preoccupy the dentist in a diagnostic sense, the supporting tissue response usually determines the success of the restorations. This fact is of particular importance in cases of amelogenesis imperfecta and patients with a history of malnutrition. The complexity of clinical treatment is customized to fit the esthetic, functional, and psychological needs of the individual patient. Concomitant dental interdisciplinary attention is common, such as periodontic treatment with restorative dentistry.

Questionable abutments that are classified in the congenital or growth group are usually treated by the following:
1. Orthodontics or oral orthopedics, or both
2. Interceptive periodontics
3. Restorative dentistry

The clinical treatment is better served by the dentist and to the greater satisfaction of the patient if the restorative

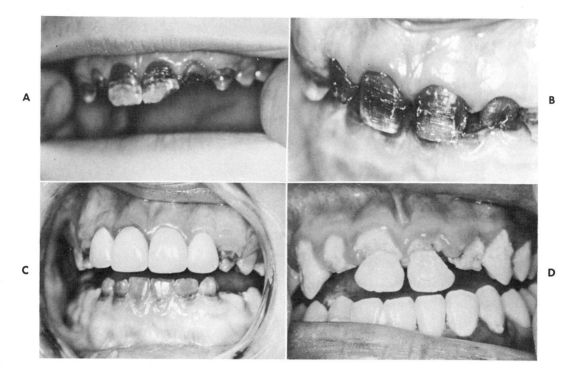

Fig. 6-57. A, Twelve-year-old patient with tetracycline stain. Drug was administered 2 weeks after birth for a congenital cardiac condition. A greater percentage of teeth with tetracycline stains appear to be more susceptible to incisal fracture than are teeth without the stain. **B,** Tooth preparation showed extent of dentin discoloration. Traditional pulpal location during preparation is unavailable to dentist, that is, color alteration near the pulp. **C,** Placement of acrylic-veneer crowns as a provisional measure is a definite psychologic advantage to patient and prevents further fracture. Further treatment can progress as growth of patient permits. **D,** Inordinate caries rate involves a decisive treatment plan with alternate methods of treatment presented to patient. A maxillary tooth–supported full denture may be most pragmatic treatment in patients with uncontrolled caries. (From Malone, W. F., and Sarlas, C. H.: Dent. Clin. North Am. **13**(2): 461, April 1969.)

dentist and allied dental specialty combine their knowledge *prior* to institution of any treatment. Although cases in this classification are known to be arduous, an unfavorable prognosis is infrequently transmitted to the patient. This communication is extremely important in light of the economic involvement and time expenditure for these patients. Euphoric claims of predictable results are unwarranted and present an undesirable situation at the conclusion of treatment.

A discussion of the more routinely observed questionable abutments should provide some guidelines to treatment. They will be reviewed separately, with the exception of endodontically treated teeth, which is discussed in Chapter 21.

CARIOUS TEETH

The use of carious teeth for or as an abutment is determined by the amount and distribution of the remaining healthy tooth structure. The removal of carious tooth structure is performed in a predetermined sequence termed a "caries-control program." The DMF rate (Fig. 6-57,

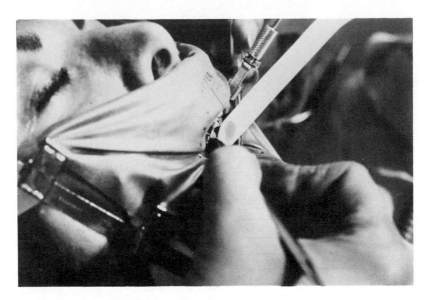

Fig. 6-58. Rubber dam usage is a beneficial and necessary adjunct to satisfactory caries-control procedures.

D), age of the patient, and other abnormalities of calcification in the dentition should be recorded.

There is no contraindication for the use of abnormalities or teeth severely affected by caries as abutments provided that they possess sufficient tooth structure to support a retainer and have an acceptable supporting structure. Polycarious teeth rarely provide enough tooth structure for intracoronal retainers, and these teeth are generally considered more susceptible to repeated carious attacks. The coronal portion of teeth with mineralization disturbances and high-DMF-rate patients are commonly restored with full coverage to provide adequate mechanical retention with satisfactory tooth preparations.

Strict recall programs are a mandate. This is particularly true for young adults. In summary, the clinical approaches to uncontrolled caries are as follows:

1. Caries-control program
   a. Prophylaxis and fluoride treatments
   b. Dietary consultation
   c. Operative dentistry (mechanical excavation of caries with rubber dam in place, Fig. 6-58) for quadrant amalgam restorations as seen in Chapter 5.
2. Endodontic and periodontic consultation
3. Cast-metal restorations where indicated after amalgam placement
   a. Teeth of prime importance receive treatment, the canines and terminal molars
4. Recall system strictly maintained

OCCLUSAL-PLANE CORRECTION

If teeth egress beyond their normal occlusal plane, construction of a fixed prosthesis with an acceptable occlusal plane can be nearly impossible. A malposed tooth that has gravitated or supraerupted into a space where the antagonist has been lost is a common problem in fixed prosthodontics. The offending tooth must be reduced to a satisfactory occlusal plane *prior* to the preparation of it and the construction of the opposing prosthesis. A supraerupted tooth (Fig. 6-59) is usually a restorative handicap because of the reduced periodontal ligament and resulting bizarre bone relationships. In a large percentage of cases, intentional extirpation of the pulp may be required. Intentional extirpation of the pulp of a supraerupted mandibular molar or a gravitated maxillary molar is sometimes necessary to retain "key teeth." However, providing the retentive and resistence form during tooth preparation becomes a formidable operative task. This is attributable to the reduced occlusogingival length, possible violation of the gingival attachment, and the preparation design near furcal areas.

MALPOSED TEETH

Malposed teeth are not contraindicated for use as abutments. The deciding factors are whether a suitable retainer can be designed to accept the magnitude of forces that are directed toward a fixed partial-denture abutment. Judicious tooth reduction and placement of a perceptively designed retainer can effect a more optimal arch position that renders the tooth a more desirable unit for a fixed prosthesis. Minor tooth movement,[1] telescopic techniques,[2] and endodontics have been employed to correct problems of a malposed tooth to be used as an abutment for a fixed prosthesis.

Orthodontic treatment (although frequently impractical) is the optimum direction of treatment in most cases. However, the benefits of orthodontic treatment for minor tooth movement (Fig. 6-60, A) are commonly neutralized by the length of treatment and the inordinate expense to the patient. General dentists usually are not aware of the ramifications of moving one tooth to a desirable arch position without banding the entire arch.

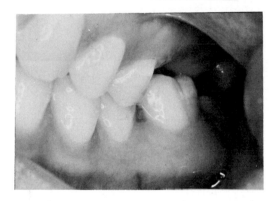

Fig. 6-59. Supraeruption of lower first molar—a formidable problem for occlusal plane establishment. Intentional extirpation of pulp or extraction, depending on wishes of patient, would be needed in cases of this nature.

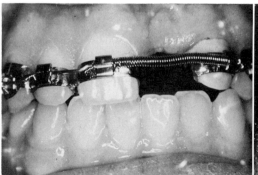 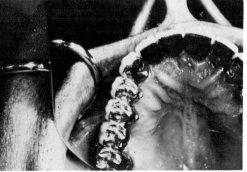

Fig. 6-60. A, Minor tooth movement usually results in a full-arch band-stabilization procedure if optimal results are to be realized and maintained. Tooth movement was deemed necessary to restore space after an incisor was avulsed. Midline orientation and symmetry are accomplished more easily with this approach. **B,** Tap-off lugs placed on lingual surfaces of full maxillary splint to facilitate its removal.

Oversimplification of tooth movement by the general dentist identifies a national curricular problem that should be entertained by interspecialty consultations.

The use of study casts with diagnostic wax-ups prior to tooth preparation will be of immeasurable assistance to the dentist. Periodic occlusal adjustment is necessary upon completion of a prosthesis when malposed teeth are used as abutments. Sand-blasted occlusal surfaces, tap-off lugs (Fig. 6-60, *B*), and interim cements will facilitate the recall procedures for removal, occlusal adjustment, and recementation of a fixed prosthesis with questionable abutments. After placement of a fixed prosthesis with malposed teeth a multiple recall system is mandate to ensure satisfactory results. A recommended time period is commonly 3 to 5 days after insertion or until recognizable interferences have been attended to.

PERIODONTALLY INVOLVED TEETH

When a potential abutment is mobile, the myriad of reasons contributing to the condition of the tooth must be reviewed before the tooth is used as part of a fixed prosthesis. Periodontal treatment should be considered prior to or concomitant with caries-control programs. Excessive bony involvement resulting in severe mobility should exclude fixed partial fabrication until functional occlusal relationships are predetermined and the potential success of periodontal therapy can be assessed.

The mechanical disadvantages inherent in the use of mobile teeth for a fixed prosthesis become readily apparent. The reduced bony root support of periodontally involved teeth further embarrasses Ante's law. Splinting would appear to compensate for this shortcoming, but the addition of sound teeth to a splint can also result in their loss if discretion is not exercised.

Restorative dentists are routinely encouraged to splint teeth with inadequate bony support to more healthy members of the dentition. However, therapeutic treatment of this nature has not been adequately supported with longitudinal studies or sufficient data to attest to the validity of these procedures. A more comprehensive approach to the problem of periodontally involved teeth is discussed by Frederickson in Chapter 24 and Francis and Porter in Chapter 2.

Preparation of the anterior teeth after periodontal surgery (Fig. 6-61, *A*) is extremely difficult. The narrowed cervical portion of the teeth (Fig. 6-61, *B*) usually enhances the possibility of pulpal involvement when an attempt is made to develop optimal esthetics. In addition, the impression materials used to duplicate the preparations are prone to tear and become distorted upon removal from the mouth. This is attributable to the larger embrasure areas (Fig. 6-61, *C*) and increased undercuts after periodontal surgery.

We hope that the justified attention to supportive tissues will develop a less vociferous and more implementive profile by the following:

1. Interception of early periodontal cases to prevent extensive treatment
2. Elimination of periodontally involved teeth beyond the dignity of a restoration
3. Preparation of gingival finish lines on a fixed prosthesis that preferably terminate at or above the soft tissue (except for esthetic needs or retentive demands)
4. Quadrant splinting if and when single units are impossible
5. Development of near optimal morphologic contours of restorative units[3]
6. Telescopic type, full arch splinting for terminal cases[4]

Splinting of teeth is performed only when necessary.[5-7] It is a costly procedure that severely limits the patient's ability to perform routine oral hygiene procedures.

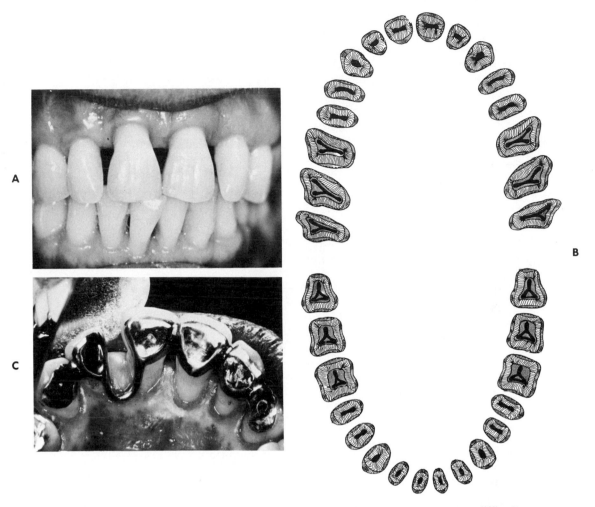

Fig. 6-61. A, Teeth that appear elongated after periodontal surgery are difficult to restore esthetically. Perceptive, early diagnosis is needed to avoid such problems. "Curtain" type of surgical procedures that are performed from lingual aspect provides a better esthetic result. **B,** Approximate outline forms of various teeth at gingival plane in upper and lower arches. It becomes apparent that full coverage restorations are difficult in periodontally involved teeth because of pulpal proximity. **C,** Pinledge splint employed to stabilize the maxillary incisors. Pinbridge stabilization for periodontal prosthodontics has never realized the success that dental profession had anticipated. Note large embrasure areas and undercuts.

One of the most crucial decisions is to use a sound terminal abutment as part of a splint to stabilize less healthy teeth. Loss of a terminal abutment can alter the entire treatment plan from a fixed to a removable prosthesis.[8]

ERODED TEETH

Teeth that have eroded are generally treated with traditional preparation, except when the labial or buccal surfaces require coverage. The gingival finish lines are placed beyond the eroded area to prevent further loss of tooth structure. This approach can arrest or hold in abeyance this insidious process. One danger in the preparation of teeth with erosion is to assume that pulpal recession has proceeded at the same rate as erosion. Although this hypothesis is not thoroughly sponsored by research, the adroit clinician will realize that the perported pulpal recession is not commonly related to the erosion process.

In cases where modifications are instituted when one surface of the tooth is prepared at a different gingival termina-tion, difficulty is experienced with esthetics and gingival tissue response. Successful margin placement depends on a minimizing of plaque retention. When compromises are necessary because of retainer design for bizarre clinical conditions, every effort should be made to fabricate restorations with smooth surfaces and acceptable contours. A harmonious transition from restoration to tooth structure should be one of the dentist's objectives to ensure a reasonable measure of success. Treatment of erosion directly challenges this specific objective. Fortu-

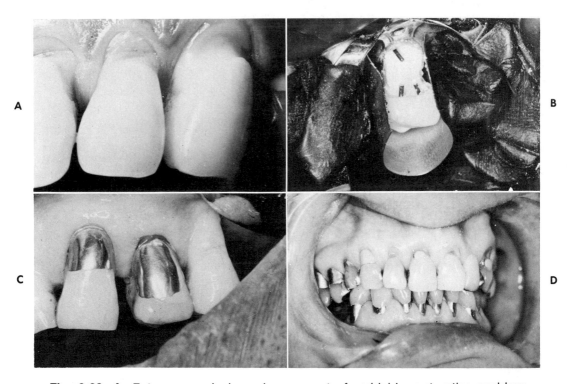

Fig. 6-62. A, Extreme cervical erosion presents formidable restorative problem. Esthetic requirements of patients commonly determine selection of intracoronal or extracoronal restoration in advanced cases. **B,** Pin amalgam placement on eroded tooth prior to tooth preparation preceding an acceptable esthetic restoration. Note extensive base prior to amalgam placement. **C,** Pin-supported amalgams from Fig. 6-60, *A,* placed prior to veneer crowns. **D,** Gold foil restorations are adequate in some cases of erosion but composites are an inept means of treatment with complex cases. Complete veneer crowns would be a more perceptive restoration in most adult patients who have extensive maxillary anterior involvement. (**A** and **C** from Malone, W. F., and Paul, J.: Ill. Dent. J. **37**(5):296, 1968.)

nately the bone support of teeth with cervical erosion is usually adequate. Patients should be informed of the many hypotheses of the etiologic aspects of erosion, such as citric fruits, brushing habits, injestion of abrasives, and malocclusion. Figs. 6-62, *A* and *B*, illustrates the placement of amalgam restorations with horizontal pin amalgams prior to tooth preparation. Polishing amalgam restorations of this nature is obviously optional. Fig. 6-62, *D*, is an example of a patient with progressive erosion who now requires full-coverage restorations. Class V amal-

gam and composite restorations can precede full-coverage preparations. Currently, amalgam is preferable to composites because of γ2 free-phase superior strength, but composites may have to be used because of esthetics.

ABRASION AND ATTRITION

Teeth that have been subjected to severe abrasion present problems for tooth preparation to obtain vertical retention of a prospective abutment. Determination of an acceptable vertical dimension is also a critical determination. Conven-

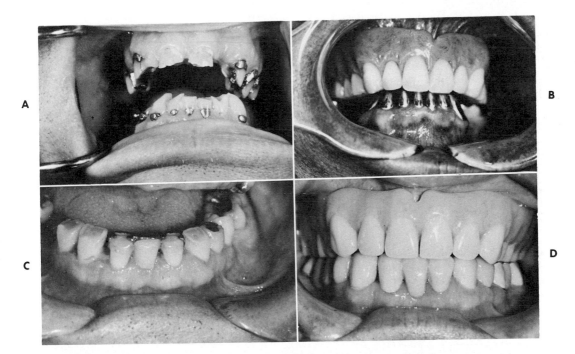

Fig. 6-63. A, Forty-seven-year-old patient whose abrasion presents a formidable restorative problem. Altered freeway space, reduced axial surfaces of the teeth, and bizarre osseous formation challenge the traditional restorative procedures. Use of telescopic crowns on abutment teeth with a fixed or removable maxillary prosthesis is one direction of treatment. **B,** Maxillary and mandibular tooth–supported denture for patient in **A** with severe abrasion. Mandibular anterior fixed prosthesis is still possibility at later date. **C,** This mandibular abrasion on 30-year-old male is always a problem when encountered by dentists. **D,** Patient in **C** with abrasion restored with mandibular fixed prosthodontics and a maxillary complete denture service. Use of acrylic teeth on maxillary denture increases longevity of mandibular restorations. (**A** and **B** from Malone, W. F., editor: Electrosurgery in dentistry, American Lecture Series, Springfield, Ill., 1974, Charles C Thomas, Publisher.)

tional fixed prosthodontics may be impossible or improbable because of a variety of factors, in addition to those mentioned above, such as patient orientation to restorative limitations.

A tooth-supported prosthesis (Fig. 6-63, *A* and *B*) with multiple telescopic copings may be the most pragmatic treatment because of technical (retentive) problems of the dentist and the economic resources of the patient. Fig. 6-63, *A*, illustrates the type of abrasion cases that usually contraindicate fixed prosthodontics. The gross abrasion accompanied by gravitation of maxillary teeth suggests a removable tooth-supported maxillary denture with a multiple mandibular coping (Fig. 6-63, *B*) type of prosthesis. Vertical-dimension determination becomes problematic (Fig. 6-63, *C*) in cases where fixed prosthodontics is the treatment of choice. Chapter 17 discusses the pros and cons for the alteration of vertical dimensions.

RESECTED TEETH FOR ABUTMENTS

Occasionally it is deemed necessary to use a tooth with a resected root as an abutment. This procedure may appear impractical upon initial examination, but clinical evidence will show selected usage is acceptable. It was previously believed the use of a sectioned tooth would reduce the support of the bridge, violate Ante's law, and curtail the longevity of the prosthesis. Such is not always the case where perceptive surgery during resection has provided an area for a cleansible gingival termination. In our opinion lower "bicuspidized" molars are more suitable for this imaginative approach.

Resected upper molars are usually a heroic practice with a guarded prognosis unless the procedure is used to provide additional support for a long-span bridge. Esthetic considerations and maintaining tissue health are common problems with resected maxillary molars (Fig. 6-64). Fig. 6-65 illustrates the difficulty a dentist would have in establishing an acceptable gingival seal and creating an environment for a satisfactory tissue response.

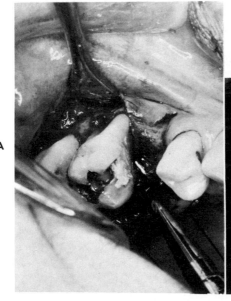
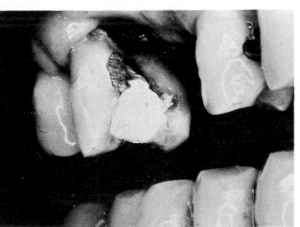

Fig. 6-64. A, Upper first molar that will be splinted to terminal molar after resection of mesiobuccal root. Tooth preparation, gingival margin, and pontic design are arduous. Teeth treated in this manner are currently being subjected to longitudinal evaluation. **B,** Postoperative picture of resected upper first molar in **A.** "Pork-chop" shape of coronal portion of core-and-dowel fabrication remains an uncleansible area with questionable esthetics.

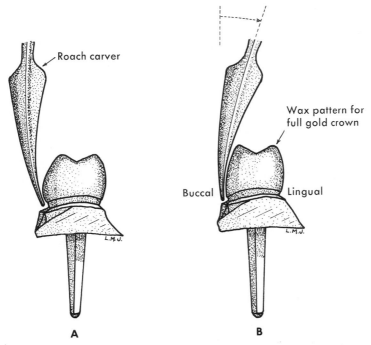

Fig. 6-65. Developing physiologic contours in wax pattern saves time and material while ensuring a more favorable tissue response. **A,** Adaptation of wax pattern margin. **B,** "Protective-deflective bulges" are avoided and can be eliminated by a change of angulation of carving instrument during wax procedure. Note flatter buccal and lingual contours compared to those in **A.** Mesial view of mandibular right first molar.

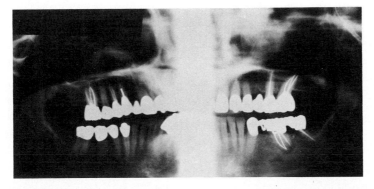

Fig. 6-66. Panoramic view of patient with resected mandibular second molar. This procedure temporarily averts a removable prosthesis but has a questionable prognosis.

The acceptable abutment is designated to withstand additional occlusal loads. A resected abutment tooth is *not* always capable of supporting the additional forces (Fig. 6-66) to which it will be subjected as part of the fixed partial denture. However, the risk is warranted if the patient agrees and the dentist believes there is a chance for the root, splinted to

an additional tooth, to preserve arch integrity.

In summary, increased biologic liabilities usually result in a proportionate increase in the failure rate of a restoration or prosthesis. Resected teeth are presently considered a biologic liability; so appropriate recall systems must be instituted to monitor these teeth.

The resected mandibular preparation or bicuspidized molar is prepared for a core and dowel (Fig. 6-67) after endodontic treatment. The suprastructure can be modified in its occlusal relationship to decrease functional forces imposed by the maxillary dentition. If the resected mandibular molar (single or double rooted) opposes a removable prosthesis, the longevity of the resected tooth is obviously more favorable.

Maxillary resected teeth are infinitely more involved because of the trifurcation of the roots. A "pork-chop" design (Fig. 6-68) is a common design for a molar whose either mesial or distobuccal root has been removed after endodontic treatment. Splinting the resected first molar to a terminal abutment (Fig. 6-69) can aid the stability and increase the prognosis of the fixed prosthesis. Removal of both buccal roots and retention of only the lingual root should be a rare procedure, but

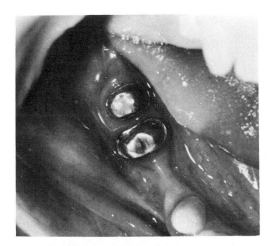

Fig. 6-67. "Bicuspidized" lower molar that will be used as a terminal abutment is an imaginative approach to avert placement of removable mandibular prosthesis. Opposing maxillary arch has undergone complete denture service lending more credence to retaining resected mandibular molar.

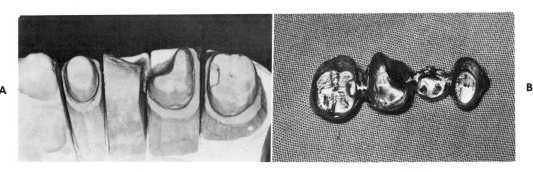

Fig. 6-68. A, Resected mesiobuccal root of upper first molar. Crown portion of coronal-radicular stabilization with "pork-chop" outline. B, Gingival and intaglio view of fixed prosthesis for prepared teeth in Fig. 6-68, *A.* Gingival contour of resected maxillary first molar is always difficult to design when coronal portion of tooth is removed. (**A,** Courtesy Drs. Lee Jameson, Ken Bray, and Ed Theiss, Maywood, Ill.)

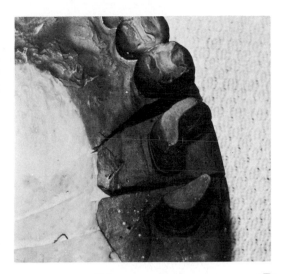

Fig. 6-69. Resected molars with core-and-dowel assembly seated. Splinting of these teeth will increase stability and allow patient to function without removable prosthesis. Procedures of this nature are heroic in nature and the patient should be so informed.

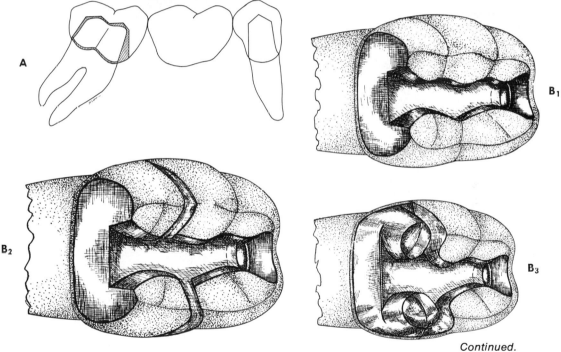

Continued.

Fig. 6-70. A, Telescopic crown for terminal abutment to attain parallelism. **B,** *1,* Outline form with a proximal slice for mesial half crown. *2,* Grooves cut buccally and lingually through occlusal fissures of lower molar. *3,* Occlusal view of preparation. *4,* Addition of proximal keyway and occlusal well gives added retention to retainer. *5,* Mesial half crown used on tilted mandibular molars to provide rigid soldered joint for fixed prosthesis. **C,** *1,* Lingual dovetail preparation for anterior incisor. *2,* Stressbreaker or "rest" preparation can be placed in retainer with rest extension from pontic. *3,* Labial surface of incisor abutment is thereby preserved. **D,** Repositioning of anterior maxillary quadrant prior to placement of a fixed prosthesis. Orthodontics is a proved adjunct to treatment prior to restorative dentistry in cases of trauma.

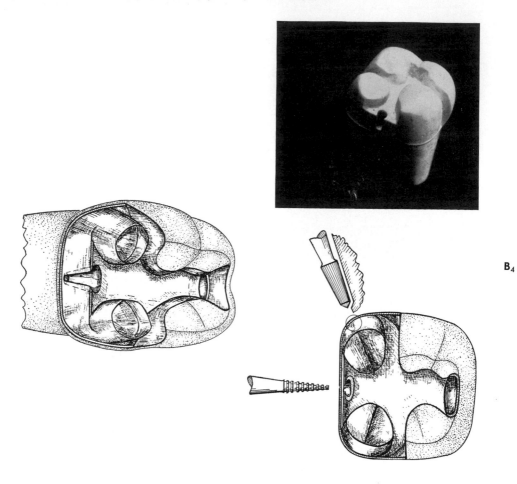

B₄

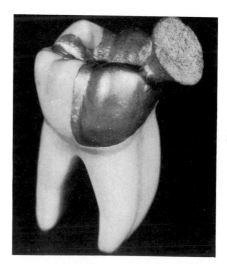

B₅

Fig. 6-70, cont'd. For legend see p. 195.

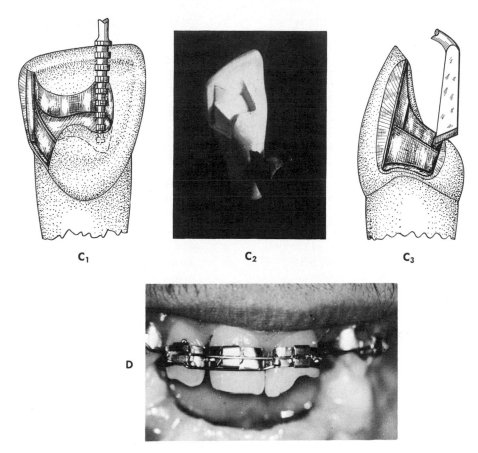

C₁   C₂   C₃

D

Fig. 6-70, cont'd. For legend see p. 195.

if it occurs, the following technical procedures are performed:

1. Core and dowel placement is mandated.
2. Overlaying crown contours should be constructed to prevent tissue stagnation.
3. Splinting the resected tooth to teeth with a more favorable prognosis is a rational approach or the longevity of the resected teeth will be drastically reduced.

Periodontists dislike the maxillary "pork-chop" appearance. They remove the coronal aspect of the teeth with the resected root *only* when absolutely necessary. This approach is also much more acceptable to the restorative dentist.

TILTED TEETH AND PARALLELISM

The most common questionable abutment observed by the dentist is a tilted tooth (Fig. 6-70, *A*), which is considered for an abutment for a fixed prosthesis. When the distal abutment has drifted beyond 23 degrees, it is nearly impossible to reduce the mesial wall parallel to the anterior abutment without endangering the pulp. The resultant prosthesis is also a cleansing problem to the patient. Tilted abutment teeth have been treated with the following techniques to obtain the necessary parallelism for a fixed prosthesis:

1. Use of a "mesial half crown" (Fig. 6-70, *B* and *C*) on the distal abutment. Modification of Tylman's

preparation includes a broader mesial proximal box for additional retention.

2. Stress breakers with the female portion on the anterior retainer, with the male portion being placed within the pontic. Modification of traditional stressbreakers with semi-attachments and precision attachments are common. These can be seen in Chapter 22.

3. Use of telescopic systems.

4. Customized attachments and techniques that are popular in various parts of the world because of the geographic location of the originator.

5. Orthodontic treatment to realign teeth in poor arch position (Fig. 6-70, *D*). This may be the best therapeutic approach when evaluated in light of longevity. All other methods still place adverse forces mesial to the long axis of the terminal abutment.

Parallelism has always disconcerted the dental student and taxed the pedagogic approaches of dental educators. Experience reduces the "mystique" of parallelism, but certain guidelines are necessary to obtain consistent results. Malposed, tilted, and rotated teeth and teeth out of the acceptable plane increase the need for more rigid adherence to guidelines and use of a stressbreaker type of prosthesis. The following guidelines can be helpful for obtaining parallelism in cases of this nature:

1. Place the central groove of the tooth preparation parallel to the crest of the ridge during occlusal reduction. This is performed on all abutment teeth regardless of arch position.

2. Place the mesial and distal proximal slice 1 mm from the contact of the adjacent tooth. Visually align these slice-depth penetration cuts to the mesial surface of the anterior abutment so that the wax pattern will draw with the distal surface of the posterior abutment. This same procedure is repeated to make the mesial surface of the distal abutment parallel to the mesial surface of the anterior abutment.

3. The next step is to *first* remove the tooth structure that is the farthest from the central groove; for example, a lingually inclined molar may require more tooth reduction on the lingual surface than on the buccal surface.

4. Take an alginate impression after gross reduction. This impression can be poured in fast-setting stone. Temporization procedures can be initiated concomitantly to prevent loss of time. Any gross or subtle undercuts noted from the model are then removed prior to impression taking.

5. The use of large intraoral mirrors and the "snap" impressions should help immeasurably to attain parallelism with a long-span prosthesis.

6. Do not reduce the most accessible surface of the potential abutment first, that is, the reduction of the mesial surface of a maxillary first molar where the maxillary second premolar is missing. This direction of preparation will decrease the chances for desirable retention and may result in loss of excessive tooth structure. If one of the abutment teeth has undergone endodontic therapy, the core and dowel or pin buildup should be placed after the preparation of the tooth possessing a vital pulp. This will facilitate the attainment of parallelism and preserve tooth structure of the teeth with vital pulps.

TELESCOPIC SYSTEMS

Telescoping consists of fitting a full-coverage substructure (primary casting or coping) to a prepared tooth and fitting a superstructure (secondary casting and in-

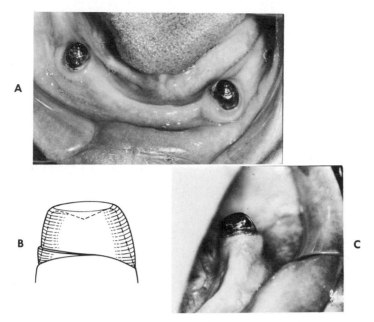

Fig. 6-71. A, Ceka attachment for mandibular canine and premolar on endodontically treated teeth. Resulting increase in retention of removable prosthesis necessitates a proportional degree of coronal-radicular stabilization. However, coronal retentive height is initially reduced to obtain a more favorable crown-root ratio. **B** and **C,** Mandibular coping for complete denture service for a premolar. Telescopic crowns for fixed prosthodontics differ from copings for removable tooth-supported prosthesis.

tegral part of the fixed prosthesis) to the primary casting. As early as 1887, telescoping bridgework was being reported in the *American System of Dentistry.*

Objectives of telescoping systems

Telescoping or sleeve coping is another popular means of placing a fixed prosthesis on a tilted tooth or malposed teeth while the vitality of the abutment is maintained. The objectives of coping in fixed prosthodontics are as follows:

1. Protect the prepared tooth
2. Provide an atmosphere for gingival health
3. Achieve parallelism to seat the fixed prosthesis

The preparation is a difficult procedure that should be performed with emphasis on the predetermined design of the fixed prosthesis related to the coping. Fig. 6-71 illustrates the difference in design of the coping for a removable prosthesis in contrast to the fixed coping (Fig. 6-70). The main difference is that the fixed copings possess less divergence and greater coronal height. See Chapter 24.

Indications of telescoping

The general indications of multiple telescopic crowns are placed in this chapter because of their increased usage for questionable abutments. We are aware of the fact that one full chapter on malposed teeth and splinting might be warranted but to increase the correlation of questionable abutments to the use of copings and splinting, we considered it more propitious to discuss both topics within this chapter. The indications are as follows:

1. A gain in parallelism on severely tipped abutment teeth for conventional fixed prosthodontics
2. An increase in retention on teeth

with short clinical crowns for individual restorations

3. Parallelism of multiple abutments for fixed restorations with the most conservative tooth removal

4. Fabrication of full-arch periodontal splinting of fixed bridges in several smaller quadrant segments, thereby facilitating construction

5. Provision of protection to an abutment during treatment restoration placement or if the permanent superstructure becomes loosened

6. Copings that will allow assessment of the supporting structures by periodic removal of secondary castings

7. Telescoping that will facilitate belated endodontic therapy without damage to secondary castings

8. Use of the telescoping system with internal grooves to supply additional retention on badly broken down teeth, thereby maintaining arch integrity (See Chapter 22)

9. A combined telescopic system that can be advantageously used in conjunction with resected teeth (Illustrations of the benefit of this system can be reviewed in Chapter 24.)

Considerations for preparation of telescopic crowns of questionable abutments

The following factors are recommended:

1. Adequate occlusal and incisal reduction to accommodate "double casting" coverage.

2. Exaggerated proximal space must be provided to accommodate the metals and maintain an adequate interproximal embrasure.

3. Esthetic consideration may dictate various designs anteriorly to accommodate facings on fixed prosthesis or tooth placement for a removable appliance, for example, coping with exaggerated shoulders on the labial or buccal side with beveled margins near the level of the gingival tissue.

4. Use of a preparation that attempts to parallel the abutment teeth to distribute the forces of occlusion more equitably; that is, some abutment teeth might require intentional pulpal extirpation for the dentist to accomplish a favorable crown-root ratio or parallelism.

SPLINTING OF TEETH
Definition

Splinting refers to any joining together of two or more teeth for the purpose of stabilization.

Rationale

There are few areas in restorative dentistry that will elicit more controversy than splinting. Academic emphasis has been rightfully placed upon the attention of the dentist to constant surveillance of the supporting structures within the oral cavity. Recent advancements in periodontal therapy have elucidated the inability of some traditional (Fig. 6-44) and heroic (Fig. 6-72) restorative procedures to support periodontal treatment. Consequently, because of disenchantment with ordinary restorative procedures, one group of dentists believes that

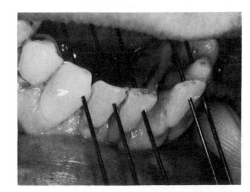

Fig. 6-72. Horizontal pin splint technique, which suggests a questionable prognosis and demanding technical implementation. (From Malone, W. F., Eisenmann, D., and Kusek, J.: J. Prosthet. Dent. **22**(5):555, 1969.)

further stabilization by the splinting of teeth is the answer, whereas another group has decided that the inherent limitations of restorative dentistry dictates a more conservative approach of "wait and see" after periodontal treatment. There is a dearth of conclusive longitudinal studies to support either direction. A separate bibliography was specifically included in this chapter because of the controversial nature of splinting.

One answer to the problem is the as-sessment of the individual case by the dentist. The treatment plan must be based upon the tissue response of a given patient. The advantages of splinting (Figs. 6-73 and 6-74) should clearly outweigh the disadvantages.[6] Another professional refinement that facilitates treatment is direct communication between the periodontist and the restorative dentist prior to any treatment. Diametrically opposed concepts of dental treatment merely disconcert and confuse the patient. Complete commitment by the pa-

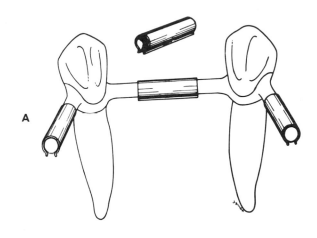

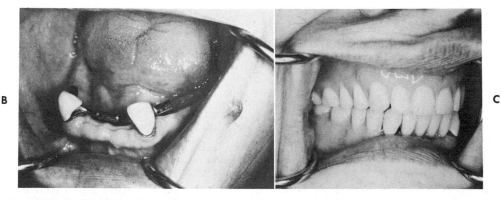

Fig. 6-73. A, Clip-bar splint used in conjunction with removable prosthesis. Sufficient supporting structure of abutment teeth is a mandate. Distal clips are only indicated if the antagonist is a removable prosthesis. **B,** Clip-bar splint at "try-in" stage. Final impression in mercaptan rubber or polyether is taken with bar in place after centric closure position determination. **C,** Clip-bar splint in **B** seated with maxillary and mandibular removable prosthesis in centric closure position. (**A** from Malone, W. F., Ensing, H., Gerhard, R. J., and Morganelli, J. E.: J. Acad. Gen. Dent. **2**(3):75, June 1970.)

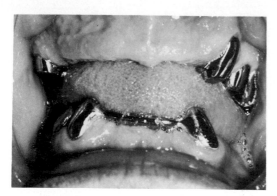

Fig. 6-74. Mandibular bar with multiple maxillary copings. Both maxillary and mandibular teeth retain vital pulps because of available interocclusal clearance. Fixed prosthodontics can be placed at a later date on mandibular arch, depending on recovery of supporting structures.

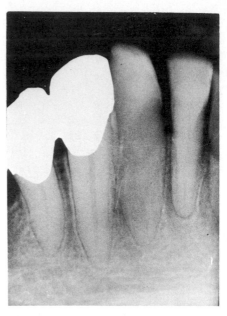

Fig. 6-75. Splinting of anterior abutment teeth of a four-unit fixed prosthesis with a telescopic crown used on posterior abutment.

tient to recall evaluations can ensure some measure of professional success.

Disadvantages of permanent splinting

1. Splinting is an arduous restorative procedure:
   a. Maintaining vertical dimension
   b. Developing acceptable occlusal patterns
   c. Fabrication of treatment restorations
   d. Design of the gingival third of restorations for optimal tissue response
2. Splinted teeth discourage patients from cleaning embrasures.
3. Splinting can be prohibitive economically.
4. Splinting commonly requires more tooth reduction for parallelism.
5. Repairs can be problematic and untimely for the patient.
6. Inflexible treatment plans can result from extensive splinting. Early perceptive diagnosis of a questionable abutment can be difficult.
7. Technical fabrication for a functional, esthetic prosthesis is involved; that is, embrasure areas must be adequate despite the obvious need of additional bulk for strength.

Advantages of splinting

1. The dentist is purported to be able to retain questionable teeth for a longer period of time.
2. It permits, in some cases, a more favorable maxillomandibular relationship by redirection of the forces during function.
3. It prevents food impaction (from the occlusal surfaces only) by eliminating the occlusal embrasure.
4. There is stabilization of teeth during or after trauma and orthodontic or periodontic treatment.

Both advantages one and two have been and are the subject of continued research.

Indications for splinting

1. Stabilization of abutment teeth for removable prosthodontics, that is,

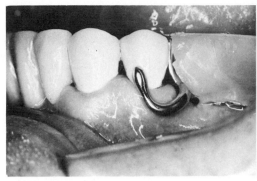
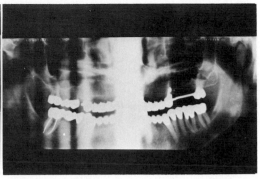

A

B

Fig. 6-76. A, Eight-unit fixed prosthesis with splinted retainers. A paralleling guide plane can be additional burden to maintaining a cleansible area. **B,** Fixed-removable maxillary splint used for a patient with moderate periodontal involvement. Ceka attachments were used as additional retentive and esthetic measure on maxillary bar splint. **(A,** Courtesy Dr. Russell Lee, Honolulu, Hawaii.)

the double abutment of both mandibular premolars (Fig. 6-75) bilaterally for a patient edentulous in the molar areas. This is particularly true if there is evidence of bone loss or the anterior abutment teeth have conic roots.

2. Prevention of supraeruption or gravitation of teeth without an antagonist, for example, splinted maxillary first and second molars where the mandibular second molar has been removed. Some dentists prefer the removal of the maxillary second molar.

3. Maintenance of satisfactory arch position, for example, splinted premolars for a fixed prosthesis with a tilted second molar restored by use of a telescopic crown replacing a first molar (Fig. 6-70, A).

4. Treatment of questionable teeth. Stabilization of periodontally involved teeth will be retained by the patient for a longer period of time. Whether these retained teeth will contribute to the loss of additional healthy abutments must be a judgment made by the dentist for a given patient. The determination of the

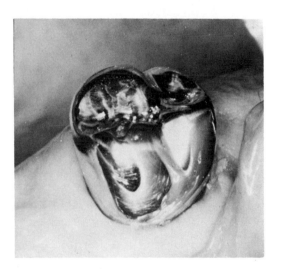

Fig. 6-77. Complete crown on maxillary molar with a mesial stabilizing guide plane for a removable prosthesis. This innocuous method of stabilization is often overlooked for a terminal abutment. (From Malone, W. F., and Sarlas, C. H.: Dent. Clin. North Am. **13** (2):461-482, April 1969.)

presence of secondary traumatic (Fig. 6-76) occlusal forces might be a justification for splinting. However, the projected effect upon the remaining dentition is crucial; that is,

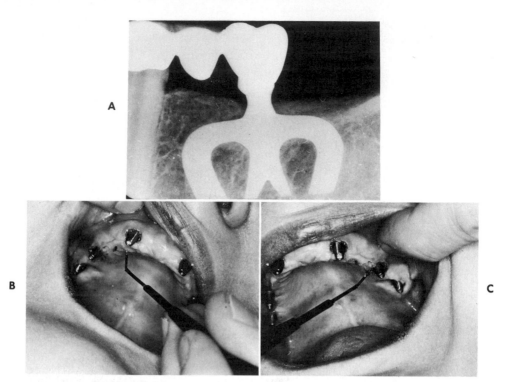

Fig. 6-78. A, Distal blade implant placed for temporary stabilization. Coronal design of these implants needs modification for better retention. Implantation has developed a more reliable profile as basic research substantiates its therapeutic use. **B,** Full maxillary arch of blade implants. Splinting is an obvious necessity in these cases. Success of these blade implants is enhanced because of complete mandibular denture. **C,** Blade implants can be placed because of anatomic necessity in a less desirable arch position. Anterior coronal portion of this full arch maxillary would be more ideal if it were in canine area instead of lateral incisor position. Redundant tissue is carefully and quickly removed from ridge adjacent to blade implant post.

excessive stress on a terminal abutment (Fig. 6-77) tooth eliminates the flexibility of any treatment plan. A removable appliance might be a less complex direction to treatment.

5. Resected teeth should be provided with additional support.
6. Patients who demonstrate excessive supportive tissue destruction after periodontal surgery. A full-arch splint may be the patient's last chance for a fixed prosthesis. Terminal splinting to allow the patient the opportunity of a fixed prosthesis is a definite justification for fabrication of a maxillary full-arch splint. Placement of a removable appliance on the mandibular arch will increase the longevity of the maxillary splint.
7. Splinting is commonly used in conjunction with implants (Fig. 6-78).

SELECTED REFERENCES

1. Dawson, P. E.: Evaluation, diagnosis, and treatment of occlusal problems, St. Louis, 1975, The C. V. Mosby Co.
2. Gordon, T.: Telescopic reconstruction: an approach to oral rehabilitation, J.A.D.A. **72:**97-105, 1966.
3. Malson, T. S.: Anatomic cast crown reproduction, J. Prosthet. Dent., **9:**106, 1959.

4. Weinberg, L. A.: A double casting of metal to metal in full coverage, J.A.D.A. **63**:821, 1961.
5. Brewer, A. A., and Morrow, R. M.: Overdentures, St. Louis, 1975, The C. V. Mosby Co.
6. Glickman, I., Stein, R. S., and Smulow, J. B.: The effect of increased functional forces upon the periodontium of splinted and non-splinted teeth, J. Periodontol. **32**:290, 1961.
7. O'Leary, T. J.: Tooth mobility—its significance in periodontics and restorative dentistry, J. Periodontol. **44**:117, 1973.
8. Brecker, S. C.: Conservative occlusal rehabilitation, J. Prosthet. Dent. **9**:1001-1016, 1959.

GENERAL REFERENCES

Abrams, A., and Coslett, G.: Occlusal adjustment by selective grinding. In Goldman, H., and Cohen, D. W., editors: Periodontal therapy, ed. 5, St. Louis, 1973, The C. V. Mosby Co.

Amsterdam, M.: Periodontal prosthesis, The Alpha Omegan **67**:21, 1974.

Amsterdam, M.: Periodontal prosthesis. In Goldman, H., and Cohen, D. W., editors: Periodontal therapy, ed. 5, St. Louis, 1973, The C. V. Mosby Co.

Amsterdam, M., and Fox, L.: Provisional splinting—principles and techniques, Dent. Clin. North Am. **3**:73, 1959.

Amsterdam, M., and Rossman, S.: The technique of hemisection of multirooted teeth, The Alpha Omegan **53**:4, 1960.

Basaraba, N.: Root amputation and tooth hemisection, Dent. Clin. North Am. **13**:121, 1969.

Bhaskar, S.: Experimental occlusal trauma, J. Periodontol. **26**:270, 1955.

Chacker, F.: Etiology of periodontal disease. In Goldman, H., and Cohen, D. W., editors: Periodontal therapy, ed. 5, St. Louis, 1973, The C. V. Mosby Co.

Chayes, H.: On the dangers of fixed bridgework, Dent. Cosmos **58**:1401, 1916.

Clark, J., Weatherford, T., and Mann, W.: The wire ligature–acrylic splint, J. Periodontol. **40**:371, 1969.

Cohen, D., and Chacker, F.: Criteria for selection of one treatment plan over another, Dent. Clin. North Am. **8**:3, 1964.

Cohn, L.: The physiologic basis for tooth fixation in precision attachment partial dentures, J. Prosthet. Dent. **6**:220, 1956.

Cross, W. G.: The importance of immobilisation in periodontology, Parodontologie **8**:119, 1954.

Cross, W. G., and Yuktanandana, I.: The role of orthodontics in periodontal treatment, Dent. Pract. **7**:388, 1957.

Friedman, N.: Temporary splinting: an adjunct in periodontal treatment, J. Periodontol. **24**:229, 1953.

Gecker, L. M.: Ortho-prosthesis and its significance in dental practice, N. Y. Dent. J. **35**:203-207, 1965.

Glickman, I.: Clinical periodontology, ed. 4, Philadelphia, 1972, W. B. Saunders Co.

Glickman, I.: Role of occlusion in the etiology and treatment of periodontal disease, J. Dent. Res. **50**(suppl. to 2):199, 1971.

Glickman, I., Stein, S., and Smulow, J.: The effect of increased functional forces upon the periodontium of splinted and nonsplinted teeth, J. Periodontol. **32**:290, 1961.

Glickman, I., and Weiss, L.: Role of trauma from occlusion in initiation of periodontal pocket formation in experimental animals, J. Periodontol. **26**:14, 1955.

Glickman, J.: Occlusion and the periodontium, J. Dent. Res. **46**:53, 1967.

Glickman, J., and Smulow, J.: Adaptive alterations in the periodontium of rhesus monkeys in chronic trauma from occlusion, J. Periodontol. **39**:101, 1968.

Glickman, J., and Smulow, J.: Alterations in the pathway of gingival inflammation into the underlying tissues induced by excessive occlusal forces, J. Periodontol. **33**:7, 1962.

Glickman, J., and Smulow, J.: The effect of excessive occlusal forces upon the pathway of gingival inflammation in humans, J. Periodontol. **36**:141, 1965.

Goldberg, H. J. V.: Changes in tooth mobility during periodontal therapy, Gen. Meeting of I.A.D.R. **40**:Abst. 261, 1962.

Goldman, H., and Cohen, D. W.: Lesions of the attachment apparatus. In Goldman, H., and Cohen, D. W., editors: Periodontal therapy, ed. 5, St. Louis, 1973, The C. V. Mosby Co.

Grupe, H.: Bruxism splint—a technique, J. Periodontol. **30**:156, 1959.

Gupta, S. C., Chawla, T. N., Kapur, K. K., et al.: Tooth mobility, 2. Its relation to traumatic bite, oral hygiene, and splinting, J. Indian Dent. Assoc. **44**:142, 1972.

Hirschfield, I.: The individual missing tooth: a factor in dental and periodontal disease, J.A.D.A. **24**:67, 1937.

Hirschfield, L.: The use of wire and silk ligatures, J.A.D.A. **41**:647, 1950.

Kahn, A. E.: Unbalanced occlusion in occlusal rehabilitation, J. Prosthet. Dent. **14**:725-738, 1964.

Kessler, M.: A variation of the "A" splint, J. Periodontol. **41**:268, 1970.

Kjennerud, I.: Development, etiology and diagnosis of increased tooth mobility and of traumatic occlusion, J. Periodontol. **44**:326, 1973.

Klavan, B.: Clinical observations following root amputation in maxillary molar teeth, J. Periodontol. **46**:1, 1975.

Krough-Poulsen, W.: Management of the occlusion of the teeth. In Schwartz, L., and Chayes, C., editors: Facial pain and mandibular dysfunction,

Philadelphia, 1968, W. B. Saunders Co., pp. 256-271.

Levine, B. F.: Basic concepts in occlusal corrections of natural teeth, J. Prosthet. Dent. **15**:732-735, 1965.

Levinson, E., and Gurr, R.: Splinting—a review and clinical investigation—preliminary report, J. Dent. Assoc. South Afr. **24**:284, 1969.

Lindhe, J., and Svanberg, G.: Influence of trauma from occlusion on the progression of experimental periodontitis in the beagle dog, J. Clin. Periodontol. **1**:3, 1974.

Lloyd, R., and Baer, P.: Periodontal therapy by root resection, J. Prosthet. Dent. **10**:363, 1965.

Lovdal, A., et al.: Tooth mobility and alveolar bone resorption as a function of occlusal stress and oral hygiene, Acta Odontol. Scand. **17**:61, 1959.

Mann, A. W.: Examination diagnosis and treatment planning in occlusal rehabilitation, J. Prosthet. Dent. **17**:73-78.

Marks, M., and Corn, H.: The integration of adult tooth movement in a comprehensive periodontal treatment program. In Ward, H., editor: A periodontal point of view, Springfield, Ill., 1973, Charles C Thomas, Publisher, pp. 75-96.

Meklas, J.: Splinting: a rationale, N. Mex. Dent. J. **21**:12, 1971.

Meyer, G. E.: Textbook of crown and bridge prosthodontics, St. Louis, 1969, The C. V. Mosby Co. pp. 151-153.

Miller, G., and Cohen, D. W.: Role of the initial preparation of the mouth in periodontal therapy. In Goldman, H., and Cohen, D. W., editors: Periodontal therapy, ed. 5, St. Louis, 1973, The C. V. Mosby Co.

Miller, H. L., and Swepston, J. H.: Rationale of rehabilitation, Texas Dent. J. **82**:4-8, 1964.

Mühlemann, H. R.: Tooth mobility—a review of clinical aspects and research findings, J. Periodontol. **38**:686, 1967.

Mühlemann, H. R., Savdir, S., and Rateitschak, K. H.: Tooth mobility—its causes and significance, J. Periodontol. **36**:148, 1965.

Mühlemann, H. R., and Zander, H. A.: Tooth mobility. III. The mechanism of tooth mobility, J. Periodontol. **25**:128, 1954.

Nyman, S., Lindhe, J., and Lundgren, D.: The role of occlusion for the stability of fixed bridges in patients with reduced periodontal support, J. Clin. Periodontol. **2**:53, 1975.

O'Leary, T. J.: Tooth mobility—its significance in periodontics and restorative dentistry, J. Periodontol. **44**:117, 1973.

O'Leary, T. J., Rudd, K. D., and Nabers, C. L.: Factors affecting horizontal tooth mobility, Periodontics **4**:308, 1966.

O'Leary, T., Shanley, D., and Drake, R.: Tooth mobility in cuspid-protected and group function occlusions, J. Prosthet. Dent. **27**:21, 1972.

Olson, R. C.: Maintaining the occlusion during full or partial reconstruction. The stop-sleeve technique, J. Am. Acad. Gen. Dent. **20**:32-34, 1972.

Ono, I.: The crushing power and masticatory area of teeth as foundations of oral hygienics, Dent. Cosmos **63**:1278, 1921.

Parfitt, G. J.: Dynamics of a tooth in function, J. Periodontol. **32**:102, 1961.

Parfitt, G. J.: Measurement of the physiological mobility of individual teeth in an axial direction, J. Dent. Res. **39**:608, 1960.

Parkinson, C. F.: Excessive crown contours facilitate endemic plaque niches, **35**:424, 1976.

Polson, A. M., Kennedy, J. E., and Zander, H. A.: Trauma and progression of marginal periodontitis in squirrel monkeys. I. Codestructive factors of periodontitis and thermally produced injury; II. Mechanically produced injury, J. Periodont. Res. **9**:100, 109, 1974.

Posselt, U.: Bite planes and splints in the treatment of bruxism, J. Can. Dent. Assoc. **29**:773, 1963.

Posselt, U.: Physiology of occlusion and rehabilitation, ed. 2, Philadelphia, 1968, F. A. Davis Co.

Pritchard, J.: Advanced periodontal disease, ed. 2, Philadelphia, 1972, W. B. Saunders Co.

Pruden, W. H.: Development of occlusion where total reconstruction is contraindicated, J. Prosthet. Dent. **16**:549-553, 1966.

Pugh, C., and Smerke, J.: Rationale for fixed prosthesis in the management of advanced periodontal disease, Dent. Clin. North Am. **13**:243, 1969.

Ramadan, A.: Temporary and permanent splints in periodontal therapy, Egypt. Dent. J. **16**:25, 1970.

Ramfjord, S.: Bruxism—a clinical and electromyographic study, J.A.D.A. **62**:21, 1961.

Ramfjord, S.: Dysfunctional TMJ and muscle pain, J. Prosthet. Dent. **11**:353, 1961.

Ramfjord, S., and Ash, M.: Occlusion, ed. 2, Philadelphia, 1971, W. B. Saunders Co.

Rateitschak, K.: The therapeutic effect of local treatment on periodontal disease assessed upon evaluation of different diagnostic criteria. I. Changes in tooth mobility, J. Periodontol. **34**:540, 1963.

Reidel, R.: A review of the retention problem, Angle Orthodont. **30**:179, 1960.

Reitan, K.: Tissue rearrangement during retention of orthodontically rotated teeth, Angle Orthodont. **29**:105, 1959.

Renggli, H. H.: Splinting of teeth—an objective assessment, Helv. Odontol. Acta **15**:129, 1971.

Report of committee IV: Treatment of periodontal disease, J.A.D.A. **45**:27, 1952.

Rosen, H., and Gitnick, P.: Separation and splinting of the roots of multirooted teeth, J. Prosthet. Dent. **21**:34, 1969.

Ross, S.: Temporary stabilization, J. Periodontol. **40**:50, 1969.

Rudd, R. K., and O'Leary, T. J.: Stabilization of

periodontally weakened teeth by using guide-plane partial dentures: preliminary report, J. Prosthet. Dent. **16**:721, 1966.

Scott, M. E., and Baum, L.: Procedure and technics for restoring "canine function" for abraded teeth, J. South. Calif. Dent. Assoc. **32**:23-28, 1964.

Selipsky, H.: Osseous surgery—how much need we compromise? Dent. Clin. North Am. **20**:79, 1976.

Shapior, M.: Orthodontic procedures in the care of the periodontal patient, J. Periodontol. **27**:7, 1956.

Silness, J.: Periodontal conditions in patients treated with dental bridges, J. Periodont. Res. **5**:60-68; III, **5**:225, 1970; IV, **9**:50, 1974.

Simring, M., and Posteraro, A. F.: Hazard and short-comings of splinting, N.Y. State Dent. J. **30**:19, 1964.

Simring, M.: Splinting—theory and practice, J.A.D.A. **45**:402, 1952.

Simring, M., and Thaller, J.: Temporary splinting for multiple mobile teeth, J.A.D.A. **53**:429, 1956.

Son, S., Hotx, P., and Mühlemann, H.: The effect of marginal gingivitis on tooth mobility, Helv. Odontol. Acta **15**:103, 1971.

Sorrin, S.: The use of fixed and removable splints in the practice of periodontia, Am. J. Orthodont. & Oral Surg. **31**:sec. Oral Surg. 354, 1945. Correction 454, July 1945.

Stallard, H.: Survival of the periodontium during and after orthodontic treatment, Am. J. Orthodont. **50**:583, 1964.

Stern, I.: The status of fixed splinting procedures in the treatment of periodontally involved teeth, J. Periodontol. **31**:217, 1960.

Sternlicht, H. C.: Principles and techniques for stabilization of loose teeth, Dent. Clin. North Am. **13**:323, 1969.

Sternlicht, H.: Tooth movement in periodontal disease, Texas Dent. J. **77**:4, 1959.

Sugarman, M. M., and Sugarman, E. F.: Bruxism and occlusal traumatism—diagnosis and treatment, Northwest U. Dent. Res. Grad. Stud. Bull. **49**:216, 1970.

Sved, A.: The problem of retention, Am. J. Orthodont. **39**:659, 1953.

Terkla, L. G.: Crown morphology in relation to operative and crown and bridge dentistry, Oregon State Dent. J. **5**:2-10, 1955.

Ward, H., and Weinberg, L.: An evaluation of peri-odontal splinting, J.A.D.A. **63**:48, 1961.

Waerhaug, J.: Justification for splinting in periodontal therapy, J. Prosthet. Dent. **22**:201, 1969.

Waerhaug, J.: Pathogenesis of pocket formation in traumatic occlusion, J. Periodontol. **26**:107, 1955.

Waerhaug, J., and Hansen, E.: Periodontal changes incident to occlusal overload in monkeys, Acta Odontol. Scand. **24**:91, 1966.

Wasserman, B., Geiger, A., and Turgeon, L.: The relationship of occlusion and periodontal disease. Part VII: Mobility, J. Periodontol. **44**:572, 1973.

Weinberg, L. A.: Force distribution in splinted posterior teeth, Oral Surg. **10**:1268, 1957.

Weisgold, A.: Temporary stabilization. In Goldman, H., and Cohen, D. W., editors: Periodontal therapy, ed. 5, St. Louis, 1973, The C. V. Mosby Co.

Wentz, P., Jarabak, J., and Orban, B.: Experimental occlusal trauma initiating cuspal interferences, J. Periodontol. **29**:117, 1958.

Yuodelis, R. A., and Mann, W. V., Jr.: The prevalence and possible role of nonworking contacts in periodontal disease, Periodontics **3**:219, 1965.

Yurkstas, A.: The effect of missing teeth on masticatory performance and efficiency, J. Prosthet. Dent. **4**:120, 1954.

Yurkstas, A., and Fridley, H. H.: A functional evaluation of fixed and removable bridgework, J. Prosthet. Dent. **1**:570, 1951.

SECTION F

Crown contours and gingival response

Complete crown restorative procedures involve the reestablishment of tooth contours, function, and esthetics while a physiologic balance of the oral musculature, the temporomandibular joint, and the periodontium are maintained. Current high-speed techniques, coupled with the inherent properties of the dental materials presently available, make the maintenance of gingival tissue integrity an arduous task. Minimal preinsertion disruption still leaves the restorative dentist with the problem of reestablishing crown contours conducive to periodontal health. Based on current research and clinical procedures this section presents guidelines for reestablishment of crown contours conducive to gingival health maintenance.

THE DENTOEPITHELIAL JUNCTION

A review of the nonpathologic dentogingival junction is provided to serve as a reminder of the natural state one must attempt to preserve and maintain during clinical restorative procedures.

Before the tooth has erupted into the oral cavity and after completion of enamel formation, the enamel surface is lined with the *reduced enamel epithelium* (containing postsecretory ameloblasts in various developmental stages[1]), and there is the *primary epithelial attachment* between the reduced ameloblasts and the enamel surface. When the tooth erupts, the reduced enamel epithelium gradually changes to a stratified squamous epithelium that joins with the proliferating oral epithelium to form the *junctional epithelium* ("Ameloblasts do not necessarily degenerate but can transform into junctional epithelial cells."[1]). The *secondary epithelial attachment* is now the junction between the junctional epithelium and the enamel surface.

The junctional epithelium is widest in the region of the gingival sulcus (15 to 30 cells) and tapers to its apical termination near the cementoenamel junction (Fig. 6-79). This tissue has a rapid cellular turnover rate whereby basal cells next to the connective tissue and those most apically located migrate coronally toward the tooth. The junctional epithelium joins the tooth surface with the connective tissue of the gingiva by means of the *epithelial attachment*. This attachment consists of an *internal basement lamina* and *hemidesmosomes* (Fig. 6-79, inset). A similar attachment system occurs on the connective tissue side, with the basal lamina being designated by the term *external basal lamina*. The attachment apparatus may be directly associated with the tooth surface, or an intervening *dental cuticle* may be present. It covers most of the cervical enamel and in proliferating apically "may terminate either over enamel, afibrillar cementum or the coronal extension of fibrillar cementum."[1]

The gingival sulcus extends from the free gingival margin to the free surface of the junctional epithelium (Fig. 6-79). The lining of the gingival sulcus may be composed of nonkeratinized oral sulcular epithelium coronally and the free surface of the junctional epithelium apically. Deepening of the sulcus can occur by the influence of local inflammation, whereby an increase in accumulating polymorphonuclear leukocytes at the coronal portion of the junctional epithelium will result in disintegration and loss of the superficial cells of the junctional epithelium.

CROWN CONTOURS—LITERATURE REVIEW

As with most clinical parameters, many articles have been written in regard to crown contours and soft-tissue response,

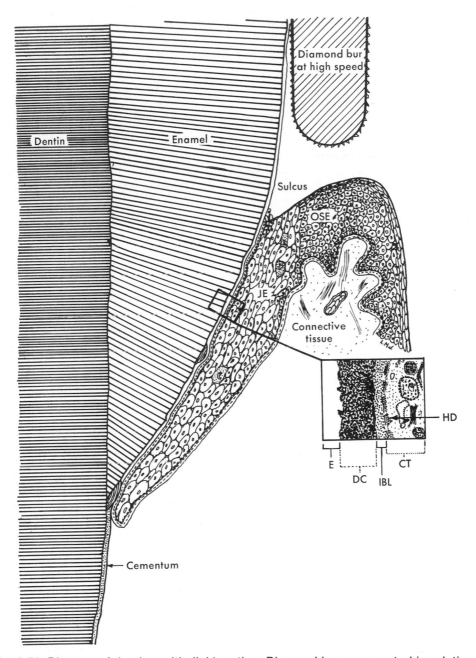

Fig. 6-79. Diagram of dentinoepithelial junction. Diamond bur represented in relative size to biologic structures. *CT,* connective tissue; *DC,* dental cuticle; *E,* enamel; *HD,* hemidesmosome; *IBL,* internal basement lamina; *JE,* junctional epithelium; *OSE,* oral sulcular epithelium.

but few research studies are available to document well-intentioned opinions. A crown is a prosthesis and precise reproduction of the natural cervical third-tooth contour within the laws of biologic compatibility and optimal use of the properties of dental materials is probably impossible.[2,3]

Some authors[4-13] have advocated food-deflecting crown contours to protect the gingival crevice from food impaction. Wheeler[3] stated that undercontouring causes recession as a direct result of trauma whereas overcontouring produces food accumulation and stagnation. Other investigators[14-20] have challenged the "deflective-protective" concept in favor of natural physiologic contours that are in harmony with muscular actions, minimize food-collection capacity, and are capable of being maintained by the patient. Morris[16] stated that an excessive crown contour "causes, rather than prevents, gingival inflammation" and should "range from flat to the most subtle of convexities."

Eissman et al.[14] emphasized physiologic tooth contouring that would expose the largest area of the crown and gingiva to the cleansing and massaging action of (1) food flow, (2) musculature, and (3) oral hygiene devices. Interproximal contours should be concave gingival to the contact area to form an obtuse angle because "embrasures with acute apices must be considered trap embrasures." The food-flow pattern is also used as the basis for placing "sluice grooves" on the lingual side of the marginal ridges directed gingivally.

Perel[19] proposed a reevaluation of restorative procedures involving class V areas and presented clinical evidence that has an application to buccolingual crown contours. He discusses three case situations that "present various forms of axial surface undercontour" (such as asymptomatic class V erosion) and clinically healthy gingiva. He suggested that undercontoured restored surfaces might be beneficial periodontally since "the accessibility of the tooth-gingiva environment to cleansing and stimulation may supersede the implied soft-tissue protection by empirically placed restorative contours." In another study, Perel[18] removed tooth structure from facial and lingual surfaces and overcontoured buccal surfaces with self-curing resin (avoiding the gingiva) on mongrel dogs. Gingival pathosis was absent around those teeth undercontoured, whereas the overcontoured teeth developed inflammation that eventually lead to hyperplasia, food-stagnation areas, decreased keratinization, and gingival fiber deterioration. Sackett et al.,[21] in a somewhat similar study on humans, cemented (with zinc polycarboxylate) standard processed acrylic overcontours (produced from 12-gage half-round wax wire patterns) on premolars of teen-age females and evaluated the results by index scoring, collecting crevicular fluid (measurement by the ninhydrin-staining technique), and standardized photographic techniques. The results showed 27 of the 42 sites tested exhibited clinical inflammatory signs and disruption of normal soft-tissue architecture, and they concluded that "alteration of normal crown form by overcontouring the buccal, axial third of a tooth may be a factor which predisposes the subjacent gingival tissues to inflammatory disease."

Yuodelis et al.,[20] stated that overcontouring to protect the gingival crevice from food during mastication "encourages the accumulation of particulate and microbial matter in an area inaccessible for cleaning by the patient." He challenged the "protective-deflective" concept, since (1) the contemporary diet is relatively soft, (2) the proprioceptive mechanism offers gingival protection from hard food items, (3) the gingiva does not encounter the bulk and total force of the milled bolus, (4) a clinical bulge is nonexistent in most human dentitions and yet gingival trauma from mastication is not exhibited (for example, deciduous dentitions with the subgingival cervical bulge), and (5) the diets of lower animals is much coarser than that of humans and yet masticatory trauma is not common. He concluded that his clinicians "endeavored to flatten the facial and lingual contours of restorations and have observed excellent gingival response, most probably because the cervical region is made more accessible for routine home care." Kornfeld[2] stated that his approach to the contour of crowns "is creation of a rather subtle deflection ridge to flatten the facial and lingual contours to a great extent" and that "a great effort is made to have a smooth, gradual transition from the restoration to the tooth structure."

Vogan[22] considered the validity of present concepts of buccolingual crown contours, citing studies that show that a "self-cleansing mechanism" plays little or no part in the prevention of periodontal disease in man. The stimulation-keratinization concept does not increase the resistance of sulcular tissue (nonkeratinized area) to gingivitis, and the food impaction theory plays little if any role in the actual pathogenesis of inflammatory periodontal disease, which is initiated by the presence of plaque. He concluded that the main requirement of crown contours "is the maintenance of a gingival environment from which bacterial plaque can be removed."

In summary, the prevalent concept concerning crown contours would indicate that the "protective-deflective" artificial contours have a tendency to initiate gingival inflammatory response by providing a protective plaque-accumulating area. Thus the area cannot fully benefit from any natural cleansing potential that the oral musculature may offer and can hinder oral hygiene procedures by making the cervical third of the clinical crown less accessible. Temporarily cementing crowns[8] (with tap-off lugs to facilitate re-moval) for a 30-day trial period can be used to ensure that proper physiologic contours have been developed.

MEASURING GINGIVAL RESPONSE

A tissue response to a dental prosthesis has traditionally be evaluated clinically by such means as color, texture, and pocket depth. Various subjective indices are used, such as the gingival index by Löe and Silness,[23] which requires the dentist to assign numerical values to varying inflammatory states. Unfortunately, once these clinical symptoms are obvious, much tissue destruction has occurred. Fluid originating from the gingival sulcus is one of the first indications of gingival inflammation.[24] Current interest in gingival crevicular fluid evolved from the work of Waerhaug,[25] who demonstrated the dynamic nature of the gingival sulcus area by placing India ink in the healthy gingival sulcus of young dogs and noting their removal by what he described as a increased "transudation of fluid."

Brill[26-32] first suggested using crevicular fluid as a measure of gingival inflammation since it provides a quantitative means to monitor the physiology of the sulcular region. While investigating the permeability of the human crevicular epithelium, Brill et al.[26] noted a greater fluid flow from patients with extensive restorative work compared to clinically healthy nonrestored marginal gingiva. Mann,[33] using a subjective index system (Parfitt), noted that high gingival scores were associated with high values of crevicular fluid flow and concluded that "these variables indicated that inflammation was the main factor contributing to the rate of fluid flow." Egelberg[34] found a correlation existed between the amount of gingival exudate collected on filter-paper strips and the area of inflammatory cell infiltration as revealed by histologic examination. He stated, "Gingival exudate measurements can be considered a method which fulfills rather great demands in regard to objectivity and sensitivity. . . ." Löe and Holm-Pedersen[24] measured crevicular fluid from 118 adults and concluded that (1) cervicular fluid flow begins prior to the appearance of clinical changes and persists for a while after clinical inflammatory changes have disappeared and that (2) "gingival fluid is an inflammatory exudate and that the absence or presence of fluid may represent the definite clinical criterion in the refined distinction between normal and inflamed gingiva."

The composition of crevicular fluid has been found to be very complex and the origin of certain constituents is not fully explained.[35] Among the substances identified are (1) immunoglobulins γG, γA, and γM,[36,37] (2) globulins α_1, α_2, and β_1, (3) albumin, (4) fibrinolytic factors, (5) lactic acid, (6) urea, (7) hydroxyproline, (8) endotoxins, and (9) lysosomal enzymes.[1,31,35,38,39,40] Interpretation of the presence of certain substances, such as in the enzyme studies, must be done with reservations since there is very little material available for analysis, contamination of the samples with saliva is an ever present problem, and the task of distinguishing between the two possible enzyme sources—cells of the host or the local microflora—is difficult.

Previously, measuring this minute crevicular fluid required the staining technique using ninhydrin (triketohydrindene hydrate, which is specific for α-amino groups).[29,41] Recently, there was developed an instrument* (Fig. 6-80) that electronically measures discrete fluid volumes by the reduction in capacitance between two sensors when in contact with a standardized filter-paper strip containing the fluid to be measured. Shern et al.[42] compared the ninhydrin-staining method and the crevicular fluid flow meter (Harco) for quantifying human crevicular fluid flow. They found that "precision, accuracy and reliability of measur-

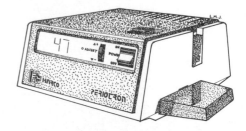

Fig. 6-80. Periotron is an instrument used to measure minute volumes of gingival crevicular fluid. Sterile filter paper strips are used to collect crevicular fluid and placed between sensor jaws to right of machine by lowering of level. On screen will appear digital reading which is converted to microliters by division of digital number of 200. (Harco Electronics Ltd., Winnipeg, Manitoba, Canada.)

ing crevicular flow proved greater using a flow meter than using the ninhydrin dye method." Suppipat[43] investigated the use of the HAR-600 Gingival Crevice Fluid Meter* in clinical research and found measuring gingival crevicular fluid to be a sensitive and objective method for evaluating the condition of the marginal gingiva (using the orifice method for fluid collection). Golub and Kleinberg[44] found that "evidence has accummulated indicating that monitoring GCF flow can be used to detect subclinical gingival pathology, quantify the severity of gingival inflammation, and objectively monitor the response of the gingivae to periodontal therapy. . . ." Egelberg and Attström[45] determined the orifice method (after Löe and Holm-Pedersen[24]; Fig. 6-81) of collecting crevicular fluid samples (using standardized sterile filter-paper strips) had less statistical variation between samples compared to intracrevicular sampling (placing the filter-paper strip deep within the sulcus). Jameson,[46] using a crevicular fluid meter (Harco; Fig. 6-80) compared human crevicular volumes from restored (full-coverage) and non-

---

*Harco Electronics, Ltd., Winnipeg, Manitoba, Canada.

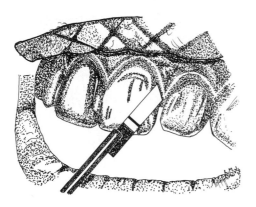

Fig. 6-81. Gingival crevicular fluid collection using sterile filter paper strip and standardized collecting procedure. Note collection site has been thoroughly dried and isolated with cotton rolls.

restored teeth using an orifice collecting technique (after Löe and Holm-Pedersen[24]; Fig. 6-81) and found a significantly greater volume of crevicular fluid from restored teeth compared to the contralateral nonrestored tooth of the same patient. He concluded, "Subclinical inflammatory changes associated with subgingival full-coverage restorations can be objectively and quantitatively measured using standardized techniques and a gingival crevicular fluid meter."

Theories regarding the origin of crevicular fluid have centered around the controversy of classifying it as a normal physiologic filtration product[25] or as an inflammatory exudate.[24] The problem has been complicated because of the variation in collection techniques, which results in some investigators recording fluid flow from clinically normal gingival tissues and others noting its absence under the same situations. Alfano[47] proposed that gingival crevicular fluid arises by two distinct mechanisms: (1) the generation of a standing osmotic gradient generated by macromolecular by-products of the bacteria present in the subgingival plaque colony and (2) the initiation of the

classic inflammatory response. Pashley[48] viewed gingival fluid production as resulting from the release of mediators of inflammation causing increased capillary pressure and leakage of plasma proteins into intersitial fluid. He postulated that "the low compliance of gingival tissue and the high hydraulic conductance of sulcular epithelium result in this interstitial fluid moving from connective tissue into the sulcus." The studies involving crevicular fluid flow are relatively new and through further research its origin will be more clearly delineated.

FACTORS AFFECTING GINGIVAL RESPONSE

Comprehensive diagnostic procedures coupled with a rational and individualistic sequential treatment plan are much discussed topics but frequently given cursory attention in restorative rehabilitation. The complete diagnosis should include (1) a clinical exam reviewing all existing conditions thoroughly, (2) radiographs, and (3) elimination of any dentally related pain, if present. Judicious judgment in formulating a treatment plan means *not* placing fixed bridgework where a tooth has been missing for many years with no adverse results, *not* using one reconstructive technique universally on all the different occlusal patterns and variations that patients present, and being aware of those clinical situations that are known to provide difficult oral rehabilitation problems (see Brecker, S. C.: J. Prosthet. Dent. 9(6):1001-1016, Nov.-Dec. 1959). Thus successful restorative procedures necessitate "scholarly diagnosis, formulating a logical treatment sequence according to relative importance, with built-in flexibility and meticulous implementation. . . ."[49]

The type of restorative material used will govern the amount of tooth reduction and influence the location of the gingival margin and the type of preparation termination (Fig. 6-82). Trivedi and Talim[50]

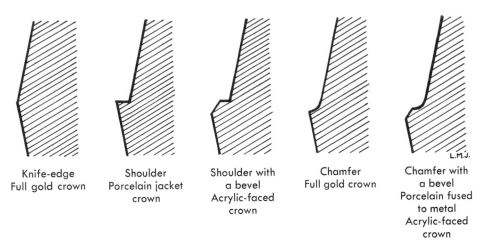

| Knife-edge
Full gold crown | Shoulder
Porcelain jacket
crown | Shoulder with
a bevel
Acrylic-faced
crown | Chamfer
Full gold crown | Chamfer with
a bevel
Porcelain fused
to metal
Acrylic-faced
crown |

Fig. 6-82. Correct selection of gingival termination to meet requirements of restorative material and of patient is prerequisite for favorable gingival response to final restoration.

studied the response of the human gingiva to amalgam, silicate cement, acrylic resin, and gold by histologic examination and concluded, "The gingival response appeared to be caused by chemical injury, unpolished restorative materials, poor marginal adaptation and inadequate oral hygiene." Waerhaug's[51] histologic evaluation of gingival response to restorative materials showed that gingival inflammation occurred from plaque and was not necessarily initiated by the nature of the material or its surface roughness. Löe[52] stated that investigations have shown "that any known type of dental restoration extending into the subgingival area causes damage to the periodontal tissues, either by providing possibilities for bacterial retention and/or by a direct irritational effect of the material per se. . . ." Wise and Dykema[53] cautioned against making any definitive clinical implications from their study, but reported that (1) there was no statistical difference between plaque-retaining capacities of heat-cured resins and porcelain, (2) porcelain had a statistically significant lower plaque-retaining capacity than did ceramometal gold (precious), and (3) acrylic resin (heat cured) had a statistically significant lower plaque-retaining capacity than that for type III gold and ceramometal gold (precious).

Those situations (Table 6-1 and Fig. 6-83) necessitating subgingival margins should be executed with meticulous care and should begin with careful probing (with a periodontal probe) of the sulcus (Fig. 6-84) around the entire perimeter of the tooth. Knowing the exact location of the sulcus bottom should be used as a guide during the instrumentation procedures for the gingival termination (Fig. 6-85). Orban et al.[54] have stated that "in removing the whole enamel of the tooth to which the epithelium is still attached, recession of the gum margin will follow." Encroachment on the attachment apparatus either by high-speed instrumentation or electrosurgical retraction procedures[55] will result in recession. This has been documented by Valderhaug and Birkeland[56] by following patients over a 5-year period of time who had crown margins placed subgingivally, at the gingival crest, and supragingivally. Their results showed that (1) initially 65% of the crown margins were subgingival compared to 41% 5 years later and (2) subgingival crown margins had an increase

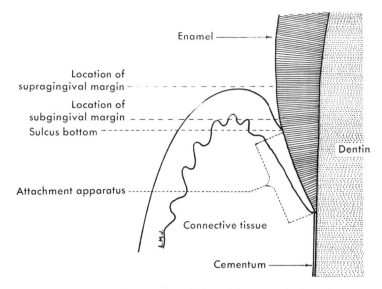

Fig. 6-83. Gingival termination in relationship to periodontal structures.

Table 6-1. Gingival termination guide*

	Supra-gingival	Subgin-gival
DMF rate		
High		X
Moderate		X
Low	X	
Age		
55 or older	X	
21 to 54	X	
Under 20 years		X
Present or projected oral hygiene		
Excellent	X	
Good	X	
Fair		X
Poor		X
Postperiodontal	X	
Cosmetic compromise anteriorly		X
Crown-root ratio		
Favorable	X	
Deficient vertically		X

*Location of the gingival termination should be determined for each individual case by the dentist.

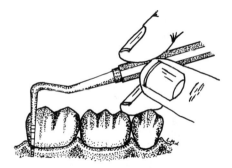

Fig. 6-84. Determine depth of sulcus around entire perimeter of tooth for proper gingival termination in those cases necessitating subgingival margins. (Glickman periodontal probe no. 26G.)

in gingival index[23] scores, pocket depth, and loss of attachment compared to supragingival placement. Similarly Newcomb[57] found that (1) "the nearer a subgingival crown margin approaches the base of the gingival crevice, the more likely it is that severe gingival inflammation will occur," and (2) "the least inflammation is observed when subgingival crown margins are placed at the gingival crest or just into the gingival crevice." Many authors[54,56-59] have provided additional research concerning the detrimental effects of subgingival margins and others[8,10,14,60-62] recommend supragingival margins whenever esthetics, DMF rate, and vertical space permit.

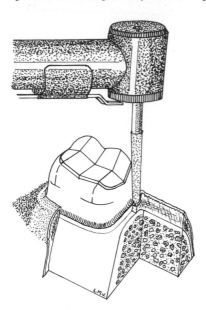

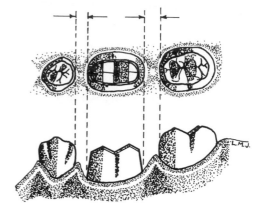

Fig. 6-87. Adequate interproximal reduction of the preparation is necessary to prevent stagnation of interdental papillae and col area.

Fig. 6-85. Careful execution of subgingival termination procedures will minimize disruption of sulcular epithelial integrity. High-speed rotary instrument should not penetrate below previously measured sulcular depth (see Fig. 6-84). (Full crown preparation on mandibular right first molar using a chamfer gingival termination.)

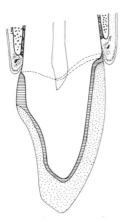

Fig. 6-86. Diagrammatic cross section of porcelain-fused-to-metal restoration on maxillary central incisor illustrating the relationship of preparation to pulpal tissue and gingival termination to sulcus. Lingual termination is chamfer, whereas labially there is a chamfer with a bevel. *Horizontally hatched area,* Precious metal substructure; *stippled area,* porcelain.

The concern for crown-margin placement is well substantiated since maxillary anterior teeth on women are the most frequently restored dental segment,[63,64] a fact that means an increased use of porcelain fused to metal[64] (Fig. 6-86) and subgingival margins (esthetic compromise anteriorly; Table 6-1). Table 6-1 was developed as a guide to margin placement and indicates the many complex factors that must be carefully evaluated by the restorative dentist before beginning treatment.

Preparation of the teeth for a prosthesis is an arduous procedure demanding physical exertion, fine technical skill, acute visual perception, and intelligent clinical judgment. Favorable gingival response is greatly dependent on proper preparations. Overcontoured crowns is generally attributed to inadequate tooth preparation,[2,62] particularly the proximal surfaces (Fig. 6-87). "If insufficient tooth structure is removed during preparation, the dental laboratory technician will overcontour the crown to obtain appropriate thickness of metal."[62] This problem is further exaggerated for veneer materials, such as procelain fused to metal,[11] which require specific thicknesses for desirable shade characteristics. Another

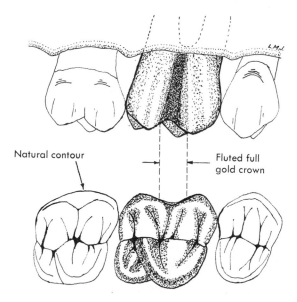

Natural contour

Fluted full gold crown

Fig. 6-88. Fluting incorporated into final cast crown contour in patient who has undergone periodontal surgery. Fluting enables accessibility for plaque removal by patient.

overlooked area is associated with preparations involving postperiodontal exposure of furcations. The preparation should be fluted by accentuation of the buccal groove, and the anatomic form thus created should be reproduced in the final crown contour (Fig. 6-88) so that adequate accessibility is provided to the patient for plaque removal.[2,3,14,20]

Minimizing disruption of the integrity of the gingiva during the preparation phase must also carry over to the retraction procedures prior to taking the impression. The less injury incurred by the attachment apparatus and the unkeratinized oral sulcular epithelium (Fig. 6-79) the more favorable the gingival response to the final restoration. Harrison[65] working with dogs and various retraction materials found that (1) mechanical and chemical retraction materials do temporarily injure the gingival sulcus epithelium and (2) a retraction cord with 8% epinephrine or 100% alum solution to control heavy bleeding or seepage may be used for retraction times of 5 to 10 minutes. Woycheshin[66] in a similar study found that (1) zinc chloride is caustic and prolonged application will cauterize tissue, (2) epinephrine applied to lacerated tissue will be absorbed and result in an increased heart rate and blood pressure, which are dangerous for patients with cardiovascular disease, hyperthyroidism, and hypersensitive individuals, and (3) application of high concentrations of epinephrine to lacerated or abraded gingival tissue should be avoided. Reiman[67] described a procedure to avoid this by exposing subgingival margins using epinephrine—impregnated retraction cord prior to placing the subgingival termination and retracting after the procedure using untreated cotton cord and an additional cotton cord treated with aluminum chloride. Nemetz[68] described a specific instrumentation procedure of judicious use of electrosurgery, proper bevel placement (for porcelain-fused-to-metal preparations), aluminum sulfate—impregnated cord and properly contoured provisional restorations.

Use of electrosurgery as a retraction procedure must follow established guidelines[52] to avoid injury[69] and ensure favorable healing. These include (1) using a fully rectified instrument, (2) proceeding through tissue in a swift and audacious manner, (3) selecting thin diameter tips[70] (minimizing heat buildup), and (4) avoiding areas with potential excessive recession because of soft- and hard-tissue architecture (specifically, lingual of maxillary molars, distobuccal root of maxillary molars, lingual of mandibular molars, and labial of anterior incisors particularly the canine eminence.[55] The contraindications for electrosurgery are (1) patients with pacemakers or systemic limitations to any surgical procedure, (2) patients in whom the healing process is belated by a debilitating disease (such as collagen disturbances), and (3) patients who have received head and neck radiation.[55]

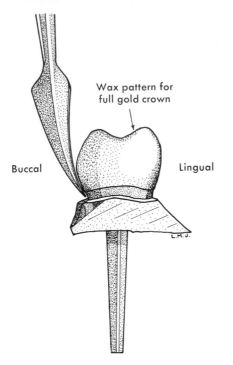

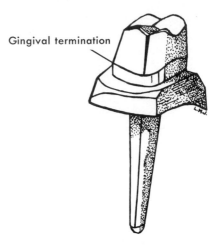

Fig. 6-90. Carefully trimmed dies provide for correct location of margin in wax pattern. Lingual view of full gold crown preparation on maxillary left first molar with knife-edge gingival termination.

Fig. 6-89. Developing physiologic buccal and lingual contours in wax pattern will save time and material and ensure favorable tissue response. Instrument shown is a Roach carver. Mesial view of mandibular right first molar.

All procedures previously discussed concerning final crown contours also apply to acrylic temporary crown contours, with particular emphasis on embrasure areas. These areas should be free of temporary cement, they should have minimal tissue contact, and they should have accessibility for oral hygiene procedures built into their design. Placing cold-cure acrylic in contact with abraded gingiva will delay healing and may ultimately affect the gingival response to the final restoration; therefore it is imperative that all coronal surfaces of the temporary be highly polished.

To ensure correct margin placement for the final restoration, it is recommended that the restorative dentist trim the prepared die (Fig. 6-89). The person preparing the tooth has the best capability for determining the precise marginal termination of the preparation (Fig. 6-90).

Creating physiologic contours is best obtained by the laboratory technician in the wax pattern (Fig. 6-88) *not* after casting during the polishing procedures. Burch[71] has established dimensional guides based on natural tooth contours for the laboratory technician to use as an aid in obtaining these contours. These include the following: (1) the lingual convexity should not protrude more than 0.5 mm beyond the cementoenamel junction, (2) proximal surfaces should be flat or slightly concave buccolingually and occlusocervically (for papillae and gingival col health), and (3) the faciolingual width should not exceed 1 mm beyond the faciolingual width at the cementoenamel junction. It is the responsibility of the dentist to inform the laboratory technician concerning the development of proper crown contours, since he only has stone representations of biologic structures.

A review of the literature on the relationship between full crown restorations and the gingiva shows that even the best margin is at least 30 μm open,[72] that plaque grows in this space,[17] some plaque bacteria even have an affinity for certain cements,[73] and histologic evaluation of gingival tissue from extensive oral rehabilitation cases may have detrimental soft-tissue effects.[74,75] A bleak picture confronts the restorative dentist; however, new and better materials and techniques are on the horizon and much has yet to be learned among patients concerning their clinically observable variation to restorative materials. Reported cases of excessive bone loss[76] without the presence of the aforementioned known etiologic factors associated with periodontal disease makes Osler's[77] assertion even more meaningful: "It is much more important to know what sort of a patient has a disease, than what sort of disease a patient has!"

Restorative dentistry is preventive dentistry when the dentist uses scholarly diagnosis, follows a logical sequence of treatment with meticulous and empathetic implementation, and follows the admonition, *Primum non nocere* (Above all else, do no harm).

REFERENCES

1. Schroeder, H. E., and Listgarten, M. A.: Monographs in developmental biology. Vol. 2, Fine structure of the developing epithelial attachment of human teeth, Basel, Switzerland, 1971, S. Karger, AG.
2. Kornfeld, M.: Mouth rehabilitation clinical and laboratory procedures, ed. 2, St. Louis, 1974, The C. V. Mosby Co., vol. 1, pp. 167-181.
3. Wheeler, R. C.: Complete crown form and the periodontium, J. Prosthet. Dent. 11(4):722-734, July-Aug. 1961.
4. Amsterdam, M., and Fox, L.: Provisional splinting—principles and technics, Dent. Clin. North Am., pp. 73-99, 1959.
5. Cohen, D. W., and Chacker, F. M.: Criteria for selection of one treatment plan over another, Dent. Clin. North Am. 8:3, 1964.
6. Coomer, O. B.: Occlusion in operative dentistry, J.A.D.A. 58:34, 1959.
7. Dummett, C. O.: Advances made in determining the local etiology of periodontitis, Periodontics 4:322, 1966.
8. Glickman, I.: Clinical periodontology—preven-
tion, diagnosis, and treatment of periodontal disease in the practice of dentistry, ed. 4, Philadelphia, 1972, W. B. Saunders Co.
9. Goldman, H. M., and Cohen, D. W.: Periodontal therapy, ed. 5, St. Louis, 1973, The C. V. Mosby Co.
10. Grant, D. A., Stern, I. B., and Everett, F. G.: Orban's periodontics—a concept-theory and practice, ed. 4, St. Louis, 1972, The C. V. Mosby Co.
11. Graver, H. T.: Restorative dentistry must be preventive dentistry, J. Prevent. Dent. 3(5): 17-29, Sept.-Oct. 1976.
12. Ingraham, R., and Koser, J. R.: An atlas of gold foil and rubber dam procedures, Buena Park, Calif., 1961, West Orange County Publishing Co.
13. Ramfjord, S.: Local factors in periodontal disease, J.A.D.A. 44:647, 1952.
14. Eissmann, H. F., Radke, R. A., and Noble, W. H.: Physiologic design criteria for fixed dental restorations, Dent. Clin. North Am. 15(3): 543-568, July 1971.
15. Hazen, S. P., and Osborne, J. W.: Relationship of operative dentistry to periodontal health, Dent. Clin. North Am., pp. 245-254, March 1967.
16. Morris, M. L.: Artificial crown contours and gingival health, J. Prosthet. Dent. 12(6):1146-1156, Nov.-Dec. 1962.
17. Parkinson, C. F.: Excessive crown contours facilitate endemic plaque niches, J. Prosthet. Dent. 35(4):424-429, April 1976.
18. Perel, M. L.: Axial crown contours, J. Prosthet. Dent. 25:642-649, 1971.
19. Perel, M. L.: Periodontal considerations of crown contours, J. Prosthet. Dent. 26(6):627-630, Dec. 1971.
20. Yuodelis, R. A., Weaver, J. D., and Sapkos, S.: Facial and lingual contours of artificial complete crown restorations and their effects on the periodontium, J. Prosthet. Dent. 29(1):61-66, Jan. 1973.
21. Sackett, B. P., Gildenhuys, R. R.: The effect of axial crown overcontour on adolescents, J. Periodontol. 47(6):320-323, June 1976.
22. Vogan, W. I.: The effect of bucco-lingual crown contours on gingival health, J. Prevent. Dent. 3(4):30-31, July-Aug. 1976.
23. Löe, H.: The gingival index, the plaque index, and the retention index systems, J. Periodontol. 38:61, 1967.
24. Löe, H., and Holm-Pedersen, P.: Absence and presence of fluid from normal and inflamed gingivae, Periodontics 3(4):171-177, July-Aug. 1965.
25. Waerhaug, J.: The gingival pocket. Anatomy, pathology, deepening and elimination, Odont. Tidskrift 60:suppl. 1, 1952.

26. Brill, N., and Björn, H.: Passage of tissue fluid into human gingival pockets, Acta Odontol. Scand. **17**:11-21, 1959.

27. Brill, N., and Krasse, B.: Effect of mechanical stimulation on flow of tissue fluid through gingival pocket epithelium, Acta Odontol. Scand. **17**:115-130, 1959.

28. Brill, N.: Influence of capillary permeability on flow of tissue fluid into gingival pockets, Acta Odontol. Scand. **17**:23-33, 1959.

29. Brill, N.: Effect of chewing on flow of tissue fluid into human gingival pockets, Acta Odontol. Scand. **17**:277-281, 1959.

30. Brill, N.: Removal of particles and bacteria from gingival pockets by tissue fluid, Acta Odontol. Scand. **17**:431-440, 1959.

31. Brill, N., and Brönnestam, R.: Immuno-electrophoretic study of tissue fluid from gingival pockets, Acta Odontol. Scand. **18**:95-100, 1960.

32. Brill, N.: The gingival pocket fluid, Acta Odontol. Scand. **20**:suppl. 32, 1962.

33. Mann, W. V., Jr.: The correlation of gingivitis pocket depth and exudate from the gingival crevice. J. Periodontol. **34**:379-387, 1963.

34. Egelberg, J.: Gingival exudate measurements for evaluation of inflammatory changes of the gingivae, Odontol. Revy **15**:381-398, 1964.

35. Cimasoni, G.: Monographs in oral science, Vol. 3, The crevicular fluid, Basel, Switzerland, 1974, S. Karger, AG.

36. Skapski, H., and Lehner, T.: A crevicular washing method for investigating immune components of crevicular fluid in man, J. Periodontol. Res. **11**(1):19-24, 1976.

37. Weinstein, E., Mandel, I. D., Salkin, A., Oshrain, H. I., and Pappas, G. D.: Studies of gingival fluid, Periodontics **5**(4):161-166, July-Aug. 1967.

38. Brandtzaeg, P., and Mann, W. V., Jr.: A comparative study of the lysozyme activity of human gingival pocket fluid, serum, and saliva, Acta Odontol. Scand. **22**:441-455, 1964.

39. Carraro, J. J., Milstein, S., Sznajder, N., and Zdrojewski, D.: Electoforesis en agar del flúido gingival de encías normales, Rev. Asoc. Odontol. Argentina **52**:77-80, March 1964; Dent. Abstr. **9**:680, Nov. 1964.

40. Gustafsson, G. T., and Nilsson, I. M.: Fibrinolytic activity in fluid from gingival crevice, Proc. Soc. Exp. Biol. Med. **106**:277-280, 1961.

41. Daneshmand, H., and Wade, A. B.: Correlation between gingival fluid measurements and macroscopic and microscopic characteristics of gingival tissue, J. Periodontol. Res. **11**(1):35-46, Feb. 1976.

42. Shern, R. J., Von Mohr, G., and Joly, O.: Crevicular fluid flow and cytopathology as objective clinical measurements, J. Dent. Res. **53**: 175, Feb. 1974.

43. Suppipat, N.: The use of the HAR-600 Gingival Crevice Fluid Meter in clinical research (unpublished master's thesis), University of Oslo, Norway, 1976.

44. Golub, L. M., and Kleinberg, I.: Gingival crevicular fluid: a new diagnostic aid in managing the periodontal patient, Oral Sci. Rev. **8**:49, 1976.

45. Egelberg, J., and Attström, R.: Comparison between orifice and intracrevicular methods of sampling gingival fluid, J. Periodontol. Res. **8**(6):384-388, 1973.

46. Jameson, L. M.: Comparison of the volume of crevicular fluid from restored and nonrestored teeth (unpublished master's thesis), Loyola University Dental School of Chicago, 1976.

47. Alfano, M. C.: The origin of gingival fluid, J. Theor. Biol. **47**:127-136, 1974.

48. Pashley, D. H.: A mechanistic analysis of gingival fluid production, J. Periodontol. Res. **2**(2):121-135, April 1976.

49. McElroy, D. L., and Malone, W. F.: Handbook of oral diagnosis and treatment planning, Baltimore, 1969, The Williams and Wilkins Co., pp. 172-176.

50. Trivedi, S. C., and Talim, S. T.: The response of human gingiva to restorative materials, J. Prosthet. Dent. **29**(1):73-80, Jan. 1973.

51. Waerhaug, J.: Histologic considerations which govern where the margins of restorations should be located in relation to the gingiva, Dent. Clin. North Am., pp. 161-176, March 1976.

52. Löe, H.: Reactions of marginal periodontal tissues to restorative procedures, Int. Dent. J. **18**(41):759-778, Sept. 1962.

53. Wise, M. D., and Dykema, R. W.: The plaque-retaining capacity of four dental materials, J. Prosthet. Dent. **33**(2):178-190, Feb. 1975.

54. Orban, B., and Mueller, E.: The gingival crevice, Am. Dent. Assoc. J. **16**(7):1206-1242, July 1929.

55. Malone, W. F.: Electrosurgery in dentistry; theory and application in clinical practice, Springfield, Ill., 1974, Charles C Thomas, Publisher, pp. 97-113.

56. Valderhaug, J., and Birkeland, J. M.: Peridontal conditions in patients 5 years following insertion of fixed prostheses, J. Oral Rehabil. **3**: 237-243, 1976.

57. Newcomb, G. M.: The relationship between the location of subgingival crown margins and gingival inflammation, J. Periodontol. **45**:151-154, 1974.

58. Larato, D. C.: Effects of artificial crown margin extension and tooth brushing frequency on gingival pocket depth, J. Prosthet. Dent. **34**(6): 640-643, Dec. 1975.

59. Marcum, J. S.: The effect of crown marginal

depth upon gingival tissue, J. Prosthet. Dent. **17**(5):479-487, May 1967.

60. Burch, J. G.: Periodontal considerations in operative dentistry, J. Prosthet. Dent. **34**(2): 156-163, Aug. 1975.

61. Kahn, A. E.: Partial versus full coverage, J. Prosthet. Dent. **10**(1):167-178, Jan.-Feb. 1960.

62. Palomo, F., and Peden, J.: Periodontal considerations of restorative procedures, J. Prosthet. Dent. **36**(4):387-394, Oct. 1976.

63. Tylman, S. D.: Theory and practice of crown and fixed partial prosthodontics (bridge), ed. 6, St. Louis, 1970, The C. V. Mosby Co., pp. 94-96.

64. Valderhaug, J., and Karlsen, K.: Frequency and location of artificial crowns and fixed partial dentures constructed at a dental school, J. Oral Rehabil. **3**:75-81, 1976.

65. Harrison, J. D.: Effect of retraction materials on the gingival sulcus epithelium, J. Prosthet. Dent. **11**(3):514-521, May-June 1961.

66. Woycheshin, F. F.: An evaluation of the drugs used for gingival retraction, J. Prosthet. Dent. **14**(4):769-776, July-Aug. 1964.

67. Reiman, M. B.: Exposure of subgingival margins by nonsurgical gingival displacement, J. Prosthet. Dent. **36**(6):649-654, Dec. 1976.

68. Nemetz, H.: Tissue management in fixed prosthodontics, J. Prosthet. Dent. **31**(6):628-635, June 1974.

69. Wilhelmsen, N. R., Ramfjord, S. P., and Blankenship, J. R.: Effects of electrosurgery on the gingival attachment in rhesus monkeys, J. Periodontol. **47**(3):160-170, March 1976.

70. Noble, W. H., McClatchey, K. D., and Douglass, G. D.: A histologic comparison of effects of electrosurgical resection using different electrodes, J. Prosthet. Dent. **35**(5):575-579, May 1976.

71. Burch, J. G.: Ten rules for developing crown contours in restorations, Dent. Clin. North Am. **15**(3):611-618, July 1971.

72. Saltzber, D. S., Ceravolo, F. J., Holstein, F., Groom, G., and Gottsegen, R.: Scanning electron microscope study of the junction between restorations and gingival cavosurface margins, J. prosthet. Dent. **36**(5):517-522, Nov. 1976.

73. Ørstavik, D., and Ørstavik, J.: *In vitro* attachment of *Streptococcus sanguis* to dental crown and bridge cements, J. Oral Rehabil. **3**:139-144, 1976.

74. Antonoff, S. J.: The paradoxes of fixed prosthodontics, J. Prosthet. Dent. **34**(2):164-169, Aug. 1975.

75. Mahajan, M.: Histological evaluation of gingiva in complete crown restorations. (Master's thesis), Loyola University Dental School of Chicago, 1976.

76. DeMarco, T. J.: Periodontal emotional stress syndrome, J. Periodontol. **47**(2):767-768, Feb. 1976.

77. Dubos, R.: Mirage of health utopias, progress, and biological changes, New York, 1959, Harper & Row, Publishers, p. 143.

7

Tissue dilation for cast metal restorative procedures

James D. Harrison and William J. Kelly, Jr.

There are several terms in general use today for exposing cavity margins when making impressions of prepared teeth to receive cast metal restorations. In this chapter, the term used is "tissue dilation" and the preceding definition is synonymous with "tissue retraction" or "tissue displacement." This procedure is one of the key factors in obtaining accurate duplication of subgingival cavity margins. One must use an exacting technique to obtain excellent and consistent results. For any tissue-dilation procedure, it is imperative that the dentist work with essentially healthy clinical gingiva if predictable results are desired.

The rationale for a tissue-dilation procedure does not start with exposing the cavity margin, since the previous management of the gingival tissue is also important to the success of the technique. The patient must have healthy gingival tissue, because inflamed tissue does not provide a proper foundation for tissue dilation. In addition, one must maintain the tissue in a healthy state after the impression is made by placing exacting treatment restorations on the prepared teeth. (See Chapter 11 on treatment bridges.)

In addition, patients needing cast metal restorations or other restorative procedures should establish a good oral hygiene program to maintain the health of the gingival tissues. If gingival surgery was indicated, the tissue should be fully matured before preparations are made and tissue dilation is done. Usually, the healing of the gingival tissue after surgery varies, but a minimum of 3 weeks should elapse before preparations and tissue-dilation procedures are done.[1] Tissue shrinkage that may occur after tissue-dilation procedures can result from a traumatic procedure or any of the preceding if done incorrectly.

CLASSIFICATION

The most widespread classification for tissue dilation is as follows:

1. Mechanical—the tissue is pushed away or dilated by strictly mechanical methods.
2. Mechanicochemical—a cord is used for mechanically dilating the tissue away from the cavity margin and is impregnated with a chemical to stop any bleeding or tissue-fluid seepage during the impression making.
3. Surgical—a small ribbon of gingival tissue is removed from the sulcus around the cavity margin by dental electrosurgery. This procedure produces a space in the tissue around the tooth, controls bleeding or seepage, and provides a trough for the impression material.

The cast metal preparations must be made as carefully as possible to minimize tissue laceration when it is necessary to

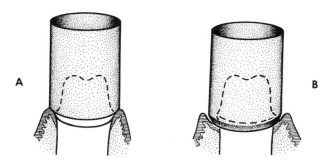

Fig. 7-1. A, Oversized copper band should be about 2 mm wider than mesiodistal width of tooth. B, Gingival surface is trimmed and contoured inward to allow band to just clear cavity margin during impression procedure.

finish the cavity margin beneath the crest of the gingival tissue. The dentist can reduce tissue laceration by (1) initially carrying the preparation margin to just above the existing tissue and by (2) creating a sulcus space by a dilation procedure. This procedure allows for improved vision and a more exacting margin refinement. If the mechanical or mechanicochemical method is used for dilation, the entire procedure will usually have to be repeated before an additional impression is made. When one uses the surgical (electrosurgical) method, the tissue-dilation procedure does not have to be repeated. Only cleansing and spot coagulation to control bleeding or seepage may be necessary. Additionally, some practitioners prefer to pack an astringent medicated cord into the surgical trough for control of seepage or bleeding.

Elastic impression materials will not displace blood, saliva, debris, or tissue; therefore the tissue must be displaced laterally or a small ribbon of tissue must be removed to expose the cavity margin before making an impression of the preparation. The tissue adjacent to the exposed cavity margin must also be dry and clean to obtain an accurate impression.

MECHANICAL TISSUE DILATION

Mechanical dilation may be used effectively, but the procedure must be done

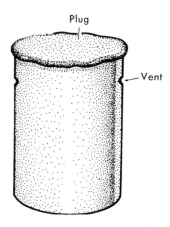

Fig. 7-2. Band with plug and vent for individual cast restorations.

carefully to minimize trauma to the tissue. Oversized copper bands can be contoured to the gingival outline and contoured inward toward the cavity margin when gently pushed over the tooth (Fig. 7-1). A resin or compound plug is placed on the top for stability and the band is vented to allow for escape of excess rubber base or silicone impression material (Fig. 7-2).

One must be careful not to push the band down with too much pressure or the tissue may be stripped away from the tooth. Since tissue dilation can be done efficiently and effectively by other methods, mechanical dilation is of minimal value today.

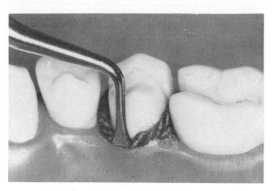

Fig. 7-3. Cord packed in sulcus with small blunt or serrated instrument.

MECHANICOCHEMICAL DILATION

This procedure uses cords impregnated with chemicals and is gently tucked into the gingival sulcus beneath the cavity margin (Fig. 7-3). Again, one must be careful to minimize trauma to prevent tissue recession. The area must be kept dry for maximum effectiveness of the styptic or hemostatic chemical in the cord. After 5 to 10 minutes the cord is gently removed and the crevice is examined to determine if the cavity margin is exposed and that any bleeding or tissue seepage has been controlled. If any bleeding or seepage is still present, the crevice must be repacked for an additional 5 minutes.

Cords impregnated with alum (various aluminum sulfates) or aluminum chloride provide a styptic action to control bleeding or seepage. If a hemostatic agent is needed, 1:1000 solution of epinephrine can usually be used with safety. However, we do not recommend the use of hemostatic agents like epinephrine in patients with cardiac problems.[2,3]

SURGICAL TISSUE DILATION

Continuous visualization of the subgingival margin has long been one of the most difficult areas in crown and bridge for the dental practitioner. Cords, chemicals, rubber or leather rings, copper,

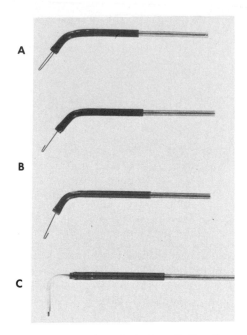

Fig. 7-4. Electrodes of choice. **A,** Continuous loop. **B,** J loops, left and right. **C,** AP 1½.

stainless steel and aluminum bands, and a host of other materials, either alone or in combination, have been employed with various success over the years.[4,5] With the refinement of the electronic circuits and techniques that are now available through dental electrosurgery, many of the impression problems, especially in securing multiple abutment preparation, can be overcome.[6]

The choice of current for subgingival margin exposure preferred by the authors is electrosection. The working electrodes will vary, depending on tooth form and tooth position in the mouth. This can be done with little or no patient discomfort in a relatively bloodless field. With each electrode the basic rules of electrosurgery must not be disregarded. The working electrode must be clean and with little or no carbonization. In precise marginal dilation, the carbonized electrode has a tendency to drag, which tears the tissue and usually results in bleeding. If a continuous loop or a modified loop is

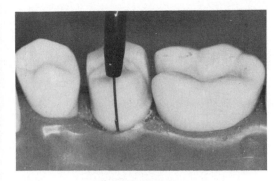

Fig. 7-5. J loop in position to establish a sub-gingival trough. Open end is 1.5 mm and is used to gage depth of trough.

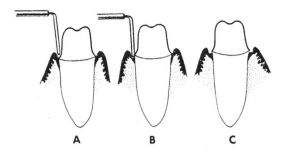

Fig. 7-6. A, Continuous-loop electrode in gingival sulcus. **B,** Electrode in position beneath cavity margin. **C,** Subgingival trough extending 0.2 mm beneath cavity margin.

used, such as the J loop, these may need to be cleaned between each pass around the tooth. The AP 1½ J loops, or the continuous loop, is most often the electrode of choice (Fig. 7-4). With the J loop, the long side of the loop is held against the tooth, and by observing the short side of the J, one can calculate the depth of the created sulcus (Fig. 7-5). To properly expose the margins using J loops, one must use a right and left J loop.[7]

The depth of tissue removal is determined by the location of the subgingival margin. The tissue trough should extend about 0.2 mm below the margin to provide definite margin detection in the impression and on the master dies. Fig. 7-6 diagrammatically illustrates making a subgingival trough by use of a continuous-loop electrode. When a continuous loop or J loop is used, there may be a small amount of tissue left beneath the margin because of the shape of the loop. This tissue tag should be removed with a single-wire or variable-tip electrode (Fig. 7-7). The variable-tip electrode wire can be pushed in or pulled out to the desired length. Fig. 7-8 illustrates electrosurgical tissue dilation on a premolar crown preparation by use of a continuous-loop electrode.

With the AP 1½ working electrode the insulated side of the electrode is carried around the tooth, removing the gingival

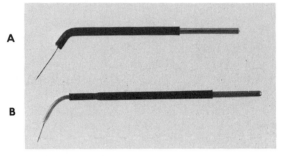

Fig. 7-7. A, Straight-wire electrode. **B,** Variable-tip electrode.

sulcular epithelium (Fig. 7-9). The 1½ designation indicates that the working tip extends 1½ mm beyond the insulation, therefore giving one a known sulcus depth. If a less depth in the subgingival trough is desired, one may remove (grind off) part of the tip to create the desired depth.

A technique that is gaining in popularity is the use of the "variable-tip" or straight-wire electrode. The crown preparation with the desired margin is performed by termination of all margins just shy of the existing soft tissue. One adjusts the single wire (variable tip) to the desired subgingival depth, and circumscribes the tooth by making several passes around the tooth *in segments;* that is, the lingual subgingival trough is established, then the buccal area followed

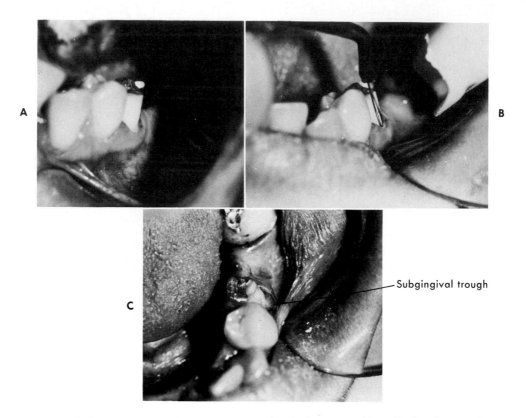

Fig. 7-8. A, Premolar veneer crown preparation before troughing. **B,** Continuous-loop electrode used for tissue dilation. **C,** Subgingival tissue trough after electrosection.

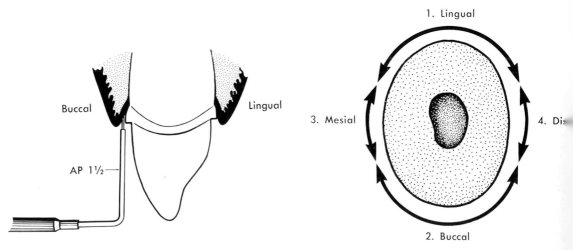

Fig. 7-9. Buccolingual view of AP 1½ in position for creating subgingival trough.

Fig. 7-10. Suggested sequence, *1-4,* to establish subgingival trough.

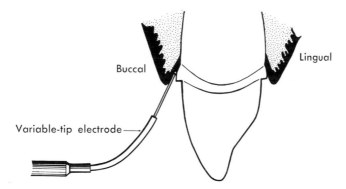

Fig. 7-11. Buccolingual view of variable-tip electrode in position for creating subgingival trough.

by the mesial and distal (Fig. 7-10). When the procedure is done in this manner, a buildup of any heat in the tissue is avoided. For most operators, it is virtually impossible to circumscribe a tooth with one or two connecting passes. If a straight-needle electrode or the variable-tip electrode is used, the operator may find that the electrode is too fine to remove enough tissue to get an adequate bulk of impression material into the sulcus. This is especially true if the end of the working electrode is held parallel with the long axis of the tooth. By angling the working electrode approximately 30 degrees and carrying the tip through the tissue until it rests against the tooth, a small wedge of tissue (worm) will be lifted out (Fig. 7-11). If bleeding does occur, it is usually interproximal and can be easily controlled by use of the same electrode and by touching the bleeding area using the coagulation current. Another method is the use of hydrogen peroxide and water, equal parts, to stop slight local hemorrhage. After the area is dried, the extended sulcus area should be debris free and easily visualized. The margins can then be finished to the desired depth, the area again flushed either with water or with water and peroxide, and the impressions secured.

In the anterior area of the mouth where the gingivae are especially thin, the angle at which the working electrode is held is modified to more nearly parallel the long axis of the tooth. Again with the segmented approach, the sulcular epithelium is removed, and if a narrow buccolingual sulcus has been created, cord may be placed prior to the impression to hold the tissue away from the tooth. It is imperative that the intermediate (temporary) restoration be properly adapted to the existing margins and that no luting material be allowed to impinge on the regenerating sulcular epithelium.

We opine that any impression must extend 0.2 mm below the cavity margin to assure accuracy. The use of electrosurgery to remove a ribbon of tissue around the cavity margin provides necessary space for adequate bulk of the elastic impression material as does the extension below the cavity margin.

After securing the final impression(s), tincture of myrrh and benzoin (50:50 solution) should be placed on any area subjected to surgery, air dried, and repeated five to seven times before the temporary or treatment restoration is placed. The tissue healing is rapid and a properly executed subgingival trough heals in 5 to 7 days.[8]

SUMMARY

The exposure of the cavity margin for making elastic impressions of cast metal restorations must be done with precision. Mechanical tissue dilation is limited in usage because of the great possibility of tissue trauma and resulting shrinkage of tissue.

The use of the mechanicochemical method with cords can be accomplished with less traumatic consequences but can be time consuming. Also, one must remember that once the cord is removed, the tissue will start returning to its original position and this movement may result in a thin layer of elastic impression material at the cavity margin. This can result in margin distortion of the individual dies because the impression lacks stability in bulk of the material at a critical area.

The use of dental electrosurgery provides a rapid, efficient method for tissue dilation, provides adequate bulk of impression material at the cavity margin, and, correctly done, does not cause any clinically significant shrinkage of the tissue.

SELECTED REFERENCES

1. Glickman, I.: Clinical periodontology, ed. 3, Philadelphia, 1964, W. B. Saunders Co., pp. 576-577.
2. Harrison, J. D.: Effect of retraction materials on the gingival sulcus epithelium, J. Prosthet. Dent. **11:**514, May-June 1961.
3. Harrison, J. D.: Current therapy in dentistry, St. Louis, 1964, The C. V. Mosby Co., vol. 1, pp. 193-195.
4. Tylman, S. D.: Theory and practice of crown and fixed partial prosthodontics (bridge), ed. 6, St. Louis, 1970, The C. V. Mosby Co., pp. 403-410.
5. Johnston, J. F., Phillips, R. W., and Dykema, R. W.: Modern practice in crown and bridge prosthodontics, ed. 3, Philadelphia, 1971, W. B. Saunders Co., pp. 183-190.
6. Malone, W. F.: Electrosurgery in dentistry theory and application in clinical practice, Springfield, Ill., 1975, Charles C Thomas, Publisher, pp. 1-15.
7. Oringer, M. J.: Electrosurgery in dentistry, ed. 2, Philadelphia, 1975, W. B. Saunders Co., pp. 419-452.
8. Harrison, J. D., and Kelly, W. J.: Tissue response to electrosurgery. In Malone, W., editor: Electrosurgery in dentistry, Springfield, Ill., 1975, Charles C Thomas, Publisher, pp. 186-206.

8

Impression materials for cast metal restorative procedures

James L. Sandrik and Hosea F. Sawyer

The historic development of modern impression materials spans a relatively brief period of time from about 1925 to the present. Prior to this period, materials such as waxes, plaster, and compound were used with varying degrees of success. It is no coincidence that the mid-1920s witnessed an immense development in the science of dental materials, for this was the period of development of the American Dental Association Council on Dental Materials and Devices. The A.D.A. was to have both a direct as well as indirect influence on the quality of materials used in dentistry. Up to this time, anyone with the financial resources could develop and introduce a material to a very receptive profession that was undergoing an immense technologic as well as intellectual development.

The nonelastomeric impression materials were used for impressions of dental problems before the introduction of some of the complex polymer impression materials used in dentistry today. Specifically, these materials are gypsum, impression compound, and zinc oxide–eugenol–based impression material.

New techniques resulting from new instrumentation demanded higher quality materials. Although plaster was capable of reproducing very fine detail as well as maintaining superb dimensional stability, its inelastic properties left a great deal to be desired.

The competitive manufacturers of gypsum critically control the setting expansion, setting time, and consistency of this material. The setting expansion, vital to the accuracy of each individual impression, is generally controlled from 0.06% to 0.5%. Mathematically, this is equal to approximately 0.005 inches (0.127 mm). It is obvious to anyone who has worked with gypsum as an impression material that it has many severe undesirable characteristics. Although it assumes an early set and can be read easily, it often is difficult to separate from a working cast. Advantageously, it is not an unesthetic material and has been made to have an acceptable taste. For the most part, the material makes an ideal mucostatic impression that will not displace loose or fibrous tissue. When used in the preparation of fixed or removable partial dentures, it is generally as an indexing material, where it may be combined with starch to produce an index that will dissolve in hot water. The use of gypsum in general must be classed as very limited.

IMPRESSION COMPOUND

Impression compound is composed essentially of natural products such as resin, copal resins, carnauba wax, and stearic acid. However, the exact composition of a particular brand is proprietary. Generally, this material is limited to edentulous primary impressions. It can sometimes be

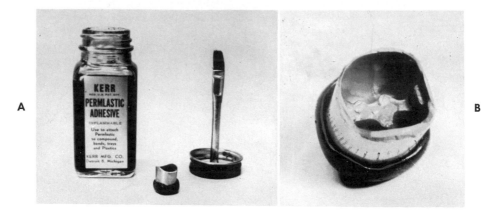

Fig. 8-1. A, Inside of band and occlusal stop painted with adhesive. **B,** Modeling compound used to close occlusal end of band before taking impression in mercaptan impression material. (Courtesy Kerr Manufacturing Co., Romulus, Mich.)

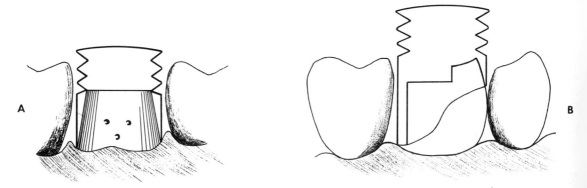

Fig. 8-2. A, Preparing band for single tooth impression. **B,** Reenforcings and closing occlusal end of band to be used for single impression. (Courtesy Kerr Manufacturing Co., Romulus, Mich.)

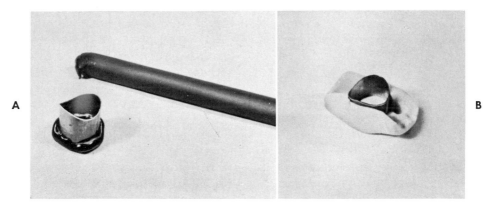

Fig. 8-3. A, Compressomatic cap fitted to curvature of gingiva prior to filling with impression material for complete crown preparation. **B,** Cap trimmed for intracoronal impression. (Courtesy L. L. Greene and N. A. Greene.)

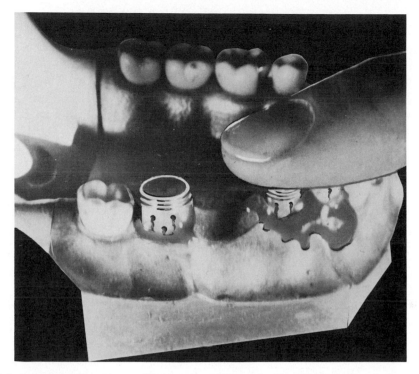

Fig. 8-4. *Left,* Filled cap in position over prepared tooth. *Right,* Bellows of cap compressed while impression material is placed into gingival crevice. (Courtesy L. L. Greene and N. A. Greene.)

removed from undercuts but generally distorts on removal. It is not appreciably esthetic or tasteful. Occasionally dentists will use this material in individualized copper bands for single tooth impressions (Figs. 8-1 to 8-4). This technique is described in detail in Chapter 21 of Tylman's sixth edition. When used in copper bands for single impressions, the material exhibits undesirable thermal expansion and contraction in addition to deleterious flow and distortion after hardening. This material in general has very limited potential or use in the practice of fixed partial dentures.

ZINC OXIDE–EUGENOL PASTES

Zinc oxide–eugenol (ZOE) pastes were developed for taking impressions of the tissues of edentulous patients. ZOE had been used for quite a number of years as a temporary filling material and was

found to be an excellent material for use as a secondary or wash impression. It registered fine detail and was nearly as dimensionally stable as plaster; however, it also is a brittle material and as such cannot be used where undercuts are present, such as in fixed prosthetics or partial denture cases.

Zinc oxide–eugenol impression paste is generally used in full dental construction for a final impression. However, it may also be used as a corrective lining in a preliminary impression. Many prosthodontists use zinc oxide–eugenol paste as a liner for a full denture base in an attempt to make a tissue-based contact. Often, because of its consistency and softness, this material can be used as an interocclusal recorder in conjunction with a bite-registration tray. Incidentally, before mixing, the material presents a very unesthetic appearance, but its main objectionable characteristics are odor, taste, and causing tissue sensitivity. It generally has a reasonable setting time, and its detailed method of hardening is described in Chapter 7 of *Skinner's Science of Dental Materials*, seventh edition, by Phillips.

In an attempt to overcome the objectionable sensitivities in certain patients, a noneugenol material is available commercially. The dimensional stability of ZOE impression materials is considered to be the best available nonelastomeric impression material.

HYDROCOLLOIDS

In 1925 agar-agar was introduced as the first elastic impression material capable of being removed from undercut areas without fracturing. Although there were and are drawbacks to the material, it was heralded as a significant advance in removable prosthodontics. However, agar hydrocolloid was not used for fixed prosthetics until the late 1930s. Two rather serious drawbacks were to accrue from the use of agar-agar as an impression material. The first was a strongly retarding effect on gypsum products, resulting in

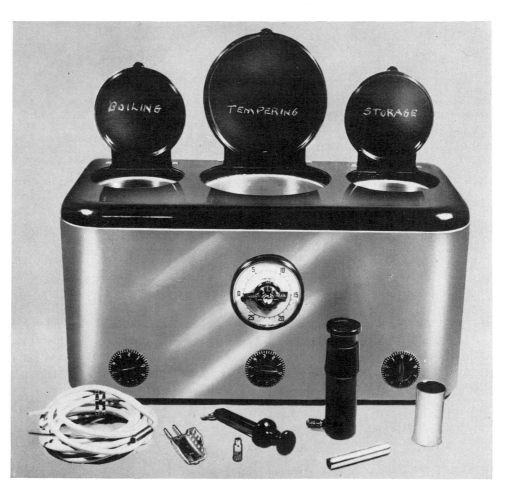

Fig. 8-5. Hydrocolloid conditioner with accessory equipment. (Courtesy Dr. Morris J. Thompson, Oklahoma City, Okla.)

casts with chalky or soft surfaces. The second was the rapid shrinkage of the impression after removal from the mouth. Both drawbacks have largely been overcome by addition of potent gypsum-product accelerators, which effectively overcame the retarding effects of the colloidal nature of agar, and the latter drawback is simply overcome by immediate filling of the impression with the cast material.

Hydrocolloid is by definition a colloid with water as a dispersion medium. There are two general types of hydrocolloids that may be used in the direct technique. One is the agar-agar type, which is reversible from the liquid to the solid and the solid to the liquid. The second is the irreversible or alginate type of material. The agar-agar type is obtained from seaweed and sets or gels at a temperature at or above mouth temperature. There are three baths necessary to prepare the impression material for the mouth (Fig. 8-5). One bath of boiling water is the liquification bath. Once the material has been liquified either in a syringe or tubes, it is placed in a storage chamber of 145° to 150° F until it is ready for use. The material in the syringe is never allowed to drop below this temperature (Fig. 8-6). However, the material to be placed in a tray is tempered in the third bath from 102° to 105° F. This is necessary because if some large bulk of material was introduced directly into the patient's mouth from the storage bath, it would not only be uncomfortable but also would burn soft tissue adjacent to the bridge being prepared. After the syringe material has been injected into the gingival crevice (Figs. 8-7 and 8-8), the tray is seated over the area to be impressioned. Before the tray is filled with hydrocolloid and placed in the storage bath, definite stops must be made in the tray to be sure that it always seats itself in the same position. The gingival crevice may be opened mechanically with cotton string or dilated with electrosurgical techniques. It is absolutely essential that

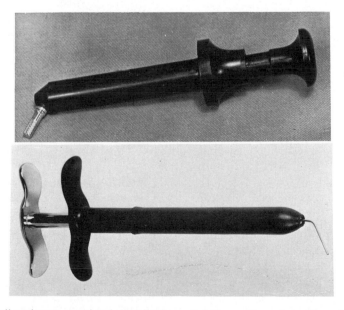

Fig. 8-6. Small syringes used to inject hydrocolloid in cavity preparation. (Courtesy Dr. Morris J. Thompson, Oklahoma City, Okla.)

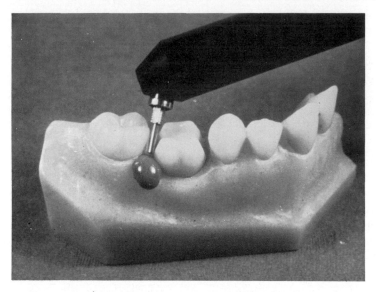

Fig. 8-7. Location of initial injection of hydrocolloid in gingival interproximal area. (Courtesy Dr. Morris J. Thompson, Oklahoma City, Okla.)

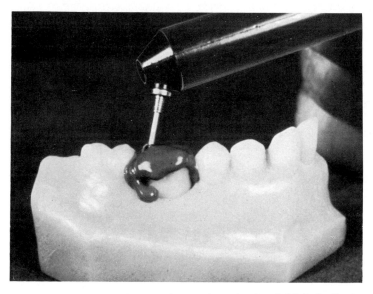

Fig. 8-8. Covering occlusal surface and rest of tooth after initial gingival application of hydrocolloid. (Courtesy Dr. Morris J. Thompson, Oklahoma City, Okla.)

all bleeding or seepage be stopped before the application of this impression material. Reversible hydrocolloid will not displace any tissue fluids or saliva. As a matter of fact, there is a tendency for the gingival crevice to close on this impression material in an attempt to squeeze it out of the sulcus while the material is setting. After the placement of the tray over the impression area (Fig. 8-9), room temperature water should be circulated initially through the impression tray, followed by colder and colder water until the agar-agar has set—approximately 5 to

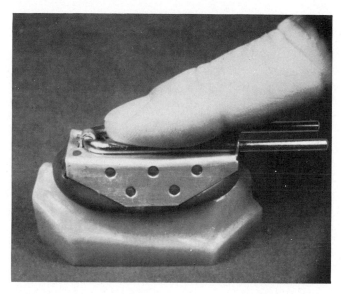

Fig. 8-9. Tray and properly tempered hydrocolloid are positioned over covered abutments and held in place without any movement until complete gelation of hydrocolloid has taken place in water-cooled tray. (Courtesy Dr. Morris J. Thompson, Oklahoma City, Okla.)

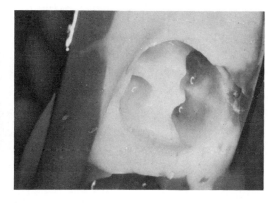

Fig. 8-10. Final hydrocolloid impression of preparation for complex inlay preparation.

Table 8-1. Mean deviations of stone casts from a master die in 0.0001 inch

	Alginate 1	Alginate 2	Agar-agar
Vertical mean	−68	−158	−9
Horizontal mean	14	32	7

6 minutes. The tray must be held immobile and firmly so that it has been seated in accord with the stops or indexing material previously placed in the tray (Fig. 8-10). The accuracy of casts made from hydrocolloid impressions designated it as a very accurate impression material when the cast is poured immediately (Table 8-1). The material is esthetic and possesses a tolerable taste and a pleasant odor. It is a team procedure and definitely should not be handled solely by the dentist.

Like agar the alginates are elastic impression materials, but here the similarity ends. They are not so accurate nor do they reproduce the fine detail that the dentist came to expect from agar. Being elastic and capable of removal from undercuts, they were a moderately acceptable substitute for agar and superior to waxes and compound.

The alginate impression materials are more convenient to use and require less elaborate equipment than does agar and for these reasons it continued to be used for some time after agar again became available. After the outbreak of World War II, the supply of Japanese kelp (the raw material used in the preparation of agar) was cut off, resulting in a severe shortage of elastic impression material.

The dimensional stability of alginate and effect on gypsum casts is similar to that experienced with agar.

The alginate hydrocolloids, however, can easily be handled by one person but are better utilized when an assistant is available. In general, the alginate hydrocolloids are used in removable partial denture construction, although dentists use it for fixed partial dentures and general restorative dentistry for their opposing models and templates for treatment restorations. In general, the material is not used with the syringe injection technique but is applied to the area to be impressioned with a wiping motion of the finger. The tray material when placed in the tray without stops is carefully seated over the impressioned area so that the impression material is not perforated. This material measures easily, smells good, is esthetic, but produces cases that are generally not acceptable bases for castings. (See Tylman's sixth edition). Some alginates are not compatable with dental stone and consequently do not produce smooth accurate cases.

ELASTOMERIC IMPRESSION MATERIALS

The elastomeric impression materials are soft and rubberlike. These materials are easily stretched, and they snap back to their relaxed state when the stress is removed. Consequently, these materials are generally called "rubber impression materials."

During the early 1950s a new material was developed that possessed an elasticity similar to the hydrocolloids but without the deleterious effects on gypsum casts. This material was developed by the Thiokal Corporation and is known as polysulfide impression material, a synthetic rather than natural product, unlike the

other impression materials that preceded it. Two pastes are mixed together (Fig. 8-11) resulting in a rapidly polymerizing or vulcanizing elastic polymer, thus the expression "elastomer." The polysulfides were considered by many to be much more convenient than agar and considerably more dimensionally stable than either of the hydrocolloids. Although they are somewhat less accurate than is agar, one need not pour the gypsum cast immediately and as such achieved almost immediate acceptance by the profession.

Polysulfide rubber

The first material to be discussed will be that of the polysulfide impression materials. Lead peroxide is used as an accelerator in the system. Consequently, these impression materials are known as the lead peroxide systems. The physical appearance before and after mixing is unesthetic, and they are smelly. This material is best used in a custom-made tray (Fig. 8-12) when the thickness of the rubber is approximately 2 to 4 mm (Fig. 8-13). The second most accurate group uses, as an alternative to lead peroxide, an organic hydroperoxide or copper hydroxide. These materials mix and behave much like their lead peroxide cousins. These materials too should be used in a custom tray where a constant thickness of material is required.

Silicone polymers

Silicone synthetic polymers were to follow shortly after the development of the polysulfides but were not acceptable for use as impression materials until the mid- to late 1950s. These new elastomers possessed two distinct advantages over the polysulfides: a more pleasant appearance (white or pink as opposed to chocolate brown) and absence of the repulsive sulfide odor. However, it was only after a considerable effort that the drawbacks of short shelf life and dimensional instability were lessened. At present, both

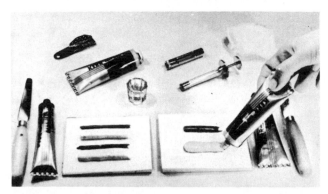

Fig. 8-11. Mercaptan impression materials, light and heavy, with complete armamentarium for their use. (Courtesy Kerr Manufacturing Co., Romulus, Mich.)

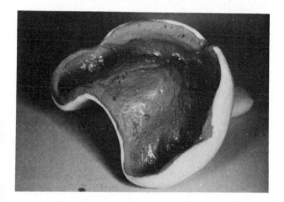

Fig. 8-12. Custom tray with heavy-body mercaptan rubber impression of patient's released diagnostic cast. Light-bodied material may be injected and placed in impression tray for reline technique.

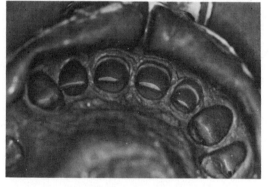

Fig. 8-13. Mercaptan rubber impression for three porcelain-fused-to-metal crowns. Note distinctive definition of labial level.

polysulfide and silicone impression materials are extensively used and capable of a high degree of acceptability and accuracy when used in light of their limitations.

Polyethers

An innovative development in elastomeric impression materials occurred in Germany about 1965. A generically distinct elastomer, polyether, was produced that was found to possess an astonishing accuracy and dimensional stability. Unlike any of the other elastomers, the polyether impression materials do not suffer from continued polymerization after removal from the mouth. As such, the long-term accuracy of impressions made from these polymers can be expected. They do suffer however from one drawback; that is, they are rather stiff when set. They are also somewhat less elastic than the polysulfides and silicones. Because of these properties, proximal tears may occur when the impressions are removed from severe undercuts. Nonetheless, the polyethers are clearly the most accurate and dimensionally stable of the elastomers and do not appear to suffer from long-term storage prior to mixing.

Although the polyether impression materials were developed in the mid-1960s, they did not become available in the U.S.A. until 1973. Since then at least one new product has been developed in this country and marketed in 1975. It is termed "polythioether" and is intended as a custom tray or primary impression material into which is placed a conventional polysulfide secondary impression material.

The polyether materials produce the most accurate casts that we have been able to make to date. The material mixes easily, and it does not have an objectionable odor. When set however, it is more rigid as compared to the other elastomers. This would be a definite disadvantage in involved periodontal cases, extreme undercuts, and previously placed fixed bridges, unless the undercuts were removed before the impression was made. Again a custom tray should be used. The mixing and spatulation of elastic materials are eloquently described in Chapter 10 in *Skinner's Science of Dental Materials*, by Phillips. Furthermore, most instructions included in each package of the material include descriptive literature that specifically explains the procedures for mixing. The polyether rubber is the only material of this group developed at this time that need not be poured immediately. All other materials will produce cases that have deviations from a master die within the first minute after removal. Because of the high degree of dimensional stability, the polyether impressions may be stored for a considerable period before being poured. None of the polyether impression materials should be stored in any type of solution because of their hydrophilic characteristics.

These materials in general have the ability to displace tissue fluids and saliva to a small degree. As the reader can see, each material has some desirable characteristics and some undesirable characteristics, and the material chosen should be the one that fits the requirements of the impression to be made.

Addition silicones

The most recent development in elastomeric impression materials is the addition silicones, incorrectly referred to as polysiloxane by some dental manufacturers. These materials were first marketed in this country in 1975. They differ from the original silicones, referred to earlier, in their method of polymerization. These materials set by means of an addition polymerization. As a result, they do not yield a by-product, such as ethyl alcohol, and have been shown to be a substantial improvement over the older silicones particularly with regard to dimensional stability.

The esthetics, manipulative properties, and other characteristics are similar to the original silicone polymers. In a recent study by Ciesco it was shown that the addition silicones have a dimensional stability similar to the polyethers. When these materials were adhesively bound to a custom tray, they demonstrated a dimensional stability statistically identical to the polyethers.

CRITERIA FOR SELECTION OF AN ELASTIC IMPRESSION MATERIAL

From the foregoing, one can see that there are several acceptable materials available for preparing gypsum casts of oral structures. The choice of the proper material for use in fixed prosthodontics is dependent on several factors, which may include cost, shelf life, accuracy (immediate and time dependent), ease of handling, and patient acceptance.

Alginate hydrocolloid, by virtue of its inability to reproduce fine detail coupled with its poor time-dependent dimensional stability, can be ruled out for use in fixed prosthodontics. Its low cost and ease of handling, however, often present a temptation that the dentist ought to avoid. On the other hand, the agar hydrocolloids possess a high degree of immediate accuracy, reproduce fine detail well, and are low in cost. The one serious drawback is the absolute requirement that the impression be poured immediately. The cost of water-cooled trays and conditioning units are trivial when compared to the cost of the polymeric materials.

Impressions that are to be sent to a laboratory where the gypsum is to be fabricated present serious problems that require careful consideration. The recently introduced polyether impression materials have eliminated the primary cause of ill-fitting cast metal restorations; that is, the time-dependent dimensional change that these materials undergo is very small and may be neglected in most instances. Once the material has set in the patient's mouth, very little change in shape is likely to occur. This behavior is attributable to the rate and extent of polymerization. Five minutes after being mixed, the polymer has completed its formation, and upon removal from the patient's mouth, polymerization shrinkage will not affect the dimensions of the impression. In addition, there is no by-product formed on polymerization. In contrast, the silicone and polysulfide materials give off water, alcohol, and other volatiles. The evaporation of these by-products is likely to result in small and unpredictable stresses that can cause the impression to slowly change shape. Because of the high degree of dimensional stability, the polyether impression may safely be sent to a laboratory without concern for dimensional change.

The relatively short working time (typically less than 2 minutes) of the polyether impression materials may be a cause of concern to some clinicians, but this is easily overcome with experience. A serious drawback and cause of some concern in specific cases is the stiffness of the set material. Although elastic, it is less so than the silicone and polysulfide materials. Severe undercuts and periodon-

tally involved patients may present some difficulty. In addition, the relatively high cost may be a consideration that has to be dealt with. However, all things considered, the superior accuracy, dimensional stability, ease of manipulation, patient acceptance, and long shelf life are extremely attractive.

Acceptable alternatives to the polyether impression materials are the silicone and polysulfide impression materials. Both are capable of very fine reproduction and very good immediate accuracy. Both suffer from time-dependent dimensional change—the silicones more so than the polysulfides. The most significant drawback to the polysulfides is the unpleasant odor and color, as well as staining potential to clothing. The polysulfide impression materials are the least expensive of the elastomers, an attractive consideration. When poured soon after removal from the mouth, they produce very suitable gypsum casts. In fact, some specific brands of this material possess excellent dimensional stability. Unfortunately, this information is not readily available to the clinician. As such, polysulfide impressions ought not to be sent to distant laboratories.

The attraction of silicone impression materials is their esthetics and patient acceptance. They are generally pleasantly colored, do not possess an unpleasant odor or taste, and are relatively easy to remove from clothing when set. As noted above, their main drawback is dimensional change with time. Like the polysulfides, some brands appear more acceptable than others. An additional drawback is the relatively short shelf life coupled with a propensity to separate in the tubes on standing. A clear liquid (the silicone monomer) may be seen to precede the white base on extrusion from the tube. This may or may not present a problem; however, it would be decidedly unwise to prepare an impression from a material that exhibited this problem.

Dimensional stability, the change in accuracy with respect to time, is an important criterion for selecting a particular elastomeric impression material. Ciesco found that when any elastomer was bound with adhesive to a custom tray the initial accuracy of all the above materials were statistically identical. In addition, he found that the dimensional stability was also significantly improved. It was only after 72 hours that differences began to become apparent. This clearly points out the importance of a properly prepared custom tray particularly for conventional polysulfide and silicone impressions that are to be sent to a dental laboratory. Although disposable or stock trays do find some utility in dental practice, they should be avoided except in those instances where casts are prepared within a few hours from the time the impression is taken.

SUMMARY

When drawbacks and advantages are carefully considered, the order of acceptability of elastic impression materials would appear to be, beginning with the most acceptable: polyether, agar, polysulfide, silicone, and alginate.

GENERAL REFERENCES

Mann, A. W.: A critical appraisal of the hydrocolloid technique—its advantages and disadvantages, J. Prosthet. Dent. 1:773, Nov. 1951.

Morrow, R. M., Brown, C. E., de Loriner, B. E., Powell, J. A., Rudd, J. M., and Rudd, K. D.: Compatability of alginate impression materials and dental stone, J. Prosthet. Dent. 25:554-566, 1971.

Myers, G. E., and Stuelsman, D. G.: Factors that affect the accuracy and dimensional stability of the mercaptan rubber base impression materials, J. Prosthet. Dent. 10:525, 1960.

Phillips, R. W.: Skinner's science of dental materials, ed. 7, Philadelphia, 1973, W. B. Saunders. Co.

Sawyer, H. F., Birtles, J. T., Neiman, R., et al.: Accuracy of casts produced from seven rubber impression materials, J.A.D.A. 87:126, July 1973.

Sawyer, H. F., Dilts, W. E., Aubrey, M. E., et al.: Accuracy of casts produced from the three classes of elastomer impression materials, J.A.D.A. 89:644, Sept. 1974.

Sawyer, H. F., Sandrik, J. L., and Neiman, R.: Accuracy of casts produced from alignate and hydrocolloid impression material, J.A.D.A. 93(4):806, Oct. 1976.

Sears, A. W.: Hydrocolloid technique for inlays and fixed bridges, Dent. Dig. 43:230, 1937.

Thompson, M. J.: Hydrocolloid, Bull. Okla. State Dent. Assoc. 38:7-24, Oct. 1949.

Tylman, S. D.: Theory and practice of crown and fixed partial prosthodontics (bridge), ed. 6, St. Louis, 1970, The C. V. Mosby Co.

9

Oral histologic considerations for treatment restorations

William F. P. Malone
John E. Flocken

The concept of treatment restorations demands that prepared teeth be covered with protective and functional interim restorations. These restorations should approach, as close as possible, the form and function of the final restoration. Perceptive fabrication of a treatment matrix for teeth prior to or during tooth preparation is essential for an optimal, predictable tissue response. The primary purpose of treatment restorations is to preserve the vitality of the pulp and secure the general comfort of the patient. A treatment restoration also serves as a healing matrix for the gingival tissue surrounding abutment teeth and the edentulous spaces.

TYPES OF TISSUE

The removal of tooth structure obviously results in varying degrees of pulpal hyperemia. Standard texts on oral histology cover the subject of cytology in more detail. However, dentists are keenly interested in the relationship between histologic responses and their profound effect upon restorative dentistry procedures.

Dental tissues are divided into two general groups: the calcified and the noncalcified. Within the calcified group are enamel, dentin, cementum, and the alveolar process. The noncalcified group includes the pulp, the periodontal liga-

ment, and supportive soft tissues (Plate 1).

Enamel

Enamel is the hard tissue that the dentist is routinely involved with and commonly reflects the degree of success or failure of his work. Enamel is generally defined as the material that covers the anatomic crown of a tooth. This calcified tissue is the hardest of animal tissues. The inner surface of the enamel cap is not a smooth surface (Fig. 9-1). It meets the underlying dentin in a series of irregular dentinal processes.[1] This histologic arrangement helps to explain the difficulty in removing enamel during the preparation of a complete crown. Enamel, however, is capable of response to external chemical and physical stimuli. Although considerable didactic attention has been given to the direction of enamel rods during preparation, assurance that enamel walls rest upon sound dentin is a primary premise for restorative dentistry. Enamel has limited inherent strength; so unsupported enamel results in fracture under the forces of mastication.

These histologic features of enamel are of particular importance for preparation. One group of dentists prefers removing all enamel during complete crown preparation because it enables the establishment of a shoulder with optimum angula-

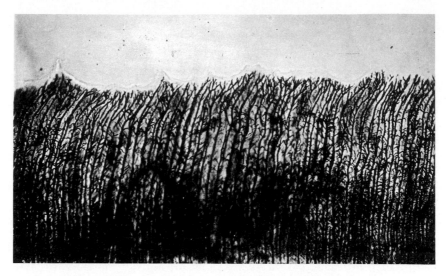

Fig. 9-1. Scalloped union between dentin and enamel.

tion at the cervical line to which the crown may then be accurately fitted. Conversely, another group of dentists claims the removal is neither necessary nor desirable. Accurate shoulder with current high-velocity instrumentation can be prepared in enamel. This approach preserves tooth structure. Also, if all the coronal anatomy is removed from the tapering root, it is difficult, if not impossible, to restore satisfactory anatomy and establish an acceptable gingival margin. The claim or merits of each group are more fully appreciated when gingival crevice and soft-tissue responses are discussed. During preparation the major cutting of the enamel surface is commonly performed with a diamond stone bathed in water. Interim coverage should adequately protect the cavosurface angles of tooth preparations.

Amelogenesis imperfecta. Amelogenesis imperfecta is a mineralization disturbance in which the maturation of the surface enamel is incomplete. The coronal portion of the teeth are truncated and commonly stained a light brownish color. Soft-tissue architecture is poor and bizarre pulpal responses are common. Vertical-dimension determination and the establishment of occlusal relationships are the usual direction of restorative treatment after the initial periodontal therapy. There is seldom caries from lack of proximal contact areas, which leaves the oral cavity relatively free of plaque. Spontaneous pulpal involvement, with the accompanied complications caused by incomplete fusion of cusps during tooth eruption, is common. Complete crowns is the usual course of restorative therapy.[2] Treatment restorations are routinely constructed in the laboratory from mounted casts prior to tooth preparation to aid the establishment of an acceptable vertical dimension.

Dentin

Dentin is a strong connective tissue substance that is calcified but is not considered brittle. The bulk form of the tooth is determined by dentin. Dentin has minute canals containing living protoplasmic extensions of the odontoblasts, which are subject to calcification during aging. The clinical significance of this lies in the fact that younger individuals tend to experience greater sensitivity during operative procedures than do older patients. There are more tubules with greater di-

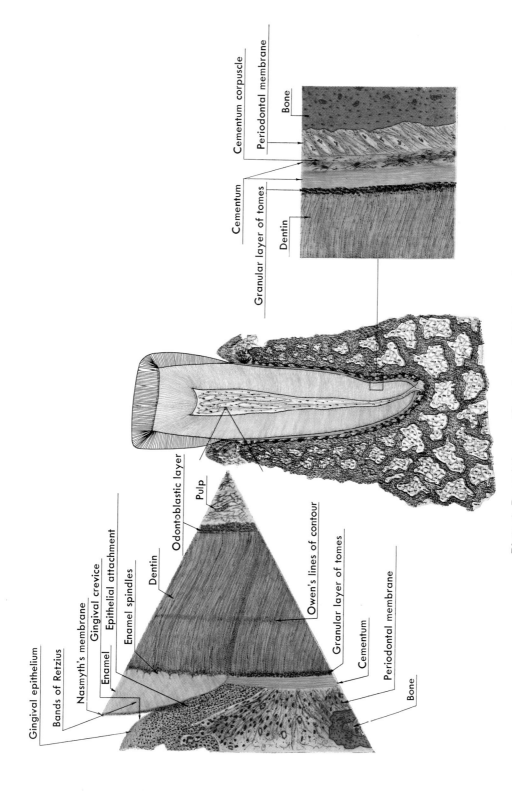

Plate 1. Dental tissues. (Drawing by E. H. Ragan.)

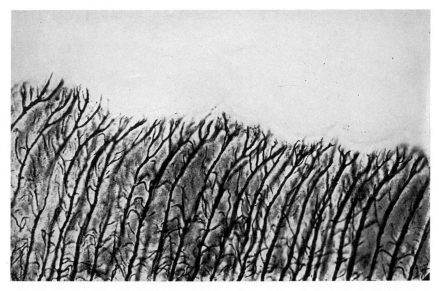

Fig. 9-2. Magnification of dentinoenamel junction showing branchings and anastomoses of dentinal tubules.

ameters and increased anastomosis near the pulp than there are near the peripheral surface that approximates the dentinoenamel junctions (Fig. 9-2). This fact explains the proportional increase in discomfort for the patient as the depth of the preparation approaches the pulp. Dentin has the ability of responding to thermal, mechanical, or other stimuli by depositing more dentin (Fig. 9-3). This secondary dentin biologically safeguards the vitality of the pulp.[3]

The concept of dentin as a vital tissue susceptible to infection is not given sufficient emphasis by dentists. If the nature of a preparation involves exposure of a considerable amount of dentin, every precaution should be taken to prevent bacterial invasion and dessication. Failure to provide adequate protection of dentin contributes to severe hypersensitivity. Alteration of osmotic pressures and changes in surface tension of the cytoplasm within the dentinal tubuli are two reasons for this predictable sensitivity. Medicaments that are used to sedate the tooth after preparation are discussed in Chapters 2 and 20.

Dentinogenesis imperfecta or opalescent dentin. Patients with dentinogenesis imperfecta possess teeth with a bluish gray opalescence (Fig. 9-4, *A*). A microscopic section of this type of dentin reveals a promiscuous distribution of tubules throughout the mass of dentin. Patients with this phenomenon are immune to caries with a pronounced recession of pulps. However, they are subject to incisal fracture and posterior abrasion. Complete crowns are indicated for these patients at an early age (Fig. 9-4, *B*). Programmed laboratory-processed treatment restorations are a preemptive measure to ensure adequate tissue response.

Cementum

Cementum retains the tooth in position by attaching the periodontal membrane fibers to the root of the tooth. Cementum receives its nourishment from the periodontal ligament. Cementum is highly responsive to variable forces. Periodontal fibers are constantly detached and new ones formed with a simultaneous laying down of new cementum that reattaches the new fibers.[4] Endodontic treatment

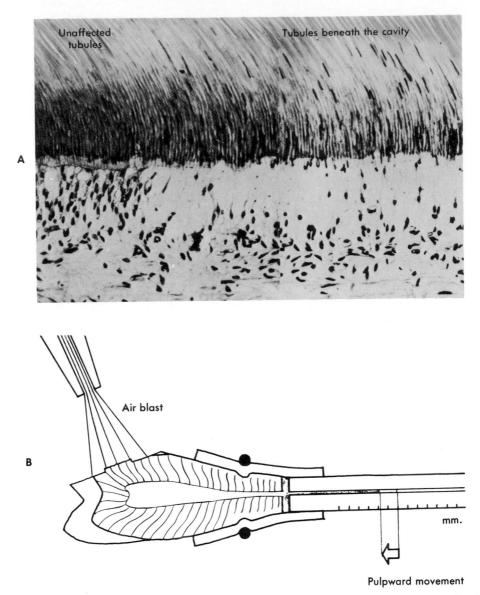

Fig. 9-3. A and **B,** Pulp and dentin adjacent to cavity exposed to airstream for 30 seconds. Odontoblast nuclei in dentinal tubules. Tooth was extracted after 5 minutes. (From Brännström, M.: Acta Odont. Scand. **18:**17, 1960.)

and orthodontic therapy are largely possible because of the biologic versatility of cementum. Thus the clinical significance of cementum in restorative dentistry is obvious. Excessive forces beyond the compensatory ability fo cementum results in resorption, bone reduction, and eventual loss of teeth. Conversely, stimu-

lating forces will initiate root adaption and readjustment to the new conditions by deposition of secondary cementum in layers of varying width.

Alveolar process

For the purposes of fixed prosthodontics it is essential that abutment teeth have

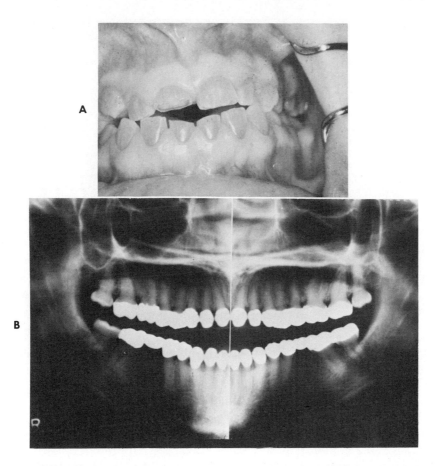

Fig. 9-4. A, Dentinogenesis imperfecta in patient 15 years old. **B,** Patient in **A** restored with complete crowns. Note absence of pulpal tissue. Posterior stops have been maintained. (Courtesy Dr. S. Drab, Villa Park, Ill.)

a "normal amount" or distribution of alveolar bone. Few teeth whose alveolar processes have been reduced by more than half of their original height are suitable for bridge abutments. In teeth out of function one will find that the supporting bone is relatively sparse with irregular, comparatively thin trabeculae, whereas the marrow spaces are enlarged (Fig. 9-5). The clinical significance of this fact becomes apparent when one remembers that placing a fixed prosthesis on teeth that have been out of function for years submits the abutment teeth to an increased load that may be beyond their endurance. A treatment prosthesis, when placed in a light occlusion, initially will assist the teeth in adapting to normal functional stresses.

Alveolar bone is highly sensitive to any changes in the magnitude or direction of transmitted forces. One must keep in mind that the vitality and ability of bone to respond to new stimuli decrease with age. Biologic efficiency decreases in its ability to meet the mechanical requirements of long-span fixed partial dentures in older patients. The utilization of provisional or treatment bridges has been a proposed method to provide a transitional period for the patients to accommodate to fixed prostheses.

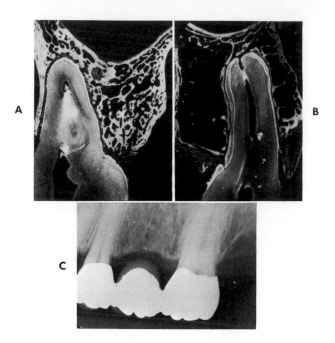

Fig. 9-5, A, Normal tooth. **B,** Functionless tooth. **C,** Adequate supportive structures increase projected longevity of any fixed prosthesis.

Noncalcified tissue

Pulp. One of the more important considerations in placing restorations on vital teeth is to preserve the normal condition of the pulp. Arteries, nerves, and veins of the pulp enter through a small apical foramen. This exposes the pulp to certain dangers. Hildebrand[5] has enumerated four irritants that definitely affect the pulp: (1) mechanical, (2) thermal, (3) chemical, and (4) microbiologic. All forms of irritation can be inflicted upon the dentition during tooth preparation. The dentist must be perceptive enough to assess the recovery ability of a potential abutment and minimize the trauma to the tooth during and after preparation.[6] Coolants during tooth preparation and sedative medicaments placed within adequate treatment bridges usually provide a satisfactory climate for pulpal repair. One source of irritation is repeated exposure of the tooth to oral fluids during fabrication of the fixed prosthesis. Com-

pletion of the tooth preparation in one visit is a decided advantage. Excessive exposure of prepared teeth to desiccation also results in increased sensitivity in each successive appointment. Prolonged use of treatment bridges seated with the more plastic, sedative type of interim sealants compresses the terminal portion of the dentinal tubuli, causing an irritating reaction in the odontoblasts. This condition is usually expressed as subacute pain in the patient. Obtundants, insulators, and general sedative sealants are effective merely as interim measures.

Periodontal ligament. The periodontal ligament is strategically located between the alveolar socket wall and the root of the teeth. It also extends coronally from the area of the gingivae. The "give" in the periodontal ligament is *not* attributable entirely to the elasticity of the fibers when force is exerted. However, when force is removed from these fibers, they return to their original length. One of the more important groups of the principal fibers to the restorative dentist is the free gingival group. It is this group of fibers that keeps the gingivae in close apposition to the crowns. Every reasonable effort to minimize trauma to this group of fibers should be exercised during tooth preparation.

Attaching the root to the alveolar process is only one function of the periodontal ligament. Another equally important function of the fibers is to sustain and dissipate the forces of mastication. The periodontal ligament possesses its characteristic arrangement as the result of functional forces rather than in anticipation of any unusual forces. If the direction or degree of forces is changed, the periodontal fibers adjust themselves to meet the altered conditions. Obviously, if all the groups of periodontal fibers are intact and function properly, the tooth is held more firmly in arch position. Misplaced lateral forces destroy this versatile, adaptive collagenous tissue. The concept of the periodontal ligament's role is one that has the root suspended in a limitless number of expansive, adaptive fibers oriented in different groups and locations. Fig. 9-6 illustrates the direction of forces to which teeth are subjected. Fixed prostheses whose span exceeds the limits of tolerable pound pressure per square inch of vertical pressure simply fail (Fig. 9-7). Exceptions to Ante's law[7,8] are rare, but if a fixed bridge opposes a removable prosthesis, the prognosis is naturally more favorable despite the span.

Gingivae. Gingival responses to any restoration are closely related to the success or failure rate of any operative treatment. Whether there is a union or intimate apposition directly below the restoration is still an academic curiosity. Where and how to terminate a gingival finish line with a minimal amount of trauma to the gingiva is, however, of paramount interest. Clinically, it is also important to know that the height of the

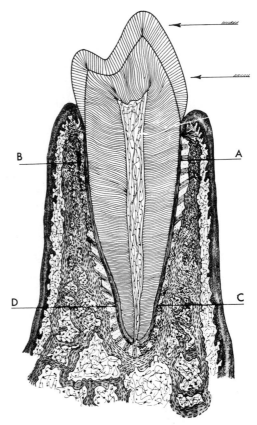

Fig. 9-6. Areas of tension, **A** and **D,** and those of compression, **B** and **C,** in periodontal membrane; center of rotation lies between apical one third and occlusal two thirds of root.

gingival tissue depends largely on the height of the gingival attachment. As stated previously, injury to the attachment directly affects the response of the soft tissue to the restorations or prosthesis. The gingivae, by their general position around the teeth, serve to protect against infection and provide stabilization[9,10] for the entire dentition (Fig. 9-8). Because of high vascularity, the gingivae heal readily. However, the level of gingival recession after tooth preparation with specific tissue-dilation methods and placement of treatment bridges is not always predictable.[11-13]

The placement of the gingival margin

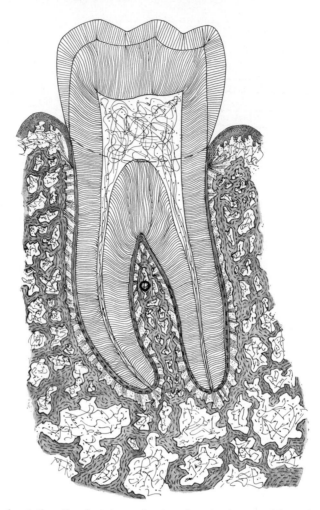

Fig. 9-7. Center of rotation lies in interradicular alveolar bone midway between crest and base.

supragingivally or subgingivally depends largely on the clinical conditions presented by the patient. If one initially decides to place the margin subgingivally, the eventual exposure of the gingival margin of a restoration and the speed with which it occurs depends on many factors, as follows: (1) the age of the patient when the restoration was placed, (2) the gingival health of the patient, (3) the projected oral hygiene of the patient, (4) occlusal relationships, and (5) the presence of any systemic disease. After a period of years, most soft tissue recedes. If, after years of service, the level of tissue is objection-

able because of esthetics, the crowns or bridges can be remade with minimal harm to the tooth or soft tissue. However, overextended or improperly shaped treatment restorations cause irreversible tissue damage. Hasty fabrication of treatment bridges is one of the main causes of adverse tissue responses during construction of a fixed prosthesis.

TREATMENT RESTORATIONS
Temporization

The placement of an interim covering on a tooth after preparation is a biologic mandate to maintain vitality. A satisfac-

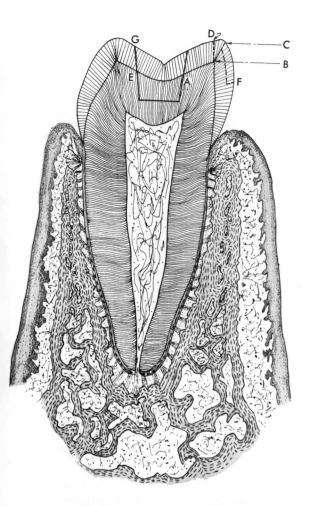

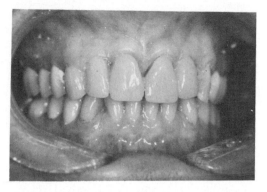

Fig. 9-9. Cold-cure acrylic temporization for anterior treatment restoration made from alginate impression prior to preparations. This material (Scutan) is nonexothermic.

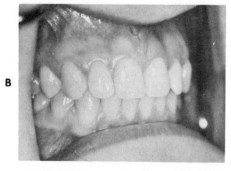

Fig. 9-8. A, Position of gingiva of adolescent in relation to coronal portion of tooth. Gingival area in highly vascular. **B,** Ideal soft-tissue appearance.

tory treatment, matrix restoration, is also necessary to ensure patient comfort and esthetics (Fig. 9-9).

There are three major problems commonly associated with the clinical fabrication of treatment restorations:

1. The time involvement necessary for the fabrication of adequate interim tooth coverage is underestimated by the majority of dentists.
2. Treatment coverage is *not* always replaced by permanent restorations within the shortest possible time.
3. There are presently no inexpensive, tissue-compatible materials that are fabricated by the dentist.

One possible measure to combat these problems is to increase the length of the appointments to prevent hastily constructed treatment restorations. Another measure is to program and coordinate appointment dates with laboratory services to accelerate the date of insertion of the final restorations. Repeated visits by the patient to recement fractured or dislodged interim-coverage restorations taxes the confidence of the patient and is an untenable economic practice for both dentist and patient.[14]

There are eight cardinal requirements for treatment restorations:

1. The pulp of the tooth must be in-

sulated from all forms of adverse stimuli. This includes prevention of leakage of saliva on recently prepared dentin to assure patient comfort.

2. Arch positions of the prepared teeth should be maintained and stabilized to prevent extrusion of teeth and promote the accuracy of the impressions.

3. Treatment restorations should not impinge upon the gingival tissues causing inflammation and unpredictable tissue recession.

4. Interim coverage should appear reasonably esthetic, particularly in the incisor and premolar areas.

5. Treatment restorations should develop occlusal function to assist in the establishment of a satisfactory maxillomandibular relationship.

6. Interim coverage should also possess sufficient inherent strength to withstand light forces of occlusion.

7. Treatment coverage should be fabricated in such a manner to permit the patient to keep the area clean and serve as a healing matrix to tissues surrounding prepared teeth and edentulous areas.

8. Construction techniques of treatment restorations should be within the realm of the average dentist. They also should be capable of being easily removed with minimal damage to the teeth and supportive structures.

The scope of all temporization procedures is large, but universally demeaned because of the intended longevity of the restoration. Nevertheless, ramifications of poorly fabricated treatment restorations commonly haunt the dentist. However, dentists who perform extensive restorative dentistry in one lengthy appointment are also subjected to a fatigue factor. This natural reaction is difficult to combat after lengthy appointments. Preformed or programmed treat-

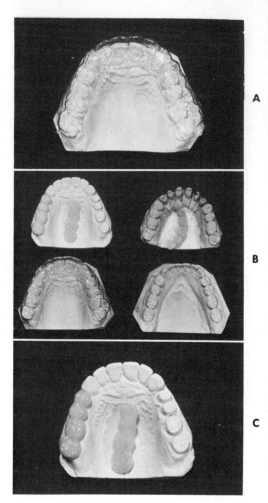

Fig. 9-10. A, Omnivac indirect system of treatment restoration fabrication. Development of esthetics and of desired occlusal relationships is facilitated. **B,** Heat-cured interim coverage from the second set of diagnostic casts. **C,** Minimal tooth preparation on cast provides latitude and direction for dentist during actual tooth preparation.

ment restorations are one way of combating the fatigue problem (Fig. 9-10).

Types of treatment restorations

Treatment restorations can be constructed as single units or as splints with or without edentulous areas. They are composed of metal (precious and nonprecious) and nonmetal materials:

1. Cast metal (precious and nonprecious)
2. Aluminum shell and copper band temporization
3. Preformed commercially processed metal crowns
4. Cellulose acetate crown matrix and polycarbonate crown forms
5. Heat-cured treatment restorations
6. Cold-cured acrylic restorations made from preoperative alginate impressions
7. Template (Omnivac) techniques
8. Post-crown technique

Various techniques can be utilized to fabricate short-term biologically acceptable interim restorations. Dentists commonly use the alginate direct-impression technique, the popular indirect Omnivac approach and commercial preformed treatment restorations. The latter technique is usually restricted to one or two units of treatment restorations.

Fixed prosthodontics have advanced in treatment restorations from the hastily placed aluminum shell crowns to the indirect-direct efficient systems. The Omnivac system represents a perceptive method that elevates temporization techniques to the level of a potential healing matrix.

Cast-metal treatment restorations. Cast-metal treatment restorations are used in conjunction with cases that are difficult to diagnose, for example, patients with maxillomandibular discrepancies that are arduous to implement. The time lapse in cases of this nature is commonly excessive. The cast-metal treatment restoration will perform concomitantly as a preemptive guideline to test the validity, reliability, and practicality of the entire direction of the treatment plan. Cases of this nature are infrequent. The use of a noble metal is prohibitive. Nonprecious metals with a high silver-chromium content is rational if the tissue response to monomer-polymer products is bizarre.

Tap-off lugs are routinely employed to assist periodic removal of these expensive cast treatment restorations. Cast-metal treatment restorations can be truly a healing matrix for prosthodontic cases with an accompanying systemic liability. Another indication for cast-metal type of interim restorations is the maintainance of vertical dimension. All terminal molars can be seated prior to any additional tooth reduction. Treatment restorations made from nonprecious metals help to retain the original interocclusal relationships. Highly polished axial surfaces enhance the tissue-compatible properties of metal. Sandblasted occlusal topography to aid occlusal determinations are also an immeasurable assistance. Duplication of the previous canine function and maintenance of posterior vertical stops can be accomplished in this manner.

Cast-metal treatment restorations would be utilized more frequently if they could be fabricated inexpensively. There is a commercial preformed metal crown that can be modified at the gingival one third. This preformed modified crown form can be invested and cast for a final restoration. This method has merit for future cast-metal healing matrices. Even nonprecious cast-metal treatment restorations remain a luxury for the ordinary fixed prosthodontic procedure. However, the superb tissue response is undeniable (Fig. 9-11).

Aluminum shell crowns. The use of the aluminum shell has been restricted to the premolar and molar area. A shell of suitable diameter is selected and festooned to adapt to the preparation and the height of the gingival crest. To secure the design of the shell to the preparation, a luting medium is placed into the shell. Whenever there are patients with a reduced interocclusal distance, a resin mixture must be placed within the shell. The shell is then removed to be further trimmed for adequate occlusal relationships. After this procedure it is cemented with a sedative-cementing medium.

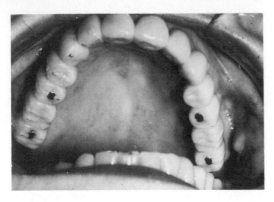

Fig. 9-11. Heat-processed suprastructure restoration for provisionally splinted teeth with telescopic crowns as substructural support. Posterior metal occlusal vertical stops for full maxillary-arch coverage help to mimic prior vertical dimension.

Aluminum shells do possess a consistency that permits a definite amount of molding to a patient's occlusion, but lacks the rigidity for acceptable marginal strength and proximal contacts. With the advent of more tissue-tolerant products, aluminum shell crowns should be infrequently used.

Copper band temporization is unacceptable because of improper tissue relationships and absence of occlusal coverage. Copper bands are desirable for an impression matrix, but seldom, if ever, for interim coverage. Interim coverage for teeth undergoing endodontic treatment are an exception to these guidelines.

Preformed commercial metal crowns. Preformed metal crown forms are employed primarily in the posterior teeth. Notable exceptions are the stainless steel crown forms used in pedodontics for fractured anterior teeth. The preformed metal crowns are a distinct improvement over its predecessor, the aluminum shell crowns or the copper band filled with a medicament. These newer products have improved occlusal and axial surfaces but still remain malleable enough to allow the patient to quickly shape the occlusion

of the treatment restoration. The cervical portion of the improved preformed crowns is also slightly constricted to enable a more tolerable tissue relationship (Fig. 9-12) to exist. Although a certain amount of recession is predictable after preparation, excessive irritation or recession can be prevented by contouring of the gingival margins. Selection of the size of the preformed crown is usually critical for satisfactory tissue response. The time-saving aspect of these preformed commercial products are their most attractive feature.

Cellulose acetate crown forms and preformed polycarbonate anteriors. The cellulose acetate crown form consists of thin, soft, and transparent material. Sizes and shape can be selected from a mold guide (Fig. 9-13). A selected crown form is trimmed and festooned to fit the preparation without impingement on the soft tissue. The translucent matrix is then filled with a resin. There are three popular types of resins currently in use:

1. Methyl methacrylate, such as Temporary Bridge Resin (Caulk)
2. Ethyl methacrylate, such as Trim (Bosworth)
3. Epimine, such as Scutan (Premier)

The materials are mixed according to the manufacturer's directions. Forms are filled and gently pressed upon the preparation, and all excess is removed concomitantly. The crown matrix is repeatedly removed and reset during the later setting stages of polymerization to control excessive distortion and to ensure removal after the resin is completely set. Final setting can then take place outside of the mouth. The cellulose shell should be peeled off when the material is set. Treatment restorations are trimmed, and occlusion is checked and polished. Binders used for cementation depend on specific clinical conditions presented by the patients.

Polycarbonate crown forms are more tolerable than their cellulose predecessor

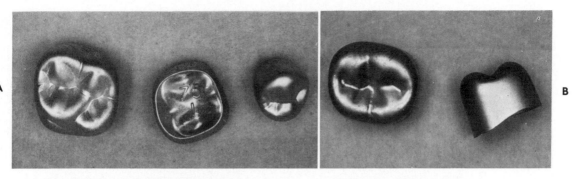

Fig. 9-12. A, Preformed metal crowns manufactured with a constricted gingival collar. **B,** Preformed metal crowns that are not so constricted gingivally. These forms are less malleable than those in **A.**

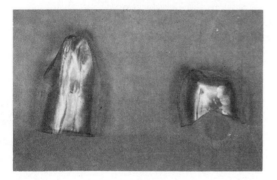

Fig. 9-13. Cellulose acetate crown forms can be filled with resin to form a suitable esthetic interim coverage for incisors and premolars. Celluloid matrix is removed before interim cementation.

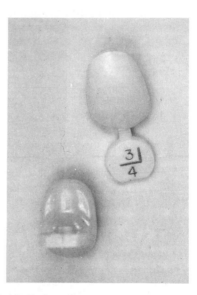

Fig. 9-14. Polycarbonate crowns are an integral part of treatment restorations. This type of interim coverage is stronger.

(Fig. 9-14). An appropriate preformed crown is selected to establish contact areas. One of the three types of resins is chosen and placed into the form. The polycarbonate crown is placed on the prepared tooth. After the resin is partly set, the crown is removed. Excess resin is trimmed, occlusion adjusted, and the crown form cemented to place. This is an excellent coverage for individual anterior teeth. Misuse is seen most often with improperly trimmed gingival margins. The polycarbonate crown form remains on the prepared tooth, whereas the cellulose crown matrix is removed prior to cementation.

Heat-cured resins for treatment bridges. Laboratory-prepared crowns are used when multiple preparations are involved and when it is impractical to use alternate methods (Fig. 9-15). Teeth are reduced on a second set of diagnostic casts to simulate tooth preparation. The technician places the desired occlusion and contact areas on mounted models. The wax is boiled off and heat-cured temporaries are fabricated. These crowns need

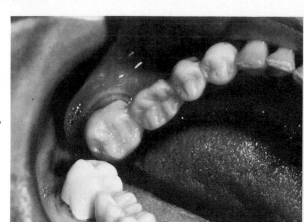
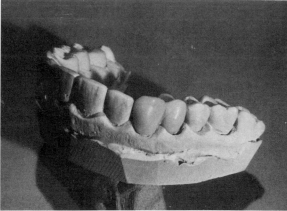

Fig. 9-15. A, Heat-cured treatment restoration for multiabutment posterior bridge. Note fluted buccal surface form of interim coverage. (Courtesy Dr. Hanne Sweetnam, Joliet, Ill.) **B,** Splinted canine and premolar with cold-cure acrylic from a preoperative alginate impression.

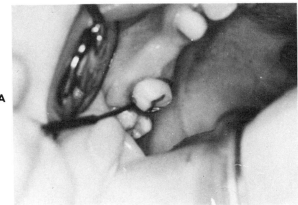
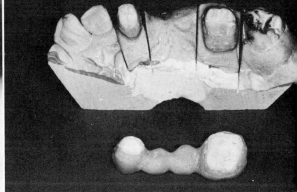

Fig. 9-16. A, Electronic tissue dilation prior to impressions. Note edentulous area where previous pontic elicited the usual unfavorable tissue response. **B,** Cold cure–alginate method of treatment restoration construction. Pontic area is not placed in contact with tissue to encourage optimum tissue response.

only slight modification prior to interim cementation.

Plastic denture teeth may be used to fabricate more esthetic, functional treatment bridges. The availability of a wide variety of shades and molds from denture teeth makes this technique adaptable for most pontic areas.[15] Utilization of plastic teeth for construction of treatment crowns

and bridges prior to actual tooth preparation is an ideal method of developing esthetics and a satisfactory occlusal plane prior to the insertion of the final prosthesis.

Laboratory expenses and the time expended for preparation of secondary diagnostic casts by the dentist may be prohibitive for a three-tooth prosthesis,

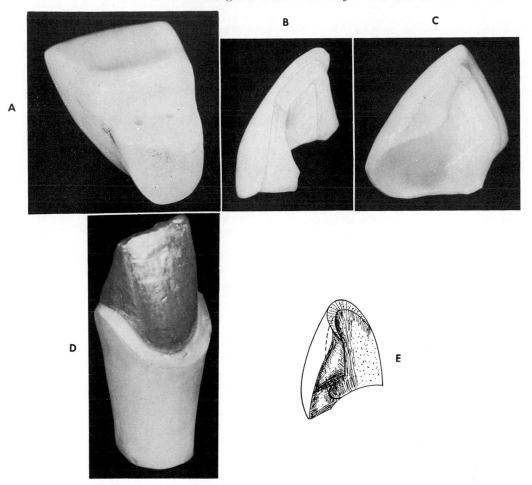

Fig. 9-17. A, Acrylic denture tooth to be prepared for treatment restoration similar to Hollenbock veneer crown. **B,** Sufficient bulk of acrylic must be removed from labial surface so that template is created for more rigid esthetic requirements. **C,** Proximal reduction and flange preparation affords sufficient bulk of acrylic resin for retention of single treatment restoration. This procedure is performed for maximum esthetics. **D,** Adequate bulk removed from labial or buccal side of stone models to permit adaptation of acrylic denture tooth. **E,** Prepared acrylic facing prior to addition of wax. Facings are flasked and processed for polymerization. Proximal flanges for a single customized treatment restoration.

but they may be a mandate prior to construction of a full maxillary periodontal prosthesis.

Cold-cure alginate impression technique (Fig. 9-16). An alginate impression of the teeth is taken on the day the preparations are made but before any reduction of teeth. The alginate impression is set aside and kept in a damp environment to pre-

vent excessive distortion. After completion of the preparations, a mixture of one of the resin materials previously used in conjunction with the cellulose crown form is placed in the section of the alginate impression corresponding to the crown preparations. The alginate impression with the resin is placed back into the mouth. A small amount of the resin material is kept in hand in order to judge the progress of the set. The impression is removed just prior to the rigid set of the acrylic. The cold-cure acrylic is then removed from the alginate impression and placed back into the mouth so that occlusion may be checked and the margins may be trimmed. By this time polymerization is nearly complete to permit the treatment matrix to be polished and cemented. Excess cement beyond the margins of the restorations are responsible for an unpredictable recession level in a great percentage of cases. Fritts and Thayer[16] employ a similar method but use a strong pliable wax in lieu of alginate.

The use of acrylic denture teeth as a method of developing maximal esthetic results prior to fabrication of the final restorations is possible. This method provides a template for the establishment of a more desirable esthetic result (Fig. 9-17). Preparation of this type of treatment restoration is not needed for routine care of patients but will be a definite aid for a dentist who is involved with a difficult case.

Template technique. With the template technique, stone models of both archs are used prior to mouth preparation. A hole can be drilled through the center of the stone cast if desired. If a fixed prosthesis is being fabricated, a denture tooth or teeth are waxed into the edentulous area. An appropriate plastic denture tooth can be used as formerly described. The template is constructed with the aid of a thermal vacuum machine that adapts a plastic sheet over the entire stone cast (Fig. 9-18). The plastic sheet is trimmed around the teeth to be prepared. After tooth preparation, the temporaries are fabricated in a manner similar to the cellulose crown technique.[17] There are incidences when the Omnivac overlay is cemented with a periodontal pack. However, the Omnivac treatment material is usually removed prior to cementation.

Post-crown technique. Interim crowns

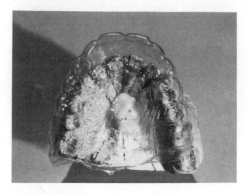

Fig. 9-18. Omnivac temporary to be used in construction of an interim maxillary splint.

for endodontically treated teeth can be an arduous task. If the tooth in question is a part of a fixed prosthesis or splint, the temporary restorative measure is usually less involved. Single treatment restorations on endodontically treated teeth that are in a critical occlusal position require additional coronoradicular stabilization.

A wire or nonprecious metal post is adapted to the canal. The selected crown form is then filled with an acrylic resin and placed over the post, including a portion of the radicular surface of the tooth. After sufficient polymerization has taken place, the crown is removed along with the temporary post, which is now set within the resin. Care must be exercised with this technique while one trims the root-coverage area properly to assure a satisfactory response. The entire assembly of makeshift dowel extension and crown form is cemented with a retentive adhesive. Esthetics and a gingival tissue healing matrix are the indication for this type of interim restoration.

Limitations of temporization. The majority of interim coverage is poor for a variety of reasons. Dentists are fully aware of inadequacies of temporaries when compared to perceptive construction of satisfactory treatment restorations. Literature that confuses the two types of coverage is undesirable. Temporization possesses problems inherent to all existing techniques and materials. The following is a succinct list of limitations of temporization:

1. *Lack of inherent strength.* Temporaries fracture in long-span coverage and with patients who possess a reduced interocclusal clearance. If the bulk is increased, the patient's discomfort and accommodation periods also increase proportionately.

2. *Poor marginal adaptation.* This inherent deficiency can be adjusted but seldom to the satisfaction of the dentist. Temporization usually defies exacting marginal finish and polish.

3. *Color instability.* This instability is apparent when temporaries are placed in the patient for an inordinate length of time.

4. *Poor wear properties.* Teeth will drift or undergo torque if the patient places heavy occlusal stress upon the interim coverage.

5. *Detectable odor emission.* Odor occurs despite the dentist's close attention to creating sufficient embrasure spaces. Resins, particularly cold-cured types, are porous and permeable to fluids.

6. *Inadequate bonding characteristics.* There are few cements that currently secure an adequate interface relationship with resins. Sedative cements are notorious for incompatibility with materials that are subject to stages of polymerization.

7. *Poor tissue response to irritation.* All present forms of interim coverage are just that. Certain techniques are merely more innocuous than others. Fortunately, various patients possess tremendous tissue-adaptation powers.

8. *Arduous cement removal.* It is not uncommon to find cement in the proximal gingival cuff and the apex of the embrasure areas. The inaccessibility of entrapped cement resists

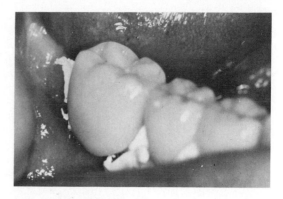

Fig. 9-19. Mandibular provisional splint placed with a sedative type of cement. Removal of all luting media interproximally is difficult. A second appointment when occlusion is adjusted is an ideal time to check for any excess of cementing media.

dislodgment. Operator concentration after lengthy appointments reduces the incidence of redundant cement, but it is not uncommon to have some luting medium lodged interproximally after placement of interim coverage (Fig. 9-19). Postoperative radiographs often help.

9. *Time expenditure for fabrication can be prohibitive.*

Radiopaque treatment restorations. The majority of treatment bridges and crowns are made of acrylic resin. Unfortunately most resins are radiolucent and cannot be detected on radiographic examination.

Treatment restorations can be dislodged during mastication, trauma, and biting habits. If this dislodgment occurs, accidental inhalation of the acrylic resin coverage becomes a real danger, such as during sleeping hours.

Although most dental materials that are accidentally swallowed usually pass through the gastrointestinal tract without difficulty, they can be delayed at various passages or aspirated into the respiratory tracts, which can become blocked. This could lead to serious or even fatal results. The need for a radiopaque resin is obvious.[18]

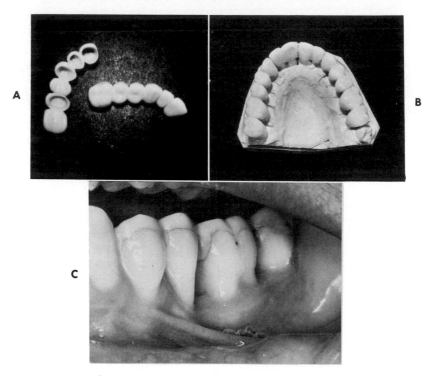

Fig. 9-20. A, Heat-cured treatment restorations for complete maxillary restoration with a fixed prosthesis. Hemisected approach reduces degree of dentist's fatigue and assists maintenance of existing vertical dimension. **B,** Assembly of heat-cured treatment restorations on master cast. Note presence of maxillary third molar to aid maintenance of existing vertical dimension. **C,** Heat-cured treatment restorations for splinted intracoronal units used in conjunction with periodontal therapy. Acrylic treatment restorations for individual units are difficult to fabricate and are more easily dislodged during mastication than are splinted units.

The first patent issued for a radiopaque dental acrylic was almost a quarter of a century ago; however, it has been difficult to manufacture an acceptable radiopaque denture resin that would not adversely affect the color, stability, or strength. In addition, the additives must be nontoxic for the patients.

Patient education is presently the only protection afforded the patient. The use of polycarboxylate cements for interim coverage has become popular. Greater adhesion provides greater stability particularly in long-span treatment bridges. Patients must be warned not to continue wearing a treatment restoration that is fractured or becomes dislodged. Physi-cians should become more familiar with all types of prostheses so that they are capable of instituting early treatment for possible aspiration in the case of accident or trauma. This has been mentioned briefly previously. The intended longevity of the interim coverage encourages hastily fabricated temporaries, not treatment restorations.

Provisional splints. This type of treatment prosthesis requires an adroitly designed, heat-cured resin that is used as a durable therapeutic restoration. Provisional splints are usually employed with advanced periodontal treatments or complex restorative dentistry (Fig. 9-20). The limitations of cold-cure splints have been illustrated graphically by various authors.[19]

Heat-cured provisional splints primarily provide the opportunity to do the following:

1. Reestablish the proper physiologic crown contour.[20]
2. Develop adequate embrasure areas prior to replacement with a more permanent type of restorative material.[21]
3. Assist gradual establishment of a satisfactory occlusion where there is disparity between the maxillary and mandibular relationship.[22,23]
4. Formulate a template to determine optimal esthetics.
5. Permit periodic removal for optimal visibility assessment of surgical recovery.[24]

This topic is covered in more depth in Chapter 24.

Longitudinal studies are needed to validate the optimal period of time to use the provisional splint. The varying capacities of patient recovery will obviously be the subjective factor so difficult to assess.

Summary

Various methods and materials are available to the dentist for the fabrication of adequate interim coverage for prepared teeth. To obtain reasonable success, the dentist must know and appreciate the materials available as well as their properties. Misuse and abuse will result in predictable failure and disappointment for the patient and the dentist. Knowledge of innovative techniques and materials will result in successful treatment restorations for the prepared teeth.

Literature that advocates prolonged use of interim coverage without specific indications for its use should be ignored. Cold-cured techniques for a provisional prosthesis or splints should be minimized. Capricious designs for the retention of questionable teeth without longitudinal studies to support introspective therapeutic procedures is worthless to the clinician. Conversely, well-fabricated treatment restorations may be one method to predict the results of teeth classified as questionable abutments.

A specific and suitable method of fabrication for treatment restorations as a healing matrix before and during periodontal therapy is described by Flocken in the following section. Certain aspects of his treatment restorations are applicable to periodontal prostheses. Longitudinal studies currently in progress will aid the dentist in the more esthetic "final" restoration.[24] Research in more durable products with desirable working properties will, we hope, render present treatment restorations obsolete.

A healing matrix

Not temporaries. It is unfortunate for dental patients and the dental profession that the word "temporary" has been commonly employed to describe such a necessary and exacting interim restoration. Treatment restorations are designed and fabricated to provide many benefits to prepared teeth, surrounding gingivae, and the restoration of occlusal function.

Irritation. The concept of temporaries infers a capricious design for the construction of these restorations. It has become commonplace for temporaries to provide minimal and, too frequently, subminimal protection to the operative site. Not only do temporaries encourage inadequate axial contours and insufficient identification and adaptation to the prepared margins, but also actually contribute to gingival irritation. The outstanding shortcoming of the "temporary concept" is the failure of removing excess sedative cement that remains within the gingival crevice after cementation of the temporary.

Healing matrix. To establish a climate for optimal tissue response, one must remove the restoration after the sedative cement sets to permit (1) the complete removal of all extraneous cement within the gingival crevice, (2) to permit identification of margins allowing the operator to trim the treatment restoration to precise margins, (3) to identify and open embrasure areas for the health of the proximal tissue, and (4) to remove all extraneous cement from the interproximal and outer axial surfaces of the treatment restorations.

After many years of trial and error it has been determined that it is impractical to rely solely on prefabricated metal or plastic temporaries to achieve the desired oral health. This is especially true in the achievement of the desired oral health with a fixed prosthesis. Crowns and bridges are restorations that provide or perpetuate a healthy oral condition. It becomes of paramount importance that treatment restorations are constructed to provide protection for the abutment teeth and their supporting tissues.

Specific technique. During the past 50 years the dental literature has over 100 references to temporary coverage. Unfortunately many suggested techniques result in gingival irritation, gingival recession, and displeased patients and dentists.

It has often been recommended that temporaries not look too good or fit too well because final restorations may not be so esthetic or adaptive. This is an insipid policy and actually results in inferior final restorations. It is incumbent on the dental profession to fabricate the finest treatment restorations. Our final restorations will become more esthetic, functional, and biologically acceptable to the dental environment. If temporaries are inadequate they produce gingival irritation and fracture and are dislodged. This permits the patient to lose confidence in the prospect of the final restoration.

Sequence of fabrication. Prior to the appointment for preparations, the diag-

nostic cast is corrected with wax. It is important to increase the gingival third of all buccal and lingual axial surfaces that are scheduled for full reduction. This will permit sufficient plastic material for final relationship with the gingival tissues after the required polishing and finishing. Treatment restorations can be fabricated by the dental assistant or laboratory technician in the interval between the completion of tooth preparation along with gingival dilation procedures and the final impression procedures.

Technique

1. Upon the arrival of the patient for the operative procedure, the corrected cast is water soaked to remove entrapped air and to facilitate removal of the cast from the alginate over-impression. If vacuum-forming equipment is available for making a clear plastic shim, this alternative method could serve both as the outer form for fabricating the treatment restoration as well as a guide for preparing the tooth.

   After the alginate over-impression of the cast is carefully made by the dental auxiliary, the impression is trimmed and stored in a humidor until tooth preparation and tissue dilation (not retraction) has been accomplished.

2. Clean the operative site of all debris. The first impression is used as a further cleanup procedure and for the construction of the treatment restoration. This impression may serve to identify the adequacy of margins and as a determinant for the parallelism of multiple preparations. This initial impression (cleanup impression) may be accomplished in several ways:
   a. A full hydrocolloid impression
   b. A full alginate impression in which alginate material is either injected or rolled into the

gingival crevice by finger pressure

c. A combination of hydrocolloid injection into the subgingival crevice with an alginate covering impression

In the interest of time and accurateness, method *c* is most desired because it is fast, inexpensive, and accurate. However, for method *c* to be accomplished three precautions are necessary:

(1) The interval of time between insertion of the hydrocolloid and final placement of the alginate over-impression must be short.

(2) Approximately ⅛ inch less water within the measuring cup is used to make a thicker alginate that then acts as a plunger to drive the hydrocolloid into the gingival crevice.

(3) The surface of the alginate must not be smoothed with a wet finger because this alters the water/powder ratio.

3. Pour the cleanup impression of the preparations in impression plaster or quick-setting dental plaster. Ordinary dental plaster may be mixed with slurry water instead of plain water to accelerate the set. The cast is better separated from the impression by air pressure after the initial set so that fracturing of the reproduction of the teeth is avoided.

4. Trim the cast. It is important to trim the mesial and distal ends at right angles to the line of teeth. Wherever possible, cut the cast in the middle of an uncut tooth. The edentulous posterior reproduction may also be trimmed at right angles to the ridge. It is mandatory that the cast be given a curettage in all areas of subgingival tooth preparation. The crevices are opened laterally with a 3½ Hollenbeck or a gingival curette to better expose the readable subgingival margins. Remove all positive blebs on the cast that would interfere or prevent the seating of this cast into the initial alginate over-impression.

5. Apply a liquid tinfoil substitute to the cast. Blow off excess and do not wait or allow the coating of tinfoil substitute to dry.

6. Proceed immediately to place 2 or 3 drops of acrylic monomer into the crevice and sift in acrylic polymer. Use vibration to ensure reproduction of gingival detail without air entrapment. If excess powder occurs, add sufficient monomer to produce liquidity.

7. Make the final trimming of the initial alginate over-impression (clear plastic matrix form). It is essential that all alginate reproductions of interproximal embrasures be pinched off with cotton pliers to ensure accurate reseating of the cast into the impressions.

8. Dry the over-impression well. Mix sufficient quantity of self-curing acrylic of the correct shade in a dappen dish to a heavy liquid consistency.

9. Carefully vibrate the fluid acrylic into the prepared areas within the over-impression. Fill the pontic areas and approximately two thirds of the abutment areas. Avoid excess acrylic in the impression of the adjacent unprepared teeth.

10. Carefully reseat the cast into the over-impression to its exact position as determined by noting the fit, anteriorly and posteriorly, of the cast against the impression. Do not overseat or compress, nor underseat. Excessive pressure will pro-

duce a subocclusal restoration. Insufficient pressure will induce a restoration in supraocclusion.

11. Secure the cast and impression assembly with a rubber band that will hold the two in position without excess squeezing of the cast into the impression.

12. Place the assembly in hot water (approximately 150 to 160° F.) in a pressure pot under a pressure of 30 pounds for 10 minutes. Use only approved safe-pressure pot equipment. Be sure the pressure pot is assembled correctly. The higher the pressure used, the better quality and harder the treatment restoration will be.

13. Remove the assembly from the pressure pot. Separate the cast and treatment restoration from the over-impression.

14. If any voids or flaws exist in the treatment restoration, fill in the deficiency by wetting the area with monomer, sift in polymer as needed, and replace into the pressure pot for 3 to 5 minutes.

15. Remove the treatment restoration from the cast by inserting the point of a knife into the cast 2 to 3 mm below the preparation. Gentle twisting of the knife blade will separate the treatment restoration from the cast.

16. Trim and polish the treatment restoration. Note that the restoration can be used to identify the margins. Trim the gingival margins to the readable margin.

17. Test fitting of the treatment restoration in the mouth is usually not required when all of the above are accomplished correctly. Little or no adjustment is required. Be sure that all interproximal areas are properly adjusted to the gingival tissues.

18. Cementation embodies special procedures: dry the treatment restoration thoroughly and mix a special sedative cement for cementation.

19. As a sedative dressing use a modified zinc oxide and eugenol (Caulk's B & T [base and temporary]) cement along with Burrough's Neosporin ointment. Neosporin ointment contains neomycin, a fungicide, and bacitracin, a bacteriostatic agent. Place approximately 1/8 inch of Neosporin ointment on the mixing pad; add 4 or 5 drops of liquid; mix and add enough powder to produce a mashed potato consistency. Line the inner aspects of the treatment restoration with a thin coating of this cement. Remove excess moisture from tooth preparation. Do not overdry the preparation. Seat the treatment restoration under normal occlusal loading. Allow the cement to set usually 4 to 5 minutes. The consistency of the sedative cement is adjusted with the Neosporin ointment to achieve this 4 to 5 minute setting time. If the cement sets sooner than 4 minutes, increase the Neosporin ointment ratio at a subsequent occasion. If setting time is longer than 5 minutes, reduce the amount of ointment used.

20. When the initial set has occurred, use a pair of Backhaus towel forceps with a cotton wood stick (Dixon Manufacturing Company) as a fulcrum to remove the treatment restoration. Baade forceps are not so effective. The sedative cement lining also serves as an excellent impression material for further identification of the margins. Trim as required. Remove all excess cement from the treatment restoration and the gingival crevices.

21. Recement the treatment restoration by reactivating the sedative cement. Dry the cement surface and apply a very thin coat (almost dry coat) of modified eugenol liquid. The prepared teeth are lightly dried and treatment restoration is replaced. The cleaned, recemented restoration will need no further adjustment.

Summary

Treatment restorations prepared by the above procedure serves as a healing matrix for the gingival tissue. They serve as a predictor of the final result. They serve as an oral hygiene training device and provide security and comfort to the patient while the final restoration is being fabricated. This technique also saves considerable time at each subsequent appointment, during which castings are fitted, joints are soldered, and porcelain is adapted prior to the final delivery. At these subsequent appointments, treatment restorations may be removed and replaced with the same ease, eliminating cleanout of old cement, recementation, cleanup, and adjustment in occlusion.

SELECTED REFERENCES

1. Tylman, S. D.: The dentino-enamel junction, J. Dent. Res. **8**:615, 1928.
2. Malone, W. F., and Bazola, F. N.: Early treatment of amelogenesis imperfecta, J. Prosthet. Dent. **6**:39, 540-544, 1966.
3. Diamond, D. D., Stanley, H. R., and Swerdlow, H.: Reparative dentin formation resulting from cavity preparation, J. Prosthet. Dent. **16**:1127-1134, 1966.
4. Kronfeld, The biology of cementum, J.A.D.A. **25**:1451, 1938.
5. Hildebrand, G. Y.: Studies in dental prosthodontics, Stockholm, 1937, Aktiebolaget Fahlcrantz Boktryckeri, vol. 1.
6. Collett, H. A.: Protection of the dental pulp in construction of fixed partial denture prostheses, J. Prosthet. Dent. **31**:637-646, 1974.
7. Ante, I. H.: The fundamental principles of fixed and removable bridge prosthesis, Dominion Dent. J. **42**:109, 1930.
8. Ante, I. H.: The fundamental principles of abutments, Michigan State Dent. Soc. Bull. **8**:14, July 1926.
9. Hagerman, D. A., and Arnim, S. S.: The relation of new knowledge of the gingiva to crown and bridge procedures, J. Prosthet. Dent. **5**:538, 1955.
10. Cran, J. A.: Development of the gingival sulcus, Aust. Dent. J. **11**(5):322-328, 1966.
11. Coelho, D. H., and Brisman, A. S.: Gingival recession with modeling-plastic copper-band impressions, J. Prosthet. Dent. **31**:647, 1974.
12. Harrison, J. P.: Effect of retraction materials on the gingival sulcus epithelium, J. Prosthet. Dent. **11**:514-521, 1961.
13. Daughlin, J. W.: The emphasis is on electrosurgery, Am. Acad. Gen. Dent. **18**:25-28, 1973.
14. Bassett, R. W., Ingraham, R., and Koser, J. R.: An atlas of cast gold procedures, Buena Park, Calif., 1964, Uni-Tro College Press, Chap. 1.
15. Tonn, J. H., and Cook, J. A.: Esthetic temporary crowns from plastic denture teeth, J. Mich. Dent. Assoc. **53**:118-120, 1971.
16. Fritts, R. W., and Thayer, K. E.: Fabrication of temporary crowns and fixed partial dentures, J. Prosthet. Dent. **30**(2):151-155, 1973.
17. Satera, A. J.: A direct technique for fabricating acrylic resin temporary crowns using the Omnivac, J. Prosthet. Dent. **29**:577-580, 1973.
18. Monar, E. J.: Why temporary restorations should be opaque, J. Calif. Dent. Assoc. **35**:12-15, 1972.
19. Loomar, D. A.: Provisional crown and bridge, J. N. J. Dent. Soc. **41**(3):10-12, 1969.
20. Deferick, D. R.: The processed provisional splint in periodontal prosthesis, J. Prosthet. Dent. **33**:553-558, 1975.
21. Kazis, H., and Kazis, A. J.: Complete mouth rehabilitation, Philadelphia, 1956, Lea & Febiger, Publishers, p. 365.
22. Malone, W. F.: The occlusal epidemic: profile of confusion, Illinois Dent. J. **39**(10):643-652, 1970.
23. Myers, G. E.: Textbook of crown and bridge prosthodontics, St. Louis, 1969, The C. V. Mosby Co., pp. 184-189.
24. Frederick, D. R.: The provisional fixed partial denture, J. Prosthet. Dent. **34**(5):520-526, 1975.

GENERAL REFERENCES

Adams, W. K.: A temporary fixed partial denture, J. Prosthet. Dent. **24**:571-572, 1970.
Amsterdam, M., and Fox, L.: Provisional splinting —principles and techniques, Dent. Clin. North Am., pp. 73-99, March 1959.
Baumhammers, A.: Temporary and semipermanent splinting, Springfield, Ill., 1971, Charles C Thomas, Publisher, pp. 99-107.
Behrend, D. A.: Temporary protective restorations in crown and bridge work, Aust. Dent. J. **12**:411-416, 1967.
Brotman, I. N.: Contoured temporary aluminum shell crown, Dent. Survey **28**:807-809, 1952.

Dill, G. C., Schmidt, J. B., and King, C. J.: A technique for temporary bridge construction, South Carolina Dent. J. **27:**22-24, 1969.

Donaldson, D.: Gingival recession associated with temporary crowns, J. Periodontol. **44:**691-696, 1973.

Donaldson, D.: The etiology of gingival recession associated with temporary crowns, J. Periodontol. **45:**468-471, 1974.

Fiasconaro, J. E., and Sherman, H.: Vacuum-formed prostheses. Part I. A temporary fixed bridge or splint, J.A.D.A. **76:**74-78, 1968.

Fischer, D. W., Schillingburg, H. T., and Dewhirst, R. B.: Indirect temporary restorations, J.A.D.A. **82:**160-163, 1971.

Greenfield, B. E.: Temporary crowns, Conserv. Dentistry **5:**71-73, 1971.

Grieder, A., and Cinnatti, W.: Periodontal prosthesis, St. Louis, 1968, The C. V. Mosby Co., pp. 269-274.

Herlands, R. E., Lucca, J. J., and Morris, M. L.: Forms, contours and extensions of full coverage restorations in occlusal reconstruction, Dent. Clin. North. Am., pp. 147-161, March 1962.

Innes, P. B., and Shroff, F. R.: Orientation of the crystallites in the surface layer of human enamel, J. Dent. Res. **47:**1029, 1968.

Jones, E. E.: Vacuformed clear resin shells, J. Prosthet. Dent. **29:**460-462, 1973.

Johnston, J. J., and Phillips, R. W.: Modern practice in crown and bridge prosthodontics, ed. 2, Philadelphia, 1965, W. B. Saunders Co., pp. 88-91.

Josephson, B. A.: Efficient acrylic temporary coverage: description of technique, N.Y. J. Dent. **36:**7-8, 1966.

King, C. J., Young, F. A., and Cleveland, J. L.: Polycarbonate resin, and its use in the matrix technique for temporary coverage, J. Prosthet. Dent. **30:**789-794, 1973.

Knight, R.: Temporary restorations in restorative dentistry, J. Tenn. Dent. Assoc. **47:**346-349, 1967.

Leff, A.: An improved temporary acrylic fixed bridge, J. Prosthet. Dent. **3:**245-249, 1953.

Meyer, J., and Gerson, S. J.: A comparison of human palatal and buccal mucosa, Periodontics **2:**284-291, 1964.

Osborn, J. W.: Directions and interrelationship of prism and cuspal and cervical enamel of human teeth, J. Dent. Res. **47**(3):395, 1968.

Richardson, E. R.: Comparative thickness of the human periodontal membrane of functioning versus non-functioning teeth, J. Oral Med. **22:**120-126, 1967.

Schmidt, J. B., Dill, G. C., and King, C. J.: Anterior temporary coverage, South Carolina Dent. J. **27:**5-8, 1969.

Selvig, K. A.: The fine structure of human cementum, Acta Odontol. Scand. **23:**423-441, 1965.

Silverman, S., Jr.: Ultrastructure studies of oral mucosa, J. Dent. Res. **46:**1433-1443, 1967.

Sochat, P. L., and Schwarz, M. S.: The provisional splint—troubleshooting, J. South. Calif. Dent. Assoc. **41:**92-93, 1973.

Skurow, H. M., and Lythe, J. D.: The interproximal embrasure, Dent. Clin. North Am. **15:**641-647, 1971.

Stahl, G. J., and O'Neal, R. B.: The composite resin dowl and core, J. Prosthet. Dent. **33:**642-649, 1975.

Talkov, L.: Temporary acrylic fixed bridgework and splints, J. Prosthet. Dent. **2:**693-702, 1952.

Talkov, L.: The copper band splint, J. Prosthet. Dent. **6:**245-251, 1956.

Tonn, J. H., and Cook, J. A.: Esthetic temporary crowns from plastic denture teeth, J. Mich. Dent. Assoc. **53:**118-120, 1971.

Willis, H.: Gold temporary crowns simplified, J. South. Calif. Dent. Assoc. **40:**51-53, 1972.

Zwarych, P. D.: The adaptation of the micro-structure of dental tissue to occlusal stress, Penn. Dent. J. (Phil.) **69:**10-14, 1965.

10

Construction of working models: soldering and bridge assembly

Gregory P. Miller

The construction of a working model is a critical step in achieving a final restoration. Dissection and fabrication of dies represents one of the more exacting and arduous procedures in cast restorations.

The following procedures can be used with either rubber base, hydrocolloid, silicone or polyether impression materials. This particular technique is one of the more efficient and less complicated methods used in the dental laboratory. In this chapter, rubber base impression material was used to illustrate the technique.

PREPARING THE IMPRESSION

After making the impression, it is necessary to remove all saliva and debris using a sable's hair brush with slow-running water. Rubber base material contains little, if any, moisture. Polyether impression materials are hydrophilic. Water immersion will distort the impression. A wetting agent is applied to the impression to reduce the surface tension. A wax pattern cleaner aerosol is used initially, whereas a no. 2 brush is used to wash the pattern with a cleaning agent. The pattern is then allowed to dry.

Straight pins with color-coated heads are placed on the buccal and lingual extensions of the impression, parallel to the borders of the prepared tooth (Fig. 10-1). If the mesial or distal borders are on a slight angle, the straight pins are placed parallel to the borders. This will enable the placing of dowel pins parallel with the borders of each preparation.

POURING THE IMPRESSION

The poured die stone forms the first layer. The thickness should be approximately 15 to 18 mm. This is usually a sufficient amount to cover the longest margin of the preparation and the serrated part of the dowel pin.

The die stone should be mixed to comply with the manufacturer's specifications. This mixture can be made with a power mixer or hand mixer (Fig. 10-2).

One pours the die stone into the impression with a vibrator, introducing small amounts each time, starting at one end of the impression and letting it fill to the other (Fig. 10-3).

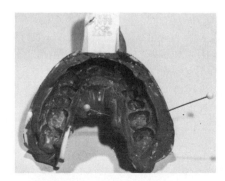

Fig. 10-1. Pins locating the prepared tooth.

Retention hooks, bent paper clips, or lock washers are placed on either side of the prepared tooth located by the straight pins. The retention hooks are inserted only halfway into the die stone; the dowel pin placement will then result in negligible distortion.

Tweezers are used for the insertion of dowel pins. The dowel pins are placed into the die stone adjacent to the straight pin (Fig. 10-4). If more than one dowel pin is needed, the pins are kept at the same height. An attempt should be made to position both flat surfaces of the pins facing the same way. This precaution will aid the trimming and seating of the dies. A minimum of 30 minutes is needed for the material to harden to stone. Straight pins can then be removed.

A small ball of wax is placed on the tips of the dowel pins to act as a location aid or guide prior to trimming of the model.

The impression is then ready for the second pour of stone. A separating medium is used to separate the two stone pours. Trisodium phosphate (soap solution) is painted on the die stone just around the dowel pin and then rinsed off.

Stone of a contrasting color is used for the second pour. One gently vibrates the impression while adding the stone, to prevent trapping of air bubbles. The dowel pins and the ball of wax at the tip of the die are covered after the final application of stone. Maximum hardness takes place after approximately 24 hours. NOTE: There is usually *no* need for boxing in the impression (Fig. 10-5).

The impression is not separated until it has been immersed in tap water for a few minutes to relieve some of the surface tension. The stone is gently separated from the impression by careful prying of

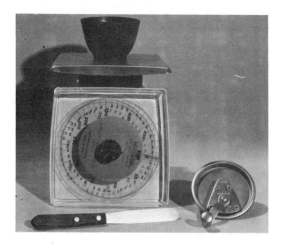

Fig. 10-2. Hand mixer and scale.

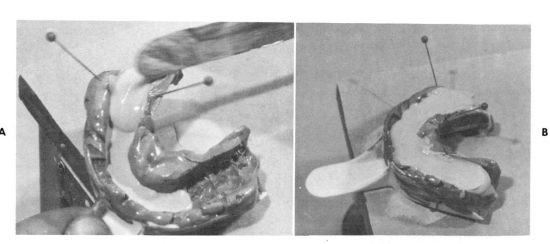

Fig. 10-3. A, Pouring the impression. **B,** Thickness of die stone, 15 to 18 mm.

the edges of the set stone with a plaster knife. The model is ready to be trimmed.

TRIMMING THE MODEL

The model is trimmed to clearly observe the definite distinction of the two stone pours on the buccal or labial surfaces. The base is trimmed until you see the ball of wax at the tip of the dowel pin. Sight of the wax will indicate the dowel pin. The second pour of stone is tapered slightly to the center of the model during the trimming of the model. This will facilitate the articulation of the models. An

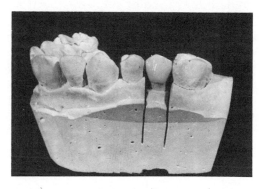

Fig. 10-6. Note distinction between two types of stone used for this technique.

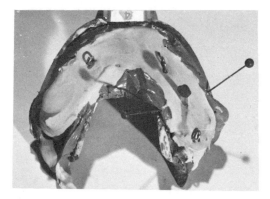

Fig. 10-4. Dowel pin placed adjacent to straight pins.

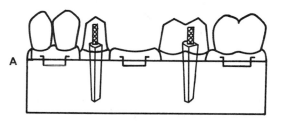

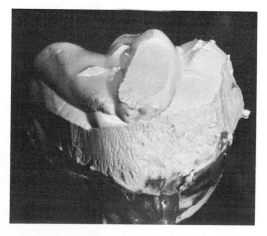

Fig. 10-5. Second pour covering dowel pins. Note that there is usually *no* need for boxing impression for second pour.

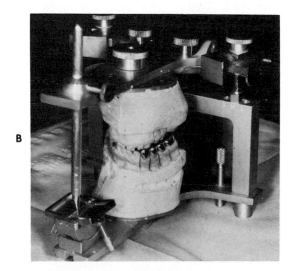

Fig. 10-7. A, Removable dies placed within model of prepared abutments. **B,** Relationship between mounted models and articulator prior to resetting of condylar and incisal components of articulator.

acrylic bur is used to cut away the stone on the lingual aspect of the model. A distinction between the two pours will become evident (Fig. 10-6). If the model is cut in this manner, it will encourage a more accurate seating of the die on the model. The slightest variations during this phase of die manipulation will alter the seating of the dies on the master model.

ARTICULATING THE MODEL

The model is mounted on an articulator by use of an appropriate interocclusal in-dex, such as the wax checkbite. One may separate the working model from the articulator base by indexing the base. Separating media will allow the distinct relationship between the working model and the articulator so that remounting the working model is possible (Fig. 10-7).

CUTTING AND TRIMMING THE DIE

A die saw with a blade thickness of 0.010 inch is commonly used to cut through the die stone. Two vertical cuts are made on the mesial and distal side of the tooth, so that it tapers slightly toward

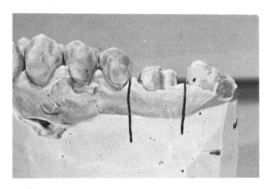

Fig. 10-8. Two vertical cuts are made on model, mesially and distally. Care is exercised to avoid cutting proximal surfaces of adjacent teeth.

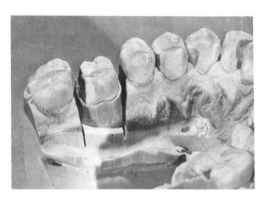

Fig. 10-9. Removable die shown after Carborundum wheel has been used to contour the base of die.

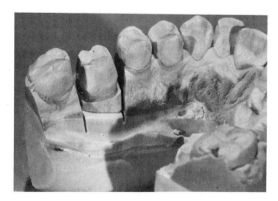

Fig. 10-10. No. 39 inverted cone bur and No. 11 scalpel blade are used to bring out high lines of gingival margin.

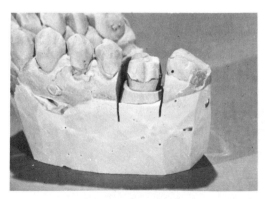

Fig. 10-11. Gingival margin has been marked, and die is ready to be waxed. A definite margin is required to wax satisfactorily prepared gingival margins.

the dowel pin. The initial cut is made through the die stone, just beyond the second pour (Fig. 10-8).

Trimming the die is the most crucial step in model preparation. Locate, recognize, and dissect the margins on the die with care. As many as six different types of gingival termination are commonly seen for crown preparation.

Immerse the die into water to restore moisture. This prevents the dies from chipping while being trimmed. When the dies are trimmed, carborundum stones mounted on a mandrel, a no. 39 inverted cone bur, and a no. 11 scalpel blade are the most common instruments used. The carborundum wheel on a handpiece is rotated counterclockwise slowly so that the

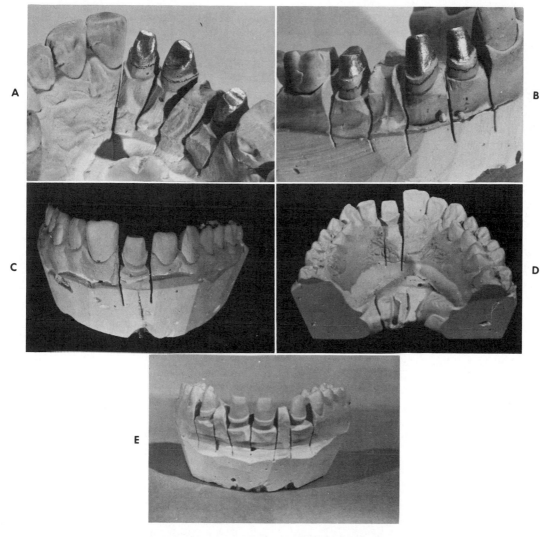

Fig. 10-12. A and **B,** These pictures illustrate buccal and lingual views of dissected dies for multiple preparation for fixed prosthesis. **C,** Labial view of die trimmed for complete porcelain crown. **D,** Lingual view of **C.** Note length of vertical cut and dissection of lingual shoulder. **E,** Master model trimmed prior to waxing after mounting on articulator. If model is trimmed excessively below shoulder, the die will be susceptible to fracture during porcelain manipulation.

excess die stone may be removed from the margins. The die dissection is terminated just short of the perceived margin (Fig. 10-9). The margins are dissected by use of a no. 39 inverted cone bur. Excessive ditching of the die with the inverted bur will create a die susceptible to fracture. Use a no. 11 scalpel blade to dissect the high lines of the margin. Insert die back on the model and prepare for waxing (Figs. 10-10 to 10-12).

SOLDERING AND BRIDGE ASSEMBLY

In the process of soldering and bridge assembly, there are a variety of concepts involved. The main objective in soldering is to produce a strong rigid joint. In addition, the solder joint must restore the natural contact and maintain the interproximal space between crowns.

Requisites of solder

Skinner and Phillips list the following requisites for a satisfactory dental solder: "(1) It must not be corroded or tarnished by the mouth fluids; (2) its melting point must be lower than that of the metal upon which it is employed, in order that the latter may not be fused during the soldering operation; (3) its color should match that of the metal employed; (4) it should flow properly and smoothly over the surface of the part being joined; (5) its physical properties should be at least as good as those of the metal, in order that the joint may not be a source of weakness."[1]

Factors for a successful soldering and bridge assembly

Cleanliness. The interproximal surface to be joined should be clean and free from metallic oxides. All wax or acrylic resin material must be either boiled out with water or completely burned off. Any foreign material will contaminate the solder. All precautions should be exercised to keep all surfaces clean. Smooth and highly polished surfaces also ensure a strong soldered joint.

Exposure of contact area. To invest the bridge in a tight metal-to-metal contact is undesirable. The metals of the bridge will expand when heat is applied. Expansion will crack the investment causing distortion of the entire fixed prosthesis. If the space to be soldered is too wide, the solder will not span the gap. A space of 0.0005- to 0.0001-inch thickness is provided between the areas to be soldered.

Flux. Flux is used primarily to cleanse and protect the surfaces against oxides. Flux may be used as either a powder or a paste. Commonly used fluxes are borax (sodium tetraborate), potassium nitrate, or potassium carbonate with pulverized charcoal.

Antiflux. Antiflux is used to confine the gold solder to a definite area. Antiflux may be graphite, carbon, or chloroform and rouge. Antiflux is strategically placed at the periphery of the joints, just prior to preheating of the invested model.

Time and temperature. The bridge assembly should be preheated to a temperature of 900° to 1,000° F. Overheating for a prolonged period of time may cause warpage. In addition, harmful sulfur dioxide gases may lead to brittleness. If the bridge assembly is heated too rapidly, distortion is also probable.

Positioning of invested bridge. The bridge is placed on the model and secured with a quick-cure resin. The resin is applied to the contact area and into the joint itself. The resin is allowed to harden for an appropriate length of time (Fig. 10-13). When the resin has set, the bridge is removed from the model. The bridge is checked for voids. Wax is added if the voids appear in the interproximal area. If voids are not covered, investment will seep in these areas. This seepage will result in a small, weakened soldered joint.

After mixing the investment to the manufacturer's specifications, slowly pour it into the inside of the crowns to prevent trapping air. Make a patty of the investment about 1 inch thick, placing the

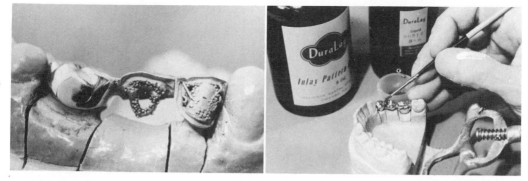

Fig. 10-13. A, Bridge assembly on model. **B,** Quick-cure resin is applied. (Courtesy The J. M. Ney Co., Bloomfield, Conn.)

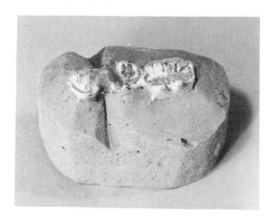

Fig. 10-14. Maximum exposure of bridge in investment is best for soldering. (Courtesy The J. M. Ney Co., Bloomfield, Conn.)

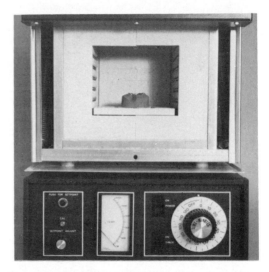

Fig. 10-15. Preheating invested model in furnace. Precaution: Do not overheat bridge (900° to 1,000° F). (Courtesy The J. M. Ney Co., Bloomfield, Conn.)

bridge with the occlusal surface up. The patty should have a periphery of ½ inch around the entire assembly. The bridge assembly should not be submerged. The margin should be invested with 1 to 2 mm of investment. Maximum exposure of metal is best for soldering. Let investment reach its final set before trimming (Fig. 10-14).

Trimming and preheating of invested model. The model is trimmed with a plaster knife. A V-shaped groove is cut on either side of the intended solder joint. The sides of the investment are rounded. This is done to develop an investment index that will add to the efficiency of the

applied soldering flame. The investment is preheated in either a furnace or a flame but not directly above the flame. It is placed off to one side by use of a tripod and wire-mesh screen. The only precaution is overheating (Fig. 10-15).

Soldering flame and selection of solder. The optimal flame and its correct use are equally important in the soldering operation. In examining Fig. 10-16 of a flame, one will notice that there are several zones. The first, zone A, indicates the air

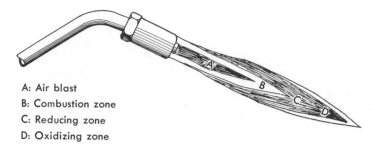

A: Air blast
B: Combustion zone
C: Reducing zone
D: Oxidizing zone

Fig. 10-16. Blowpipe flame and zones.

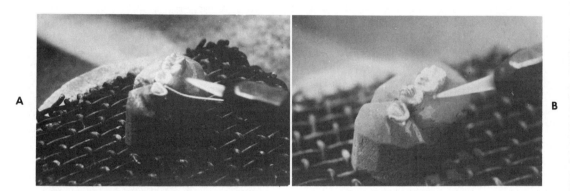

Fig. 10-17. A, Positioning of solder and flame. **B,** Flowing of solder. (Courtesy The J. M. Ney Co., Bloomfield, Conn.)

blast coming from the center of the nozzle; *B* indicates the area of partial combustion where air and the gas are mixed; zone *C* is the reducing zone or the deoxidizing flame and is usually represented as a pale blue color. This region is readily located if a piece of oxidized copper or a penny is placed in the blowpipe flame. When the metal immediately brightens in the area covered by the flame, the appropriate region has been located. This zone contains highly heated but unburned hydrogen, which, when it contacts an oxidized surface or an oxide, combines with the oxygen and leaves the surface free of oxide. The tip or the end of the flame, *D*, represents the oxidizing flame or zone and is the area of complete combustion. The application of this part of the flame to the metal surface to be soldered results in their oxidization and the necessity of applying additional flux in order to clean the surface. The proper use or misuse of the soldering flame very often determines the success or failure of a soldering operation. In addition to the use of an appropriate flame, the parts to be soldered should *not* be exposed to unnecessary heat or maintained at a high temperature for an extended period of time. The objective in soldering is to make the solder flow where it is required as quickly as possible and at as low a temperature as is consistent with the soldering operation. Solder should be selected for each particular appliance so that its maximum melting range will be approximately 120° to 140° F. below the initial melting point of the metals to be soldered. The fusing range of solder from the solid to the liquid state should not exceed 100° F.[2]

Soldering the bridge. After the bridge is preheated, it is placed on a soldering

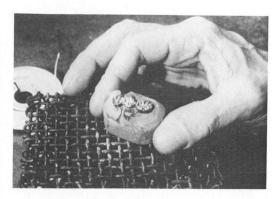

Fig. 10-18. Allow bridge to bench-cool before removing investment. (Courtesy The J. M. Ney Co., Bloomfield, Conn.)

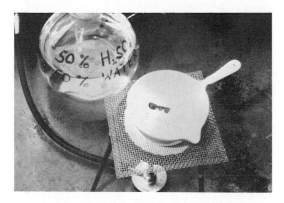

Fig. 10-19. Pickling the bridge; 50% sulfuric acid, 50% water. (Courtesy The J. M. Ney Co., Bloomfield, Conn.)

screen. A small amount of paste flux is placed into the joint and also on the tip of the solder. With the reducing zone of the flame, the bridge is heated until it becomes a dull red color. It is then ready to be soldered. The solder is introduced from the occlusolingual surface. Because solder flows by capillary action, it is essential to keep the solder joint small. Solder will also flow to the highest concentration of heat; so the torch is positioned to distribute the flame equally on the desired solder joint (Fig. 10-17). After soldering is done, the bridge is allowed to bench-cool for heat treatment prior to removing investment. This will aid the development of maximum heat hardness of the metal and, with hope, will discourage warpage (Fig. 10-18).

Pickling. A solution of one part sulfuric acid and one part water is commonly used. The water is never poured into acid. The acid is slowly poured into water. The bridge is placed in a porcelain dish and slowly heated until the surface of the gold is free of oxides (Fig. 10-19). Special tweezers, which are not soluble in pickling acids, are used. The acid is then rinsed off the bridge. Finishing and polishing of the bridge is then initiated.

SELECTED REFERENCES

1. Skinner, E. W., and Phillips, R. W.: The science of dental materials, ed. 6, Philadelphia, 1936, W. B. Saunders Co.
2. Tylman, S. D.: Theory and practice of crown and fixed partial prosthodontics (bridge), ed. 6, St. Louis, 1970, The C. V. Mosby Co., pp. 692 to 694.

GENERAL REFERENCES

Jelenko, J. F.: Crown and bridge construction: a handbook of dental laboratory procedures, ed. 6, New York, 1974, The Jelenko Co.

Johnston, J. F., Phillips, R. W., and Dykema, R. W.: Modern practice in crown and bridge prosthodontics, ed. 3, Philadelphia, 1971, W. B. Saunders Co.

Martinelli, N.: Dental laboratory technology, St. Louis, 1970, The C. V. Mosby Co.

Ney, J. M.: Ney Crown and bridge manual, Hartford, Conn., 1972, The J. M. Ney Co.

11

Pontics for fixed prosthodontics

Paul D. Dinga

A pontic is defined as the suspended member of a fixed partial denture or bridge, replacing the lost natural tooth, restoring its function, and usually occupying the space of the missing natural tooth. The pontic is connected to the bridge retainers, which are attached to the remaining natural teeth. The union of the pontic and the retainer is usually accomplished by means of a rigid connection such as a soldered joint. Special cases require that the union between pontic and retainer be nonrigid, such as a key and keyway, or a rigid union using telescoping retainers.

CLASSIFICATION

Pontics can be classified in several ways. The shape of a pontic that contacts tissue can be used for purposes of classification, that is, conical or conical extension, spheroid, and ridge lap (Fig. 11-1). The materials used in pontic makeup is another method of classification, such as a combination of metal alloy with porcelain, combination of metal alloy with acrylic, and metal alloy by itself. The metals referred to here are gold alloy and nonprecious alloys. For all practical purposes a classification that takes into account most of the data on pontics is simple but best clarifies the classification of pontics.

Included in this classification are pontics designed and created by the manufacturer, which may or may not need to be altered by the dentist. They are lug- or backing-retained facings and Trupontics

made of porcelain or acrylic; pin-retained facings or Trupontics made of porcelain or acrylic (Figs. 11-2 to 11-4); and tube-retained denture tooth pontics made of porcelain or acrylic. In addition, there are the custom-made or dentist-technician–created pontics. The latter makes use of porcelain, acrylic, and metal alloys to create a pontic that most closely fits the requirements of pontic design (Fig. 11-5).

REQUIREMENTS

To fulfill its requirements satisfactorily, a pontic must (1) restore the function of the tooth it replaces, (2) meet the demands of esthetics and comfort, (3) be biologically acceptable to the tissues, (4) ensure its sanitation, and (5) prevent tissue inflammation of underlying residual ridge mucosa. These requirements form the base from which pontic construction begins.

A better term for pontic construction is pontic design. Studies have shown that of the existing pontic materials that come into contact with the residual ridge, none is superior to another in preventing tissue inflammation. Surface smoothness coupled with a convex surface buccolingually and mesiodistally in light contact with the residual ridge is what is required to prevent a tissue lesion under pontics.

PONTIC DESIGN

The specifications for pontic design are described by Stein.[7]

Posterior pontic design. A correctly de-

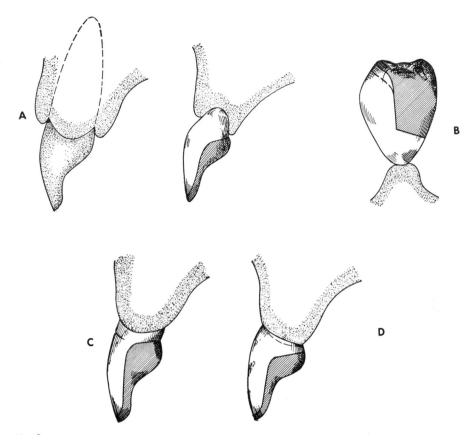

Fig. 11-1. A, Conic extension type of pontic used anteriorly for immediate replacement type of bridge. **B,** Spheroid type of pontic used posteriorly for lower arch. **C,** True ridge lap type of pontic no longer used for any situation. **D,** Variation of ridge lap type of pontic, developed so that lingual contour may be in harmony with adjacent teeth.

signed posterior pontic should have the following characteristics: (1) all surfaces should be convex, smooth, and properly finished; (2) contact with the buccal contiguous slope should be minimal (pinpoint) and pressure free (modified ridge lap); (3) the occlusal table must be in functional harmony with the occlusion of all of the teeth; (4) the buccal and lingual shunting mechanisms should conform to those of the adjacent teeth; and (5) the overall length of the buccal surface should be equal to that of the adjacent abutments or pontic (Fig. 11-6 to 11-8).

Anterior pontic design. A correctly designed anterior pontic should have the following characteristics: (1) all surfaces should be convex, smooth, and properly finished; (2) contact with labial mucosa should be minimal (pinpoint) and pressure free (lap facing); esthetics may require a long area of contact to prevent the black appearance if the residual ridge is excessively resorbed; (3) the lingual contour should be in harmony with adjacent teeth or pontics* (Figs. 11-9 to 11-11). These specifications, which when visualized mentally by dentist and technician, make up what was classified earlier as a custom-made pontic. An additional specification that the dentist must keep in

---

*Stein, R. S.: Pontic–residual ridge relationship, J. Prosthet. Dent. **16:**251, 1966.

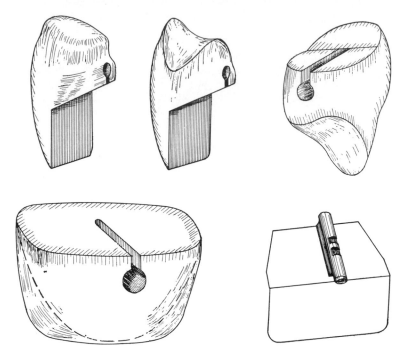

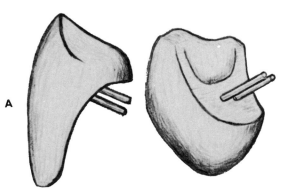

Fig. 11-2. Lug-retained and backing-retained pontics.

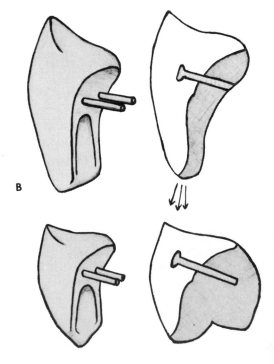

Fig. 11-3. A, Pin-retained pontic facings. **B,** Typical Harmony long-pin facing pontics for anterior and bicuspid restorations. Note compound arch form of backings made possible by integral hollow grinding of facings, which provides adequate metal protection for porcelain. (Courstesy Dr. Donald Smith, Los Angeles, Calif.)

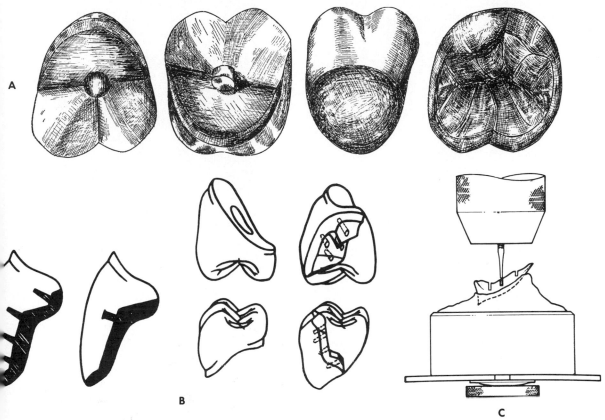

Fig. 11-4. A, Porcelain tube tooth used in posterior pontic. **B,** Converting denture teeth into pontic facings by employing reverse-pin principle of retention. Holes drilled into porcelain; pins cast as part of gold back give retention to facing. Same principles applied to posterior teeth. **C,** Drilling holes in porcelain facing, with precision drill. (**A** from Odell, A. W.: Dent. Cosmos **66:**958, 1924. **B,** From Shooshan, E. D.: J. Prosthet. Dent. **9:**284, 1959. **C,** From Shooshan, E. D.: J. Prosthet. Dent. **9:**284, 1959.)

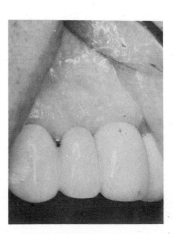

Fig. 11-5. Stein type of pontic used for an anterior fixed prosthesis. Note tissue response.

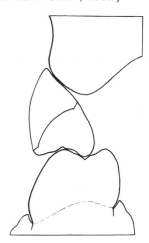

Fig. 11-6. Posterior pontic design illustrating contiguous relationship of pontic to alveolar ridge.

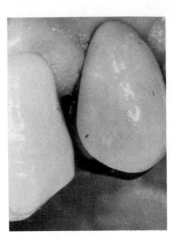

Fig. 11-7. Posterior pontic design illustrating overall length of buccal surface equal to that of adjacent abutments. (Courtesy R. Sheldon Stein, Boston.)

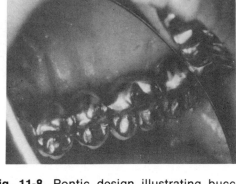

Fig. 11-8. Pontic design illustrating buccal and lingual shunting mechanisms conforming to those of adjacent teeth. (Courtesy R. Sheldon Stein, Boston.)

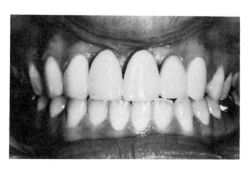

Fig. 11-9. Anterior pontic design illustrating long area of contact to prevent black-space appearance. (From Stein, R. S.: J. Prosthet. Dent. **16:**251, 1966.)

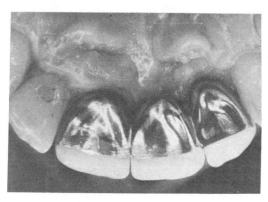

Fig. 11-10. Anterior pontic design illustrating lingual contour in harmony with adjacent teeth. (Courtesy R. Sheldon Stein, Boston.)

the mind is that the gingival portion of a pontic is never terminated against unattached mucosa (Fig. 11-12).

The details involved in the laboratory procedure of pontic design are not within the realm of this chapter, other than to mention that the wax-ups result in metal castings, allowing for sufficient thickness of porcelain or acrylic. This is important both from the standpoint of color esthetics and functional breakage of the acrylic or porcelain. The processing of acrylic and bonding of porcelain to metals is de-

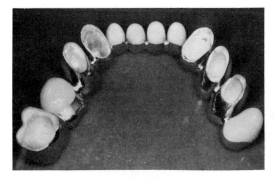

Fig. 11-11. Anterior and posterior pontic design illustrating all surfaces to be convex and smooth. (Courtesy R. Sheldon Stein, Boston.)

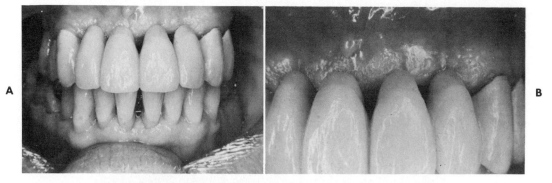

Fig. 11-12. Pontic design for periodontal prosthesis. **A,** Full arch. **B,** Anterior segment. (Courtesy Charles Bagley Porter, New Orleans, La.)

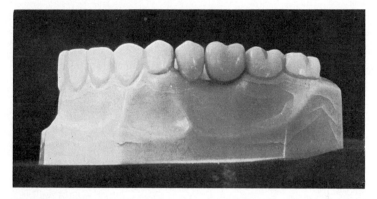

Fig. 11-13. Bicuspid and molor facings narrowed mesiodistally in gingival third. Note gingival embrasures.

scribed in the chapter on crown construction.

In view of what has been described on pontic design, it would seem that the use of facings and Trupontics, designed and created by the dental supply companies, would be somewhat limited for fixed partial dentures. Since this technique is still widely used and written about, the following steps are suggested as guides to this type of pontic construction.

PONTIC CONSTRUCTION

First, select a facing or Trupontic that most closely resembles the labial or buccal contour of the adjacent teeth (Fig. 11-13). Make this selection with the idea that minimal grinding will be required. These facings and Trupontics are de-signed to be interchangeable in case of functional breakage. When this selection is made depends on the type of retainers that will be used for the fixed partial denture. Where full coverage is used, the pontic selection is made after the retainers are completed. Where inlays and three-quarter crowns are used, the pontic selection is made from the study casts.

Second, place facings or Trupontics in as near an ideal position as possible on the stone cast. If any grinding is required at this point, it will be at the embrasure area of the anterior pontics or mesiodistally of the posterior pontics. Lute, then, the facings or Trupontics to the stone cast from the lingual with minimal sticky wax (Fig. 11-14). Lubricate the buccal surface of stone cast and facing. Apply plaster

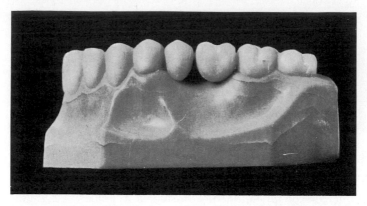

Fig. 11-14. Same region as shown in Fig. 11-13, with facings held in position with wax, ready for pouring of plaster core.

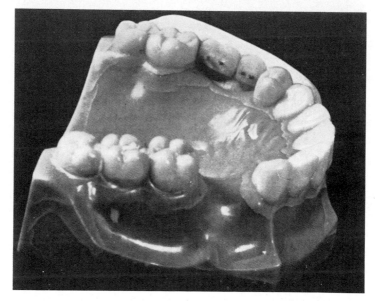

Fig. 11-15. Plaster core with facings held in position after removal of wax on lingual surface.

carefully to cover the labial or buccal surface of lubricated model and facings (Figs. 11-15 and 11-16). Plaster should extend 0.5 mm beyond the occlusal or labial edge of the facing and be thick enough with a handle to avoid breakage. The core, as it is called, becomes the base for firing porcelain onto the facing or trupontic in accordance with the pontic design mentioned earlier. The core is removed and if the gingival section of the core, where facing or Trupontic rested, is

fuzzy, careful reshaping with a Bard-Parker knife is called for.

The firing of porcelain is the third step. The details of how this is done are purposely omitted because the procedure is a delicate one and at this point the expertise of a ceramist should be enlisted. The main reason for firing porcelain onto a facing or Trupontic is to develop convex surfaces mesiodistally and labiolingually or buccolingually in relation to the residual ridge; do this while avoiding firing

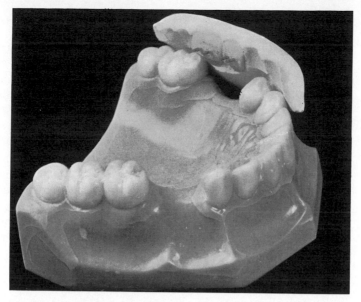

Fig. 11-16. Plaster core and facings, separated from working model.

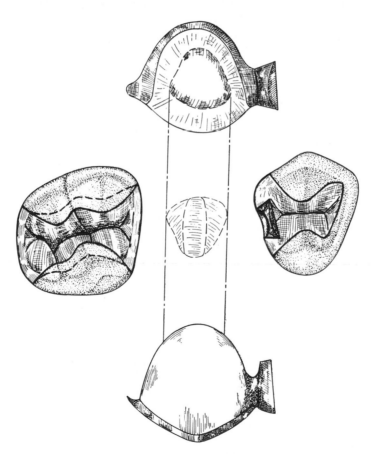

Fig. 11-17. Only narrow oval part of pontic, buccolingually, touches mucosa of ridge; remainder is convex mesiodistally. (From Smith, D. E., and Potter, H. R.: Dent. Dig. **43:**16, 1937.)

the porcelain into the pinholes and grooves of the facing or Trupontic into which the backing is to be fitted (Fig. 11-17).

The fitting of the lug or backing is the fourth step. They are made of burn-out plastic or are cast to metal. The lug is preferred for ease of handling. The lug is placed into the groove of the facing or Trupontic and ground flush with the lingual of the latter and gingival surface of the former. Obviously, this step is not necessary when pin-retained facings and Trupontics are used. The combination is placed into position on the stone model, and the plaster core is then placed in position to hold the facing or Trupontic in its position. It is important, now, that the articulation be examined for space between the occlusal portion of the trupontic and opposing teeth and for space between the incisolingual surface of facing and incisal edges of lower teeth (the case of lower anterior pontics does not present this problem except in certain types of

occlusion). Where space is insufficient for proper thickness of wax and subsequent metal to protect the pontic from fracture, the delicate process of hollow grinding comes into play. This also applies to the mesial and distal surfaces where sufficient thickness for the soldered connection must be taken into account.

To repeat, the use of commercially manufactured Trupontics and facings have obvious limitations, no matter how they are altered. They have become obsolete in fixed partial dentures for the following reasons: (1) the demand for esthetics is not met, and (2) their so-called replaceable value is lost during hollow grinding (Figs. 11-18 and 11-19).

The fifth step is waxing and contouring. With the facing or Trupontic, along with the plaster core in place on the stone model, lubricate the area well, and wax as any conventional pattern would be (Fig. 11-20). The width of the wax patterns of a long-span prosthesis should conform to Ante's law, whereas the wax patterns of a

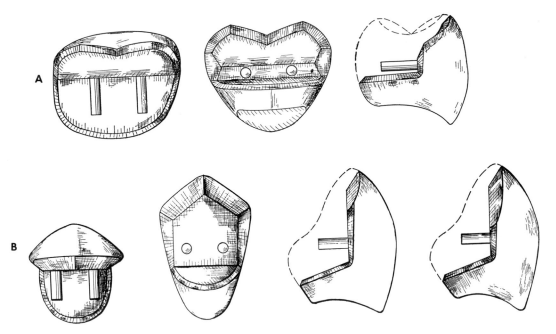

Fig. 11-18. A, Molar pontic. **B,** Bicuspid pontic; right pontic hollow ground.

short-span prosthesis should follow the specification outlines for the modified ridge lap earlier.

The final step of investing and casting and assembling the metal casting to the pontic is a laboratory procedure that does not differ from procedures involving any other wax pattern. Where pin facings are used, graphite pins are placed into the pinholes of the pattern (Fig. 11-21). These are removed from the casting with small round burs of the same diameter of the pins.

SPECIAL SITUATIONS

There are special situations in fixed partial dentures where the requirements for a pontic cannot be fulfilled. One such

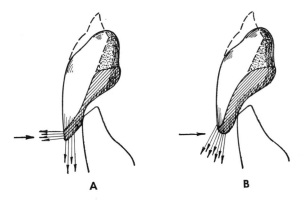

Fig. 11-19. Methods of beveling incisal edge. **A,** Incorrect. **B,** Correct. (Courtesy Dr. Donald Smith, Los Angeles, Calif.)

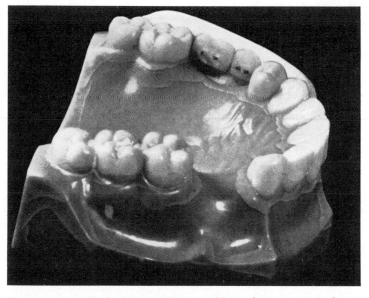

Fig. 11-20. Plaster core with facings held in position after removal of wax on lingual surface.

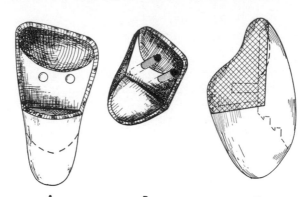

A   B   C

Fig. 11-21. A, Completed porcelain facing. **B,** Lingual portion contoured in inlay wax. Wax pattern has two graphite points inserted in pinholes. **C,** Cross section shows casting fitted to porcelain portion of pontic.

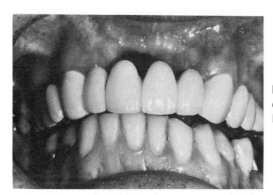

Fig. 11-22. Pontic design for patient with inordinate bone loss where the "smile" or lip line is not a deterrent to esthetics.

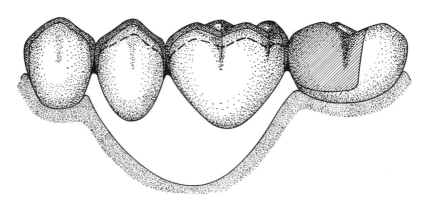

Fig. 11-23. Position of lower pontics where ridge is excessively resorbed. (Courtesy Dr. Donald Smith, Los Angeles, Calif.)

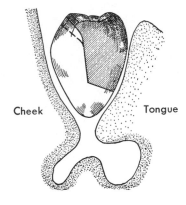

Cheek · Tongue

Fig. 11-24. Cross section of pontic shown in Fig. 11-23. (Courtesy Dr. Donald Smith, Los Angeles, Calif.)

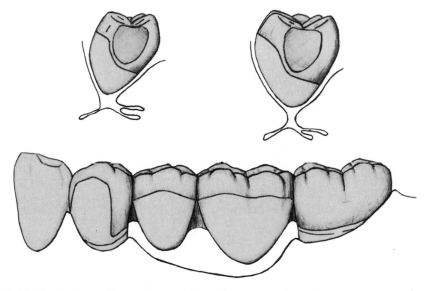

Fig. 11-25. Typical condition of excessive ridge resorption with Harmony pontic form permits contact of cheek and tongue beneath tips to facilitate hygiene. (Courtesy Dr. Donald Smith, Los Angeles, Calif.)

situation is the excessively resorbed residual ridge. The position of the pontic is shown below (Figs. 11-22 to 11-25).

Another case is that of the patient whose collection of calculus is excessive in the lower anterior region. The design for pontics is to keep them well off the residual ridge where esthetics will allow (Figs. 11-26 to 11-28).

The following figures show that carefully glazed porcelain pontics and carefully polished acrylic resin pontics had calculus deposits 1 month after insertion. A recommended design to avoid tissue stagnation is shown in Fig. 11-26.

Still another case is that of the patient with shallow mucobuccal folds adjacent to the bicuspid and molar pontics. The accumulation of debris because of inadequate food clearance is shown in Fig. 11-29. Reshaping pontic form is shown in Fig. 11-30, or a designing pontic as shown in Fig. 11-31, permits proper food clearance. The high muscle attachment, which

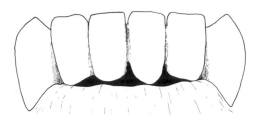

Fig. 11-26. Recommended design of lower anterior pontics for patients who have excessive calculus formation. (Courtesy R. Sheldon Stein, Boston.)

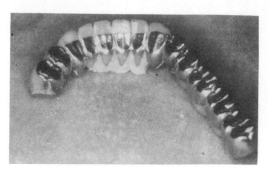

Fig. 11-27. Carefully polished acrylic resin pontics have calculus deposits 1 month after insertion. (Courtesy R. Sheldon Stein, Boston.)

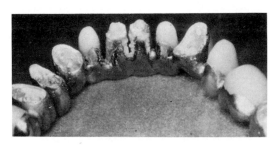

Fig. 11-28. Carefully glazed porcelain pontics have collected calculus deposits after 1 month. (Courtesy R. Sheldon Stein, Boston.)

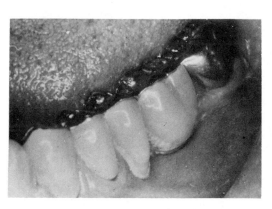

Fig. 11-29. Shallow mucobuccal folds adjacent to the bicuspid and molar pontic. The accumulation of debris attributable to inadequate food clearance is apparent. (Courtesy R. Sheldon Stein, Boston.)

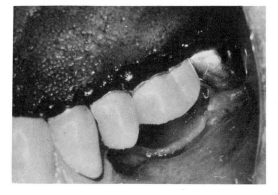

Fig. 11-30. Removal of pontic body reveals severe inflammation brought about by food entrapment. Pontic form reshaped to a "sanitary" design permits proper food clearance. (Courtesy R. Sheldon Stein, Boston.)

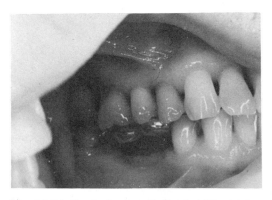

Fig. 11-31. Posterior pontic design illustrating patient with shallow mucobuccal fold. (Courtesy R. Sheldon Stein, Boston.)

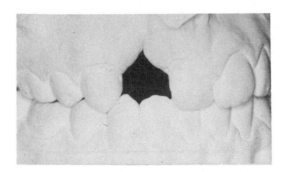

Fig. 11-32. Patient with cleft palate prior to placement of fixed prosthesis. (From Malone, W. F., and Sarlas, C. H.: Dent. Clin. North Am. **13**:480, April 1969.)

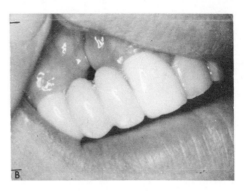

Fig. 11-33. Patient with cleft palate showing placement of fixed prosthesis. (From Malone, W. F., and Sarlas, C. H.: Dent. Clin. North Am. **13**:480, April 1969.)

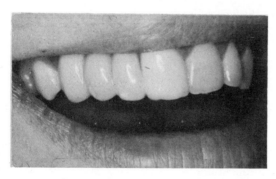

Fig. 11-34. "Smile" line of a patient with cleft palate after placement of fixed prosthesis. (From Malone, W. F., and Sarlas, C. H.: Dent. Clin. North Am. **13**:480, April 1969.)

limits the depth of the mucobuccal fold is shown very clearly in Fig. 11-31.

The case of a patient with a cleft palate is another special situation. Here the photographs speak for themselves (Figs. 11-32 to 11-34).

Lastly, the immediate fixed partial denture is most easily resolved by the use of acrylic alone, since the residual ridge resorption is difficult to ascertain. A final prosthesis is constructed later.

SUMMARY

Pontics have been classified into four different designs, that is, conical root extension, spheroid, ridge lap, and modified

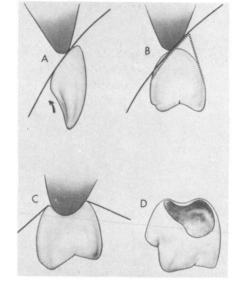

Fig. 11-35. A and **B,** Properly designed convex undersurfaces of pontics allow dental floss to maintain oral hygiene regardless of length of contacting surfaces *(dotted line).* **C,** Dental floss suspended on contiguous extremities of a ridge-lap pontic defeats purpose for which it is intended. Mucosa is scraped by floss, and food particles are forced into surface irregularities of concave undersurface of pontic. **D,** Mucosal view of pontic where food particles commonly accumulate.

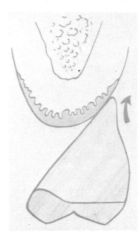

Fig. 11-36. Root contour of facial aspect of pontic should be included when adjacent tooth contours show an apical positioning of gingival margin. (From Stein, R. S.: J. Prosthet. Dent. **16:**251, 1966.)

ridge lap. The ideal design is now known to be the modified ridge lap with pinpoint contact on the facial contiguous slope of the residual ridge. The ideal design should include a surface smoothness and a fine finish. No distinguishing advantage is observed with porcelain, acrylic resin, or gold. The key to successfully constructed pontics lies in properly designed convex surfaces. Fig. 11-35, *A* and *B*, shows properly designed convex undersurfaces of pontics, which allow dental floss to maintain oral hygiene regardless of the length of the contacting surface (dotted line). Fig. 11-35, *C*, illustrates dental floss suspended on contiguous extremities of a ridge-lap pontic defeating the purpose for which it is intended. The mucosa is scraped by the floss, and food particles are forced into the surface irregularities of the concave undersurface of the pontic in Fig. 11-35, *D*. Where adjacent tooth contours show an apical positioning of gingival margins, a root contour of the facial aspect of the pontic should be included (Fig. 11-36).

SUGGESTED REFERENCES

1. Allison, J. R., and Bhatia, H. L.: Tissue changes under acrylic and porcelain pontics, J. Dent. Res. **37:**66, 1958.

2. Ante, I. H.: The fundamental principles, design and construction of crown and bridge prosthesis, Dent. Items Interest **1:**215, 1928.
3. Columbus Manufacturing Company: The complete Steele's technique, Columbus, Ohio, 1969, Columbus Manufacturing Co.
4. Gade, E.: Hygiene problem of fixed restorations, Int. Dent. J. **13:**318, 1963.
5. Shooshan, E. D.: Reserve pin-porcelain facing, J. Prosthet. Dent. **9:**284, 301, 1959.
6. Smith, D. E., and Potter, H. R.: The pontic in fixed bridgework, Dent. Dig. **43:**16, 1937.
7. Stein, S. R.: Pontic–residual ridge relationships, J. Prosthet. Dent. **16:**251, 1966.
8. Malone, W. F., and Sarlas, C. H.: Prosthodontic considerations in ephedodontics, Dent. Clin. North Am. **13:**461, April 1969.

GENERAL REFERENCES

Allison, J. R., and Bhatia, H. L.: Tissue changes under acrylic and porcelain pontics, J. Dent. Res. **37:**66-67, 1958.
Ante, I. H.: Construction of pontics, J. Can. Dent. Assoc. **2:**482, 1936.
Beke, A. L.: The biomechanics of pontic width reduction for fixed partial dentures, J. Acad. Gen. Dent. **22**(6):28-32, Nov.-Dec. 1974.
Boucher, C. O.: Occlusion in prosthodontics, J. Prosthet. Dent. **3:**635, 1953.
Boyd, H. R., Jr.: Pontics in fixed partial dentures, J. Prosthet. Dent. **5:**55, 1955.
Brecker, S. C.: Clinical approach to occlusion, Dent. Clin. North Am., pp. 163-182, March 1962.
Brice, S. E.: Construction of lower anterior pontics without display of gold, J.A.D.A. **27:**575, 1940.
Brill, N.: Influence of occlusal patterns on movements of the mandible, J. Prosthet. Dent. **12:**255, 1962.
Brill, N., Schubeler, S., and Tryde, G.: Aspects of occlusal sense in natural and artificial teeth, J. Prosthet. Dent. **12:**123, 1962.
Brodie, A. G.: Occlusion, N.Y. J. Dent. **29:**60, 1959.
Brotman, D. N.: Contemporary concepts of articulation, J. Prosthet. Dent. **10:**221, 1960.
Bruce, R. W.: Clinical applications of multiple unit castings for fixed prostheses, J. Prosthet. Dent. **18**(4):359, 1967.
Bruce, R. W.: Evaluation of multiple unit castings for fixed partial dentures, J. Prosthet. Dent. **14:**939-943, 1964.
Cavazos, E., Jr.: Tissue response to fixed partial denture pontics, J. Prosthet. Dent. **20**(2):143-153, 1968.
Chasens, A. I.: Effect of traumatic occlusion on the periodontium and associated structures, and treatment by selective grinding of the natural dentition, Dent. Clin. North Am., pp. 63-77, March 1962.
Clayton, J. A.: Roughness of pontic materials and dental plaque, J. Prosthet. Dent. **23:**407, 1970.

D'Amico, A.: Origin and development of the balanced occlusion theory, J. South. Calif. Dent. Assoc. **28**:317, 1960.

D'Amico, A.: Functional occlusion of the natural teeth of man, J. Prosthet. Dent. **11**:899, 1961.

D'Amico, A.: New concept of functional occlusion of natural teeth in restorative dentistry, Texas Dent. J. **80**:4, 1962.

Draper, D. H.: Forward trends in occlusion, J. Prosthet. Dent. **13**:724, 1963.

Engelberger, A., Rateitschak, K. H., and Mühleman, H. R.: Diagnosis and treatment of functional disturbances of the masticatory system, Dent. Abstr. **6**:150, 1961.

Ewing, J. E.: Reevaluation of the cantilever principle, J. Prosthet. Dent. **7**:78, 1957.

Fedi, P. F., Jr.: Cardinal differences in occlusion of natural teeth and that of artificial teeth, J.A.D.A. **64**:482, 1962; Inform. Dent. **44**:3601, 1962.

Gibson, T. D.: Theory of centric correction in natural teeth, J. Prosthet. Dent. **8**:468, 1958.

Göransson, P., and Parmlid, Å.: The pontostructor method and a new impression technique, J. Prosthet. Dent. **15**:900-907, 1965.

Graf, H.: Occlusal contact patterns in centric relation and centric occlusion, Int. Assoc. Dent. Res. **40**:81, 1962 (abstr.).

Granger, E. R.: Occlusion in temporomandibular joint pain, J.A.D.A. **56**:659, 1958.

Granger, E. R.: Establishment of occlusion, the articulator and the patient, Dent. Clin. North Am., pp. 527-529, Nov. 1960.

Harbard, W. C.: A simple accurate technic for immediate bridges, Dent. Dig. **50**:500, 1944.

Harmon, C. B.: Pontic design, J. Prosthet. Dent. **8**:496, 1958.

Hedges, P. G.: Occlusion as it relates to fixed restorations, J. Prosthet. Dent. **13**:499, 1963.

Henry, P. J.: Pontic form in fixed partial dentures, Aust. Dent. J. **16**:1, 1971.

Hirshberg, S. M.: The relationship of oral hygiene to embrasure and pontic design, J. Prosthet. Dent. **27**:26, 1972.

Hood, J. A., Farah, J. W., and Craig, R. G.: Stress and deflection of three different pontic designs, J. Prosthet. Dent. **33**:54, 1975.

Jackson, G. E.: Functional consideration of the problems of occlusion, Dent. Clin. North Am., pp. 355-368, July 1959.

Jankelson, B.: Dental occlusion and the temporomandibular joint, Dent. Clin. North Am., pp. 51-62, March 1962.

Jankelson, B.: Considerations of occlusion in fixed partial dentures, Dent. Clin. North Am., pp. 187-203, March 1959.

Karlström, S.: Pontostruktormetodiken sedd i kasuistikens belysning (A follow-up examination of fixed bridges produced by the pontostructor method), Svensk Tandlak. Tidskr. **45**:439-465, 1952; Int. Dent. J. **3**:264-267, Dec. 1952 (abstr.).

Klaffenbach, A. O.: Bridge pontics with porcelain tips or saddles, Dent. Dig. **38**:238, 1932.

Klaffenbach, A. O.: The role of crown and bridge prosthesis in the field of restorative dentistry, J.A.D.A. **25**:536, 1938.

Koivumaa, K. K.: Cinefluorographic analysis of the masticatory movements of the mandible, Suom. Hammaslääk. Toim. **57**:306, 1961.

Kurth, L. E.: Monoplane concept of occlusion, Dent. Clin. North Am., pp. 199-209, March 1962.

Legett, L. J.: Bridge pontics, Int. Dent. J. **8**:45, 1958.

Lindblom, G.: A new "pontic" construction for fixed bridges, Dent. Cosmos **75**:230, 1933.

Linkow, L. I.: Contact areas in natural dentitions and fixed prosthodontics, J. Prosthet. Dent. **12**:132, 1962.

Lucia, V. O.: Gnathological concept of articulation, Dent. Clin. North Am., pp. 183-197, March 1962.

Ludwick, W. E.: Construction of immediate temporary bridge, J.A.D.A. **33**:486, 1946.

Meyer, F. S.: Generated path technique in reconstruction dentistry, part II: fixed partial dentures, J. Prosthet. Dent. **9**:432, 1959.

Miska, M. G.: Simplified maxillary posterior pontic construction, N.Y. Dent. J. **28**:276, 1958.

Moulton, G. H.: Importance of centric occlusion in diagnosis and treatment planning, J. Prosthet. Dent. **10**:021, 1960.

Perel, M. L.: A modified sanitary pontic, J. Prosthet. Dent. **28**:589, 1972.

Pine, B.: Pontics for gold-acrylic resin fixed partial dentures, J. Prosthet. Dent. **12**:347-348, 1962.

Podshadley, A. G.: Gingival response to pontics, J. Prosthet. Dent. **19**(1):51-57, 1968.

Podshadley, A. G., and Harrison, J. D.: Rat connective tissue response to pontic materials, J. Prosthet. Dent. **16**:110-118, 1966.

Posselt, U.: Physiology of mastication; report of a seminar, J. West. Soc. Periodontol. **9**:40, 1961.

Posselt, U.: Recent trends in the concept of occlusal relationship, Int. Dent. J. **11**:331, 1961.

Posselt, U., and Posselt, A.: Some correlations between the occlusal pattern, function and pathology of the masticatory system, Parodontologie **13**:3, 1959.

Posselt, U.: Occlusal relationship in deglutition and mastication, European Orthodont. Soc. Tr. **34**:301 (disc. pp. 311-315), 1958.

Posselt, U.: Occlusal rehabilitation, Dent. Pract. Dent. Rec. **9**:255, 1959.

Poulton, D. R., and Aaronson, S. A.: Relationship between occlusion and periodontal status, Am. J. Orthodontics **47**:690, 1961.

Pruden, W. H., II: Occlusion related to fixed partial denture prosthesis, Dent. Clin. North Am., pp. 121-136, March 1962.

Pruzansky, S.: Applicability of electromyographic procedures as a clinical aid in the detection of occlusal disharmony, Dent. Clin. North Am., pp. 117-130, March 1960.

Ramsey, W. O.: Disorders of the mandibular articulation, J. Maryland Dent. Assoc. **2**:9, 1959.

Ruhlman, D. C., and Richter, W. A.: A method for pontic stabilization in fixed partial denture construction, J. Prosthet. Dent. **17**(4):401-405, 1967.

Schield, H. W.: The influence of bridge pontics on oral health, J. Mich. Dent. Assoc. **50**(4):143, 1968.

Schuyler, C. H.: Factors of occlusion to be observed in everyday practice, J.A.D.A. **57**:221, 1958.

Schuyler, C. H.: Considerations of occlusion in fixed partial dentures, Dent. Clin. North Am., pp. 175-185, March 1959.

Schuyler, C. H.: Evaluation of incisal guidance and its influence in restorative dentistry, J. Prosthet. Dent. **9**:374, 1959.

Schuyler, C. H.: Factors contributing to traumatic occlusion, J. Prosthet. Dent. **11**:708, 1961.

Schweitzer, J. M., Schweitzer, R. D., and Schweitzer, J.: Free-end pontics used on fixed partial dentures, J. Prosthet. Dent. **20**(2):120-238, 1968.

Schweitzer, J. M.: Masticatory function in man; mandibular repositioning, J. Prosthet. Dent. **12**:262, 1962.

Selberg, A.: An exposition of pontics and their construction for fixed bridges, Illinois Dent. J. **9**:440, 1940.

Silverglate, L.: A simplified reverse-pin porcelain facing technique, J. Prosthet. Dent. **18**:54, 1967.

Silverman, S. I.: Physiology of occlusion, Dent. Clin. North Am., pp. 3-17, March 1962.

Smith, D. E.: Improved porcelain facing design for fixed prosthesis, J. South. Calif. Dent. Assoc. **23**:34, 1955.

Staffanou, R. S., and Thayer, K. E.: Reverse pin-porcelain veneer and pontic technique, J. Prosthet. Dent. **12**:1138, 1962.

Stallard, H.: Physiology of chewing, J. Dist. Columbia Dent. Soc. **34**:9, 1959.

Stein, S. R.: Pontic-residual ridge relationship: a research report, J. Prosthet. Dent. **16**:251-285, 1966.

Stern, R. H.: Dental occlusion; an evaluation of the canine function theory, J. South. Calif. Dent. Assoc. **30**:348, 1962.

Stuart, C. E.: Why dental restoration should have cusps, J. South. Calif. Dent. Assoc. **27**:198, 1959.

Stuart, C. E., and Stallard, H.: Principles involved in restoring occlusion to natural teeth, J. Prosthet. Dent. **10**:304, 1960.

Tinker, E. T.: Sanitary dummies, Dent. Rev. **32**:401, 1918.

Tylman, S. D.: Anatomic form and function as registered and related to restorative dentistry, Illinois Dent. J. **25**:221, 1956.

Vaughan, H. C.: Occlusion and the mandibular articulation, Dent. Clin. North Am., pp. 37-50, March 1962.

Weinberg, L. A.: Prevalence of tooth contact in eccentric movements of the jaw: its clinical implications, J.A.D.A. **62**:402, 1961.

Whiteside, W. D.: Practical mandibular anterior pontic, J. Prosthet. Dent. **9**:119, 1959.

Wing, G.: Pontic design and construction in fixed bridgework, Dent. Pract. Dent. Rec. **12**:390, 1962.

Zander, H. A.: Principles of occlusal adjustment, J. Tennessee Dent. Assoc. **41**:303, 1961.

12

Methods of recording interocclusal relationships

Richard N. Pipia

In this day of prevention, it is the dentist's occupation to project his services to the patient from the first time that the patient visits his office as a child until the patient's old age. The patient's occlusion will change throughout his lifetime; some of it will be normal and some abnormal, but our knowledge and services should all be directed toward maintaining a single normal range for each individual. "Prevention," in its truest sense, is the prevention of our having to use therapy by ensuring that the patient's masticating apparatus is maintained within its normal ranges.

It is of utmost importance for the dentist not to confuse his methods of mechanical occlusal therapy with the normal ranges of nonpathologic change that occur within a person's life. It is one thing to institute occlusal therapy for a degenerating dentition, but the dentist must have the ability to recognize and perceive occlusal breakdown before it advances or deviates from the norm. Normal occlusion depends on the individual, and the dentist must possess the knowledge of what that norm is for each of his patients before he makes his occlusal therapy follow a stereotype for each individual. "Normal" is difficult to define because it is subjective; however, in this day of advancing dental services and information we must at least make an effort to differentiate it from what would be termed "ideal."

A study of interocclusal records enhances the knowledge of the dentist as to how the upper and lower dental arches are related when the teeth come together in a static relationship. Simply, it is the record or "bite" of an individual that allows the dentist to record the mandibular teeth in a relationship to the maxillary teeth, thus enabling the dentist to transfer the models of his patient's teeth to an articulator for either a restorative or an occlusal analysis procedure.

The interocclusal record, or "bite," that a dentist makes of his patient's dental arches is a very important diagnostic and treatment procedure that enables the dentist to design a treatment plan geared specifically to his individual patient's needs. If the interocclusal record is made inaccurately, such inaccuracy will be incorporated into the dentist's occlusal analysis and this error will ultimately be transferred to all of his dental restorative procedures. The dentist's knowledge of his patient's centric relation occlusion (CRO), or centric occlusion (CO), mandibular movements, the degree of orodental breakdown, and how the dental arches are related in function, will give the necessary information to decide the correct restorative procedures and the best interocclusal records necessary for each procedure.

All occlusal forces, when the mandible reaches the terminal hinge-axis position (CRO) and when final closure is made, should be directed toward the long axis of the teeth and be distributed on as many teeth as possible. Sicher[1] states that there are basically two movements of the mandible, the rotational or hinge movement about a horizontal axis passing through the rotational centers of the heads of the condyles and a translatory or sliding movement. The rotational or the hinge-axis position of the mandible is a limiting position that can be repeatedly located, recorded, and used in an individual with any degree of accuracy; it is the only reference point at which the interocclusal record is made to study or rebuild the occlusion of an individual when all other centric closure factors are lost. The teeth of an individual must be so aligned to permit the mandible to reach this position without destructive forces being placed on either the teeth or their supporting structures. The hinge-axis position is reached by individuals at the end of the swallowing cycle and at different brief times during mastication; so any occlusal interferences to the teeth occurring as the mandible reaches this position will result in occlusal wear, destruction of bone, mobility of teeth, and, coupled with periodontal disease, the eventual loss of the teeth.

Ramford and Ash[2] suggest that it is of utmost importance that, after final closure is reached, the centric holding cusps of the teeth hold that position, maintaining the occlusal vertical dimension of the face, and not move or slide forward to any degree. However, there is a natural tendency for the mandible to move forward as it seats against the upper dental arch. If there is not a sufficient number of centric holding positions of the teeth to maintain the centric position of the jaws, this movement or slide from the terminal hinge-axis position (CRO) to a more habitual anterior centric occlusal position (CO) is called "long centric." This slide is not only forward or anteroposterior, but is also "wide" or buccolingual. The extent of this "long and wide centric," prematurities in the occlusion, occlusal wear, and loss of supporting bone structures causes a decrease in the vertical dimensions with subsequent breakdown of the teeth and supporting structures.

Each individual may exhibit a normal amount of long and wide centric position that is compatible to that person without causing detrimental effects and that can be maintained throughout life without causing serious harm. I would say that this slide probably increases with age, and that it should be a constantly monitored situation on the part of the dentist. However, most of the restorative procedures constructed on patients are done by the dentist utilizing a centric occlusion (C.O.) interocclusal record because it is necessary to fabricate the restorations to an existing stable occlusion.

It is necessary to understand that a centric occlusion record of a patient's occlusion is a duplicate of that patient's "bite" (maximum intercuspation of teeth) as he presents himself to the dentist for a restorative treatment. The centric occlusion record makes it possible for the dentist to fabricate a restorative procedure for a particular patient without changing anything in the patient's occlusion. Evaluation through occlusal analysis must be done prior to any restorative procedures to see that the patient's occlusion meets all the requirements that Ramford and Ash[3] suggest for a "normal" or nonpathologic occlusion, defined as one in which the patient exhibits no facet wearing of teeth, no vertical destruction of supporting bone, no looseness of teeth, and no evidence of periodontal breakdown and that the patient has a comfortable interference-free bite with a stable, relaxed centric closure position. Equilibration procedures (see Chapter 19 on the discussion of equilibration) may be necessary to ensure the previous requirements.

The materials generally used in the fabrication of interocclusal records are (1) zinc oxide and eugenol paste washes (such as Kerr's bite registration paste); (2) waxes such as base-plate wax, Aluwax, and preformed wafer horseshoe wax bites (such as copra wax wafers); (3) plastics; (4) nonrigid polyether interocclusal materials (such as Optasil); and (5) combinations of the previous materials.

The general requirements of a material to be used in the registration of interocclusal records should be that the material does not displace the teeth during intercuspation, it should have little or no dimensional change upon setting, the material should give an accurate record of the occlusal surfaces and incisal edges of the teeth to be registered, and the material should remain rigid after setting. Ideally, the material should have so little resistance form that it would not affect the normal closing pattern of the mandible or cause abnormal movement of the teeth during closure.

For a high degree of accuracy, one should check all interocclusal records in the patient's mouth several times to be absolutely sure that the closing pattern of the patient was recorded; more than one record may be desired or even necessary. The safest way to store the interocclusal record is to put it on the models of the teeth and store it in a box prior to mounting on an articulator, or store it on the mounted models after the mounting procedure has been performed. Strohaver[4] did an excellent comparative study of centric-relation position records and found that the zinc oxide and eugenol paste washes, at the present time, come closest to meeting all the requirements of an ideal material to be used for interocclusal records. It can very accurately reproduce the incisal and occlusal form of teeth, it has very little or no resistance texture, and it remains rigid with little or no dimensional change after setting. It is also a material that can be easily reassembled if the interocclusal record is broken or damaged in any way.

Waxes have the distinct advantage when used as an interocclusal record material because they do not accurately reproduce the incisal and occlusal forms of the teeth. Wax tends to spread out laterally as the teeth close into the material, thus not correctly registering the incisal or occlusal form (Fig. 12-1). Waxes have considerable dimensional change caused by any fluctuation in temperature. Further, the texture and nature of the wax material tends to cause a patient to close in an undesirable pattern, with the further possibility of its moving the teeth into abnormal positions.

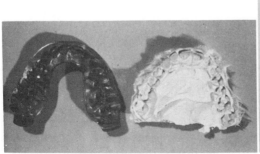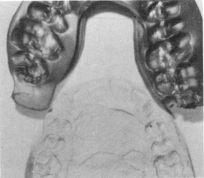

Fig. 12-1. Comparison of accuracy of a wax and a zinc oxide and eugenol centric occlusion interocclusal records of the same dental arches. Note how wax spreads out laterally and how zinc oxide and eugenol interocclusal record is trimmed to only incisal edges and cusp tips of teeth in higher magnification picture.

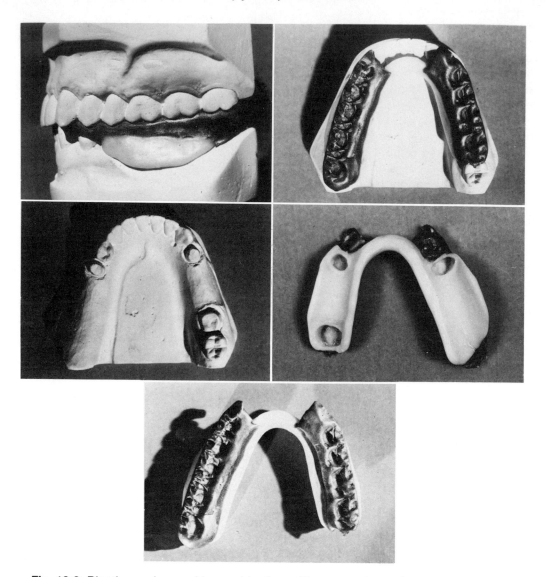

Fig. 12-2. Plastic can be used in combination with wax or zinc oxide and eugenol for an interocclusal record needed for partially edentulous areas. The plastic provides rigid frame for a more accurate recording material.

In partially edentulous areas, and in all areas where the occlusal height of opposing teeth is greater than 6 mm, plastic can be used in combination with Aluwax or zinc oxide and eugenol pastes as an interocclusal medium (Fig. 12-2). Plastics are very rigid and nonbreakable. They are fairly accurate in reproducing the incisal and occlusal edge forms of teeth. However, they have a great deal of resistance to closure and, like waxes, can alter the closing pattern of the mandible. Plastics have a considerable amount of dimensional change after setting. A further disadvantage to using plastics as an interocclusal record is that they can abrade or break the models of either prepared or natural teeth, thus having a dramatic and deleterious effect on the restorative procedure.

Another group of materials to be discussed are the nonrigid polyether materials that can be used for interocclusal records. These materials are extremely accurate in registering the incisal and occlusal forms of teeth, and they have very little dimensional change upon setting. However, these materials have certain distinct disadvantages in that they remain nonrigid after setting and have resistance to compression, which could alter the way that the dentist's models seat into this type of interocclusal record material. These materials do show a great deal of promise and should be reevaluated in the future for possible use, especially when used in conjunction with some type of rigid delivery system to the patient.

The dentist's understanding of occlusion, diagnosis, and treatment planning will give him the proper means and methods of restoring his patients' teeth, and of choosing the desired interocclusal record and to be used for each procedure, using either the patient's centric relation or centric occlusion mandibular position. The registration, whether it be in centric relation or centric occlusion of an individual, has a great many subjective qualities. As previously stated, the dentist must be on guard at all times not to transfer inaccuracies from other patients when fabricating his interocclusal records for a particular patient. The techniques for making these types of interocclusal records are varied and will be subsequently shown.

Method of registering a patient's centric occlusion position

The best method to date used to measure a patient's centric occlusion and centric relation position that is both accurate materially and least subjective as far as the dentist's interpretations of his recordings are concerned involves the use of a zinc oxide and eugenol paste wash and a metal-wire delivery frame as described by Huffman and Regenos[5] for the regis-

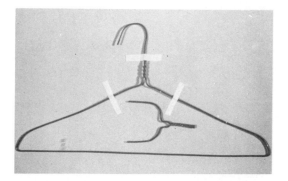

Fig. 12-3. Tape designates areas of metal coat hanger to be cut in order to form frame that is to be used for zinc oxide and eugenol interocclusal records.

trations. Prior to the registration of the centric occlusion position, it is best to have the patient open and close his mouth several times in a relaxed manner and observe exactly the closing pattern of the individual. Do not consider the whole mouth in your observation at this time. Select several teeth on both sides of the dental arches to evaluate how certain inclined planes of these teeth are meeting when the person's mouth is closed in the maximum intercuspation position. If these inclined planes come together in a repeated and exact same position, then the dentist could be confident that this is the centric occlusion position of his patient and that he may proceed with the dental registration.

The "neck" part of an ordinary coat hanger can be cut, shaped, and used for the metal-wire delivery frame (Fig. 12-3). The wire frame is then covered with a glass-fiber type of mesh that will crush into as many small-sized particles as possible (Formulator Mesh). Cut and contour the mesh to fit approximately 3 to 4 mm beyond the buccal surface and incisal edges of the maxillary and mandibular teeth, with the posterior part of the frame terminating at the most posterior tooth. Attach the mesh to the wire frame with a little soft periphery wax (Surgident). Next, trim the mesh so that it extends 3 to

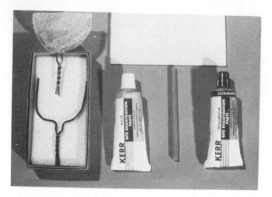

Fig. 12-4. Materials used for a zinc oxide and eugenol interocclusal record; note how formulator mesh is cut, contoured, and attached with wax to fit metal frame.

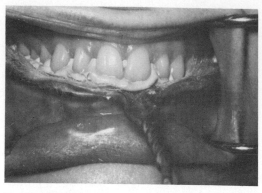

Fig. 12-5. Full-arch zinc oxide and eugenol centric occlusion interocclusal record using contoured metal wire frame.

4 mm beyond the wire frame. It would be a good idea to trim the frame prior to the patient's arrival with the use of his study models. Later when the patient is in the dental chair, seated in a semiupright position or at about a 45-degree angle, finish contouring the frame to the patient's mouth.

After the mesh is cut and contoured and attached to the metal-wire frame with wax (Fig. 12-4), mix equal amounts of zinc oxide and eugenol bite registration paste and smear the paste on the top part of the frame to a depth of about 2 mm in thickness and covering the entire frame. On the underside, or the mandibular side of the frame, add the same amount of paste in a horseshoe pattern, but do not cover the entire frame or the part where the tongue will rest.

At this point the frame is prepared for the dentist to carry through with the registration. Carry the frame to the patient's mouth, but before seating it, ask the patient to open and close his mouth several times to make sure that the patient is aware of his correct centric occlusion pattern. Warn the patient that while the frame is in his mouth he must not bite on the wire part of the frame for this would be a great source of error in the finished registration. Seat the frame and ask the

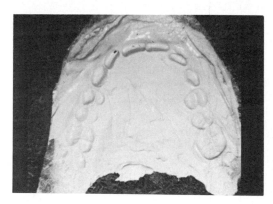

Fig. 12-6. Picture of trimmed zinc oxide and eugenol interocclusal record out of mouth.

patient to close into the paste on the frame, being sure to question the patient if his teeth are in the exact same position that they were in before the registration and instruct the patient to remain closed until the paste is set firmly. See Fig. 12-5.

When the paste has set, remove the wire frame from the mesh while the patient is still in a closed position and then, by holding the frame against the maxillary teeth, ask the patient to open his mouth and gently tease off the record from the maxillary arch (Fig. 12-6).

With a Bard-parker surgical blade remove all excess material that is registered interdentally, as well as any other tissue-impingement areas; these areas may pre-

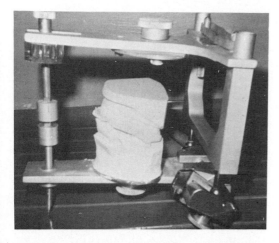

Fig. 12-7. Centric occlusion interocclusal record is used to relate maxillary cast to mandibular cast in final mounting procedures of patient's models on articulator; Whip-Mix Articulator is used in this instance.

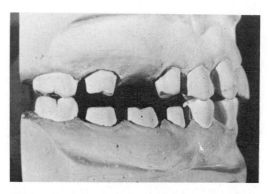

Fig. 12-8. Zinc oxide and eugenol may not build up to great distances that may exist in some prepared cases, and other means of occlusal registration may be necessary, such as using wax in combination with zinc oxide and eugenol pastes.

vent the patient's models from seating properly. Before dismissing the patient, check the models taken previously to see how they relate to the interocclusal record, and recheck the interocclusal record in the patient's mouth to assure that a proper registration of his occlusion was successful. It is of utmost importance at this time for the doctor to understand that he registered his patient's occlusion with the teeth in full contact or in maximal intercuspation and that the centric-occlusion interocclusal record must show perforations in it designating the areas of tooth contact. If this record is not perforated (hold it up to the light to see), then it is quite possible that the patient did not close his teeth together, and the interocclusal record will be in a vertically open position and was done incorrectly. See Fig. 12-7.

If a centric-occlusion interocclusal record is made of a patient's prepared mouth for restorative procedures and the interocclusal space for clearance between preparations is greater than a range of 4 to 6 mm, a combination wax and zinc oxide and eugenol paste interocclusal record should be made because the zinc oxide

and eugenol paste alone does not build up to a 6 mm height. If this is the case, a sheet of base-plate wax can be cut, contoured, and softened to fit the maxillary arch; then request the patient to close in centric occlusion. In the areas of the greatest interocclusal space or edentulous areas, Aluwax can be used to build up to these areas, or a zinc oxide and eugenol paste wash could be used over the wax (Fig. 12-8).

Procedure for registering a patient's interocclusal record in centric relation occlusion

I would define the centric relation position of an individual as being the physiologic position of the condylar heads of the mandible, resting in the most posterosuperior position in the maxillary glenoid fossae from which the arch of closure and all other mandibular positions are initiated. Stuart[6,7] says that "in this position the jaw has a definite recordable opening and closing axis" and that mandibular centricity is related to the hinge axis.

Determining this position can be done in three ways: (1) with pantographic tracings of an individual, as used with a fully adjustable articulator (such as the Stuart and Denar articulators); (2) the use of a plastic anterior jig, as Lucia[8] suggests, to guide the mandible back to its most posterosuperior position; and (3) wax interocclusal records made by the dentist to determine, to the best of his ability, the position of centric relation. Kantor, Silverman, and Garfinkel[9] did a study of recording the centric relation positions of patients and found various degrees of success using these particular methods.

No matter by what means or methods the centric relation position is to be determined on the patient, it is of utmost importance that the teeth do not come into contact while making these centric-relation interocclusal records. For once the teeth come in contact, propriosensations of the teeth could initiate mandibular deflections that could prevent the mandible from going back to its centric relation position. The most accurate centric-relation interocclusal record must be taken at the minimal vertical opening of the jaws while the patient is in a reclining position in the dental chair. Contrary to the centric-occlusion interocclusal records, where maximum intercuspation of teeth is desired, the centric-relation interocclusal record is exactly opposite and must not perforate the registering materials at all.

Registering a patient in the centric relation position when doing a pantographic tracing on a fully adjustable articulator is a necessary part of the tracing. However, a problem that can arise is that the dentist can open the vertical dimension with the clutches used in the pantograph to such a degree (7 to 8 mm of vertical opening) that the condyle heads will subluxate or could go forward to a more anterior position, making it impossible for the centric relation position to be accurately recorded in the tracing.

Registering a patient in his centric relation position with a wax interocclusal record is subjective in nature and is governed entirely by the dentist's manipulation of the mandible and his clinical evaluation as to when he has successfully registered his patient's centric relation position. The problems that can arise when making a wax centric-relation interocclusal record are that (1) the patient can close through the wax and come into tooth contact, with the possibility of mandibular deflections arising; (2) the dentist, when forcing the mandible back, may apply more pressure on one side of the mandible than on the other side, thus not being sure that equal bilateral forces brought the condylar heads back into their most posterosuperior position, or as Dawson[10] says, "One-handed techniques push the mandible back but do not consistently get the condyles up"; and (3) the stability of the wax should be a very guarded situation as not to change dimensionally after the interocclusal record is made. Wax, by its previously stated nature, is not the choicest of materials to be used for this procedure.

The last and probably most consistently accurate method of registering a patient in centric relation position is by the use of an anterior plastic jig in conjunction with a zinc oxide and eugenol paste impression of the incisal and occlusal forms of the teeth. Huffman and Regenos[11] suggest that this procedure be done by taking the most stable quick-setting plastic available, rolling it while it is in a doughy state to approximately 1 inch in length and ¼ inch in width and depth, and, while this plastic is still in a soft and doughy state, mold it on the lingual and labial surfaces of the midline between the maxillary central incisors of the prepared teeth, and then gently guide the patient's mandible back and tell the patient to close into the plastic jig without the posterior teeth coming in contact. See Figs. 12-9 and 12-10.

The dentist can judge if the posterior teeth are not in contact by checking to see that there is approximately 1 mm of ver-

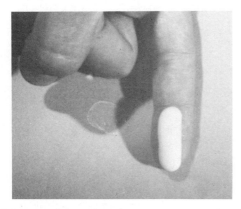

Fig. 12-9. Doughy quick-setting plastic on finger.

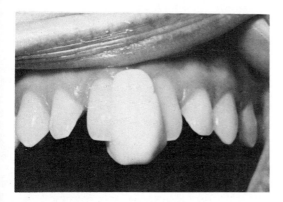

Fig. 12-10. Plastic seated in midline of maxillary central incisors.

tical opening of the posterior teeth. It is not important at this time for the patient to be guided into the centric relation position because the jig will be adjusted so that the mandible will guide itself into its proper position in the glenoid fossae. See Fig. 12-11.

After the plastic jig has hardened, remove it from the teeth and grind the excess lingual plastic formed by the incisal edges of the mandibular central incisor teeth (Fig. 12-12).

Replace the plastic jig in its proper position in the patient's mouth and, with blue articulating paper, adjust the jig so that the only point of contact with one of the mandibular teeth is made into the lingual surface of the plastic jig (but have one mesial or distal corner of one lower central incisor articulate with the jig). See Figs. 12-13 and 12-14.

Again, by using blue articulating paper on the lingual side of the jig, have the patient close. Readjust the jig with a large round bur until you finally reach a point on the lingual surface in which the mandibular teeth cannot go back posterosuperiorly any more. At this point, it is relatively safe to assume that the heads of the condyles are being seated in their most posterosuperior position in the glenoid fossae. See Fig. 12-15.

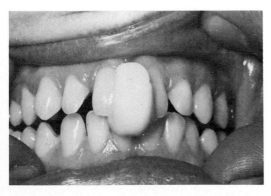

Fig. 12-11. Patient closing into unset plastic at minimal vertical opening.

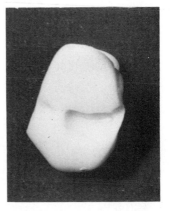

Fig. 12-12. Lingual view of set plastic jig before adjustments.

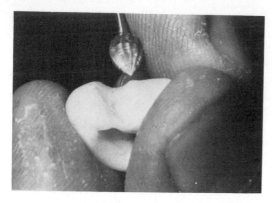

Fig. 12-13. Preliminary adjustment by grinding off excess plastic where mandibular anterior incisors are occluded.

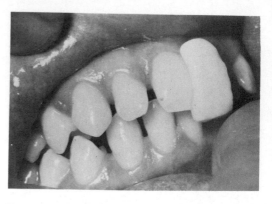

Fig. 12-16. Adjusted anterior plastic jig in centric relation position of patient at minimal vertical opening.

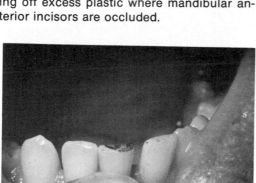

Fig. 12-14. Mesial corner of mandibular right central incisor selected to occlude with plastic jig.

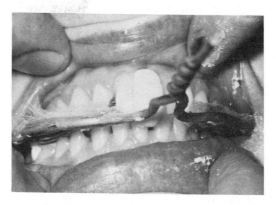

Fig. 12-17. Centric relation interocclusal record using wire frame and anterior plastic jig with zinc oxide and eugenol paste wash seated in patient's mouth.

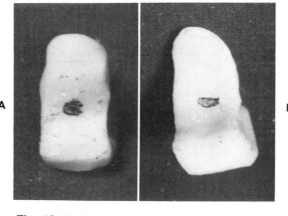

A   **B**

Fig. 12-15. Intermediate carbon mark on top picture, **A,** with final articulated carbon mark on lingual surface of jig designating centric relation position of patient in lower picture, **B.**

Be on guard not to grind the jig in excess or the teeth will come in contact posteriorly. Also, be careful not to make the jig too thick which would cause an excessive vertical opening. Once confident that the jig has been constructed properly to make the mandible reach its terminal position, use it in conjunction with the zinc oxide and eugenol paste wash for the final centric-relation interocclusal record (Fig. 12-16).

With the same procedure outlined in the making of centric-occlusion interocclusal records, the anterior plastic jig can be used for making a centric-relation

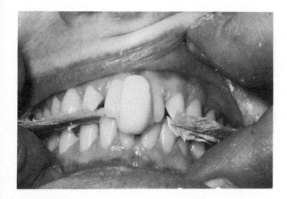

Fig. 12-18. Centric relation interocclusal record with wire frame removed.

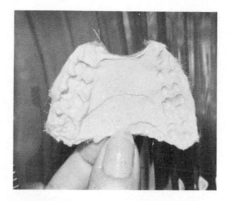

Fig. 12-19. Zinc oxide and eugenol centric relation interocclusal record; note that there are no perforations through paste by posterior teeth and that all tissue impingement areas of interocclusal record have been trimmed, leaving only cusp tips on right.

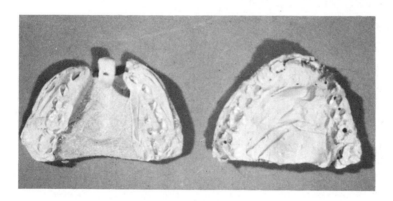

Fig. 12-20. Comparison of centric relation and centric occlusion interocclusal record; note mandatory perforations through centric occlusion record designating full intercuspation of teeth.

interocclusal record. Cutting a V-shaped section out of the anterior section of Formulator Mesh enough to allow the anterior jig to fit into the area is all that is necessary to change the technique from a zinc oxide and eugenol centric-occlusion interocclusal record to a centric-relation interocclusal record.

Seating and then holding the jig in place with one hand, while seating the frame with the zinc oxide and eugenol paste on it in the patient's mouth with the other hand, have the patient close his jaws into the exact same mandibular position previously adjusted into the anterior

plastic jig. Hold the patient's mandible in this position to prevent it from moving forward while the paste is hardening. Once hardened, remove the frame and the interocclusal record and adjust it for accuracy as was outlined previously when making a centric-occlusion interocclusal record. See Figs. 12-17 to 12-21.

Procedure for registering patient's centric relation position of the mandible using the wax "tap-in" method

In this procedure, as well as the one outlined previously using the anterior plastic jig, it is advisable to have the pa-

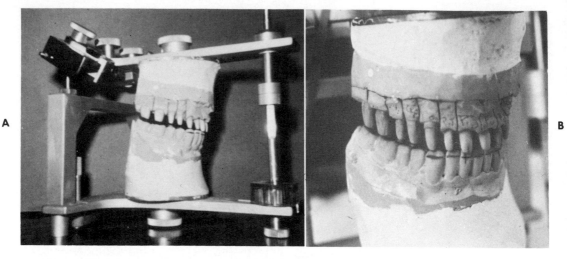

Fig. 12-21. Views of prepared maxillary dental arch mounted on a Whip-Mix Articulator. **B,** Note line on mandibular anterior teeth designating desired length of finished anterior crowns.

tient in a reclining position in the dental chair to make the terminal hinge recording easier and more consistent. A sheet of firm thin wax is then cut and contoured around the maxillary dental arch in such fashion that all incisal edges and occlusal surfaces of the teeth can be registered in the wax. Dawson,[12] however, suggests that only the registration of the posterior teeth be incorporated in the interocclusal record.

Before the registration is made, it is advisable to have the patient open and close his mouth several times to fatigue his muscles enough so that he will have minimum resistance to the mandible reaching its terminal or hinge-axis position.

After the wax is contoured and lightly pressed against the maxillary teeth (care should be taken not to force the cusps or incisal edges of the teeth through the wax), the patient's mandible is then held by the chin with the dentist's thumb resting against the labial surfaces of the lower anterior teeth and the index finger under the chin, or by Dawson's[13] method of holding the mandible bilaterally with both hands. The dentist's thumbnail

should be slightly extended over the incisal edges of the lower anterior teeth to prevent the mandibular teeth from coming into full closure with the maxillary teeth and thus perforating the wax (Fig. 12-22).

The dentist must then direct the mandible in an upward-rearward direction, and by having the patient tap lightly into the maxillary teeth, he can guide the mandible into its hinge-axis position. Tylman[14] suggests that "during the closure the patient brings the tip of the tongue up and back, touching the palate posteriorly," conditioning the patient to permit the heads of the condyles to seat into their most functional terminal position.

After feeling secure that this position has been achieved, remove the wax and chill it, and then repeat the procedure to ensure accuracy. In the final stages of registering this terminal hinge position, it is advisable for the dentist to remove his hands from the patient's mouth and have the patient gently close into this wax "bite" to see if there has been any possible misdirected force initiated by the dentist; the patient, once guided properly

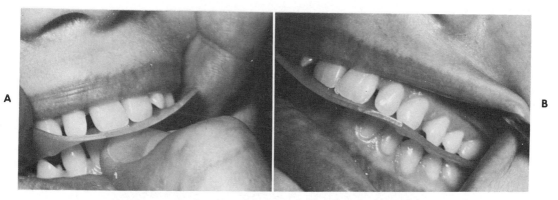

Fig. 12-22. Wafer wax method to register patient in centric relation position. **A,** Wax wafer from midsagittal view with thumb placed on teeth to prevent penetration of wax. **B,** Posterior view of interocclusal record.

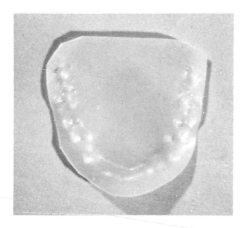

Fig. 12-23. Centric relation wax interocclusal record using "tap-in" method of registration.

into the terminal hinge position, will very often reach that same position unguided (Fig. 12-23).

It is of utmost importance that the wax not be perforated in this procedure because the proprioceptive sensations of the teeth could guide the mandible into deflected positions, causing inaccuracy; several wax bites may be necessary to achieve the desired results. Once achieved the wafer-wax centric-relation interocclusal record should be utilized as quickly as possible in the mounting procedure on the articulator to prevent distortion of the wax and possible error.

The main criticism of this technique is that it is extremely subjective on the part of the dentist as to when the terminal hinge position is reached, and he could easily guide the mandible backward and upward with a nonuniform direction and force on the condyles and not correctly establish the terminal hinge-axis position. Lastly, the thin wafer bite wax can be distorted easily if not used at once for the mounting procedures.

Procedure for lateral checkbite in adjustment of semiadjustable articulator for amount of progressive sideshift and angle of eminentia

In this day of advanced knowledge of mandibular movements and occlusion there have evolved a number of semiadjustable articulators like the Whip-Mix (Fig. 12-24) and the New Hannah articulator (refer to Chaper 13) that are capable of reproducing certain factors of occlusal morphology and mandibular movements, making it possible for the dentist to give his patients a more exact and functionally correct restorative procedure. Hickey, Lundeen, and Bohannan[15] believe that the Whip-Mix articulator has a given limit to its adjustability but is similar in operation to actual jaw movements and can be used successfully

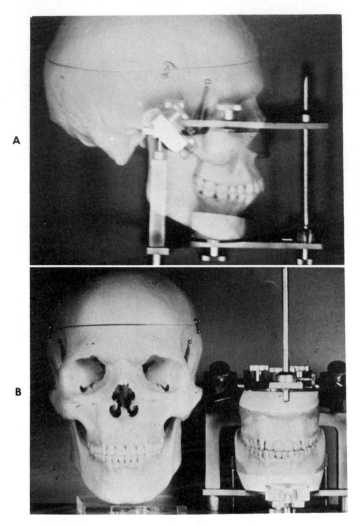

Fig. 12-24. A, Lateral view of semiadjustable Whip-Mix Articulator superimposed on human skull. **B,** Anterior view of mounted models duplicating natural occlusion. (Courtesy Whip-Mix Corp., Louisville, Ky.)

for fixed and removable restorations. Two of the factors of occlusal morphology, the angle of the eminentia and the amount of progressive sideshift (Bennett's movement, laterotrusion), can be determined and transferred to the articulators with the use of a wax lateral checkbite of the patient to be restored or occlusally corrected (Fig. 12-25).

The wax to be used for this procedure should be relatively firm and should be approximately 3 to 4 mm in thickness.

The wax is then contoured and fitted against the maxillary teeth so that only the occlusal surfaces and incisal edges of the teeth to be registered are forced into the wax without perforating it. The patient's mandible is then grasped on either side by the dentist with his thumb and forefinger and moved to either a right or left working position (buccal cusps of the upper teeth in alignment with the buccal cusps of the lower teeth), and the patient is instructed to close into the working

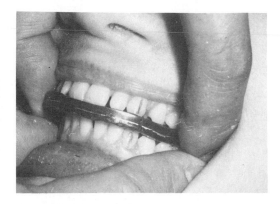

Fig. 12-25. Left lateral working-wax checkbite in a left lateral mandibular working movement used to adjust progressive sideshift and angle of eminentia on Whip-Mix Articulator.

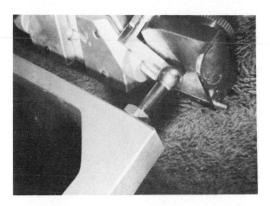

Fig. 12-26. Progressive sideshift lateral metal L bar and superior metal plate designating angle of eminentia in relation to condylar head of Whip-Mix Articulator.

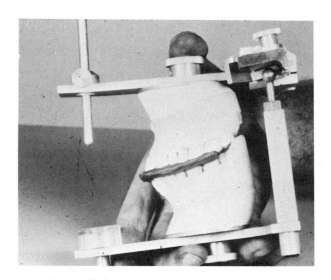

Fig. 12-27. A working-wax checkbite used to set condylar elements of Whip-Mix Articulator. (Courtesy Whip-Mix Corp., Louisville, Ky.)

position. It is of utmost importance for the patient to close into the wax enough to capture the entire occlusal table of the maxillary and mandibular arches while in the working position. The cuspids on both the upper and lower arch could be marked with a pencil to act as a guideline for that position, and as the patient's mandible is brought sideways into its proper alignment, he should be instructed to close into the wax but not hard enough for the cuspids to come into con-

tact. Very often it is less confusing for the patient to be told to move his mandible toward one shoulder or another; it would also help if the dentist tapped on the desired shoulder to indicate in which direction the patient is to move his mandible. The dentist's thumb and forefinger around the chin of the patient should act as a guide for achieving the desired direction.

The condyle that rotates about on a vertical axis in the fossa is called the "working" or the "pivoting" condyle, whereas the one on the opposite side is called the "balancing" or "orbiting" condyle.

The working checkbite is a registration of the balancing condyle as it essentially moves forward, downward, and medially from the glenoid fossa, and by making a right or left working checkbite of a patient, one can determine the amount of progressive sideshift of that patient as well as the direction of travel of the balancing condyle as it is moving away from the glenoid fossa. This direction in which

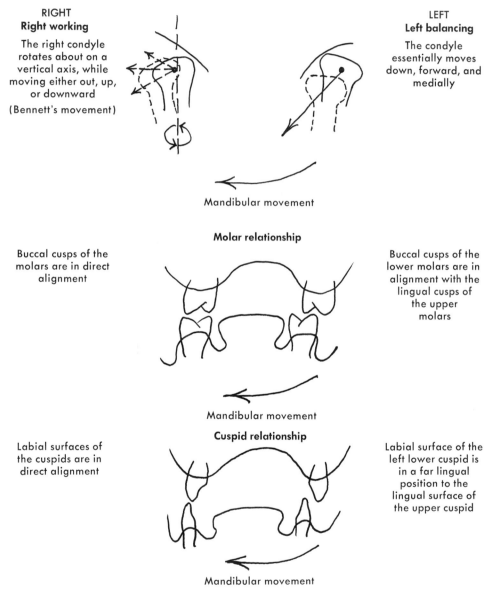

RIGHT
Right working

The right condyle rotates about on a vertical axis, while moving either out, up, or downward

(Bennett's movement)

LEFT
Left balancing

The condyle essentially moves down, forward, and medially

Mandibular movement

Molar relationship

Buccal cusps of the molars are in direct alignment

Buccal cusps of the lower molars are in alignment with the lingual cusps of the upper molars

Mandibular movement

Cuspid relationship

Labial surfaces of the cuspids are in direct alignment

Labial surface of the left lower cuspid is in a far lingual position to the lingual surface of the upper cuspid

Mandibular movement

Fig. 12-28. Diagram of mandibular condyles in a right working movement; opposite being the same for left working position. Also note relationship of molar and cuspid teeth in that position.

the balancing condyle moves is essentially representing the influence of the angle of the eminentia, the contour of the medial wall of the glenoid fossa, the position of the articulator disc in relationship to the articulating surface of the condylar head, and the influence of the musculature as it draws the condylar head away from its rest position (Figs. 12-26 and 12-27).

When the mandible moves to the right side of the maxilla and the buccal cusps of the upper teeth are in alignment with the buccal cusps of the lower teeth (buccal-upper/buccal-lower), then this side is called the working side. In this right working position, the teeth on the left side of the mandible move lingual, inward, and downward to the upper left arch and are not in contact, and this is called the balancing side (buccal-lower/lingual-upper). The opposite is true when the mandible moves to the left side of the maxilla, making this the working side.

Some of the most detrimental forces that can be placed on the teeth are contacts on the balancing side because these forces are lateral forces and are not directed toward the long axis of the teeth. These forces tend to move a tooth in a buccolingual manner, causing the destruction of supporting bone and looseness of teeth.

The movements of the mandible are not always pure movements because the working condyle can move in, out, or downward of the glenoid fossa while it pivots on its vertical axis. Ramford and Ash[16] term the lateral shift of the mandible toward the working side the "progressive sideshift," or "Bennett's movement," and it can be measured by the distance that the working condyle moves. The angle that the balancing condyle moves away from the midsagittal plane in a downward, forward, and inward manner is called "Bennett's angle."

Bennett's movement can be coupled with an immediate sideshift that is only seen in pantographic tracings of mandibular movement, and there is a question as to whether it is normal or is of pathologic origin increasing with age and occlusal disharmony (Fig. 12-28).

After mounting the patient's models on an articulator with a face-bow transfer of the upper arch and the proper interocclusal record to mount the lower cast to the lower member of the articulator, the right and left working checkbites are used to adjust condylar elements of the articulator. The right working checkbite is used to adjust the left balancing condylar elements and vice versa. The advantage of a fully adjustable articulator and of doing a pantograph with subsequent adjustments of the condylar elements is that the angle of the eminentia and the amount of Bennett's movement is corrected in a gradual curve on the fully adjustable articulator and not in a straight line as represented by a semiadjustable articulator.

SELECTED REFERENCES

1. Sicher, H.: Oral anatomy, ed. 6, St. Louis, 1975, The C. V. Mosby Co., pp. 173-191.
2. Ramford, S. P., and Ash, M. M.: Occlusion, Philadelphia, 1968, W. B. Saunders Co., pp. 63 and 253-259.
3. Ramford, S. P., and Ash, M. M.: Ibid., pp. 89-91.
4. Strohaver, R. A.: A comparison of articulator mountings made with centric relation and myocentric position records, J. Prosthet. Dent. **28:**379-390, Oct. 1972.
5. Huffman, R. W., and Regenos, J. W.: Principles of occlusion, London, Ohio, 1973, H & R Press, pp. IV-B-24 to IV-B-33.
6. McCollum, B. B., and Stuart, C. E.: A research report, South Pasadena, Calif., 1955, Scientific Press, pp. 11-13.
7. Stuart, C. E., and Stallard, H.: Why an axis, J. South. Calif. State Dent. Assoc. **32**(6):204-205, June 1964.
8. Lucia, V. O.: A technique for recording centric relation, J. Prosthet. Dent. **14:**492-499, 1964.
9. Kantor, M. E., Silverman, S. I., and Garfinkel, L.: Centric-relation recording techniques—a comparative investigation, J. Prosthet. Dent. **28:**593-600, Dec. 1972.
10. Dawson, P. E.: Evaluation, diagnosis, and treatment of occlusal problems, St. Louis, 1974, The C. V. Mosby Co., p. 57.

11. Huffman, R. W., and Regenos, J. W.: Principles of occlusion, London, Ohio, 1973, H & R Press, pp. IV-B-24 to IV-B-33.
12. Dawson, P. E.: Evaluation, diagnosis, and treatment of occlusal problems, St. Louis, 1974, The C. V. Mosby Co., pp. 62-68.
13. Dawson, P. E.: Ibid., pp. 54-61.
14. Tylman, S. D.: Theory and practice of crown and fixed partial prosthodontics (bridge), St. Louis, 1970, The C. V. Mosby Co., pp. 975-981.
15. Hickey, J., Lundeen, H. C., and Bohannan, H. M.: A new articulator for use in teaching and general dentistry, J. Prosthet. Dent. **18**:425-437, Nov. 1967.
16. Ramfjord, S. P., and Ash, M. M.: Occlusion, Philadelphia, 1968, W. B. Saunders Co., pp. 18-19.

GENERAL REFERENCES

Andrews, L. F.: The six keys to normal occlusion, Am. J. Orthodont. **62**(3):296-310, Sept. 1972.

Caplan, J.: Functional bite technique in crown, inlay and fixed bridgework, Dent. Survey **39**:48-52, July 1963.

Cohn, L. A.: Two techniques for interocclusal records, J. Prosthet. Dent. **13**(3):438-443, May-June 1963.

Emmert, J. H.: A method for registering occlusion in semi-edentulous mouths, J. Prosthet. Dent. **8**(1): 94-99, Jan. 1958.

Evans, R. L.: The gnathological concepts of Charles E. Stuart, Beverly B. McCollum and Harvey Stallard, Georgetown Dent. J. **36**:96, 1970.

Glickman, I., Pameijer, J., and Roeber, F. W.: Intraoral interocclusal telemetry. Part I: A multifrequency transmitter for registering tooth contacts in occlusion, J. Prosthet. Dent. **19**(1):60-67, Jan. 1968.

Glickman, I., Pameijer, J., and Roeber, F. W.: Intraoral occlusal telemetry. Part II: Registration of tooth contacts in chewing and swallowing, J. Prosthet. Dent. **19**(2):151-159, Feb. 1968.

Granger, E. R.: Principles of obtaining occlusion in occlusal rehabilitation, J. Prosthet. Dent. **13**(4): 714-718, July-Aug. 1963.

Kapur, K. K., and Yurkstas, A. A.: An evelution of centric relation records obtained by various techniques, J. Prosthet. Dent. **7**(6):770-786, Nov. 1957.

LaVere, A. M.: Lateral interocclusal positional records, J. Prosthet. Dent. **19**(4):350-358, April 1968.

Millstein, P. L., Kronman, J. H., and Clark, E. R.: Determination of the accuracy of wax interocclusal registrations, J. Prosthet. Dent. **25**(2):189-196, Feb. 1971.

Millstein, P. L., Kronman, J. H., and Clark, E. R.: Determination of the accuracy of wax interocclusal registrations, Part II, J. Prosthet. Dent. **29**(1): 40-45, Jan. 1973.

Nuttall, E. B.: Establishing posterior functional occlusion for fixed partial dentures, J.A.D.A. **66**:342-348, March 1963.

Ricketts, R. M.: Occlusion—the medium of dentistry, J. Prosthet. Dent. **21**(1):39-60, Jan. 1969.

Sheppard, I. M., and Sheppard, S. M.: Denture occlusion, J. Prosthet. Dent. **20**(4):307-318, Oct. 1968.

Stuart, C. E.: Accuracy in measuring functional dimensions and relations in oral prosthesis, J. Prosthet. Dent. **9**(2):220-236, March-April 1959.

Stuart, C. E.: Good occlusion for natural teeth, J. Prosthet. Dent. **14**(4):716-724, July-Aug. 1964.

Stuart, C. E.: Why dental restorations should have cusps, J. South. Calif. State Dent. Assoc. **27**(6): 198-200, June 1959.

Stuart, C. E., and Stallard, H.: Diagnosis and treatment of occlusal relations of the teeth, Texas Dent. J. **75**:430-435, Aug. 1957.

Swaggart, L. W.: Occlusal harmony in complete denture construction, J. Prosthet. Dent. **7**(4): 434-435, July 1957.

Thomas, P. K.: Syllabus on full mouth waxing technique for rehabilitation tooth-to-tooth cusp-fossa concept of organic occlusion, ed. 2, School of Dentistry, Post-Graduate Education, University of California, San Francisco Medical Center, 1967.

Trapozzano, V. R.: An analysis of current concepts of occlusion, J. Prosthet. Dent. **5**(6):764-782, Nov. 1955.

Trapozzano, V. R.: Occlusal records, J. Prosthet. Dent. **5**(3):325-332, May 1955.

Watt, D. M.: Classification of occlusion, Dent. Practitioner **20**(9):305-308, May 1970.

13

The Hanau-Teledyne 154-1 and Denar Mark II articulator systems

David L. Koth

The purpose of this chapter is to describe the use of two relatively new articulator systems: the Hanau-Teledyne 154-1 and the Denar Mark II. These instrumentation systems are useful additions to the existing armamentarium of fully adjustable and semiadjustable articulators that are commercially available to the student and dentist.

These instrument systems are not necessarily recommended as superior to others; each, however, has individual characteristics making it more or less adaptable to specific restorative procedures. Clinical and research data demonstrate that these articulator systems may be used with confidence by any student or dentist who understands completely the principles of occlusion and the complexity of all the organ systems involved in the process of mastication.

Articulators have been variously classified,[3,5,9] and much investigation comparing their relative accuracy has been carried out.[1,10-14] The Hanau-Teledyne 154-1 and Denar Mark II articulators are included together here because they are arcon, semiadjustable articulators. As such they are additions to the Whip-Mix and TMJ articulators, which are two popularly known in this classification. Figs. 13-1 to 13-4 illustrate the Hanau-Teledyne 154-1 and Denar Mark II instruments.

CLASSIFICATION AND CAPABILITIES OF ARTICULATORS
Classification

The dental articulator is a mechanical equivalent of the lower half of the head. As a basis for understanding the relative placement of this instrument into the myriad of dental articulators available, an augmented classification patterned after Heartwell and Rahn[5] will be used.

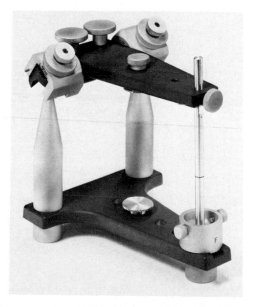

Fig. 13-1. Hanau-Teledyne 154-1 Articulator with incisal cup for customizing incisal guidance.

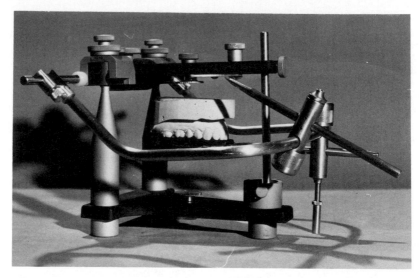

Fig. 13-2. Hanau-Teledyne 154-1 Articulator with face-bow applied.

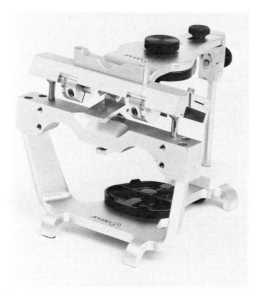

Fig. 13-3. Denar Mark II Articulator with incisal platform.

Class I. Instruments that will receive and reproduce pantograms and graphic tracings in three planes. These articulators are four-dimensional instruments, as they reproduce the timing of Bennett movement. Time is a dimension.

Class II. Instruments that will not receive and reproduce pantograms and graphic tracings in three planes. Some of these instruments will adjust to particular tracings on a pantogram but none has adjustments for the working-side (rotating) condyle or complete timing adjustments. Class II instruments may be further divided into four types:

Type 1. *Hinge type.* Capable of opening and closing in a hingelike movement. Many of these instruments have built-in, nonadjustable eccentric movements.

Type 2. *Arbitrary.* Designed to adapt to certain theories of occlusion.

Type 3. Adjustable to the opening and closing movements and the protrusive and right and left jaw positions, or movements. This category includes the instruments referred to popularly as "semiadjustable" articulators, divided into the following:

Ball and axle or shaft type. In these instruments the condylar elements are reversed from their human counterpart. The condyle, represented usually as a ball, moves with the upper member of the articulator and the angle of the eminentia is represented on the lower member.

Arcon. In these instruments the equivalent condylar guides are placed in the upper member. The condylar elements

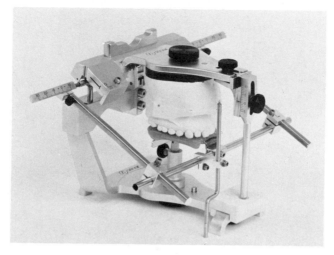

Fig. 13-4. Denar Mark II Articulator with face-bow applied.

are placed in the lower member. The Hanau-Teledyne 154-1 and Denar Mark II are properly identified as class II, type 3, arcon.

Type 4. Instruments designed and used primarily for complete denture construction.

Examples of articulators. The following outline gives examples of each class and type of articulator:

Class I
McCollum Gnathoscope
Stuart Instrument
Granger Gnatholator
Ney Articulator
Denar 5A
Cosmax
Simulator

Class II
Type 1
Stephens
Gariot
Hageman Balancer
Gysi Simplex and Adaptable
Cresant
Type 2
Maxillomandibular articulator by Monson
Type 3
Ball and Axle or Shaft
Dentatus
Gysi Trubyte—when used with face-bow mounting

Hanau H, Hanau University series (except 130-21), Hanau 145-2
House
Arcon
Hanau-Teledyne 154-1
Whip-Mix
Hanau 130-21
Denar Mark II
TMJ
Special type—Transograph
Type 4
Stansbery Tripod
Kile Dentograph
Dupli Functional

Fully adjustable articulators

To aid in visualization, one can describe the mandibular movements in three planes—horizontal, sagittal and coronal—which are mutually perpendicular (Fig. 13-5, *A*). Rotational movements of the mandible occur about axes that are perpendicular to the plane in which the motion is described (Fig. 13-5, *B*).

A completely adjustable articulator is capable of accepting a hinge-axis (kinematic) face-bow transfer, or a face-bow transfer in which anatomic averages are used for location of the transverse hinge axis. Condylar control areas capable of adjustment to posterior anatomic deter-

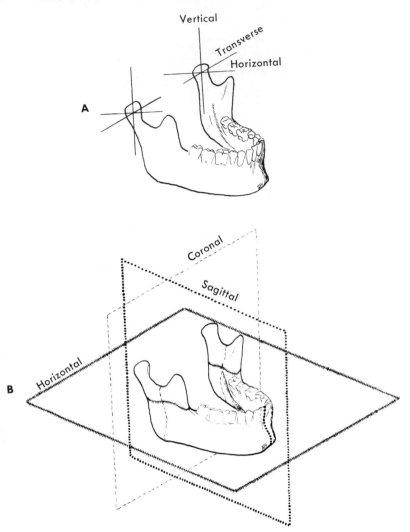

Fig. 13-5. Planes and axes relating to mandibular movements.

minants (which are right and left condylar movements) are recorded directly from the patient by a pantographic tracing. These areas consist of the following[4]:

1. Vertical axis of rotation (intercondylar distance), located in millimeters from the midsagittal plane
2. Protrusive condyle path, expressed in degrees from the horizontal reference plane
3. Orbiting condylar path, expressed in degrees from the horizontal reference plane

4. Immediate sideshift, expressed in millimeters from the centric position of the mandible
5. Progressive sideshift, expressed in degrees from the sagittal plane
6. Sagittal displacements of the rotating condyle
   a. Up or down, expressed in degrees from the horizontal plane
   b. Backward or forward, expressed in degrees from the coronal plane

In addition to the posterior controls, a fully adjustable articulator has provisions to duplicate the third determinant of mandibular movement, which is the total occlusion, and is reproduced on the instrument by recording the horizontal and vertical overlap of the anterior teeth.

It is not the purpose of this chapter to describe in detail what effects these determinants of movement may have on the occlusal surfaces of the dentition. For the purpose of understanding the Hanau-Teledyne and Denar Mark II articulator systems, the determinants that may be recorded will be described briefly. The interested reader should study some of the general references that explain the gnathologic concepts of occlusion.

Capabilities of Hanau-Teledyne 154-1 and Denar Mark II articulator systems

Transfer of relationships. To arrive at a correct static relationship of casts in the articulator, one must transfer certain basic relationships from the patient to the articulator. The transfers include for these systems the following methods:

Face-bow application to patient. Two methods are described for the Hanau-Teledyne, one with a third reference from the patient (anterior reference point) and one with an arbitrary reference. The Denar Mark II is described with earpiece face-bow and arbitrary posterior reference point.

Correct transfer of face-bow record to instrument. Again two methods are described.

Establishment of correct maxillomandibular relationship by means of an accurate centric interocclusal record.

Condylar adjustments. In this chapter these adjustments are described with lateral eccentric checkbites.

Incisal guide preparation. From patient's anterior determinants in conjunction with condylar controls.

Application of relationships. The above procedures are now discussed as applied to these articulator systems, as well as the

significance these relationships describe to the occlusal surfaces of the teeth.

Two essential steps are necessary to orient the maxillary cast on the articulator. First, the transverse (hinge) axis must be located kinematically or by anatomic average measurements. Second, an anterior point of orientation is selected to form a horizontal plane of reference through this point and the transverse axis.

Face-bow transfer. The face-bow transfer in the Hanau-Teledyne 154-1 system is based on the anatomic average location of the transverse hinge axis. In this system the external auditory meatuses are used as the transverse axis (posterior reference points). The anterior point of orientation is either the infraorbitale or the center of the articulator. The upper cast also may be transferred by a kinematic face-bow.

In the Denar Mark II system the posterior reference points may be described by means of the transverse axis or by the average anatomic measurement. In the Denar system the average anatomic measurement may be transferred from the external auditory meatuses or, by use of external marks, located by a "reference-plane locator" and is approximately 12 mm anterior to the middle of the upper border of the external auditory meatus. The anterior reference point is also determined by the reference-plane locator and is approximately 43 mm superior to the incisal edges of the upper anterior teeth.

Raising or lowering the face-bow mounting does not affect centric occlusion. However, it does affect eccentric interocclusal condylar readings, which in turn influence cusp inclines. As the plane of occlusion is elevated, the condylar readings decrease.[15] The relationship of the maxillary cast is important in the sagittal plane and also in the relationship of the occlusal plane to the angle of the eminentia. Because these factors do affect the cusp inclines, it is probably better to transfer the three points directly from the patient's hinge axis and infraorbital notch, rather than use the middle of the articulator. However, both methods will be described in this chapter.

After the maxillary cast is accurately mounted on the upper member of the articulator, the mandibular cast is oriented by means of the centric interocclusal record; thus a static relationship between the maxilla and condyles and mandibular fossa can be obtained. From this static starting position the dynamic eccentric movements are imitated by means of eccentric interocclusal records or pantographic tracings.

Posterior determinants. The posterior controls of both systems are adjusted by means of eccentric checkbites (lateral checkbites). The intercondylar distance (vertical axis) is also determined by means of these checkbites instead of direct measurement in the Hanau-Teledyne 154-1. In this adjustment this articulator differs from other semiadjustable arcon articulators, which measure the intercondylar distance directly from the face-bow. The rationale for this is explained later in this chapter. The Denar Mark II may be augmented, with adjustable intercondylar distance as an accessory benefit.

Intercondylar distance (vertical axis). This has its primary effect on the horizontal plane. As the intercondylar distance increases, the ridge and groove directions move distally on the mandibular posterior teeth and mesially on the maxillary posterior teeth. Conversely, as the intercondylar distance decreases, the ridge and groove directions move mesially on the lower posterior teeth and distally on the maxillary posterior teeth. The intercondylar distance also affects the concavity of the maxillary anterior teeth. As the intercondylar distance increases, the concavity of the maxillary teeth must be greater.[6]

Progressive sideshift (Bennett angle).

Because of the nature of checkbite recordings, this is the only accurate movement of the orbiting condyle that can be recorded. It also is the only movement of this type that the Hanau-Teledyne 154-1 articulator is capable of reproducing; immediate sideshift cannot be incorporated in this instrument. The Denar Mark II is adjustable for immediate sideshift (Bennett shift); this is integrated within the progressive sideshift adjustment. The progressive sideshift of the mandible has a primary effect on the buccolingual inclination of posterior cusps. It also influences the direction of the ridges and grooves of posterior teeth, primarily the tooth contacts on the orbiting side. The greater the sideshift, the more mesial are the ridge and groove directions on the mandibular posterior teeth, and the more distal are the ridge and groove directions on the maxillary posterior teeth. It also has an effect on the lingual concavity of the maxillary anterior teeth; the greater the progressive sideshift, the greater the maxillary lingual concavity must be.[6]

Protrusive condylar path. Because the protrusive path is set by means of a lateral (orbiting side) checkbite, the protrusive path described by the articulator will usually be somewhat steeper than it actually is (Fisher's angle). Also, because of the nature of checkbites, it will be described as a straight line instead of a convex curve relative to the horizontal plane. The protrusive condylar path has its primary effect on the protrusive inclines of the posterior teeth (mesial inclines of the mandibular cusps and distal inclines of the maxillary cusps).[6]

Anterior determinants of occlusion. The mandible is suspended beneath the cranium like a tripod, with the back legs being the right and left temporomandibular articulations, or the posterior determinants and the third leg being the total occlusion including the anterior teeth. The occlusion is the third determinant of mandibular movement and is called the "anterior determinant of mandibular movement."[4]

In the Hanau-Teledyne 154-1 and Denar Mark II articulators, the anterior determinant is set either by adjustment of the incisal guide in consideration of the horizontal and vertical overlap of the anterior teeth, or by customizing an anterior tray on the mandibular member with quick-setting acrylic and the incisal pin of the upper member, a recommended procedure in fixed prosthodontics when the anterior teeth must be prepared.

After studying this brief description of the determinants of mandibular movement, as they apply to these instruments, the reader should be aware of the potential limitations or advantages of these systems relative to other systems.

THE HANAU-TELEDYNE 154-1 ARTICULATOR SYSTEM
Rationale for fixed intercondylar distance

According to Teledyne Dental, Hanau Division,[2] the following rationalization applies to the fixed intercondylar distance:* The Teledyne Articulator is a semiadjustable articulator of the arcon type and has a fixed intercondylar width of 9 cm. A 9 cm intercondylar width is also referred to as an intercondylar distance of 45 mm from the midline. This Teledyne concept is based on the theory

*Quoted text from here to p. 317.

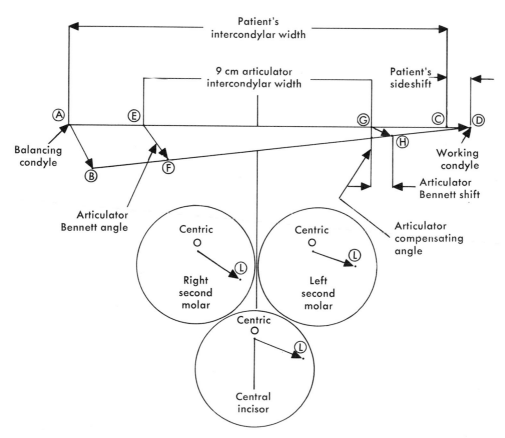

Fig. 13-6. Composite patient and articulator relationship in a left lateral excursion as viewed in horizontal plane (Teledyne Articulator 154-1).

that an adjustable intercondylar width is not necessary and that an adjustable posterior wall will provide the necessary mechanical means to reproduce the patient's mandibular cuspal path.

Fig. 13-6 illustrates a composite patient and articulator relationship in a left lateral excursion as viewed in the horizontal plane.

As the patient's working condyle shifts from centric at *C* to the working point at *D*, the patient's balancing condyle migrates forward, downward, and inward from its centric position at *A* to its balancing point at *B*.

The translation of the working and balancing condyles dictates the mandibular cusp path. Three movements are depicted as the central incisor and the right and left second molars as moving from "centric" to points *L* in this *left lateral excursion.*

Line *A-C* is the patient's intercondylar width, and points *E-G* on this line represent the fixed 9 cm articulator intercondylar width. As line *A-C* translates to its working and balancing points, it becomes line *B-D*, and points *E-G* will have migrated to *F-H* respectively.

One will note that if the articulator points *E-F* are aligned with a medial guiding wall and points *G-H* with a posterior guiding wall, the patient's *A-B* and *C-D* may be removed and the articulator will then continue to maintain the mandibular cusp paths from centric to *L*.

The articulator has an adjustable Bennett angle that is rotated on the balancing side to contact and form a medial guiding wall for the condyle movement between points *E* and *F*.

The rationale of a fixed 9 cm is directed at the posterior wall of the articulator.

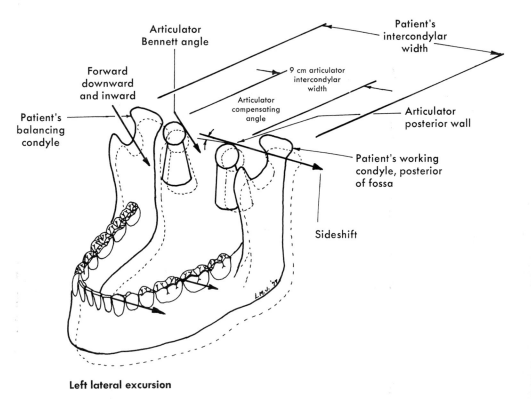

Left lateral excursion

Fig. 13-7. Composite sketch of patient and articulator condyles in a left lateral excursion.

This wall is termed the "compensating angle" and is rotated on the working side to contact and form a continuous posterior guiding wall for the condyle sideshift from point *G* to point *H*.

Fig. 13-7 also shows the mandible in a left lateral excursion. Integral to and between the mandibular condyles are articulator condyles at a 9 cm intercondylar width.

The patient's working condyle shifts to the side, guided by the superior and posterior portion of its fossa. Concurrent with this Bennett shift of the working condyle is the forward, downward, and inward movement of the balancing condyle as it is guided by the superior and medial surfaces of its fossa.

This composite sketch of a patient and articulator contains two articulator condyles that move integral to the working and balancing condyles. As the patient's working condyle shifts to the side, the articulator condyle simultaneously shifts to a mechanical equivalency, guided by the posterior and superior wall of the articulator. The degree of angulation at the continuous guiding surface of the posterior articulator wall is related to the vertical plane and is termed the "compensating angle."

The patient's balancing condyle migrates forward, downward, and inward while the articulator condyle follows its mechanical equivalent, guided by its superior and medial (Bennett angle) walls.

In summation, the posterior wall of the articulator is adjusted to form a continuous guiding surface for the repositioning of the working condyle and effectively provides a mechanical equivalent of an articulator intercondylar adjustment. The transfer means from the patient to the articulator terminal working and balancing positions is by lateral interocclusal records.

The Hanau-Teledyne 154-1 semiadjustable articulator system possesses the same possible inaccuracies as any other semiadjustable articulator, that is, the lack of adjustment for timing of mediotrusion, superior wall shape, laterotrusion direction, and immediate sideshift. Accepting these inherent possible inaccuracies and realizing the possible necessity for more than a nominal intraoral adjustment. The specific applications of this articulator system will be described.

The face-bow supplied with the system is a modified Snow type with ear inserts. The face-bow orientation may be recorded with or without a third facial reference point. For use without the third point, a bite plane support is included to center the incisal edges of the maxillary teeth in the articulator. It is, however, preferable to use a third facial point to more accurately align the maxillary cast in space. In this instance the anterior reference point is the infraorbitale and roughly relates the maxillary cast to the Frankfort plane in the articulator. For this purpose an orbital indicator is supplied with the system.

If one anticipates any alteration of the vertical dimension, either in obtaining a centric registration or in restoring the occlusion, a hinge-axis face-bow transfer is recommended. The technique for this is described in Chapter 28. For the mounting of this orientation a hinge-axis transfer template is provided.

To obtain the advantages of any articulator system a complete understanding of its components is necessary. To aid the reader in this understanding, an attempt will be made to completely describe the system and then follow through with a step by step procedure following the basic system's components.

Specific steps in setting the Hanau-Teledyne 154-1 articulator

Earpiece face-bow preparation

1. The biteplane is covered with compound or a material of choice to a

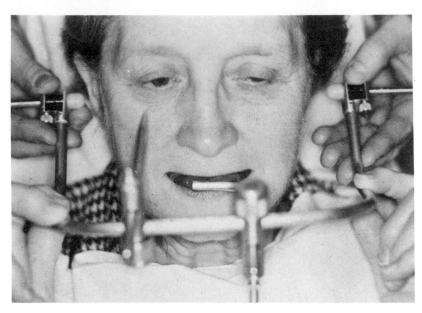

Fig. 13-8. Face-bow application to patient before adjustments are centered.

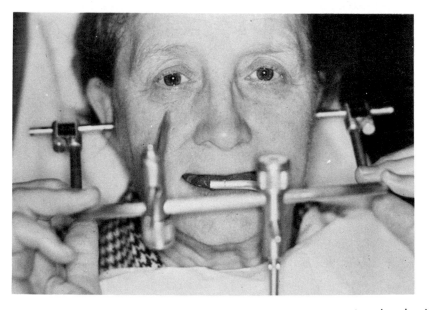

Fig. 13-9. Face-bow application to patient after adjustments are centered and anterior reference point is secured.

thickness suitable for obtaining an occlusal imprint of the maxillary teeth.

2. Slightly loosen the two frame thumbscrews and slide the scales outward to abut the nylon earpieces with the frames. The nylon earpieces are threaded onto the scales and may be removed. Loosen the clamp thumbscrew to permit free movement of the biteplane clamp on the bow.

Earpiece face-bow application with infraorbital pointer (Figs. 13-8 and 13-9)

3. The softened impression material on the biteplane is seated against the maxillary teeth to create distinct cusp imprints without metal contact and with the stem of the biteplane extending approximately parallel to the sagittal plane. This index is then chilled while the biteplane is firmly held in position by the mandibular teeth. The imprint of the maxillary occlusal surface will be used only to transfer the maxillary cast to the articulator and no attention need be given to the mandibular relation when making this registration.

4. The face-bow is then brought gently over the face with the stem of the biteplane entering the loose biteplane clamp. Hold both frame thumbscrews between the thumbs and middle fingers. Place the forefingers on the ends of the earpieces and slide the scales to enter the nylon earpieces into the meatus of the ear. Simultaneously slide the frames laterally to symmetrically adjust the scales while maintaining a comfortable, yet secure suspension of the nylon earpieces in the meatus. Tighten both frame thumbscrews to maintain this symmetry of suspension.

5. Grasp the frontal portion of the face-bow and tighten the clamp thumbscrew securely to lock the bow to a biteplane relationship. The orbital pointer, previously placed on the earpiece face-bow, is placed into gentle contact with the infraorbitale as shown. This contact should just touch the patient's skin and make no indentation. The clamp thumbscrew is tightened securely to lock this third reference to the face-bow, biteplane, and external auditory meatus relationship. Release the two frame thumbscrews and withdraw the scales with nylon earpieces from the meatus. Remove the entire face-bow assembly from the patient.

6. After the face-bow relationship has been established from the patient, three interocclusal records are needed and are most conveniently obtained at this appointment. The records necessary are centric interocclusal and right and left lateral. They may be obtained as described in Chapter 12.

The earpiece face-bow application is the same without the orbital pointer, except that there is no anterior reference point.

Articulator preparation with infraorbital pointer. Compare outline that follows step 9.

7a. Adjust the *right* and *left* condylar inclinations to 0 degrees and tighten condylar thumbscrews.

b. Loosen the compensating thumbnuts and adjust the *right* and *left* compensating angles to their stops at their most positive angulation. Tighten the compensating thumbnuts.

c. Loosen the Bennett thumbnuts and adjust the *right* and *left* Bennett angles to 20 degrees. Do not tighten the Bennett thumbnuts.

d. Adjust the incisal pin to align the registration groove with the underside of the upper member and tighten the incisal thumbscrew.

e. Apply a thin coating of petroleum jelly on the condylar elements and to all of articulator surfaces that will be exposed to the stone mounting medium.

f. Attach disposable mounting inserts to the upper member and cast support to the lower member.

Earpiece face-bow transfer with infraorbital pointer (Fig. 13-10)

8. Attach the earpiece face-bow assembly by equally adjusting the scales to suspend the nylon earpieces securely over the auditory pins of the condylar guidances.

9. Adjust the elevating jack until the orbital pointer just touches the orbital indicator as shown in Fig. 13-10. Be certain the incisal pin touches the bottom of the incisal cup without interference from the

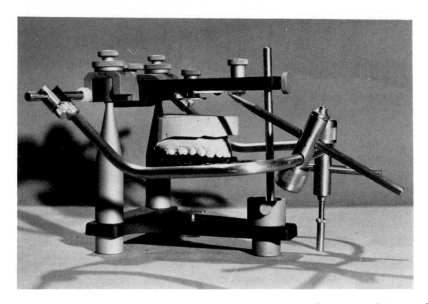

Fig. 13-10. Face-bow transfer to articulator using anterior reference pointer on face-bow and orbital indicator on upper member of articulator. Cast support will take the place of lower mounting insert.

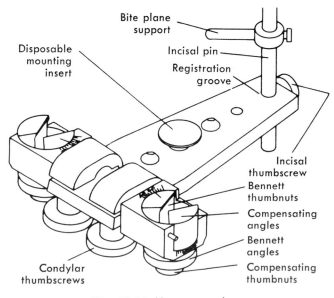

Fig. 13-11. Upper member.

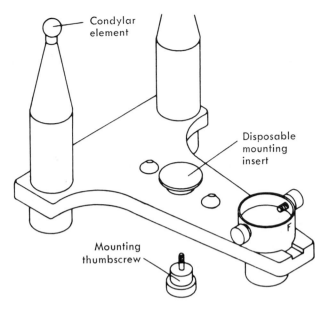

Fig. 13-12. Lower member.

maxillary cast. Adjust the cast support so that it is supporting, but do not force the biteplane. Mix a thin mix of fast-setting stone being sure stone engages the disposable mounting insert and the two circular bosses on the maxillary member. Upon completion of set of mounting, remove face-bow and cast support. Replace cast support with disposable mounting insert.

Articulator preparation without infraorbital pointer (Figs. 13-11 and 13-12). Compare previous steps 7 to 9 with steps 10 to 12.

10a. Adjust the *right* and *left* condylar inclinations to 0 degrees and tighten condylar thumbscrews.

b. Loosen the compensating thumbnuts and adjust the *right* and *left* compensating angles to their stops at their most positive angulation. Tighten the compensating thumbnuts.

c. Loosen the Bennett thumbnuts and adjust the *right* and *left* Bennett angles to 20 degrees. Do not tighten the Bennett thumbnuts.

d. Adjust the incisal pin to align the registration groove with the underside of the upper member and tighten the incisal thumbscrew.

e. Apply a thin coating of petroleum jelly on the condylar elements and to all of articulator surfaces that will be exposed to the stone mounting medium.

f. Attach disposable mounting inserts to the upper member and lower member by the mounting thumbscrews.

Earpiece face-bow transfer without infraorbital pointer (Fig. 13-13)

11. Attach the earpiece face-bow assembly by equally adjusting the scales to suspend the nylon earpieces securely over the auditory pins of the condylar guidances.

12. Rotate the suspended face-bow over the upper member and align the incisal edge index of the upper centrals on an approximate plane with the landmark groove on the incisal pin. Raise the biteplane support to contact the stem of the biteplane, and tighten the thumbscrew to maintain this alignment.

13. Swing the face-bow back and seat and securely lute the maxillary cast in the occlusal index of the biteplane.

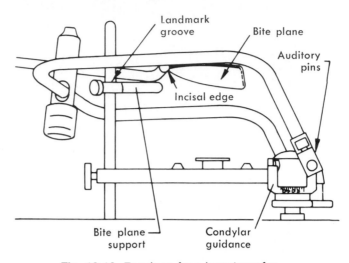

Fig. 13-13. Earpiece face-bow transfer.

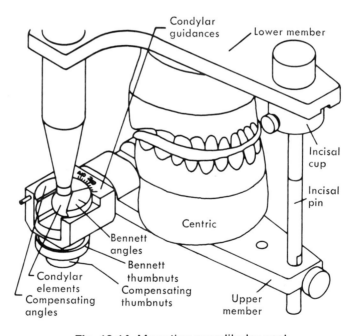

Fig. 13-14. Mounting mandibular cast.

14. A mixture of stone is heaped onto the maxillary cast and over the disposable mounting insert and the two circular bosses on the upper member.

15. The face-bow is then swung over to contact the stem of the biteplane with the biteplane support. Complete the mounting with a spatula, making certain that the two circular bosses on the upper member are covered by the stone. Remove excess material to provide for the convenient removal and accurate reattachment of the cast to the upper member.

16. Upon complete set of the mounting, remove the face-bow and biteplane support.

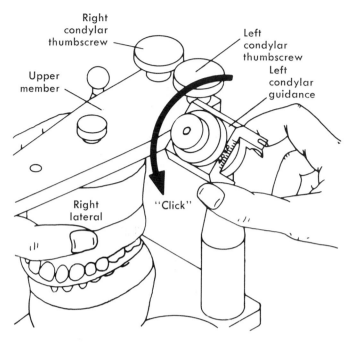

Fig. 13-15. Left condylar inclination.

Mounting mandibular cast (Fig. 13-14)

17. Accurately seat and lute the centric interocclusal record between the maxillary and mandibular casts.

18. A mixture of stone is heaped onto the mandibular cast and over the disposable mounting insert and the two circular bosses of the lower member.

19. The lower member is then inverted and the condylar elements are gently entered into the condylar guidances and to their most retruded positions. Pivot the lower member forward to lower the incisal cup into contact with the incisal pin. Use the forefingers to rotate the *right* and *left* compensating angles to an approximate parallelism with the vertical plane. This locks the condylar elements between the Bennett and compensating angles and assures a centric position of the articulator during the setting of the stone mounting. Complete the mounting with a spatula, removing excess material to provide for removal and accurate reattachment of the cast to the lower member.

20a. Upon complete set of the mounting, rotate the Bennett angles to approximately 20 degrees, remove the centric interocclusal record and carefully lift the lower member from the condylar guidances. Place the lower member in an upright position on the workbench.

b. Continue rotating both Bennett angles to 45 degrees and secure their adjustment by tightening the Bennett thumbnuts.

c. Loosen the compensating thumbnuts and rotate both compensating angles to approximately 0 degrees. Tighten the compensating thumbnuts.

d. Raise or remove the incisal pin to prevent contact with the incisal cup during subsequent adjustments.

e. Release the *right* condylar thumbscrew and remove the *right* condylar guidance. This prevents mechanical interference in step 18.

Adjustment of condylar guidances

21. Seat the *right* lateral interocclusal record between the maxillary and mandibular casts (Fig. 13-15). Grasp the

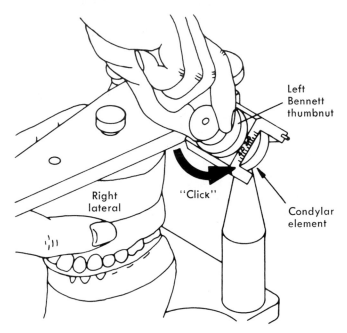

Fig. 13-16. Left Bennett angle.

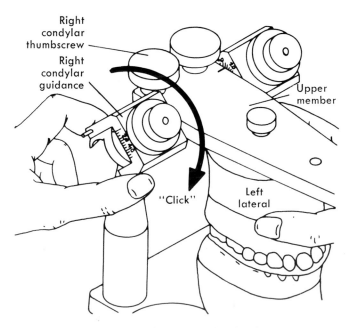

Fig. 13-17. Right condylar inclination.

maxillary cast and immobilize it and the upper member in this relation record.

a. Release the *left* condylar thumbscrew and adjust the *left* condylar guidance inclincation to contact the condylar element (Fig. 13-15). Tighten the *left* condylar thumbscrew. The suggested method of adjustment is to place the lower member onto a hard and rigid workbench that will act as a sounding board and amplify the "click" of the condylar element as it contacts the condylar guidance. The adjustment may also be made by sight and feel.

b. Release the *left* Bennett thumbnut and rotate the *left* Bennett angle to contact the condylar element (Fig. 13-16). Tighten the Bennett thumbnut.

22. Remove the upper member and reattach the *right* condylar guidance, adjusting the condylar inclination to 0 degrees.

23. Remove the *right* lateral record and seat the *left* lateral interocclusal record between the maxillary and mandibular casts (Fig. 13-17). Grasp the max-

illary cast to immobilize it and the upper member in this lateral relationship.

a. Release the *right* condylar thumbscrew and adjust the *right* condylar guidance inclination to contact the condylar element (Fig. 13-17). Tighten the *right* condylar thumbscrew.

b. Release the *right* Bennett thumbnut and rotate the *right* Bennett angle to contact the condylar element (Fig. 13-18). Tighten the *right* Bennett thumbnut.

c. Release the *left* compensating thumbnut and rotate the *left* compensating angle into contact with the condylar element (Fig. 13-19). Tighten the *left* compensating thumbnut.

24. Remove the *left* lateral interocclusal record and replace it with the *right* record (Fig. 13-20). Hold the maxillary cast firmly in this *right* lateral interocclusal record, release the *right* compensating thumbnut, and rotate the *right* compensating angle into contact with the condylar element. Tighten the *right* compensating thumbnut and remove the *right* lateral record.

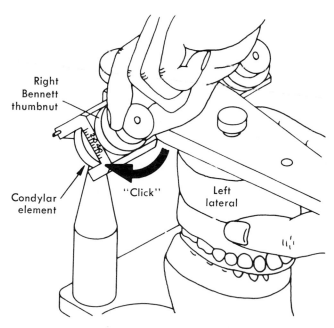

Fig. 13-18. Right Bennett angle.

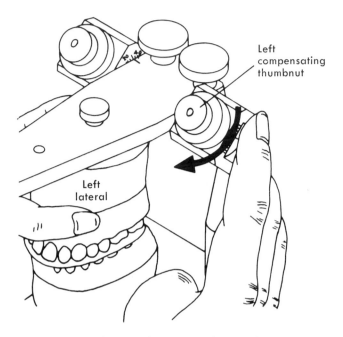

Fig. 13-19. Left compensating angle.

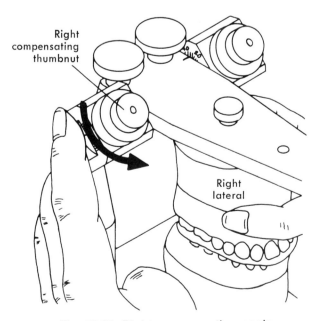

Fig. 13-20. Right compensating angle.

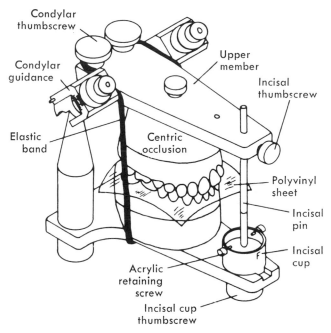

Fig. 13-21. Incisal guide preparation.

Incisal guide preparation (Fig. 13-21)

25a. Carefully engage the upper member, bringing the casts into centric position.

b. Apply an elastic band over the articulator posterior to the casts and loop it around the condylar thumbscrews. This assists the condylar elements to maintain constant contact with the condylar guidances during excursions from and returning to centric.

c. Loosen the incisal cup thumbscrew and adjust the incisal cup anteroposteriorly to approximate its center to the incisal pin. Tighten the incisal cup thumbscrew.

d. Lower the incisal pin into contact with the incisal cup and tighten the incisal thumbscrew securely.

e. Lubricate the spheric or ovoid end of the incisal pin and the interior of the incisal cup with a thin coating of petroleum jelly.

f. Firmly attach the two acrylic retaining screws at the side of the incisal cup.

g. Place a 4 × 4 inch piece of 0.0015 inch polyvinyl sheet between the maxillary and mandibular casts to resist abrasion of the stone cusps during the fabrication of the acrylic incisal guide.

Fabrication of acrylic incisal guide (Fig. 13-22)

26. Quick cure acrylic is mixed. Raise and hold the upper member to permit filling the incisal cup, completely immersing the two acrylic retaining screws.

27. After mixing, the upper member is lowered to enter the incisal pin into the acrylic. Immediately make excursions as prescribed in a, b, and c below. The incisal pin must never be used to make lateral excursions from centric as to do so will negate the Bennett shift and Bennett angle, causing the working condyle only to rotate.

a. Gently guide the maxillary cast into a full and straight protrusive by applying thumb pressure at the anterior teeth and promptly return to centric (Fig. 13-23).

b. From this centric position, gently guide the maxillary cast into a full right lateral by thumb pressure at the right side

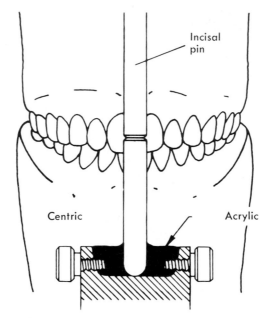

Fig. 13-22. Fabrication of incisal guide table. Incisal pin placed in acrylic resin in centric position.

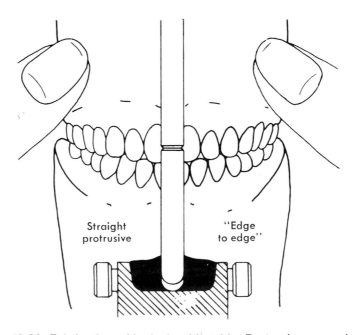

Fig. 13-23. Fabrication of incisal guide table. Protrusive excursion.

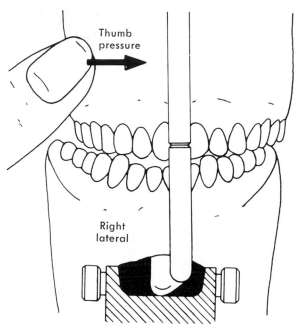

Fig. 13-24. Fabrication of incisal guide table. Right lateral excursion.

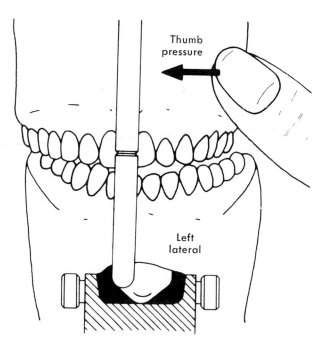

Fig. 13-25. Fabrication of incisal guide table. Left lateral excursion.

of the cast to ensure that the Bennett shift is acceptable and then return to centric (Fig. 13-24). The Bennett angle on the nonworking side will be followed automatically.

c. The maxillary cast is then guided through a full left lateral excursion with its return to centric (Fig. 13-25). Thumb pressure applied to the left side of the cast will provide the full utilization of the condylar guidance settings. The incisal pin will be observed to displace the acrylic, and the three excursions must be repeated every 15 seconds until the material has set.

28. Upon complete set of the acrylic resin, the frontal area of the plastic may be relieved with a stone to permit free opening and closing of the upper member at a centric relation.

29. Always apply thumb pressure at the side of the maxillary cast during lateral excursions to ensure that the Bennett shift on the working side and the Bennett angle on the nonworking side are acceptable. Pressure at the front of the cast will assure protrusion.

General notes. The maxillary or mandibular casts may be removed from the upper or lower member at any time and returned to their exact positional relation by virtue of the disposable mounting insert combined with the circular bosses.

The molded acrylic incisal guidance may be removed from the incisal cup by removing the two acrylic retaining screws and lifting it out of the cup.

The articulators are not 100% identical and reattachment of the maxillary or mandibular casts or the acrylic incisal guidance must be made on the same articulator. Etch the articulator serial number on the casts and incisal guidance. Also record the condylar inclination, Bennett angle, and compensating angle for possible reattachment of the case.

It is repeated that the incisal pin must never be used to make excursions from centric. To do so will negate the Bennett

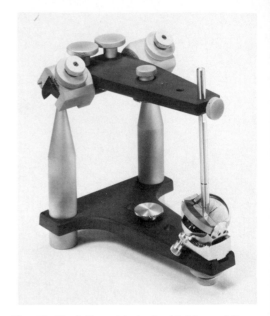

Fig. 13-26. Adjustable incisal table and its related incisal pin.

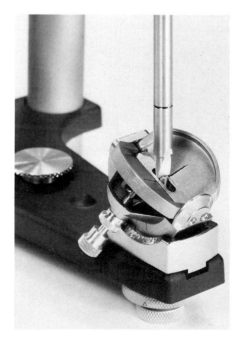

Fig. 13-27. Long centric adjustable incisal guide and its related incisal pin.

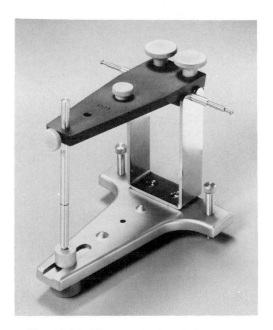

Fig. 13-28. Hinge-axis transfer template.

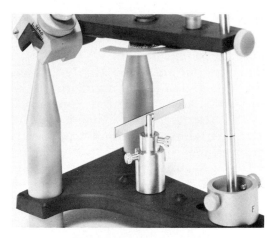

Fig. 13-30. Cast support.

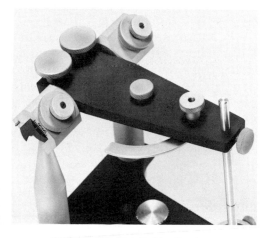

Fig. 13-29. Orbital indicator.

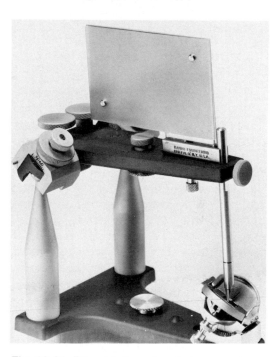

Fig. 13-31. Broadrick occlusal plane analyzer.

shift and Bennett angle causing the working condyle to rotate only.

Optional accessories

The *adjustable incisal guide* and the *related incisal pin* (Fig. 13-26) provide adjustment of incisal guidance in protrusive and right and left lateral excursions to aid in harmonious cuspal interdigitation of edentulous as well as dentulous cases.

The *long centric adjustable incisal guide* and the *related incisal pin* (Fig. 13-27) allow freedom of movement in centric occlusion. A vertically adjustable horizontal plane, when elevated above the surface of the incisal guide table, introduces a horizontal area on which the incisal pin functions before encountering lateral or protrusive inclines.

The *hinge-axis transfer template* (Fig. 13-28) permits the transfer of a true hinge axis–maxillary arch relationship record with any kinematic bow.

The *orbital indicator* (Fig. 13-29) permits orientation of the maxillary cast in the articulator when the infraorbital notch is used as a third anatomic point of reference during face-bow application and transfer.

The *cast support* (Fig. 13-30) supports the biteplane during face-bow transfer when a maxillary cast is mounted to the articulator in an upright position.

The *Broadrick occlusal plane analyzer* (Fig. 13-31) is used for analyzing the curve of Spee and in developing an acceptable curve of occlusion.

THE DENAR MARK II ARTICULATOR SYSTEM

This articulator system was developed to meet a need at the undergraduate level of dental education. Dental educators realize that the arcon type of articulator is most demonstrable when teaching courses in occlusion. It is, however, a two-piece instrument. Because of this, it is not ideally suited for carrying out extensive restorations, especially removable prostheses. The Mark II articulator incorporates a very positive lock so that it can be, essentially, a one-piece instrument.

The foregoing specification was considered to be paramount. Second, a very positive centric latch was needed, because neophytes to arcon instruments have difficulty mounting casts in centric. Third, a rigid, sturdy, and precision-manufactured instrument was requested.

To produce a system that is affordable to the student, and the dentist who wants a very adaptable articulator that is not fully adjustable, certain priorities of adjustments were arranged. After input from many dentists was received, the following priorities were detailed in descending order: protrusive adjustment, immediate sideshift, progressive sideshift, intercondylar distance adjustment, rear-wall adjustment, top-wall adjustment.

Presently the Denar Mark II articulator has adjustments for protrusive movement, 0 to 60 degrees in increments of 5 degrees; immediate sideshift, 0 to 4 mm with a Vernier scale in 0.2 mm increments; progressive sideshift, 5 to 15 degrees in increments of 5 degrees; incisal adjustment, made either by molding an acrylic custom table or by an adjustable mechanical table.

The rear wall is set to an average anatomic posterior inclination of 25 degrees. The intercondylar distance may be adjusted from 52 to 66 mm from the midline, if desired, by use of the intercondylar width adjustment accessory. Research[1] indicates this to be acceptable for the majority of patients.

The Mark II system was also developed to fill a need existing among practicing dentists and laboratory technicians. This need was expressed as a desire for a relatively uncomplicated class II, type 3, arcon articulator that was anatomically accurate and could provide a positive centric lock.

A desirable feature of the Mark II system is its similarity in design to some of the fully adjustable articulators and their accessories. This feature allows the user a less confusing transition to the so-called fully adjustable articulators, if that transition is desired.

The Denar Mark II articulator system possesses the same possible inaccuracies as other semiadjustable articulators, that is, the lack of adjustment for timing of mediotrusion, superior wall shape, and lateral movement. It does, however, provide for adjustment to immediate sideshift. In acknowledgment of these inherent possible errors and the realization of the possible necessity for more than a nominal intraoral adjustment, the specific applications of this instrument system are now discussed.

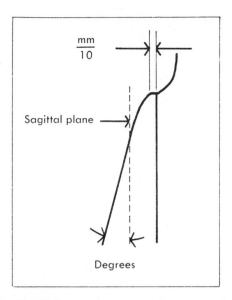

Fig. 13-32. Component condylar movements in mandibular sideshift. Immediate sideshift is expressed in tenths of a millimeter, and progressive sideshift is expressed in degrees. (Courtesy Denar Corp., Anaheim, Calif.)

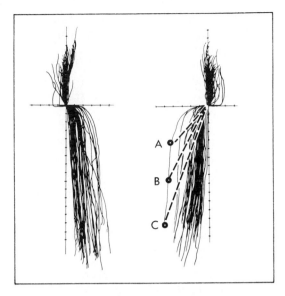

Fig. 13-33. Composite illustration of protrusive, orbiting, and rotating paths of condylar movement of right and left temporomandibular joints of 50 patients. (Courtesy Denar Corp., Anaheim, Calif.)

Immediate and progressive sideshift adjustments (Bennett shift)

The Denar Mark II semiadjustable articulator has the capability of simulating the mandibular sideshift (Bennett shift) integrating the component condylar movements: the immediate sideshift and the progressive shift. The immediate sideshift is expressed in units of tenths of a millimeter, and the progressive sideshift is expressed in degrees (Fig. 13-32).

The immediate sideshift of the mandible has primary influence on the width of the central groove of posterior teeth. The progressive sideshift has its principal influence on the balancing inclines of posterior cusps on the orbiting side and on the direction of the ridges and grooves of posterior teeth, primarily on the orbiting side. Fig. 13-33 illustrates the protrusive, orbiting, and rotating path records of the right and left temporomandibular joints of 50 patients (100 TMJ records).[7] The X and Y axes are calibrated in increments of 1 mm. The orbiting path is divided

essentially into two components: immediate sideshift and progressive sideshift. According to this research, with few exceptions, once the immediate sideshift has occurred, the progressive sideshift records are approximately parallel to each other and are inclined approximately 5 to 7 degrees to the sagittal plane. The biggest variable is in the immediate sideshift component of the orbiting path.

Points *A*, *B*, and *C* on one orbiting path represent three different condylar positions at which lateral checkbite positional records may be taken on one patient. It should be noted that if an articulator possessing a progressive sideshift and not an immediate sideshift adjustment were set to each of the three condylar positions *A*, *B*, and *C* as shown in Fig. 13-33, it would produce three different progressive sideshift inclinations corresponding to the three dotted lines in Fig. 13-33.

If an articulator possesses immediate sideshift as well as progressive sideshift adjustments, the progressive could be set to an average anatomic dimension of 6 degrees, and one immediate sideshift adjustment setting will intersect all three condylar checkbite records (*A, B,* and *C*), which could reduce the amount of irritation that otherwise might be introduced in the occlusion. The Denar Mark II articulator has this capability; therefore, when adjusting the Mark II articulator to lateral checkbite records, always set the progressive sideshift adjustment to the 6-degree average anatomic dimension for this diagnostic procedure.

Application of Denar Mark II articulator system

Face-bow/ear-bow application. The Denar Mark II Facebow/Earbow is used to register the correct position for the patient's maxillary cast to be mounted in the articulator. In other words, the face-bow/ear-bow records the relation of the patient's maxillary dental structures to the horizontal reference plane and transfers this relationship to the articulator.

The use of the Denar Facebow/Earbow involves three overall procedures:
1. Locating three reference points on the patient's face
2. Assembling the face-bow/ear-bow on the patient
3. Transferring the face-bow/ear-bow to the articulator

Locating three reference points on patient's face. The components of the face-bow kit needed are the reference plane locator and reference plane marker. These two items are used to locate three anatomic reference points on the patient's face. Of these three points, two are posterior and one is anterior.

Average measurement may be used to locate the posterior reference points whenever the vertical dimension of the casts on the articulator is not altered, or, in other words, when the mandibular cast is to be transferred to the articulator by means of an interocclusal record taken at the correct vertical dimension and the

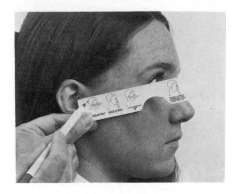

Fig. 13-34. Use of reference-plane locator to establish arbitrary posterior reference points.

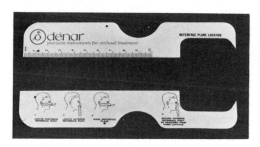

Fig. 13-35. Reference-plane locator.

vertical is not going to be changed on the articulator.

Place the *reference plane locator* along the right side of the patient's face. It should extend from the middle of the upper border of the external auditory meatus to the outer canthus of the eye.

There is a small hole in the upper posterior area of the locator. When the locator is in proper position, use a felt-tipped pen to gently mark through the hole onto the face (Fig. 13-34).

Make the mark on both sides of the patient's face.

The position of the *anterior reference point* is measured up 43 mm from the *incisal edges* of the central or lateral incisors, toward the inner canthus of the eye. The notched area of the reference plane locator is used to make this measurement. The notch is 43 mm in length (Fig. 13-35).

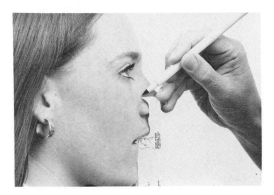

Fig. 13-36. Use of reference-plane locator to establish anterior reference point.

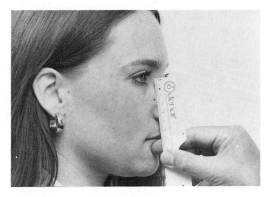

Fig. 13-37. Measurement between inner canthus of eye and anterior reference point is recorded.

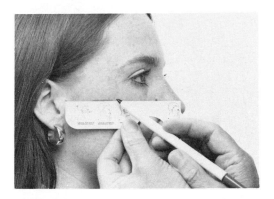

Fig. 13-38. Use of reference plane locator to establish horizontal reference plane.

Rest the lower edge of the notch on the incisal edge of the right central or lateral incisor. On an edentulous patient measure up from the low lip line. The *low lip line* is the lower border of the upper lip when it is in repose. In either case, mark the anterior reference point below the inner canthus of the right eye where the top point of the locator touches the patient's face (Fig. 13-36).

Measure the distance between the anterior reference point and the inner canthus of the eye (Fig. 13-37). Record this measurement in the patient's file for future reference. In this way, if the anterior teeth are removed or modified, one can locate the same anterior reference point by measuring downward from the fixed immovable inner canthus of the eye.

The final step is to mark the *horizontal reference plane* on the right side of the patient's face. Line the ruler up between the anterior and posterior reference points. Hold the ruler just out of contact with the patient's skin so that it will not displace the skin, and then draw a short line on the side of the face. This line represents the horizontal reference plane (Fig. 13-38).

Notice that the horizontal reference plane is identified on the face of the patient by two posterior reference points in the area of the terminal hinge axis and one anterior reference point located 43 mm above the incisal edges of the maxillary anterior teeth or low lip line of the patient.

Face-bow application to patient. The components of the kit needed are the bite fork, anterior crossbar, reference rod, reference rod clamp, and the right and left face-bow side arms with nylon earplugs at the ends of the posterior reference slides (Fig. 13-39).

Attach the bite fork to the crossbar so that the reference rod clamp is to the patient's right, and the U-shaped part in the bite fork is above the crossbar (Fig. 13-40). Then load the upper surface of the bite fork with properly conditioned

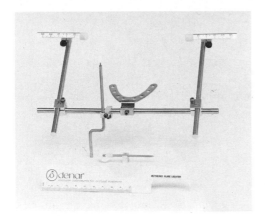

Fig. 13-39. Components used for face-bow application to patient.

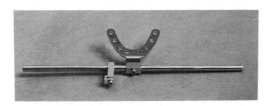

Fig. 13-40. Bite fork and reference rod clamp applied to crossbar.

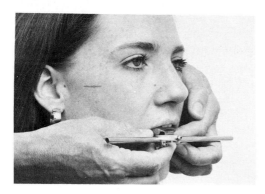

Fig. 13-41. Application of bite fork assembly to patient.

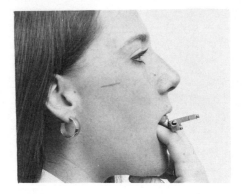

Fig. 13-42. Bite fork assembly being supported by patient.

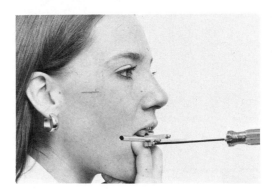

Fig. 13-43. Reference rod clamp is placed parallel with horizontal reference plane.

recording material of your choice. Place the loaded bite fork in the patient's mouth to get a light indexing impression of the maxillary teeth. When the bite fork is first placed in the mouth, be certain to align the crossbar so that it is parallel to the coronal and horizontal planes of the pa-

tient. Also be careful not to depress or displace any mobile teeth: all you really need is a slight impression of the tips of the cusps (Fig. 13-41).

Remove the bite fork from the patient's mouth, and place the maxillary cast, if available, in the bite fork to confirm accurate seating. If the maxillary cast seats accurately in the bite fork, begin assembly of the face-bow record.

Place the bite fork assembly back in the patient's mouth, indexing it to the maxillary teeth. Have the patient hold the bite fork in place (Fig. 13-42). One way to accomplish this is by having the patient bite on the index and middle fingers of the left hand. Alternatively position cot-

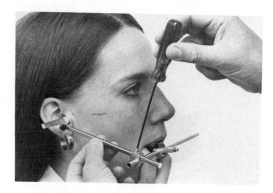

Fig. 13-44. Attaching side arm to crossbar.

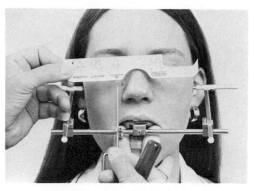

Fig. 13-45. Use of reference-plane locator in conjunction with reference rod to properly relate maxillary dental structure to anterior reference point.

ton rolls on the occlusal surface of the lower posterior teeth and instruct the patient to maintain the bite fork in place with gentle biting pressure.

Adjust the reference rod clamp so that it is parallel to the reference plane marked on the patient's face (Fig. 13-43).

The face-bow side arms are now attached. Note that they are marked right and left and refer to the patient's right and left. Make sure that the scales on the posterior reference slides are adjusted to their zero positions.

Face-bow application. Attach the nylon earpieces on both posterior reference slides and begin attaching the side arms (Fig. 13-44). First locate the right side arm on the crossbar so that the lockscrew on the crossbar clamp faces upward. The posterior reference pin, at the end of the posterior reference slide, should only lightly touch the posterior reference point. Secure the side arm clamp to the anterior crossbar. Attach the left side arm similarly.

Ear-bow application. The nylon earpieces should be on both posterior reference slides. Position the right side arm on the crossbar so that the lockscrew on the crossbar clamp faces upward. The nylon earpiece should fit snugly in the external auditory meatus. Secure the side arm clamp tightly. Attach the left side arm similarly.

The face-bow/ear-bow is now record-

ing the relationship of the maxillary dental structure to the posterior reference points.

To relate the maxillary dental structure to the anterior reference point, insert the reference rod into its clamp, bringing it up from underneath the clamp, with the step in the rod facing toward the patient's right (Fig. 13-45). Hold the reference plane locator between the thumb and index finger of the left hand so that the instructions on the back may be read. The semilunar notch on the locator's inferior surface should be placed over the bridge of the nose. Note the small hole in the center of the locator. Turn the locator down flat with the instruction side facing downward, and index the hole on the locator over the small dowel-like projection on the upper extremity of the reference rod. The operator's eye should be positioned approximately 6 inches in front of the locator. By line of sight adjust the locator by inclining it anteroposteriorly and mediolaterally until a projection of its broad surfaces passes through both posterior reference points, as indicated by the posterior reference slides (Fig. 13-46). The anterior reference point marked on the patient's face may be above or below the reference plane locator.

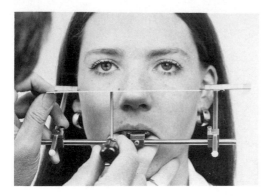

Fig. 13-46. Final position of reference-plane locator in relating reference rod.

Progressive sideshift	5°
Protrusive adjustment	30°
Incisal pin and table	0°
All other settings	0°

Fig. 13-47. Proper articulator settings for zeroing out articulator before face-bow transfer. (Courtesy Denar Corp., Anaheim, Calif.)

Adjust the height of the reference rod so that a projection of the locator's broad surfaces passes through the anterior reference point as well as the posterior reference points (Fig. 13-46). With the left hand pull the locator to the side so that the reference rod is wedged in its clamp. With the wrench in the right hand tighten the clamp to secure the reference rod in its support.

Transferring face-bow/ear-bow to articulator

To prepare the articulator to accept the face-bow, set the immediate sideshift adjustments to 0 degrees, the progressive sideshifts to 5 degrees and protrusive condylar paths to 30 degrees. The vertical dimension of the incisal pin should be set to 0 degrees (Fig. 13-47).

Next, secure a mounting plate to the upper bow of the articulator and a maxillary cast support to the lower bow (Fig. 13-48). The maxillary cast support fits

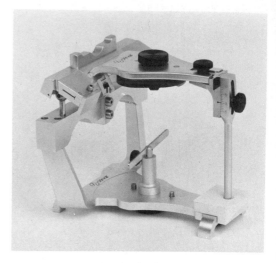

Fig. 13-48. Maxillary cast support applied to lower bow of articulator.

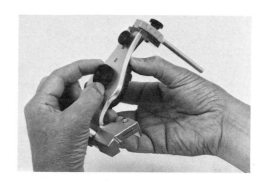

Fig. 13-49. When attaching a mounting plate to articulator bow, one should turn it in same direction as locking screw.

onto the lower bow of the articulator in lieu of a mounting plate.

When attaching a mounting plate to the bow of an articulator, always turn the mounting plate in the same direction the lockscrew is turned as the mounting plate is secured to the articulator bow (Fig. 13-49). A small piece of utility wax should be secured to the anterior margin of the mounting plate (Fig. 13-50). This wax area will facilitate removal of the mounting stone from the mounting plate when the laboratory procedures are complete.

Face-bow transfer. If the face-bow/ear-

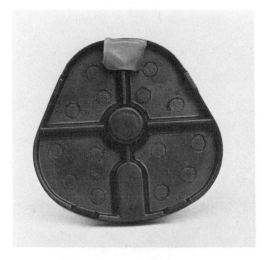

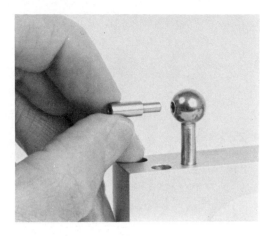

Fig. 13-52. Use of mounting studs for hinge-axis face-bow transfer.

Fig. 13-50. Small piece of utility wax applied to anterior margin of mounting plate will facilitate removal of mounting stone.

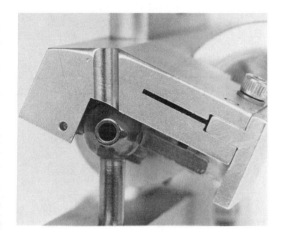

Fig. 13-51. Indices for attaching face-bow/ear-bow on lateral aspects of condyle (face-bow transfer) and condylar housing (ear-bow transfer).

bow is used as a face-bow (the posterior reference pins are oriented to the posterior reference points marked on the side of the patient's face in the area of the terminal hinge axis), the face-bow will be attached to the articulator by indexing the posterior reference pins into the face-bow indexes on the lateral aspects of the condyles (Fig. 13-51).

   Ear-bow transfer. If the face-bow/ear-

bow is used as an earbow, the nylon earplugs are removed for attachment of the bow to the articulator and the posterior reference pins are indexed into the earbow index holes on the lateral aspects of the fossae (Fig. 13-51).

   If the face-bow was oriented on the patient to posterior reference points located precisely with a hinge axis locator, noticeable readjustment of the posterior reference slides of the face-bow to accommodate it to the articulator could introduce a slight mounting error. To minimize this error, mounting studs are inserted into the lateral aspects of the condylar elements to minimize the amount of adjustment of the posterior reference slides (Fig. 13-52). This is the method illustrated.

   Attach the face-bow (or ear-bow) assembly to the articulator by equally adjusting both posterior reference slides so that both scales give the same reading when the posterior reference pins are firmly seated in their respective condylar or ear-bow index holes. This is done by indexing both posterior reference pins in their respective holes. Observe the settings to which the slides are adjusted. The sum of these settings divided by 2 is the setting to which the posterior reference slides are adjusted for proper trans-

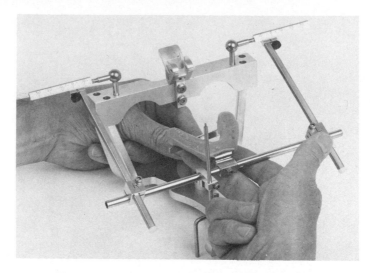

Fig. 13-53. Adjusting maxillary cast support.

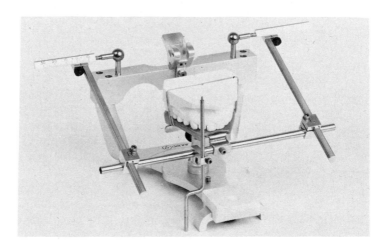

Fig. 13-54. Maxillary cast secured to bite fork.

fer of the face-bow to the articulator. (For example, the sum of +30 and −10 = +20, which divided by 2 = +10.)

The maxillary cast support is adjusted so that the support crossbar firmly contacts the undersurface of the bite fork without lifting the reference rod from its bearing surface (Fig. 13-53).

Mounting the casts in articulator

In addition to casts, interocclusal records are necessary to mount the mandib-ular cast in the articulator and to adjust the fossal controls of the articulator: a centric interocclusal record, one right and one left lateral checkbite record, and, if desired, a protrusive record. The selection of the method and material used for obtaining these records is left to the preference of the operator.

Maxillary cast. First secure the maxillary cast to the bite fork with sticky wax or with a light elastic band (Fig. 13-54).

With the mounting plate secured in the

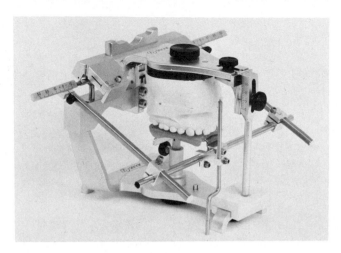

Fig. 13-55. Maxillary cast luted to maxillary bow. It is imperative that condyles maintain centric position and that incisal pin touches incisal platform.

upper bow of the articulator, fill the mounting plate with stone and apply stone to the top of the cast. Be sure the mounting stone completely fills the recesses of the mounting plate. The cast is secured to the mounting plate with a one-mix or two-mix procedure.

One-mix procedure. Use one mix of fast-setting mounting stone to secure the maxillary cast to the mounting plate. With experience a neat mounting can be achieved with this technique.

Two-mix procedure. Use one mix of fast-setting stone to completely fill the recesses of the mounting plate and to tack the cast to the mounting plate. After the stone is set, remove the mounted cast from the articulator and use a second mix of fast-setting stone to complete the mounting. The two-mix procedure is recommended to easily obtain a neat mounting.

Bring the upper bow down on top of the cast, so that the stone bonds the two together. Engage the centric latch. *Throughout this procedure be certain the condyles maintain centric position and the incisal pin touches the incisal platform* (Fig. 13-55). When the stone has set,

remove the maxillary cast support from the articulator.

With the face-bow application (not the ear-bow), it is usually easier to fill the mounting plate with stone and stock a pile of mounting stone on the maxillary cast if the maxillary bow is removed and inverted on the working surface beside the face-bow/mandibular bow assembly (Fig. 13-56).

Mandibular cast. With the maxillary cast in the articulator, separate the upper bow from the lower bow and turn the upper bow upside down. Orient the mandibular cast to the maxillary cast by accurately seating and luting the centric interocclusal record between the two casts. Secure the casts assembly with sticky wax or a light rubber band (Fig. 13-57). For greatest accuracy the casts should be related by hand. If the centric interocclusal record was taken at an increased vertical dimension, estimate the distance that the vertical dimension was increased by the centric interocclusal record and adjust the vertical dimension of the incisal pin to this dimension.

Fill the lower bow mounting plate with fast-setting stone and put an appropriate amount of stone on the base of the man-

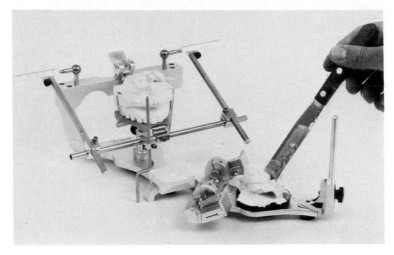

Fig. 13-56. Stacking stone in mounting plate when using face-bow application.

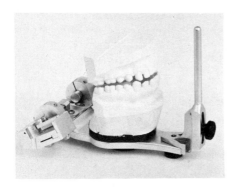

Fig. 13-57. Mandibular and maxillary casts secured to interocclusal record.

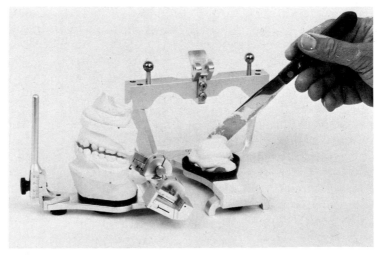

Fig. 13-58. Filling mandibular-bow mounting plate with stone. An appropriate amount of stone is added to base of mandibular cast.

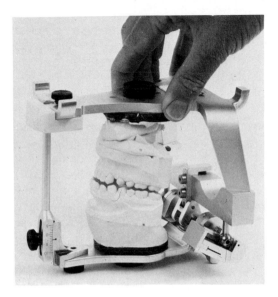

Fig. 13-59. Mandibular bow inverted and seated into maxillary bow. It is imperative that condyles be seated in centric position and that incisal pin is on incisal table.

dibular cast (Fig. 13-58). Invert the lower bow and seat it on top of the upper bow. *Make sure the condyles are seated in their fossae* (Fig. 13-59). *Make sure the incisal table is on the incisal pin.* Lock the centric latch to its most closed portion. Complete the mounting of the mandibular cast with the one-mix or two-mix procedure previously described.

An alternate method of mounting the mandibular cast is to first load the mounting plate with fast-setting stone and then put an appropriate amount of stone on the base of the mandibular cast. Next, grasp the maxillary bow and support the centrically related casts with the thumb, index, and middle fingers as illustrated in Fig. 13-60. Invert the maxillary bow-casts assembly over the mandibular bow and firmly seat the condyles in their fossae. Close the articulator until the incisal pin contacts the incisal table. While maintaining this hand grasp, have an assistant move the centric latch to its most closed position. After the initial set of the mounting stone has occurred to support the mandibular cast, the fingers are removed from the assembly. Subsequently the

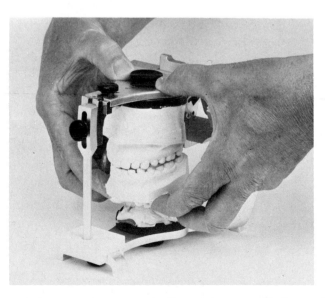

Fig. 13-60. Alternate method of mounting mandibular cast.

mounted mandibular cast is removed and the mounting is completed with the two-mix method.

Setting the articulator to checkbite records

To set the articulator to checkbite records, it is necessary to mount both the maxillary and mandibular casts. Right and left lateral checkbite records and a protrusive record also are needed. (Alternate techniques require fewer checkbite records and use average anatomic dimensions for those condylar path dimensions not recorded and measured.)

The characteristics of the patient's orbiting paths of movement will be diagnosed and recorded from the two lateral checkbite records. The inclinations of the protrusive condylar paths will be diagnosed and recorded with the protrusive checkbite record.

Simulating the orbiting condylar path. First remove the maxillary bow from the articulator and confirm that both progressive sideshift adjustments are set to the 6-degree settings. The reason for this setting was explained in the previous section on the immediate and progressive sideshift adjustments.

Next, loosen the protrusive and imme-diate sideshift adjustment lockscrews on both sides of the articulator (a total of four screws). Set the protrusive condylar paths to 0 degrees and move the medial fossa walls medially to the limit of their range of movement. Do not tighten the lock-screws.

Seat the right lateral checkbite record on the mandibular cast. Firmly seat the maxillary cast in the checkbite record by grasping the maxillary cast as illustrated in Fig. 13-61 or by applying pressure to the top of the upper bow to immobilize the maxillary cast (since the Mark II articulator has the rotating condylar paths built to average anatomic dimensions, impingement of the rotating condyle against its rear and superior fossa walls may sometimes prevent complete seating of the maxillary cast in the checkbite record). At this time the left condyle is positioned inward, downward, and forward from its centric position (Fig. 13-62). Increase the inclination of the left protrusive condylar path until the superior wall of the fossa contacts the top of the condyle (Fig. 13-63). Secure the protrusive condylar path in this position by tightening the lockscrew.

Move the left medial fossa wall later-

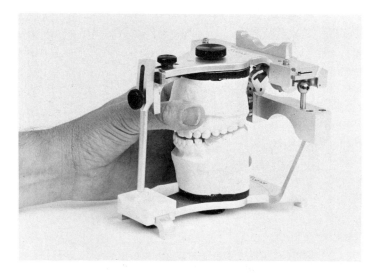

Fig. 13-61. Placing maxillary cast into lateral checkbite.

ally until it contacts the condylar element. Lock the immediate sideshift adjustment lockscrew.

NOTE: These three articulator adjustments, the immediate sideshift, the progressive sideshift, and the protrusive inclination of the superior fossa wall, establish the character of the orbiting path on the left side of the articulator.

Use the left lateral checkbite record and follow the same procedure to adjust the settings of the right articulator fossa

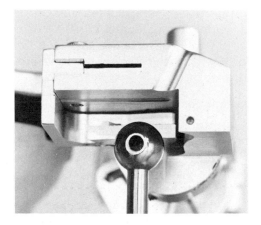

Fig. 13-62. Illustrating inward, downward, and forward position of nonworking condyle when maxillary cast is seated into lateral checkbite.

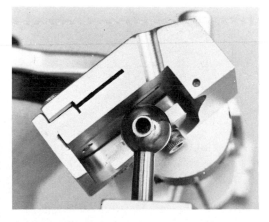

Fig. 13-63. Inclination of nonworking condyle is increased until superior wall of fossa contacts the condyle.

and to diagnose the character of the orbiting path of the right condyle.

Record the articulator settings on the patient's record.

NOTE: It is the adjustment of the right medial fossa wall medialward that allows for a mandibular sideshift to the left as the right condyle moves medially to bear and move against its medial fossa wall. Therefore, when the operator writes on the patient's record "right immediate shift 0.6 mm," the reference is to the articulator adjustment on the right side of the articulator and not to the side to which the mandible moves. The right articulator adjustment will allow for a mandibular sideshift to the left. The articulator's right side is the right side of the articulator as viewed from the rear of the articulator. A medialward adjustment of the right medial fossa wall (right immediate sideshift adjustment of the articulator) allows for a mandibular sideshift to the left.

Simulating the protrusive condylar paths. The inclinations of the protrusive condylar paths are diagnosed in the following manner.

Loosen the lockscrews of the protrusive adjustment on both sides of the articulator. Set the protrusive condylar path inclinations to 0 degrees. Do not tighten the lockscrews. Seat the protrusive checkbite record on the mandibular cast and seat the maxillary cast in the checkbite record. Apply downward pressure to the maxillary cast or upper bow to stabilize the maxillary cast in the record. Note that the condyles do not contact their superior fossa walls. Increase the inclinations of the protrusive condylar path on both fossae until the superior fossa walls contact their respective condyles. Lock the protrusive adjustment lockscrews. The inclinations of the patient's protrusive condylar paths have now been diagnosed. Record the protrusive condylar path settings on the patient's record.

Incisal table adjustments with custom incisal tables

There are two custom incisal tables that fit Denar articulators. They are shown in Accessories (pp. 348 to 350). Part no. D41 is used with articulators with long centric adjustment on the foot of the incisal pin. Part no. D41AB is used with articulators having the rounded foot on the incisal pin.

To use either of the custom incisal tables, first attach a small amount of cold-cure acrylic to the posterior portion of the incisal table. Part no. D41 has a machined precision stop on its anterior portion to maintain the correct vertical dimension, and care should be taken to ensure that no acrylic is positioned on the top of the stop. Also the long centric adjustment at the foot of that incisal pin should be turned so that the rounded end will more efficiently mold the acrylic. This is done by adjustment of the foot so that its anterior extremity is flush with the anterior surface of its dovetail support.

When the acrylic has reached a rather firm consistency, the articulator is moved in right lateral, left lateral, and protrusive excursions, allowing the anterior teeth that are kept in contact to guide these excursive movements and thereby function-ally generating a custom incisal guide. This recording is transferred to the incisal table and a small fleur-de-lis is generated in the cold-cure acrylic (Fig. 13-64). This is later perfected with a vulcanite bur.

The custom incisal table can be used to best advantage in adjusting to the vertical and horizontal overlap relation of the anterior teeth. This is particularly true in adjusting the incisal guidance of the articulator to natural teeth, which exhibit varying amounts of horizontal overlap of the teeth that bear the horizontal load in the protrusive, right lateral, and left lateral excursive movements. The custom incisal table is recommended for fixed prosthetic procedures involving the anterior teeth.

Treatment procedures

The rationale for using the diagnostic data obtained from protrusive and lateral checkbite records is as follows.

When the protrusive inclination of the superior fossa wall is adjusted to the lateral checkbite record, a characteristic of the orbiting condylar path is diagnosed. This characteristic is associated with the balancing inclines of posterior teeth on the orbiting side—the mesial aspects of the lingual inclines of the mandibular buccal cusps and the distal aspects of the buccal inclines of the maxillary lingual cusps.

When the protrusive inclination of the superior fossa wall is adjusted to the protrusive checkbite record, the inclination of the patient's protrusive condylar path is diagnosed. This inclination of the superior fossa wall is associated with the protrusive contacts of posterior teeth—the mesial aspects of mandibular cusps and the distal aspects of maxillary cusps.

The orbiting-path inclination of the superior fossa wall adjusted to lateral checkbite records is always equal to or greater than the protrusive-path inclination of the superior fossa wall adjusted to the protrusive checkbite record.

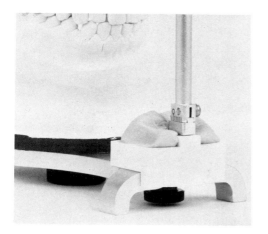

Fig. 13-64. Illustration of customized incisal guide table.

Fixed restoration and removable partial denture restorations

Adjusting the protrusive inclination of the superior fossa to an angle that is slightly less than the patient's protrusive condylar path (5 to 10 degrees less) when a restoration is produced will prevent the fabrication of protrusive contacts, or balancing contacts on the orbiting side of posterior teeth in the laboratory. When the restoration is seated in the patient's mouth and the patient's condyle tracks a steeper protrusive and orbiting condylar path, the posterior teeth will separate in both the protrusive excursion and in the lateral excursion on the orbiting side.

The Denar Company has recently made the following modifications to the Mark II Articulator:

The protrusive slot in the superior fossa wall has been eliminated. This was done because it was believed that errors could be introduced during lateral excursions, since the vertical dimension was slightly increased as the condyle moved from the slot to the flat portion of the housing.

The posterior wall of the fossa has been fitted with a setscrew. This allows forward and backward movement of the mandibular member by adjustment. It is adjustable in increments of 0.25 mm. This supplement to the articulator is available as an accessory called CR/CO adjustment.

The centric latch has been improved for a more positive resistance to lateral movement. This was done because it was perceived that resistance to lateral movement might be decreased by removal of the protrusive slots from the superior fossa wall.

Accessories

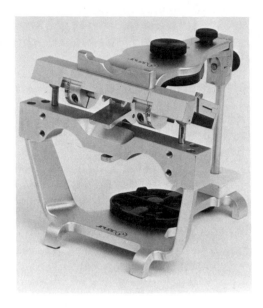

Denar Semiadjustable Articulator
Mark II Articulator (includes #300042 pin and
D41AB platform)

Mark II-41 Articulator (includes #110092 pin
and #41 platform)

Mark II-46 Articulator (includes #110092 pin
and D46 platform)

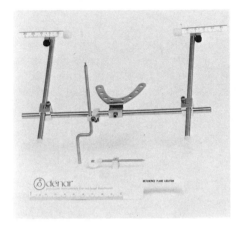

Earbow/Facebow D31AB

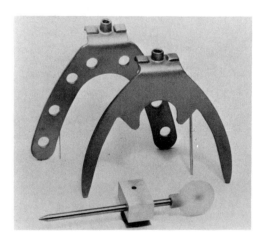

D146 Bite Fork—Standard

D148 Bite Fork—Edentulous

D145 Anterior Reference Pointer

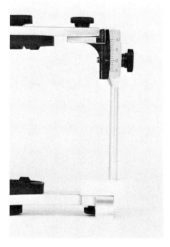

The P/N 300042 Adjustable Pin functions with
the D41AB Incisal Platform, which has a detent
in its superior surface.

Accessories—cont'd

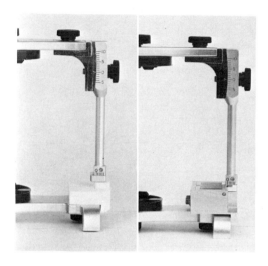

The P/N 110092 Adjustable Incisal Pin functions with the D46 Adjustable Incisal Table and the D41 Custom Incisal Platform.

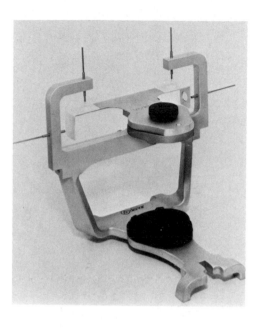

D142 VeriCheck

The VeriCheck is used to verify the accuracy of centric relation records.

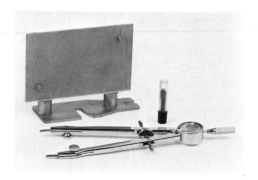

D122 Broadrick Occlusal Plane Analyzer

Used for analyzing the curve of Spee and in developing an acceptable curve of occlusion (compensating curve).

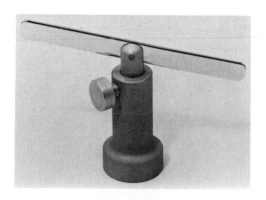

D102 Maxillary Cast Support

Accessories—cont'd

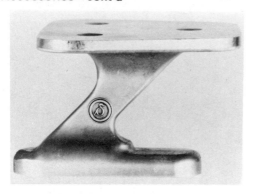

D13 Remount Record Jig

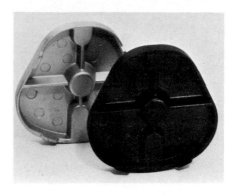

D14 Mounting Plates (2)
D15 Mounting Plates (12)
D14 Mounting Plates, Teflon (2)
D15T Mounting Plates, Teflon (12)

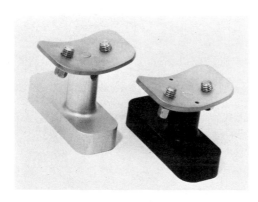

D118 Pantograph Mounting Fixture

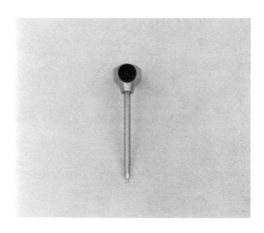

D180 Dawson Fossa-Guide Pin

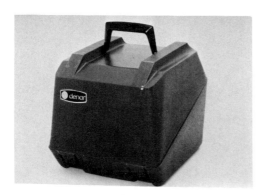

D121 Articulator Case

DISCUSSION

The theoretical purpose of a dental articulator is to provide the dentist with a theoretical replica of the stomatognathic system. Then indirect restoration of the dental arches may be accomplished without the necessity of adjustment when these restorations are placed intraorally.

To achieve this laudable accomplishment, several theories of stomatognathic function, many with their select instruments, have evolved. From these theories, many disparate, much has been discovered. A knowledge of the physiology of occlusion that is cohesive enough so that it may be taught, at least in broad principles, now exists. Within these broad principles there still exist several clinical techniques that, however credible, are based primarily on clinical empiricism. These clinical disciplines have in turn led to the development of many instruments called "dental articulators." Most of these instruments have been noted in this chapter.

None of these instruments should become a substitute for the basic knowledge of the very complex process we call masticatory function. The evolution of any theory of occlusion is based on the background and ideas of the minds behind it. This in turn depends on ideas of how the human masticatory system functions. Experience dictates caution in accepting any specific "ideal" form of treatment that would supposedly be of equal value for every patient.

Optimal dental treatment consists of applying basic knowledge and instrumentation to achieve a desirable clinical treatment. Knowledge and instrumentation occur consecutively; therefore instrumentation should never be placed first. On the other hand, since articulators are necessary in the process of oral rehabilitation, we must strive to become proficient in the use of such instruments as we are capable of understanding and in which we are willing to trust.

At the present time there is no instrument system or "occlusal theory" that can guarantee a desirable result with an unlimited prognosis for every patient. For now we must use one or more of the several tools available in combination with knowledge, experience, and good judgment, always realizing that proper treatment of the patient is paramount, this being our final proof of success.

SELECTED REFERENCES

1. Bellanti, N. D.: The significance of articulator capabilities. Part I. Adjustable vs. semiadjustable articulators, J. Prosthet. Dent. **29**:269-275, 1973.
2. Beu, R. A: Personal communication, Teledyne Dental Hanau Division, Dec. 1974.
3. Boucher, C. J.: Swenson's complete dentures, ed. 6, St. Louis, 1970, The C. V. Mosby Co., pp. 272-291.
4. Guichet, N. F.: Occlusion, a teaching manual, Anaheim, Calif., 1970, Denar Corp.
5. Heartwell, C. M., Jr., and Rahn, A. O.: Syllabus of complete dentures, ed. 2, Philadelphia, 1974, Lea & Febiger.
6. Huffman, R. W., Regenos, J. W., and Taylor, R. R.: Principles of occlusion, laboratory and clinical teaching manual, Ohio State University, Columbus, Ohio, 1969, H. & R. Press.
7. Lundeen, H. C., and Wirth, C. G.: Condylar movement patterns engraved in plastic blocks, J. Prosthet. Dent. **30**:866-875, 1973.
8. Schweitzer, J. M.: Restorative dentistry—half century of reflections, J. Prosthet. Dent. **31**:22, 1974.
9. Thomas, C. J.: A classification of articulators, J. Prosthet. Dent. **30**:11-14, 1973.
10. Villa, H. A.: Requirements in articulators, contraindicated features, J. Prosthet. Dent. **9**:619-623, 1959.
11. Villa, H. A.: Requirements of articulators for lateral movements, J. Prosthet. Dent. **9**:422-427, 1959.
12. Villa, H. A.: Requirements of articulators for protrusive movements, J. Prosthet. Dent. **9**:215-219, 1959.
13. Weinberg, L. A.: An evaluation of basic articulators and their concepts. Part I. Basic concepts, J. Prosthet. Dent. **13**:622-644, 1963.
14. Weinberg, L. A.: An evaluation of basic articulators and their concepts. Part II. Arbitrary, semi-adjustable articulators, J. Prosthet. Dent. **13**:645-663, 1963.
15. Weinberg, L. A.: Evaluation of the face-bow mounting, J. Prosthet. Dent. **11**:32, 1961.

GENERAL REFERENCES

Boucher, C. O.: Current clinical dental terminology, St. Louis, 1963, The C. V. Mosby Co.

Christensen, F. T.: Effect of incisal guidance on cusp angulation in prosthetic occlusion, J. Prosthet. Dent. **11**:48, 1961.

Christiansen, R. L.: Rationale of the face bow in maxillary cast mounting, J. Prosthet. Dent. **9**:388, 1959.

D'Amico, A.: Functional occlusion of the natural teeth of man, J. Prosthet. Dent. **11**:899, 1961.

Granger, E. R.: Practical procedures in oral rehabilitation, Philadelphia, 1962, J. B. Lippincott Co.

Huffman, R. W., Regenos, J. W., and Taylor, R. R.: Principles of occlusion, laboratory and clinical teaching manual, Ohio State University, Columbus, Ohio, 1969, H. & R. Press.

Kornfeld, M.: Mouth rehabilitation, ed. 2, St. Louis, 1974, The C. V. Mosby Co.

Lucia, V. O.: Modern gnathological concepts, St. Louis, 1961, The C. V. Mosby Co.

McCollum, B. B., and Stuart, C. E.: A research report, South Pasadena, Calif., 1955, Scientific Press.

Posselt, U.: The physiology of occlusion, Philadelphia, 1962, F. A. Davis, Co.

Ramfjord, S. P., and Ash, M. M., Jr.: Occlusion, ed. 2, Philadelphia, 1971, W. B. Saunders Co.

Sicher, H.: Temporomandibular articulation; concepts and misconceptions, Oral Surg. **20**:281, 1962.

Tanaka, H., and Beu, R. A.: A new semiadjustable articulator. Part I. Concept behind the new articulator, J. Prosthet. Dent. **33**:10-16, 1975.

Tanaka, H., Finger, I., and Porter, M. M.: A new semiadjustable articulator. Part II. Adjustment of a new-concept articulator, J. Prosthet. Dent. **33**:158-168, 1975.

14

Procedure for transfer to articulator using adjustable hinge-axis face-bow and interocclusal records

George H. Moulton

The modern practitioner must be a diagnostician and must apply his knowledge and judgment to the plan of treatment. The study of casts that have been anatomically related to one another in the articulator is essential to diagnosis based on scientific knowledge. The dental profession's major objective is to prevent dental disease and disorders. Such diagnostic procedure makes possible early recognition of disorders to which we may apply preventive measures.

When prevention is impossible, early diagnosis should reduce treatment needs to the minimum, thus avoiding more complex conditions requiring major and costly treatment at a later date.

The practicing dentist's decision can be based on scientific knowledge; he is, however, confronted with the fact that there are differences of opinion regarding application of current knowledge. Controversy over advantages of certain equipment makes selection of instruments, face-bows, and articulators difficult for him. Unfortunately, the result may be to focus too much attention on a particular design or mechanical aspect, rather than on the underlying anatomic and physiologic principles that apply. Success of treatment depends primarily on a thorough understanding of principles and diligence in carrying out exacting procedures, rather than on mechanical devices per se.

The anatomic and physiologic principles related to the physiology of occlusion have been discussed in detail in other chapters. It is my intent here to offer a procedure based on those principles, applicable to both diagnostic and treatment needs.

The instruments selected are by no means the only ones that might be employed successfully. The articulator (Fig. 14-1) has been selected because it adapts to the direct use of intraocclusal records, thus permitting a procedure involving a minimum number of required steps. Extensive and careful evaluation of clinical results fails to indicate any inadequacy when compared to other instruments or procedures. Mindful that we must make certain decisions based on current knowledge, we now accept the fact that we can record and demonstrate an opening and closing axis of the mandible. This is the most important rationale for the use of a face-bow in the transfer of the maxillary cast in correct anatomic relationship within the articulator.

McCollum[1] stated: "There is one and only one position in which the hinge axis is constant to both the mandible and maxilla." This position is the terminal hinge position of the mandible, or, more specif-

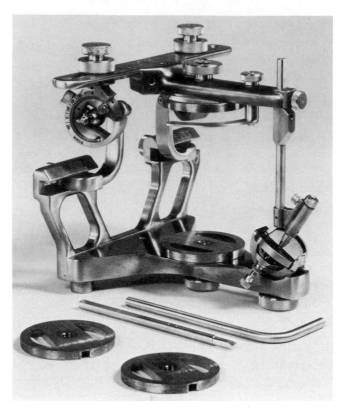

Fig. 14-1. Hanau University Articulator, Model 130-28.

ically, of the condyles in their fossae. It is also described as the most posterosuperior position of the condyles. I must emphasize that this should be a physiologically acceptable position and should not be obtained by force or by introducing drugs or anesthetics. This is the same condylar-fossa relationship that will again be emphasized in obtaining an interocclusal record of centric occlusion, thus relating maxilla and the mandible to the same axis. Granger[2] stated: "The fact that the hinge axis is constant to the mandible and therefore determines the arc of closure on which teeth meet in every contacting position is of fundamental importance. If it were merely a question of centric closure it would be relatively unimportant." Granger goes on to summarize very well the concept of the hinge axis and the rationale for the use of a hinge-axis face-bow when he says: "The object of any articulator mounting is to reproduce on a mechanical instrument the same relation of the teeth to the axis of the articulator as the teeth in the mouth occupy to the axis of the condyles." The component parts of the articulator condyles are, therefore, also in their terminal hinge positions during the transfer procedure.

Proponents of the rigid (Snow) face-bow discount the importance of the hinge axis, and some question its existence. Instead of locating an axis by trial and error, one fixes an arbitrary landmark by measuring a point 13 mm on a line from the tragus of the ear to the ala of the nose. The styluses of the face-bow are then placed over these landmarks. Schuyler[3] stated: "We have been told that the face bow as advocated by Snow is valueless. Careful use of it would seem to accomplish at least 90% of the requirements. An effort

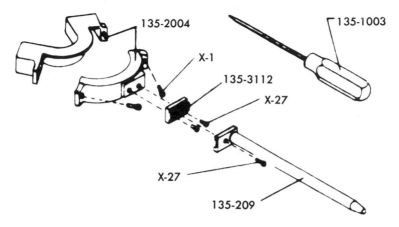

Fig. 14-2. Plain clutch tray 135-108.

to reproduce most accurately the axis is commendable."

Faced with these two schools of thought, the operator not planning to use the hinge-axis face-bow to determine the opening and closing axis should find it helpful to at least palpate the condyles while in their terminal position and mark the approximate center of the condyle. This has been found to be in closer approximation to the recorded axis than the arbitrary landmarks. The adjustable bow also makes it possible to accommodate to the frequent lack of symmetry noted between the two condylar areas.

Because most of the scientific data available at this time seems to support the use of an adjustable hinge-axis face-bow, this instrument has been chosen to describe this initial procedure in the transfer of the maxillary cast to the articulator.

LOCATION OF THE HINGE AXIS

The plain clutch tray 135-108 (Fig. 14-2) is adaptable to most lower arches and is available only in this size and contour. This tray may be altered as required, or a special individualized tray may be cast.

Optionally available is a clutch tray of similar size and contour except that it contains a built-in central bearing screw and has a companion central bearing plate (Fig. 14-3). This central bearing clutch tray is obtainable through a dental dealer and is specified as No. 135-109.

Step 1. The clutch tray consists of a labial and lingual section assembled by screws X-1. The clutch plate 135-3112 is securely attached with two screws X-27 to the flat on the labial of the tray section 135-2004 with the identification mark on the clutch plate at top right. Then attach the clutch stem 135-209 with screw X-27, noting that the identification marks of matched assembly coincide (Fig. 14-2).

Step 2. The assembled clutch tray is securely cemented to the mandibular arch, with the stem extending approximately parallel to the occlusal and sagittal planes. It is essential that the tray be anchored firmly to the dentition to prevent even the slightlest movement.

Step 3. The face-bow (Fig. 14-4) is prepared for maximum adjustability as follows: remove the condylar pointers 135-208 and slide condylar sleeves 135-3606 flush with locknuts 135-3421 and tighten. Position the square section of sliding frames 135-201L and 135-202R by rotating thumbscrew 135-205 to align the indicating marks with the edge of fixed frame 135-2003. Adjust the thumbscrew 135-3011 to lower the condylar sleeves about ¼ inch from their closed positions.

Step 4. The condyle areas are digitally

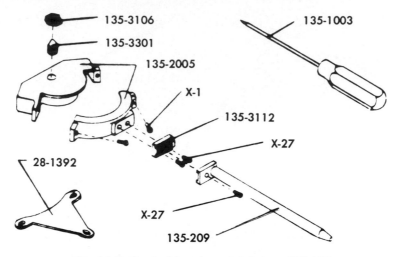

Fig. 14-3. Central bearing clutch tray 135-109.

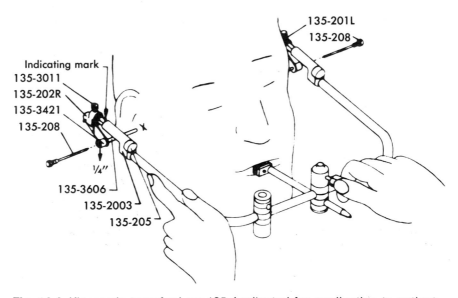

Fig. 14-4. Kinematic transfer bow 135-4 adjusted for application to patient.

located and temporarily marked on the patient. The face-bow is brought gently over the face with the stem of the clutch tray entering the loose clamp on left side of the bow. With the ends of the condylar sleeves pointing toward, and equidistant from, the temporary condyle markings, the bow is held while the clamp is tightened securely with the wrench.

Step 5. Release locknuts 135-3421 and

withdraw condylar sleeves 135-3606 with a rotating motion to permit insertion and threading of the condylar pointers 135-208 to their stops at condylar sleeves. Slide the condylar sleeves with a rotating motion to bring the pointer into proximity, without touching, to the patient's skin. Inward and outward movement of the condylar pointers must be accomplished only by movement of the con-

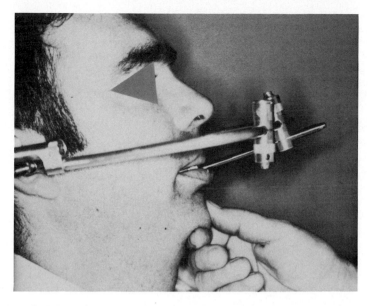

Fig. 14-5. Guiding closure to maintain condyles in terminal hinge position.

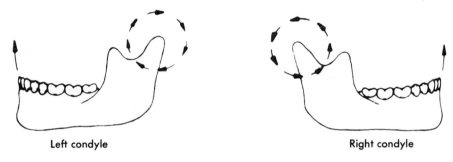

Left condyle   Right condyle

Fig. 14-6. Condyle pointer movement in relationship to hinge axis.

dylar sleeves, not the condylar pointers, which must remain undisturbed during the axis-location procedure.

Step 6. The patient is instructed to open and close within a limited range, not more than 2 cm. The condylar pointers will be observed to move in arcs when not in line with the exact hinge axis. Particular precautions must be taken to prevent incorporation of a protrusive component in the opening and closing movements of the mandible. The operator may have to guide this opening and closing movement to maintain the terminal hinge position (Fig. 14-5). This guidance is usually done by the thumb and forefinger placed on the chin to guide the movement. Force of any kind is contraindicated. Having the patient occasionally protrude and then retrude will help the dentist in developing the clinical "feel" of determining condylar position. It is also advisable to have the patient sit in an upright position with his mandible parallel to the floor. Observe the direction of movement of the condylar pointers only on the closing stroke of the mandible. Fig. 14-6 will aid in making adjustments of the condylar pointers in the correct direction. Anteroposterior adjustments of the condylar pointers are made by turning thumbscrews 135-205, and ad-

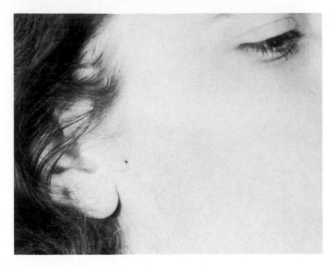

Fig. 14-7. Axis reference marking.

justments of the pointers above and below the hinge axis are made by the thumbscrews 135-3011.

The farther away the pointers are from the hinge axis, the longer will be the pointer stroke. The pointer stroke will shorten with the approach to the hinge axis. When the pointers are opposite the hinge axis, all movement of the pointers will have been transposed into a strictly rotational axis.

Step 7. When the condylar pointers have ceased to move and are observed to only "hinge" or rotate at fixed points on the face, without a protrusive influence, these points are considered as the kinematic axis.

The condylar pointers are now disengaged and withdrawn slightly to permit application of a marking medium to the points, and they are again engaged to mark the skin (Fig. 14-7). Permanent marks may be obtained by tattooing.

Step 8. To permit safe and convenient removal of the face-bow from the patient, the condylar pointers are removed from the condylar sleeves. With the wrench, loosen the clamp supporting the bow and withdraw the entire face-bow from the clutch stem. The clutch stem, clutch

plate, and two-tray assembly screws are removed in that order to permit the labial and lingual sections of the tray to be removed from the teeth.

Relating the maxillary cast to the terminal hinge position of the mandible

Step 9. The face-bow is preadjusted as in step 3.

Step 10. The prongs of the bitefork are covered on both sides with softened wax or any material of the operator's choice. The softened material is seated against the occlusal surface of the maxillary dentition to create a positive index, with the stem of the bitefork extending approximately parallel to the occlusal and sagittal plane and chilled while the bitefork is firmly held by the lower teeth. This index of the upper occlusal surface will be used to transfer the maxillary cast to the articulator.

Step 11. The preadjusted face-bow is brought gently over the face with the stem of the bitefork entering the clamp of the bow. With the ends of the condylar sleeves pointing toward and equidistant from the hinge-axis markings, the bow is held in this position while the clamp is securely tightened with the wrench.

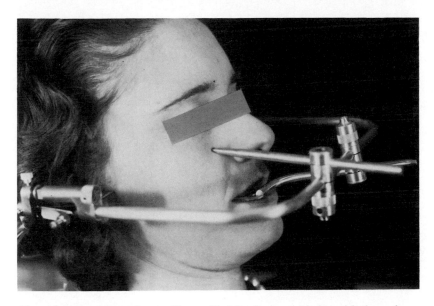

Fig. 14-8. Face-bow in position with bite fork and infraorbital marker.

Step 12. Loosen locknuts and withdraw the condylar sleeves to permit inserting the condylar pointers and screwing them to their stops at the condylar sleeve ends. Slide the condylar sleeves to bring the pointers to the skin while adjusting the thumbscrews for a precise coincidence of the pointers to the hinge-axis markings on the skin. When the condylar pointers contact the skin in this exact location, the condylar-sleeve locknuts are securely tightened. Observe that the bitefork remains firmly seated against the maxillary teeth.

Step 13. The orbital pointer is inserted in the second clamp, and with the pointer lightly touching the face at the infraorbital notch, simultaneously hold the bow and tighten the clamp securely (Fig. 14-8). Observe that the condylar pointer locations have remained consistent with the hinge-axis markings.

Step 14. The condylar pointers are unscrewed from their condylar sleeves and removed. The assembled face-bow with the bitefork and orbital pointer attached is carefully withdrawn from the patient without disturbing any of the adjustments. The condylar pointers are then replaced in the sleeves in their exact original positions.

Transfer of the maxillary cast to the articulator

Step 15. The articulator is prepared as follows, with no undue force or mechanical aids being used (Fig. 14-9).

1. Release centric locks 130-3109, rotate condylar guidances 130-137 to a minus protrusive of approximately 25, and remove the upper member of instrument.
2. The right and left condylar shaft supports 130-2018 and 2019 on the lower member are adjusted symmetrically to 55 mm.
3. Incisal guide 130-108 is set at 10 degrees.
4. Petroleum jelly, oil silicone, or Teflon is applied to all surfaces exposed to the mounting medium.
5. Mounting plate 130-2012 is attached to the upper member.
6. Median of the scribed lines on the straight incisal pin 130-3007 is adjusted flush with the lower surface of the upper member.

Step 16. Remove the calibrated shafts

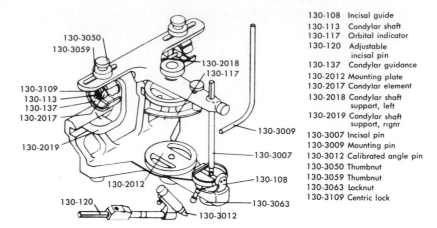

130-108 Incisal guide
130-113 Condylar shaft
130-117 Orbital indicator
130-120 Adjustable
        incisal pin
130-137 Condylar guidance
130-2012 Mounting plate
130-2017 Condylar element
130-2018 Condylar shaft
         support, left
130-2019 Condylar shaft
         support, right
130-3007 Incisal pin
130-3009 Mounting pin
130-3012 Calibrated angle pin
130-3050 Thumbnut
130-3059 Thumbnut
130-3063 Locknut
130-3109 Centric lock

Fig. 14-9. Hanau University Articulator, Model 130-28: identification of parts.

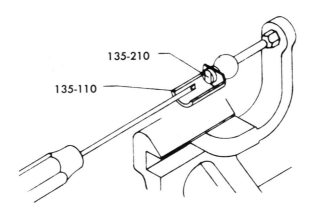

Fig. 14-10. Attachment of axial cribs.

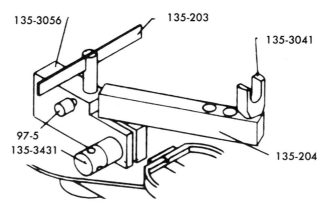

Fig. 14-11. Mounting support.

and firmly attach the axial cribs 135-110 with thumbscrews 135-210 (Fig. 14-10).

Step 17. Tightly attach mounting block 135-3056 to the lower member of articulator (Fig. 14-11). Lockscrew 135-3431 is loosened by wrench (previously used on face-bow clamps) to permit the lateral adjustment bar 135-204 to rotate freely. Thumbscrew 97-5 is loosened to lower pivot 135-203. This cast support has an extension that is removed and used only in the event of a steep mounting of the cast, which may require vertical adjustment in excess of that otherwise afforded.

Step 18. Axial aligners 135-107 are placed over the condylar pointers of the face-bow and are locked by thumbscrews 130-3013 when they abut the condylar sleeves (Fig. 14-12). The face-bow is positioned so that the axial aligners are resting firmly in the axial cribs while the third point of suspension, the bitefork stem, rests in the bitefork swivel 135-3041 (Fig. 14-13). The bitefork swivel is

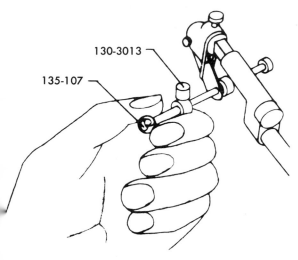

130-3013

135-107

Fig. 14-12. Axial aligners placed on condylar pointers.

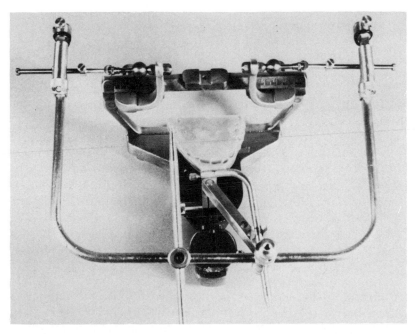

Fig. 14-13. Adjustment of the extendible condylar shafts to correct intercondylar distance.

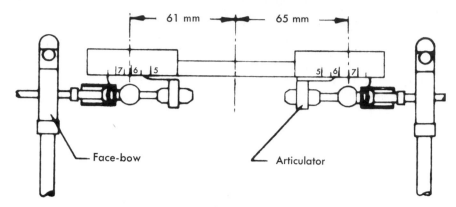

Fig. 14-14. Gaging by contacting of condylar pointers with thumbscrews on condylar shafts.

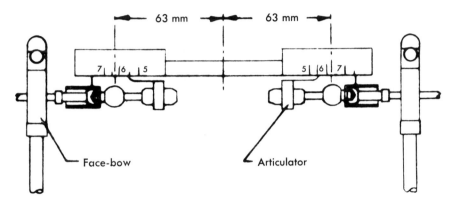

Fig. 14-15. Symmetric adjustment of intercondylar distance.

placed in the appropriate hole of the lateral adjustment bar.

To permit suspension of the axial aligners in the cribs, it may be necessary to increase, or decrease, the original 55 mm setting of the condylar shaft supports.

Step 19. Carefully increase the intercondylar distance to contact the condylar pointers with the detent in thumbscrews on the end of the condylar shaft (Fig. 14-14).

Step 20. The total sums of the scale reading on the frame of the lower member are added and then divided by two and noted. (Example [Fig. 14-15]: the left scale registering 65 is reduced to 63. The right scale registering 61 is increased to 63.)

Step 21. When the detents in the center of the thumbscrew on the ends of both condylar shafts equally touch without strain the condylar pointers of the facebow, the lockscrew 135-3431 is securely tightened by wrench (Fig. 14-11).

Upon tightening, verify the symmetry of an unstrained adjustment by lightly lifting the bitefork stem in and out of the bitefork swivel 135-3041. No drag or lateral displacement must be observed, and any evidence of improper alignment requires repeating the two preceding steps.

Step 22. The cast support is now raised until the pivot contacts both sides of the bitefork and is locked by the thumbscrew to prevent any vertical displacement caused by the additional weight of a maxillary cast and the mounting medium (Fig. 14-13). An extension has been provided if the steepness of the cast requires additional vertical adjustment for this support.

Step 23. The condylar guidances on the upper member are set at 0 degrees lateral to the calibration at underside of upper member by releasing and then tightening thumbnut 130-3050 (Fig. 14-16).

Replace the upper member of articulator by increasing or decreasing the intercondylar distance of the right and left condylar guidances by thumbnut 130-3059 to permit entry of the condylar elements 130-2017 into their respective condylar guidance slots. Orbital indicator on upper member may be rotated to prevent any mechanical interference. Tighten the centric locks to restrict the instrument to opening and closing movements only. The protrusive of condylar guidances is set at 30 degrees.

Step 24. Increase the intercondylar distance of the right and left condylar guidances to contact the flats of the condylar elements with the end shoulders of the condylar shafts 130-133 (Fig. 14-17). The flattened end of the incisal pin must be exactly coincident with the center groove of the incisal guide when the condylar guidances are tightened. Note that no perceptible sideshift of the condylar shafts in their elements exists.

Step 25. The mounting pin 130-3009 is inserted in place of the incisal pin and the bent end of this mounting pin is seated on a stable contact of the bitefork stem (Fig. 14-18). The upper member is simultaneously adjusted vertically until the orbital pointer is level with the horizontally adjustable orbital indicator on the articulator.

The orbital indicator is removed from the articulator and the maxillary cast is now mounted by the usual technique, with the mounting pin as the vertical static stop instead of an incisal pin.

Step 26. The maxillary cast, ground flat on its mounting side and properly V notched on its peripheral mounting border for the "split-cast" method, is lubricated with a thin coating of petroleum jelly or other separating medium. Boxing

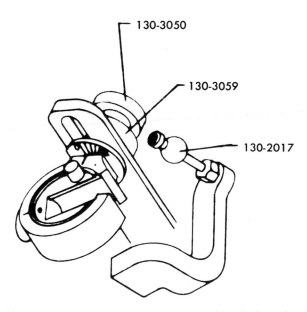

130-3050

130-3059

130-2017

Fig. 14-16. Condylar guidance set at 0-degree lateral and placed over condylar element.

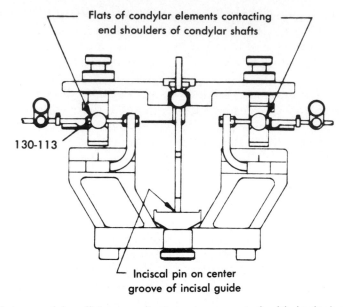

Fig. 14-17. Intercondylar distance adjustments corrected with incisal pin on center groove of incisal guide.

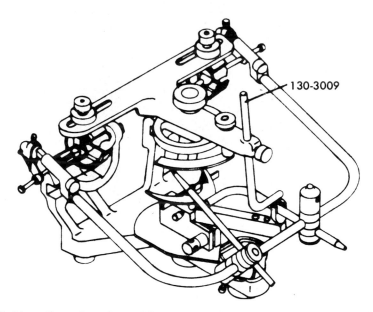

Fig. 14-18. Mounting pin adjusted in contact with stem of bite fork to align orbital pointer with orbital indicator.

wax may be wrapped around it to provide a form into which the countersection is poured.

The cast is then securely seated and luted to the index on the bitefork to main-tain the accurate relationship to the hinge axis.

Step 27. The upper member of the ar-ticulator is swung back, and a mounting medium of suitable consistency is placed

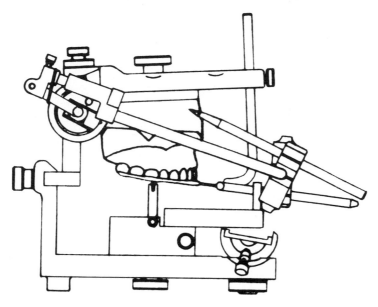

Fig. 14-19. Maxillary cast mounting to upper member of articulator, using "split cast" method.

on the cast. The upper member is swung forward to embed the mounting plate and bring the mounting pin to the static stop on the bitefork stem.

Complete the mounting with a spatula and remove excess material to expose top surface of the mounting plate for convenient removal and accurate reattachment of the cast to the instrument (Fig. 14-19).

Step 28. Upon complete set of the mounting medium, remove the face-bow, axial cribs, face-bow mounting block, and mounting pin.

Step 29. Trimming of the maxillary mount is completed to present a sharply defined line at the junction to the cast and to eliminate any possible interference with the function of the instrument.

Step 30. The adjustable incisal pin 130-120 is now attached with the indicating line on the vertical portion aligned flush with the lower surface of the upper member (Fig. 14-20).

The calibrated angle pin 130-3012 is adjusted to the median line and locked. Release the locknut of the incisal guide slightly and, while tilting the guide an-

teroposteriorly, observe that there is no vertical displacement of the upper member. Should there be, it is eliminated by raising or lowering the vertical portion of the pin and tightening the thumbscrew to maintain its position. When so adjusted, the relocating collar is brought into contact with the underside of the upper member and securely locked. Subsequent removal and replacement of the incisal pin is facilitated by this preset collar, assuring exact repositioning. Reset the incisal guide to 0 degrees and lock. Attach a mounting plate to the lower member.

FACE-BOW SELECTION

Most practitioners agree that an opening and closing axis can be demonstrated by the use of a hinge-axis face-bow. A modified hinge-axis face-bow, formerly model 135-4, is shown in Fig. 14-21. There is no denying that a relatively small percent of practitioners actually use the hinge-axis face-bow to determine the opening and closing axis.

Another type, and in greater use, is the nonadjustable (Snow) face-bow (Fig.

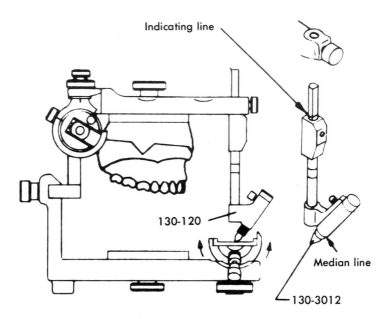

Fig. 14-20. Adjustable incisal pin attached to upper member.

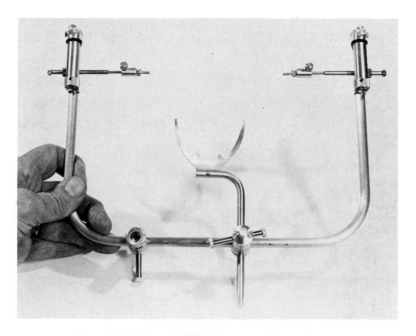

Fig. 14-21. Model 135-6 hinge-axis face-bow.

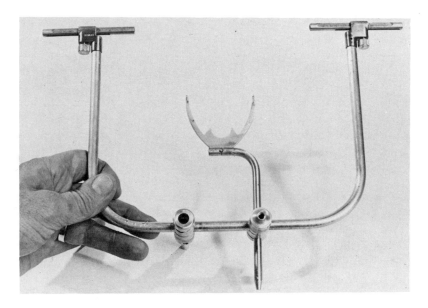

Fig. 14-22. Nonadjustable (Snow) face-bow.

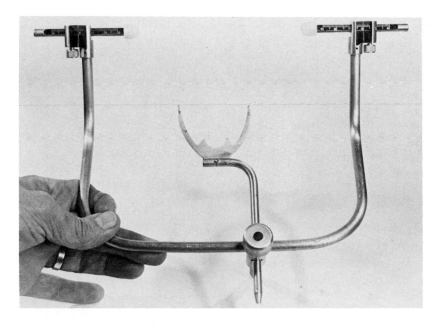

Fig. 14-23. Earpiece face-bow.

14-22). This face-bow is intended to relate to an opening and closing axis determined by an arbitrary landmark 13 mm anterior to the tragus of the ear on a line from the tragus to the outer canthus of the eye. Despite its nonadjustable limitation, we would rather attempt to relate the styluses of this face-bow to the axis, determined by palpating the condyles while in their terminal hinge position. This procedure will more nearly approximate the axis as determined by the hinge-axis face-bow than that determined by an arbitrary landmark previously described.

Another development is the earpiece face-bow, using yet another arbitrary landmark, which has also been found to be more accurate by some investigators (Fig. 14-23).

In viewing the options we have, it seems reasonable to stress the need for being anatomically correct while at the same time using procedures that are as direct and simplified as possible. The practicing dentist is concerned with the degree of accuracy that assures clinically acceptable treatment.

Within this context I believe that any face-bow that is used intelligently, approximating as accurately as possible the same axis location as can be determined by the trial-and-error method by use of the hinge-axis face-bow, is acceptable. This is an individual judgment decision. The principles and procedures to follow undoubtedly determine to a far greater degree the accuracy of the total transfer procedure and therefore whether or not the treatment is clinically acceptable.

CENTRIC OCCLUSION OR CENTRIC RELATION

The next step in our transfer procedure is to relate the mandibular cast to the already transferred maxillary cast. For emphasis, the quote from Granger[2] is repeated. "The object of any articulator mounting is to reproduce on a mechanical instrument the same relation of the teeth to the axis of the articulator as the teeth in the mouth occupy to the axis of the condyles." In this concept, the condyles must again be positioned in their terminal hinge position when the interocclusal record for transfer of the mandibular cast is made. This is the same condylar position described for recording the opening and closing axis of the mandible, and the axis position to which we related the maxillary cast. This interocclusal record is called a "centric relation record" or a "centric occlusion record." I prefer the term "centric occlusion," in that crown and bridge prosthodontics is concerned with the dentulous patient. After completion of the mounting procedure and removal of the interocclusal record, the occlusion of the teeth resultant of mandibular closure with the condyles remaining in their terminal hinge position is my preferred definition of centric occlusion.[4] It is from this relationship that a study of occlusion must begin, as the resultant closure may bring all teeth into harmonious relationship (Fig. 14-24) to one another, or it may identify a deflective occlusal contact (Fig. 14-25). If a deflective occlusal contact exists, one can observe a slide to maximum intercuspation (Fig. 14-26). This resultant relationship is eccentric occlusion. It has also been termed "acquired centric" or "dual occlusion," and has been described by others as a failure of centric occlusion to coincide with centric relation.

The requirement that this interocclusal record represents a mandible-to-maxilla relationship with the condyles in their terminal hinge position has often been the cause of confusion and controversy. This record should not be thought of in terms of whether or not it represents a functional relationship. Whether or not a patient occludes in this terminal position during function is not germane to the procedure. This record, and those used to set

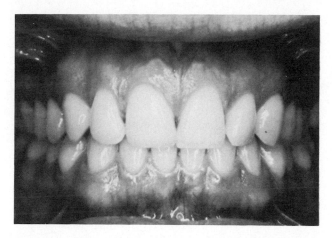

Fig. 14-24. "Ideal" occlusion. Condyles in their terminal hinge position.

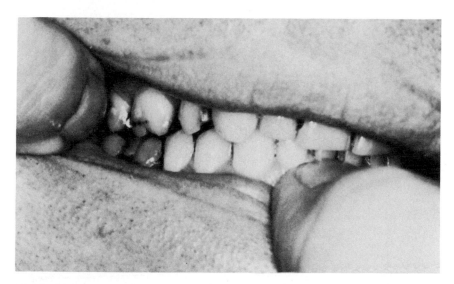

Fig. 14-25. Closure to deflective occlusal contact. Condyles in their terminal hinge position.

an instrument, must result in a duplication, in an articulator, of all tooth relationships (within functional range) that occur in the mouth. The tooth contact made in the terminal position is one of these relationships. Whether or not to restore in this position is a diagnostic decision based on at least several factors. Above all, this decision should not be confused with the required record, to transfer and to set an articulator.

PREPARATION OF INTEROCCLUSAL RECORD

Regular pink base-plate wax is used to obtain the recordings. Some advocate the use of other materials. The importance of the materials per se is not paramount, but rather the concept of correct relationships that are to be registered. In preparing for a wax record it is essential that the "wax" is uniformly softened, preferably in a water bath (Fig. 14-27). One or more thick-

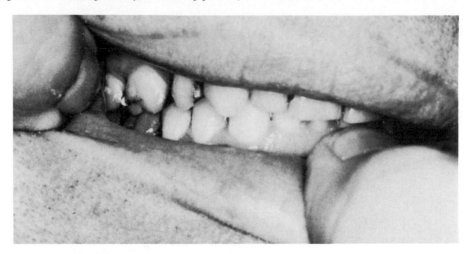

Fig. 14-26. Mandible deflected; condyles translated; maximum intercuspation; eccentric occlusion.

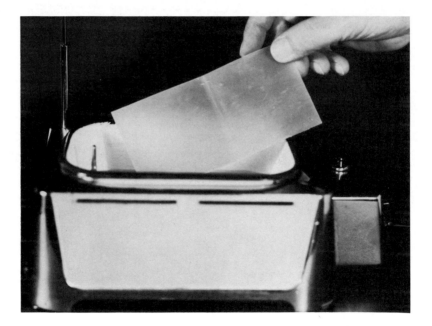

Fig. 14-27. Wax uniformly softened in water bath.

nesses of 0.002-inch tinfoil should then be interlayed between the doubled-over sheet of wax (Fig. 14-28). For the protrusive, also right and left lateral records, two thicknesses of the foil are recommended because of the greater bulk. The purpose of the tinfoil is to give reinforcement to the softened wax so that its form can be maintained throughout the various procedures. Collapsing or bending of the prepared checkbite during registration would result in its contacting other than the occlusal surfaces of the cast. The object is to use the least amount of indexing (Fig. 14-29). The index should involve the minimum of tooth surface, thus avoiding wax contact with soft tissue. To do so would inhibit accurate

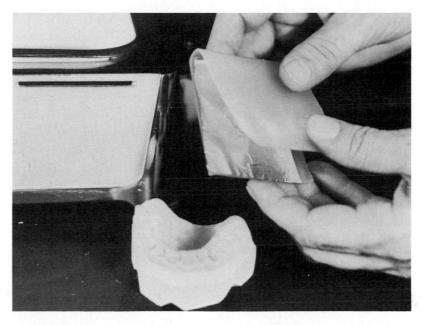

Fig. 14-28. 0.002-inch tinfoil interlayed between doubled-over sheet of wax.

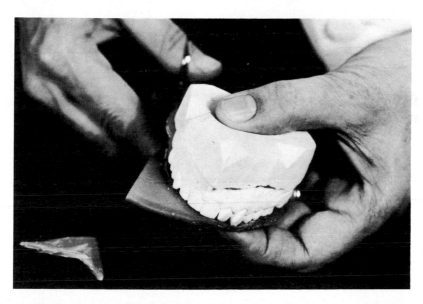

Fig. 14-29. Preliminary fitting and trimming wax record to correct dimension.

seating of the record into a stone cast. The tinfoil will also discourage actual tooth contact, which is not desirable, especially if deflective occlusal contacts exist.

Although one doubled sheet of base-plate wax is usually adequate in thickness

for centric relation registration, this must be determined by observation of the interocclusal distance between the teeth in each relationship to be recorded (Fig. 14-30). The instructions are the same for the preparation of all wax records.

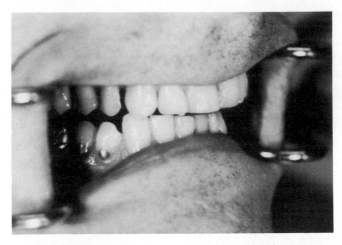

Fig. 14-30. Predetermination of required thickness of wax record.

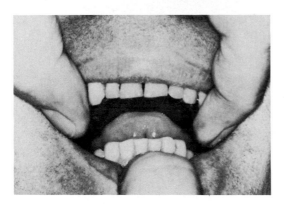

Fig. 14-31. Relating wax record to maxillary arch.

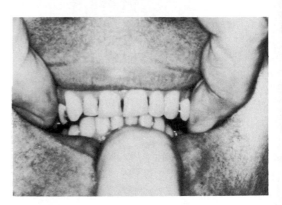

Fig. 14-32. Making centric occlusion record. Index produced; condyles in terminal hinge position.

Recording centric occlusion

The prepared record is then carried to the mouth. The record is placed on the occlusal surfaces of the maxillary teeth (Fig. 14-31). The patient is "talked" into allowing guided closure and is told to tap his teeth on the wax (Fig. 14-32). This is not a relaxed state that would result in an inferior position of the condyle. The patient is doing the opening and closing movement; therefore the muscles are bringing the condyles in a superior as well as a posterior fossa relationship. This exercise should have been carried out several times before introduction of the wax record into the mouth so that the patient is familiar with these instructions. He is told *not* to bite into the wax but to gently tap his teeth on the wax. Detailed though it is, this will avoid a common error, particularly if a deflective occlusal contact exists. This procedure will result in obtaining an index of both maxillary and mandibular teeth in the uniformly softened wax. If in doubt as to the terminal position of the condyle, it is well to have the patient fully protrude, and then retrude. With the thumb and forefinger on the patient's chin, the operator can "sense" the condylar position. The record can then be air-chilled, removed, and placed in room-temperature water. All excess should be trimmed (Fig. 14-33). The record is replaced on the teeth as dictated by the index and is rechecked for accuracy.

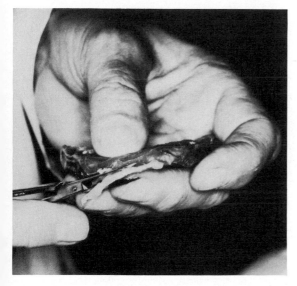

Fig. 14-33. Trimming excess from record prior to rechecking for accuracy.

TRANSFER OF MANDIBULAR CAST IN CENTRIC OCCLUSION

Step 31. The articulator is inverted and the mandibular cast is placed on the maxillary cast without the aid of the centric relation record (Fig. 14-34). Measure and note the X dimension (distance).

Step 32. Accurately seat and lute the centric occlusion record between the maxillary and the mandibualr casts. Adjust the calibrated angle pin so that the distance X is the same as previously determined when the centric relation record was not in place. This procedure compensates for the thickness of the centric record when it is later removed (Fig. 14-35).

Step 33. The lower member of the articulator is swung back slightly and a mounting medium of suitable consistency is placed on the cast. The lower member is then swung over to embed the mounting plate as well as to bring the incisal pin into contact with the incisal guide, with the operator being absolutely certain that the condylar elements are

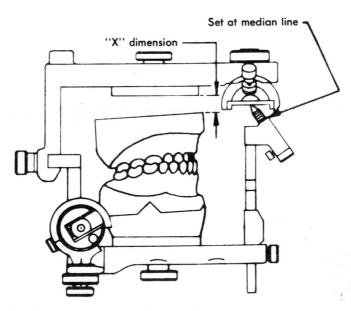

Fig. 14-34. Mandibular cast related to maxillary cast. Condyle element locked in terminal position. Articulator inverted to facilitate mounting and "X" measurement.

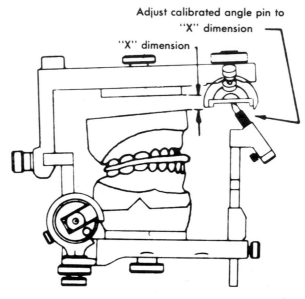

Fig. 14-35. Mandibular and maxillary casts related to interocclusal record of centric occlusion and calibrated angle pin adjusted to previous "X" measurement.

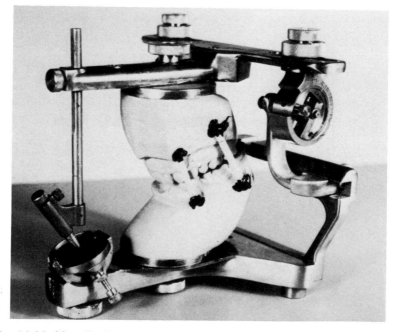

Fig. 14-36. Mandibular and maxillary casts luted together for mounting.

locked against their stops in a centric position (Fig. 14-36).

Step 34. Upon completion of the mounting, the interocclusal record is removed and the calibrated angle pin is raised out of contact with the incisal guide.

RECORDS FOR SETTING THE ARTICULATOR

The transfer procedure at this point has accomplished the positioning of the casts in the correct anatomic relationship to the opening and closing axis of the articulator. The relationship to the axis of the condyles of the patient has been reproduced within the articulator. Both the mandibular and maxillary casts are related to the terminal hinge position, the only position in which the hinge axis is constant to both the maxilla and mandible. The interocclusal record of centric occlusion can be removed, and opening and closing movements and the initial occlusion can be studied. The next step is to make additional records of eccentric records that will be used to set the instrument to reproduce protrusive and lateral movements of the mandible. Granger[2] stated: "The object of an artic-

ulator setting is to reproduce the paths of motion of this axis."

Interocclusal record of protrusive relationships

The first interocclusal record used to set the articulator is the record of the protrusive relationship, an end-to-end relationship of the incisors. This record will normally represent the maximum translatory movement of the condyles within normal limits of function. If this record should be one of tooth relationships beyond the normal functional range, it is unlikely that it would be accepted by the articulator. The protrusive record must also be one of wholly protrusive movement, and not one in which a degree of lateral movement is incorporated. Observation of the midline relationship will assure accuracy. This record is then used to set the condylar slant.

Setting articulator to protrusive record

Step 35. Centric and protrusive locks of the condylar guidances are released and the lateral of condylar guidances is set at 10 degrees.

Step 36. The maxillary and mandibular

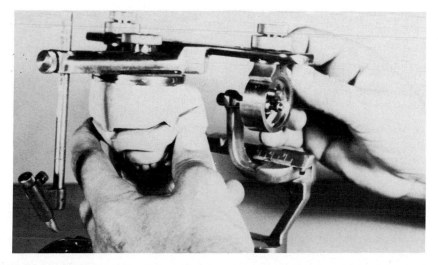

Fig. 14-37. Setting of condylar slant to protrusive record, split-cast procedure.

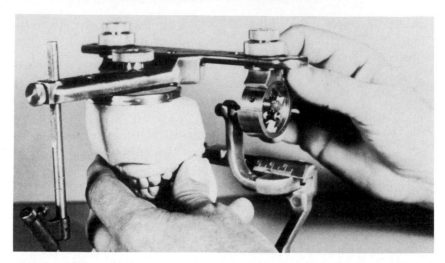

Fig. 14-38. Completion of setting to protrusive record; absolute readaptation assures accuracy.

casts, with the protrusive record accurately interposed, are related. Some operators prefer to lute them together.

Step 37. The upper member is engaged into the split cast (Fig. 14-37), and the right, then left, protrusive condylar guidances are adjusted until an absolute readaption to the cast occurs (Fig. 14-38). Without deforming the recording surface of the protrusive record, one hand may rest lightly upon the upper member of the instrument, directly over the maxillary cast, in producing a sense of feel during the adjustment.

Step 38. Protrusive adjustments are locked to retain this position. The protrusive record is then removed.

Right and left lateral interocclusal records

An interocclusal record is prepared for recording the lateral relationship. The approximate thickness of wax required to produce an index is estimated by observing the interocclusal distance in the lateral relationship.

The right and left lateral relationships that must be recorded should represent the maximum amount of condylar movement within the functional range. This

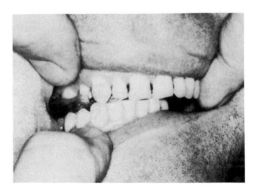

Fig. 14-39. Making interocclusal record of right lateral relationship.

position is the end-to-end relationship of the opposing cuspids or a comparable position if the cuspids are missing or malpositioned. This relationship should also be one of lateral movement only and should not contain any protrusive or translatory movement of the working condyle. If a protrusive movement of the working condyle is incorporated into the lateral record, the working condyle will not remain in its terminal position when setting the instrument. If this occurs, a new lateral record should be made. It is recommended that the patient practice, with the operator's guidance, placing the

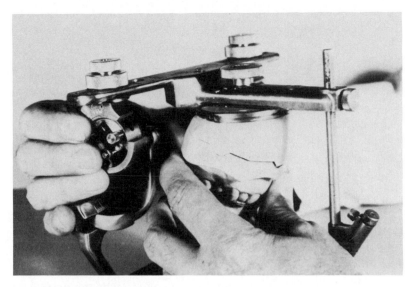

Fig. 14-40. Setting condylar element to lateral record.

teeth in this lateral position prior to introducing the wax record. Even then the operator will note that he must carefully guide the patient to this position. To determine the accuracy, a perpendicular line drawn on the labial surface of the maxillary and mandibular cuspids may help (Fig. 14-39). One can then determine, with the record in position, whether or not this line is still continuous and therefore not incorporating a protrusive movement. Determination is also made that the recorded relationship is not beyond the functional range. This is emphasized because of the fact that the condyles are capable of assuming positions that a mechanical instrument cannot reproduce. The uniformly softened record is then carried to the mouth in the same manner as described for the protrusive record and the two lateral records (right and left) are made.

This record will have recorded the movement of the axis of the condyle. After setting of the instrument we are therefore able to reproduce the path of motion of this axis. One may speak of this movement as a "lateral movement" or a "Bennett movement." As Granger[2] has stated: "The term condyle path refers to the protrusive paths of the menisci on the fossae. Bennett movement refers to the lateral paths of the menisci in lateral excursions of the mandible." McCollum[1] stated: "The influence of the Bennett path on cusps of teeth is an intricate and most interesting study. Primarily the Bennett movement influences the position of the cusps in their mesial-distal relationship, due to the fact that a jaw without Bennett movement moves laterally on a shorter radius than one with some or considerable side-shift."

Each lateral record is then used to set the appropriate condylar element. The following instructions must be rigidly adhered to.

Right lateral relation record

Step 39. The right lateral record is accurately seated between the maxillary and mandibular casts.

Step 40. Loosen the thumbnut for lateral adjustment on the balancing side, left of the articulator.

Step 41. Bring the components of the mount into light contact (Fig. 14-40) and rotate the left guidance slowly, increasing

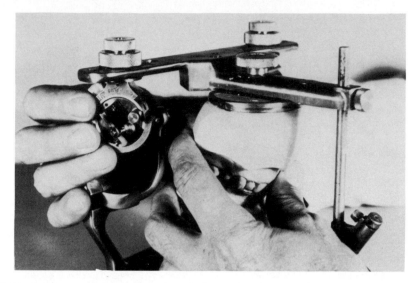

Fig. 14-41. Setting to lateral record complete; absolute readaptation required to assure accuracy.

Working side   Balancing side

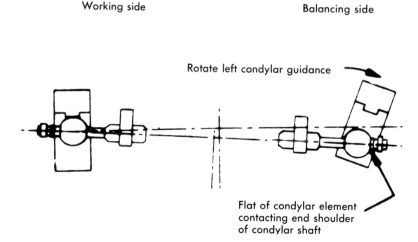

Fig. 14-42. Right lateral relation with flats of condylar element contacting end shoulder of condylar shaft on balancing side.

the angle of lateral, until the split cast falls into place (Fig. 14-41). In setting to the right and left lateral record, you may need to make a slight change in the protrusive setting to accurately relate the two split-cast components of the mounting. When this is observed, slightly counterrotate the guidance to contact the condylar element with the end shoulder of the condylar shaft and tighten the thumbnut, retaining this lateral adjustment (Fig. 14-42). Remove the lateral record.

Balancing side   Working side

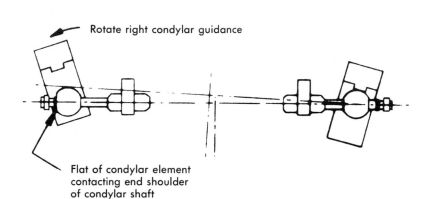

Rotate right condylar guidance

Flat of condylar element
contacting end shoulder
of condylar shaft

Fig. 14-43. Left lateral relation with flats of condylar element contacting end shoulder of condylar shaft on balancing side.

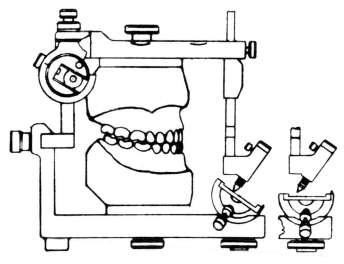

Fig. 14-44. Teeth in protrusive relationship. Incisal guide pin (on left) tilted to make contact with incisal pin.

Left lateral relation record

Step 42. The left lateral record is accurately seated between the maxillary and mandibular casts.

Step 43. Loosen the thumbnut for lateral adjustment on the balancing side, right of the articulator.

Step 44. Bring the split casts into light contact and rotate the right guidance slowly, increasing the angle of lateral record, until the split cast falls into place.

When this is observed, slightly counterrotate the guidance to contact the condylar element with the end shoulder of the condylar shaft and tighten the thumbnut (Fig. 14-43). Remove the lateral record.

ADJUSTMENT OF INCISAL GUIDE

Step 45. The components of the split-cast mounting are now permanently luted together.

Step 46. With the casts in occlusion, the

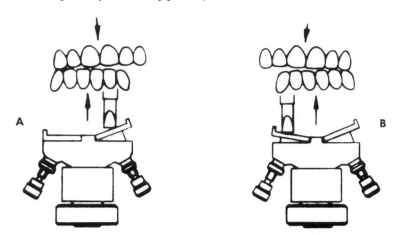

Fig. 14-45. A, Mandible in right lateral relationship; wing of guide is raised to contact pin. **B,** Mandible in left lateral relationship; wing of guide is raised to contact pin.

calibrated angle pin is lowered into contact with the incisal guide and the lockscrew is tightened. If insufficient teeth are present to maintain a previously determined vertical dimension, the angle pin is turned back to the median scribed line at which it had originally been set.

Step 47. The locknut of the incisal guide is loosened, and the incisors are brought into edge-to-edge contact. The incisal guide is then tilted anteroposteriorly to make contact with the end of the incisal pin and the locknut is tightened to maintain this position (Fig. 14-44).

Step 48. The casts are now brought into a right lateral excursion and the lateral wing of the incisal guide is raised to contact the edge of the incisal pin and locked (Fig. 14-45, *A*).

Step 49. The casts are then brought into a left lateral excursion and the lateral wing is raised to contact the edge of the incisal pin and also locked (Fig. 14-45, *B*).

Step 50. Record all of the settings for future reference—intercondylar, protrusive, lateral, and incisal guidance.

CHECKING THE ACCURACY OF THE TRANSFER

Previous instructions have described the notching of the maxillary cast and the lubrication of this cast prior to mounting as a part of the split-cast procedure. Several factors must be emphasized to assure accuracy in the setting of the instrument. After the maxillary cast is separated from the upper member of the articulator, the maxillary cast is then related to the mandibular cast as dictated by each of the interocclusal records. This relationship must be carefully maintained while the instrument is set to each record. Do not allow the maxillary cast to be displaced from the index of the interocclusal record. The component of the maxillary mounting attached to the upper member of the articulator is then closed into approximation with the maxillary cast. The appropriate settings, or articulator adjustments, should result in complete readaptation of the split-cast components. The resulting relationship should be as precise as before separation. If, in the attempt to set the instrument, the two component parts do not readapt, there is an error in the transfer procedure. Too many have assumed that a small discrepancy is of little importance. This, of course, is not true. The success of this procedure is dependent on adherence to rigid requirements. Failure to readapt as described suggests an error in the record of centric occlusion (or centric relationship). The experienced operator is less likely to have an error in the face-bow transfer of the maxillary cast or in the protrusive or lateral records.

Anatomic and physiologic principles have been applied to the clinical procedure of transfer of casts to an articulator. This procedure satisfies both diagnostic and treatment needs. The instruments selected meet all the requirements to produce the successful clinical result.

SELECTED REFERENCES

1. McCollum, B. B.: Considering the mouth as a functioning unit as a basis of a dental diagnosis; a research report, South Pasadena, Calif., 1955, Scientific Press.
2. Granger, E. R.: Functional relations of the stomatognathic system, J.A.D.A. **48**(6):638, 1954.
3. Schuyler, C. H.: Factors of occlusion applicable to restorative dentistry, J. Prosthet. Dent. **3**:772, 1953.
4. Moulton, G. H.: The importance of centric occlusion in diagnosis and treatment planning, J. Prosthet. Dent. **10**:921, 1960.
5. Teteruck, W. R., and Lundern, H. C.: The accuracy of an ear face-bow, J. Prosthet. Dent. **16**: 1039, 1966.

15

Anatomy of the stomatognathic system related to crown and fixed partial prosthodontic therapy

Parker E. Mahan

The stomatognathic system may be defined as the combined structures of the mouth and jaws. It includes the upper and lower teeth, hard and soft palate, tongue, cheeks, maxillae, mandible, temporomandibular joint, and the muscles that move the mandible. All these structures are either directly or indirectly involved in the diagnosis of occlusal and dental restorative problems. The dentist must have an understanding of the detailed anatomy and function of the stomatognathic system if he is to maximize his success in dental diagnosis and treatment planning. In this chapter, emphasis is placed on stomatognathic anatomy.

The temporomandibular joint demonstrates the correlation of structure and function in a manner that cannot be exceeded by any other joint in the body. These paired joints allow a remarkable freedom of motion of the mandible and still serve to guide and, in some positions, to limit its movement. When one is studying functional positions of the mandible, he must consider the fact that the medial structures of one joint are reinforced by the lateral structures of the opposite joint, and vice versa. The temporomandibular joint does not function as a ball-and-socket joint, but it articulates as a ball on a hill. The condyle most closely approximates and functions against the posterior

incline, the crest, and, in some patients, the anterior incline of the articular eminence. It does not function against the depth or posterior incline of the glenoid fossa. As shown in Fig. 15-1, the articular surface of the glenoid fossa extends from a point anterior to the crest of the eminence to the squamotympanic fissure. This articular surface is not cartilage but is comprised of a fibrous protein, collagen. The collagen fibers in the articular surface are specifically arranged so that they exit from the bony surface perpendicular to that surface and then turn 90 degrees to run parallel to the surface. This arrangement of fibers is admirably suited to withstand forces of friction dur-

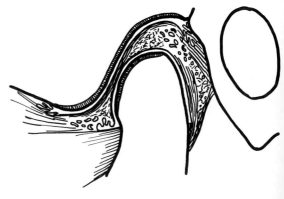

Fig. 15-1. Sagittal section through medial half of human temporomandibular joint.

ing translation of the condyle. It has been demonstrated that, in the healthy temporomandibular joint, the meniscus is tightly attached to the condyle at its medial and lateral poles and that translation occurs in the superior cavity of the joint.[1] The superior surface of the meniscus therefore glides across the articular surface of the eminence and glenoid fossa.

The superior cavity is lined at its periphery by a synovial membrane, which secretes the small amount of synovial fluid that lubricates the cavity. In the anterior and posterior of the cavity the synovial villi are arranged in long folds extending from medial to lateral. When the condyle translates down onto the eminence, the villi in the posterior of the cavity unfold to allow the meniscus to translate with the condyle. Lymphatic capillaries are associated with the synovial villi and function to provide the aqueous phase of the synovial fluid.

The meniscus of the healthy temporomandibular joint does not contain cartilage but is comprised of collagen. The collagen fibers of the meniscus are oriented anteroposteriorly in the superior and inferior surfaces but run in all three directions in space and are enmeshed together so as to provide a flexible and yet very strong pad in the posterior portion just above the condyle.[2] The medial half of the anterior border of the meniscus is attached to the superior belly of the lateral pterygoid muscle. When sectioned in the sagittal plane, the anterior portion of the meniscus is shaped like a foot with a heel, as shown in Fig. 15-1. The foot portion contains many blood vessels and Golgi tendon organs. Batson[3] has described a venous plexus that surrounds the periphery of the meniscus in which blood can be shunted back and forth during function to partially compensate for the volume vacated by the condyle. The central part of the meniscus lying between the posterior slope of the eminence and the condyle

and that part over the medial pole of the condyle are very thin. Zola[4] has found the thickness in these areas to be only 0.4 to 0.2 mm, depending on the force applied to the vernier gage. This indicates that the medial pole and anterior slope of the condyle may approximate the temporal bone very closely during function. The portion of the meniscus located just superior to the condyle is thicker than the central portion and, in the adult, is avascular. Just posterior to this region the meniscus bends down posteriorly over the condyle and contains a very rich vascular network. Griffin and Sharpe[5] have demonstrated that this vascular knee contains glomus cell anastamoses connecting the small arteries and veins. At the vascular knee the meniscus forms two distinct strata of connective tissue fibers separated by loose areolar tissue. The superior stratum of this bilaminar zone is very rich in elastin and is attached to the tympanic plate of the temporal bone. The protein, elastin, is a truly elastic fiber that will assume its initial length when applied tension is released. It is, in fact, essential that the attachment of the meniscus to the tympanic plate be loose or elastic if the meniscus translates forward with the condyle. The inferior stratum of the bilaminar zone is comprised mainly of collagen and it attaches to the posterior aspect of the neck of the condylar process. Since the meniscus in the healthy joint moves with the condyle there is no need for elasticity or laxity in this attachment of the meniscus. The collagen capsule of the joint extends from the condylar attachment of the inferior stratum to the tympanic plate of the temporal bone to complete the posterior aspect of the joint.

The inferior cavity of the joint lies between the meniscus and the condyle and is also surrounded at its periphery by synovial membrane. The synovial tissues are confined to the periphery of the cavities and do not extend over the superior and inferior surfaces of the meniscus.

The attachment of the heel of the meniscus foot to the condyle is often higher than the attachment of the inferior stratum of the bilaminar zone in the posterior. The inferior belly of the lateral pterygoid muscle attaches to the condyle neck in a fovea just inferior to the articular surface and makes this anterior high attachment necessary.

The articular surface of the condyle is very small when compared with that of the glenoid fossa and articular eminence. In the sagittal projection it extends from the pterygoid fovea only to the superior crest of the condyle (Fig. 15-1). This surface is also collagen, not cartilage as seen in other joints of the body. Its fibers are arranged parallel to the surface of the condyle. The secondary cartilage of the condylar process lies just beneath this layer of collagen. The presence of fibroblasts in the articular surface makes growth of the condyle by apposition possible. The fibroblasts may differentiate into chondroblasts to form new cartilage by appositional growth and the chondrocytes of the condylar cartilage can also undergo mitosis to provide new cartilage by interstitial growth. The persistence of the condylar cartilage accounts for the renewed growth of the mandible, resulting in a class III or prognathous relationship commonly seen in acromegalics.

The capsule of the temporomandibular joint is not so well defined and organized as the capsules of the larger joints of the body. Its lateral aspect is reinforced by the band of collagen fibers known as the temporomandibular ligament. This ligament extends from the zygomatic arch, down and posteriorly to the lateral aspect of the neck of the condylar process. Since it attaches in such a manner, it allows translation of the condyle down and forward without need for increasing its length because it functions much like the arm on a pendulum as the condyle moves forward. The remainder of the lateral wall of the capsule and the lateral half of its anterior wall are remarkably flimsy and poorly organized. The anterior wall becomes a loose meshwork of fibers in the lateral half and is deficient completely in the medial half where the superior belly of the lateral pterygoid attaches to the meniscus. The medial and posterior walls are complete but are also loosely organized. The medial, posterior, and lateral walls of the capsule are innervated by a large branch from the auriculotemporal nerve, which extends superiorly from the nerve as it crosses posterior to the condyle neck.[6] The posterior deep temporal nerves supply a small portion of the lateral and anterior walls of the capsule and the masseteric nerves supply the remainder of the anterior wall and a small portion of the medial wall. The pressures created in the bilaminar zone of the joint meniscus have been shown to become negative when the condyle translates forward out of the fossa and to become positive when the condyle moves back into the fossa.[7] The maximum pressure measure was +16 mm of mercury with the usual range being about +1 or −1 mm of mercury. These are not remarkably high pressures when one considers that the pressure in the alveoli of the lungs varies from +3 to −3 mm of mercury during normal breathing. Several studies have shown that 60% to 70% of subjects studied translate their condyles anterior to the crest of the articular eminence on wide opening of the jaws.[8,9] These are subjects who have not experienced temporomandibular joint pain syndrome or subluxation of the condyle with locking in the forward position. The concept that such extreme mobility of the condyle indicates joint dysfunction has not been validated by these studies. McLeran[9] has also demonstrated that many subjects with asymptomatic joints show considerable asynchrony of movement of the condyles during jaw function. The condyles in his subjects were shown to "hunt" toward and away from the articu-

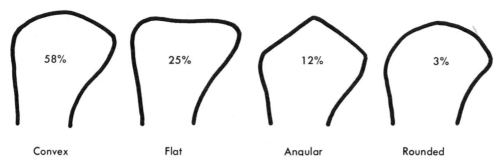

| 58% | 25% | 12% | 3% |

| Convex | Flat | Angular | Rounded |

Fig. 15-2. Four shapes of human condyles viewed in frontal plane with their incidence reported by Yale. (Yale, S. H., Allison, B. D., and Hauptfuehrer, J. D.: Oral Surg. **21**:169, 1966.)

lar eminence in a bizarre fashion as they translated out of the fossa. In some subjects one condyle would move forward at the first increment of opening while the opposite condyle would drop down and back. The concept that the condyle glides down and over the eminence smoothly along its surface seems to be in error in many cases.

The shapes of the frontal projection of thousands of mandibular condyles have been studied,[10] and their analysis has shown that there are four shapes to be considered (Fig. 15-2). The majority of human condyles (58%) are slightly convex superiorly with a radius of curvature greater than the distance from the medial to lateral poles. The next largest proportion (25%) of condyles are flat superiorly. Approximately 12% are pointed or angular in shape, and approximately 3% are bulbous or rounded in shape with a radius of curvature less than the distance from the lateral to medial poles. The surface of the articular eminence that most closely approximates the condyle is consistently congruent with the surface of the condyle.[11] The two condyles of a patient may be asymmetric; a combination of flat condyle on one side with a convex condyle on the other is most common. One never finds a rounded or bulbous condyle on one side associated with any other shape of condyle in the absence of any

bony abnormality.[11] The shape of the condyle would directly affect the nature of the Bennett shift of the mandible. A subject with an angular condyle functioning in an angular fossa would move his mandible inferiorly to a noticeable degree when making a lateral sideshift, whereas a person with a flat condyle would not necessarily drop inferiorly at all during the lateral sideshift. The patient with an angular condyle would be able to function with very steep cusps since a downward deflection of a condyle in the Bennett shift moves the teeth apart, especially on the working side.

It has been shown (Fig. 15-3) that the temporomandibular joint meniscus is tightly bound to the lateral and medial poles of the condyle independently of the capsule.[1] The capsule attaches below the meniscus at both sites and is not tightly bound between temporal bone and condyle poles. If the medial and lateral attachments of the meniscus to the condyle have not been damaged, it follows that the meniscus is placed on stretch from the condyle poles to the tympanic plate by elastin fibers and unfolded synovial membrane during wide opening of the mouth. Excessive tension will damage these fibers, especially in frail, small women. The dentist should keep these points in mind when applying great forces to seat crowns and bridges, during extraction of lower molars, when working with a rubber dam for extended periods of time, and when placing and removing impression trays. A significant percentage of temporomandibular joint pain syndromes have been shown to be initiated by dental treatment.[12]

The sphenomandibular and styloman-

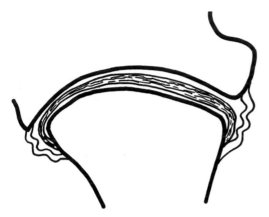

Fig. 15-3. Frontal section through human temporomandibular joint showing independent attachments of meniscus and capsule at condylar poles.

dibular ligaments span the temporomandibular joint. The sphenomandibular ligament extends from the spine of the sphenoid bone to the lingula on the mandibular foramen in the medial wall of the ramus. It represents the remnant of Meckel's cartilage, the primary cartilage of the mandibular arch. The stylomandibular ligament extends from the styloid process to the posterior border of the ramus near the angle. These ligaments are now considered to function by limiting jaw movement at maximum opening positions.

Many muscles of the head and neck have an influence on the movement and position of the mandible. The masseter, temporalis, medial (internal) pterygoid, and lateral (external) pterygoid are described as the muscles of mastication. Of these, the masseter, temporalis, and medial pterygoid serve to elevate the mandible when they shorten. The lateral pterygoid, however, when shortening in conjunction with other muscles, including the opposite lateral pterygoid, serves

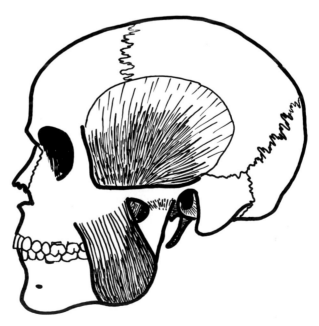

Fig. 15-4. Human skull showing only masseter and temporalis muscles.

to depress, protrude, or shift the mandible laterally.

The masseter extends from the zygomatic arch to the lateral surface of the mandibular ramus with its fibers generally directed downward and backward (Fig. 15-4). The posterior part of the muscle is divided into a superficial and a deep portion. The superior part contains many tendinous strands, and one therefore observes bulging of the masseter on forceful jaw closure, mainly in the lower half of the muscle. The fibers of the masseter are arranged at an angle to the long axis of the muscle between layers of tendon. This arrangement of numerous, short fibers between layers of connective tissue affords the masseter great power of contraction.

The temporalis muscle takes origin from the temporal fossa on the side of the skull and from the inner surface of the temporal fascia. (Fig. 15-4). Its anterior fibers are directed vertically running deep to the zygomatic arch to attach to the anterior border, apex, and deep surface of the mandibular coronoid process. The fibers covering the anterior margin of the ramus extend almost to the level of the occlusal plane and are extremely sensitive to pressure. Impingement of a thick denture flange against the anteromedial aspect of the mandibular ramus will elicit excruciating pain in the temporalis fibers. The deep portion of the anterior temporalis fibers often attaches by a separate tendon to the interal oblique line on the medial aspect of the ramus low enough to affect insertion of the needle for mandibular block anesthesia. The middle and posterior fibers of the temporalis become increasingly oblique so that the most posterior fibers run forward horizontally and bend downward in front of the articular eminence. They attach to the coronoid process as far down as the depth of the mandibular notch. The fibers of the temporalis muscle are divided by tendinous plates as in the masseter but are much

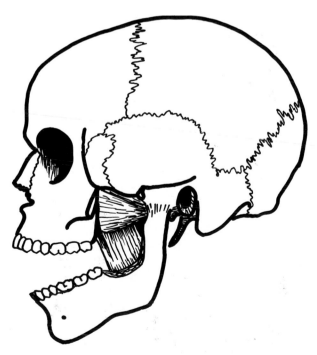

Fig. 15-5. Human skull showing relationship of lateral pterygoid muscle to medial pterygoid muscle.

longer than those of the masseter. The temporalis muscle serves mainly as an elevator of the mandible. Its most posterior fibers, functioning around the root of the zygomatic process, serve to retrude the mandible to some extent.

The medial pterygoid muscle is located deep to the mandibular ramus and functions as a counterpart of the masseter (Fig. 15-5). It takes origin in the pterygoid fossa and on the medial surface of the lateral pterygoid plate of the sphenoid bone. It extends downward, backward, and outward to insert on the medial aspect of the angle of the mandible. The most anterior fibers of the medial pterygoid muscle often extend down onto the pyramidal process of the palatine bone and maxillary tuberosity so as to produce a definite facet in the posterior border of an upper arch impression. These fibers, when present, will often displace denture flanges during functional movements of the mandible. The fibers of the medial pterygoid are arranged internally the same as those of the masseter, but the medial pterygoid is not so powerful as the masseter.

The lateral pterygoid muscle is more intimately related to the temporomandibular joint than the other muscles of mastication (Fig. 15-5). Its large, inferior head takes origin on the lateral surface of the lateral pterygoid plate and extends upward, outward, and backward to insert in the pterygoid fovea on the neck of the condyle. The small, superior head takes origin from the horizontal portion of the greater wing of the sphenoid, medial to the infratemporal crest. It extends horizontally backward and outward to attach to the anteromedial corner of the temporomandibular joint meniscus and the pterygoid fovea. When both lateral pterygoids shorten simultaneously, they either depress or protrude the mandible. If the mandibular elevators are only partially relaxed, the mandible is protruded. If the elevators are relaxed and the digastrics

are contracted with a fixed hyoid bone, the mandible is depressed. If only one lateral pterygoid is contracted, it serves to move the mandible laterally to the opposite side. Recent studies in both monkey and man[13,14] have demonstrated that the superior and inferior heads of the lateral pterygoid function as antagonistic muscles. Wire electromyograph recording electrodes implanted in the two heads of the muscle show electrical activity in the inferior head on opening in the masticatory cycle and activity in the superior head on closing. This finding indicates that the medial and lateral attachment of the meniscus to the poles of the condyle are the only factors that maintain the functional relationship of meniscus to condyle as the condyle translates down on the eminence in mouth opening. The superior head does not assist anterior movement of the meniscus, since it does not contract on opening. This also means that a tight attachment of the meniscus at the condyle poles is required to prevent meniscus-condyle dyscoordination with clicking or popping sounds on mouth opening.

The suprahyoid muscles extending from the skull and mandible to the hyoid bone serve to elevate the hyoid bone or to depress the mandible. They include the digastric, geniohyoid, mylohyoid, and stylohyoid. If the infrahyoid muscles are contracted so as to immobolize the hyoid bone, contraction of the suprahyoids depresses and retracts the mandible. If the mandible is fixed by contraction of the elevators, the suprahyoids elevate the hyoid bone and the larynx.

The muscles of facial expression are normally very thin, weak muscles that serve to move only the soft tissues of the face. Some of these muscles indirectly extend from the bones of the upper face to the mandible but under normal circumstances are not important in moving or positioning the lower jaw.

• • •

The temporomandibular joint in man functions in a manner that resembles a ball on an inverted hill rather than a ball in a socket. The mandibular condyle moves anterior to the articular eminence during wide opening of the jaws in most individuals. It also moves away from and toward the surface of the eminence during functional movement of the mandible with a considerable degree of freedom. The meniscus is tightly attached to the medial and lateral poles of the condyle in the healthy temporomandibular joint, and its attachment to the tympanic plate is made up of elastic tissue. This anatomic arrangement allows the meniscus to translate with the condyle while rotating posteriorly around its polar attachments on mouth opening. Contraction of the superior head of the lateral pterygoid on mouth closure serves to rotate the meniscus anteriorly as the condyle translates back into the glenoid fossa.[14]

The central part of the meniscus is avascular in the adult but its periphery is richly supplied with blood vessels. Boyer and others[15] have demonstrated a great complexity and quantity of blood vessels in the periphery of the meniscus in the monkey, which is very similar to that of man. Glomus-cell arteriovenous anastomoses have been demonstrated in this vascular area of the human meniscus.

The major nerve innervating the temporomandibular joint capsule is a large branch from the auriculotemporal nerve, which approaches the joint from the posterior aspect of the neck of the condyle. The posterior deep temporal and masseteric nerves also supply the capsule.

The two condyles of a patient are often asymmetric, but one never finds a rounded or bulbous condyle on one side associated with a flat, oval, or angular condyle on the opposite side in the absence of a pathologic condition in the joint.

The upper portion of the masseter muscle is comprised of a large proportion of tendinous strands, whereas the lower part is mainly made up of muscle fibers. This explains the fact that bulging of the masseter usually occurs in the lower half of the muscle when it is forcefully contracted in jaw closure. The anterior fibers of the temporalis, located just buccal to the maxillary tuberosity, are extremely sensitive to pressure and any impingement of denture flanges against these fibers will cause extreme pain in the muscle. The deep part of the anterior temporalis attaches by a separate tendon on the medial aspect of the ramus low enough to obstruct the path of insertion of the needle in a mandibular block injection. Piercing this muscle and tendon may divert the needle from the region of the lingula and inferior alveolar nerve, causing failure of the anesthesia. The posterior fibers of the temporalis are directed horizontally and serve to retrude the mandible to some extent. The anterior fibers of the medial pterygoid muscle often extend down onto the maxillary tuberosity so as to produce definite facets in the posterior border of upper arch impressions and to displace denture flanges during wide opening of the jaws. The superior belly of the lateral pterygoid muscle attaches to the medial, anterior corner of the temporomandibular joint meniscus but does not contract on mouth opening. Only tight attachments of the meniscus to the condyle poles stabilize the meniscus during translation of the condyles.[13,14] The muscles of facial expression indirectly extend from the bones of the upper face to the mandible but under normal circumstances are not important in elevating the lower jaw.

SELECTED REFERENCES

1. Choukas, N. C., and Sicher, H.: The structure of the temporomandibular joint, Oral Surg. **13:** 1203, 1960.
2. Thilander, B.: The structure of the collagen of the temporo-mandibular disc in man, Acta Odont. Scand. **22:**135, 1964.
3. Batson, O. V.: The anatomist looks at the tem-

poromandibular joint, Trans. Am. Acad. Ophthalmol. Otolaryngol. **60**:413, May-June 1956.

4. Zola, A.: Morphologic limiting factors in the temporomandibular joint, J. Prosthet. Dent. **13**: 732, 1963.

5. Griffin, C. J., and Sharpe, C. J.: The structure of the adult human temporomandibular meniscus, Aust. Dent. J. **5**:190, 1960.

6. Thilander, B.: Innervation of the temporomandibular joint capsule in man, Trans. Roy. Schools Dent. Stockh. Umea, no. 7, 1961.

7. Findlay, I. A.: Mandibular joint pressures, J. Dent. Res. **43**:140, 1964.

8. Frommer, H., and Parker, L. A.: Roentgenographic temporomandibular joint survey, Oral Diag. Pathol. **16**:1326, 1963.

9. McLeran, J. H., Montgomery, J. C., and Hale, M. L.: A cinefluorographic analysis of the temporomandibular joint, J.A.D.A. **75**:1394, 1967.

10. Yale, S. H., Allison, B. D., and Hauptfuehrer, J. D.: An epidemiological assessment of mandibular condyle morphology, Oral Surg. **21**:169, 1966.

11. Emmering, T. E.: A new approach to the analysis of the functional surfaces of the temporomandibular joint, Oral Surg. **23**:603, 1967.

12. Moulton, R.: Oral and dental manifestations of anxiety, Psychiatry **18**:261, 1955.

13. McNamara, J. A., Jr.: The independent functions of the two heads of the lateral pterygoid muscle, Am. J. Anat. **138**:197, 1973.

14. Lipke, D. P., Gay, T., Gross, B. D., and Yaeger, J. A.: An electromyographic study of the human lateral pterygoid muscle, J. Dent. Res. **56**(spec. issue B):B230, June 1977, abstr. 713.

15. Boyer, C. C., and others: Blood supply of the temporomandibular joint, J. Dent. Res. **43**:223, 1964.

GENERAL REFERENCES

Boucher, L. J.: Anatomy of the temporomandibular joint as it pertains to centric relation, J. Prosthet. Dent. **12**:464-472, 1962.

Brodie, A. G.: Occlusion from the standpoint of the fundamental sciences, Illinois Dent. J. **6**:6, 1937.

Fagerstrom, K. G., and Brodie, A. G.: Cranial and facial growth in the pig as revealed by metallic implants and serial roentgenology, Int. Assoc. Dent. Res. Preprinted Abstracts, no. 250, 1963.

Gasser, R. F.: The development of the facial muscles in man, Am. J. Anat. **120**:357, 1967.

Hase, R. R.: Anatomical carving in crown and bridge prosthodontia, J. Philippine Dent. Assoc. **15**:17, 1961.

Hockstein, I.: Arch form—a study of various dimensions and relationships in the maxillary arch, Am. J. Orthodont. **48**:554, 1962 (abstr.).

Lauritzen, A. G.: Function, prime object of restorative dentistry; a definite procedure to obtain it, J.A.D.A. **42**:503, 1951.

Lindblom, G.: Balanced occlusion with partial reconstructions, Int. Dent. J. **1**:84, 1951.

Meyer, F. S.: Bridges cast to functional occlusion, Minneapolis Dist. Dent. J. **15**:9, 1932.

Meyer, F. S.: Cast bridgework in functional occlusion, J.A.D.A. **20**:1015, 1933.

Monson, G. S.: Occlusion as applied to crown and bridgework, J. Natl. Dent. Assoc. **7**:399, 1920.

Morris, M. L.: Artificial crown contours and gingival health, J. Prosthet. Dent. **12**:1146, 1962.

Moulton, G. M.: Esthetics in fixed bridge prosthodontics, J.A.D.A. **52**:36, 1956.

Piątowska, D.: [Anatomical structure of the gingiva], Czas Stomat. **21**(10):1169-1173, Oct. 1968.

Pound, E.: Applying harmony in selecting and arranging teeth, Dent. Clin. North Am., pp. 241-258, March 1962.

Sicher, H., and DuBrul, E. L.: Oral anatomy, ed. 6, Saint Louis, 1975, The C. V. Mosby Co.

Thilander, B.: Innervation of the temporo-mandibular disc in man, Acta Odont. Scand. **22**:151, 1964.

Tinker, E. T.: Predetermination of occlusal surfaces of teeth, J.A.D.A. **18**:1046, 1931.

Tylman, S. D.: Discussion of the biologic factors involved in the fixed partial denture, J. Can. Dent. Assoc. **23**:67-75, 1957.

Wilson, W. H., and Lang, R. L.: Practical crown and bridge prosthodontics, New York, 1962, McGraw-Hill Book Co., Inc.

16

Stomatognathic physiology related to crown and fixed partial prosthodontic therapy

Parker E. Mahan

Posselt[1,2] studied the limits of motion of the human mandible at many increments of jaw opening from tooth occlusion to maximum opening. He recorded these limits with intraoral needle-point tracings at different vertical openings, one above the other, to produce a solid form that demonstrated the movement space of the mandible. A midsagittal section through a typical movement space is shown in Fig. 16-1. It has been found that an arc, *BC*, exists for the mandible in which it rotates about an axis running through or near the condyles when they are seated up in the glenoid fossae. This arc is known as the centric relation closure arc and can be demonstrated on most patients using a hinge-axis face-bow procedure. The center of this arc is the terminal hinge axis or kinematic point. When a patient has opened to point *C* in the centric relation closure arc the condyles can no longer remain up in the glenoid fossae but must translate down and forward. The mandibular reference point will therefore be deflected at point *C*; the arc *CD* represents a combination of translation and rotation of the condyles. This movement, then, has a constantly changing center of rotation. At point *D* the mandible has reached maximum opening. The curve *DE* represents the maximum, protruded closure arc. The

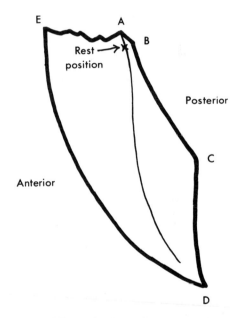

Fig. 16-1. Midsagittal section through mandibular movement space as described by Posselt. (Posselt, U.: Acta Odont. Scand. **10:** 10, 1952.)

condyles are located forward, in many cases, anterior to the eminence during this closure. The irregular path from *E* to *A* represents the movement of the mandible from the maximum protruded occlusal position back to maximum intercuspation of the teeth. The irregular path is produced by the deflection of the mandible by opposing inclines of the teeth as they move over each other.

SLIDE FROM RETRUDED CONTACT TO MAXIMUM INTERCUSPATION

Posselt found that 88% of the subjects in his study, when closing in the centric relation closure arc, first occluded their teeth at a retruded contact position (B); the mandible was then deflected up and forward to maximum intercuspation of the teeth at point A. He found that this slide from retruded contact to maximum intercuspation had a horizontal component of 1.25 ± 1 mm and a vertical component of 0.9 ± 0.75 mm relative to the sella-nasion line measured at the lower incisors. Many other investigators have studied the magnitude and direction of the slide. Beyron[3] found that 90% of 46 adult Australian aborigines had a slide that averaged approximately 1 mm; Kydd and Sander[4] found that all 14 of their subjects had a slide. Hodge[5] studied 101 young male adults and found that only 57 percent of them had a slide. These men had at least 28 natural teeth and most of them had no dental restorations. Hodge measured the horizontal, vertical, and lateral component of the slide and found that although 57% of the subjects had an anteroposterior component to their slide, only 15% had a measurable lateral component. Lateral deviation in the slide is often associated with temporomandibular joint pain syndrome.[6-9]

The lower incisor teeth close up and forward at an angle of approximately 38 degrees to a perpendicular from the Frankfort plane during the last millimeter of closure.[10] This natural angle of closure serves to move the lower anterior teeth forward a distance almost equal to their vertical movement in the last millimeter of jaw closure. Therefore, adjusting the occlusion in a patient with a long anteroposterior slide may require very little removal of tooth structure on the opposing cuspal inclines. The distal inclines of

lower teeth occlude against the mesial inclines of uppers in the slide. Since the lower teeth are moving forward in this final increment of jaw closure, tending to move these occluding inclines apart, interfering tooth substances that actually deflects the mandible is greatly minimized. When a jaw registration in the maximum intercuspation position is transferred to most adjustable articulators, there is one movement that the patient can make that the instrument cannot duplicate or simulate. That movement is the slide from retruded contact to maximum intercuspation. A dental patient will often close into the maximum intercuspation position when he is not guided or trained by the dentist.[11] When many occlusal surfaces are to be restored in an arch, the cuspal inclines that occlude in the slide may need excessive adjustment in the mouth after the restorations are seated when maximum intercuspation registration was established on the articulator so that the slide could not be simulated.

When the anterior teeth of a patient who has a slide are being restored on a nonadjustable instrument or simple hinge device, the maximum intercuspation registration will introduce less error than the retruded contact registration. This is true because the lower anterior teeth usually move up and forward to contact the lingual surface of the uppers at the end of the slide. When a retruded contact registration has been established on an adjustable instrument, the anterior teeth can be waxed so as to establish contact along the slide in the cingulum area of the upper incisors and cuspids.

Several studies using radio transmitters in fixed bridge pontics so that the keying contacts are closed by metal restorations in opposing teeth when the jaws are closed in specific occlusal positions have produced interesting results. One study[12] showed that four out of five subjects closed into retruded contact position

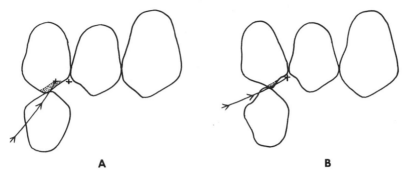

Fig. 16-2. Upper cuspid, first and second bicuspid with centric relation closure arc of lower second bicuspid indicated. **A,** Relationship that increases anterior horizontal overlap with occlusal adjustment. **B,** Relationship that does not alter anterior horizontal overlap with occlusal adjustment.

when swallowing and cleansing the mouth. All five of the subjects closed into maximum intercuspation position while chewing peanuts and rye bread and when swallowing and cleansing the mouth. The movement back to retruded contact has also been observed in subjects when swallowing a bolus of food they have masticated while wearing extraoral needle-point tracing devices.[13] Interferences in the slide are very often associated with temporomandibular joint pain syndrome.[6-9] The fact that retruded contact position is rarely used in normal function does not prevent interferences in this position from playing a role in temporomandibular joint dysfunction.

When attempting to adjust a patient's occlusion prior to extensive crown and bridge restoration, one may observe that in one patient this adjustment will create an increased horizontal overlap of anterior teeth whereas the next adjustment will not alter this measurement.[10] This observation can be explained as shown in Fig. 16-2. In Fig. 16-2, A, the lower second bicuspid closes along the centric relation closure arc (arrow) until it contacts the upper second bicuspid at its cusp tip. It then slides up and forward to the cross (+) over the marginal ridges of the upper bicuspids. When the mesial incline of the upper bicuspid is adjusted by

removal of the stippled area, the jaws can then close so that the lower bicuspid moves to the cross on the centric relation closure arc. In this case the horizontal overlap of the incisors has been increased by the distance between the crosses. In Fig. 16-2, B, the lower bicuspid closes along the centric relation closure arc until it contacts the distal aspect of the upper second bicuspid cusp tip. It then trips over this cuspal incline and moves to the cross (+) over the marginal ridges of the upper bicuspids. When the upper bicuspid has been adjusted to eliminate the slide, in this case the lower bicuspid moves to the same occlusal position it had before the adjustment, and the horizontal overlap of the anterior teeth is not altered.

It has been shown that the slide from retruded contact to maximum intercuspation in children is quite similar to that found in the adult.[14,15] Ingervall[14] has demonstrated that the only statistical difference between the slide in 10-year-old girls and that in 20-year-old women is a larger lateral component in the girls. These data indicate that during the mixed dentition stage when the permanent teeth are erupting into position in the dental arch, lateral interferences are created that tend to be corrected with time alone.

INTEROCCLUSAL DISTANCE AND MOVEMENT FROM REST POSITION TO MAXIMUM INTERCUSPATION

In 1908 Sir Norman Bennett[16] demonstrated that the center of rotation of his mandible from maximum intercuspation to rest position was located in the region of his mastoid process. In 1956 Nevakari[17] studied this movement in 75 dental students. He was interested in finding out whether or not this movement was a pure hinge movement with its center in or near the condyle. He found the average location of the center of rotation of this movement in his subjects to be also in the region of the mastoid process. His study further demonstrated that the condyle moves up and back approximately 1 mm during this movement so that both translation and rotation occur simultaneously. He found that the lower cuspids move up and forward at an average angle of 11 degrees to a perpendicular to the Frankfort plane in the movement from rest to maximum intercuspation. Posselt demonstrated (Fig. 16-1) that the rest position in the average patient is not a border movement but lies within the movement space on the free opening-closing path. These data indicate that the mandible is not back in the centric relation closure arc when it is in rest position.

A number of electromyographic studies of interocclusal distance have been reported. Garnick and Ramfjord[18] found that the posterior temporalis muscle usually demonstrates electrical activity when the mandible is in the clinically determined rest position. They considered the distance between the teeth when the first elevator muscle came into electrical activity on jaw closure to be the electromyographic (EMG) interocclusal distance. In their study of 20 subjects this distance averaged 3.3 mm, whereas their clinically determined interocclusal distance averaged 1.7 mm on the same subjects. They found an EMG resting range of 11.1 mm in their subjects instead of a specific rest position. Preiskel[19] studied the variations in interocclusal distance with different head positions. He found that when the head was turned down 35 degrees from the horizontal orientation, the interocclusal distance decreased; when the head was turned up 35 degrees, it increased. In each instance he found that the EMG interocclusal distance was greater than the clinically determined distance. It has not been practical to place electrodes on all of the mandibular muscles in these studies, but it has been shown, on the muscles that are accessible for recording, that the concept that the mandibular muscles are at minimial activity at the rest position is probably not true. It seems that at least the posterior temporalis is active, counteracting the pull of gravity on the lower jaw at our clinically determined rest position. It will be interesting to see, with the advent of space travel in the future, what effect weightlessness will have on the interocclusal distance.

The rest position in children with class II, division 1 malocclusions is different from that in children with normal jaw relationships. Ingervall[20] located the average rest position in 32 class II, division 1 girls and found it to be down and forward of the maximum intercuspation position. It is located down and backward from the maximum intercuspation position in normal subjects. The class II patient may hold his jaw forward for esthetic reasons or to allow the muscles of the lips and chin to function properly.

The addition of an acrylic palatal base plate to a patient's mouth will increase the resting height of the face.[21] A study of rest position in 13 dental students has demonstrated a statistical increase in rest face height and greater variation in rest position of the mandible when the subjects wore a palatal piece 2.5 mm thick. These subjects all had nearly full complements of natural teeth.

It is interesting that the interocclusal

distance was reduced to zero over a 12-year period in a patient with a paralyzed right lateral pterygoid.[22] In this instance an imbalance between the elevators and depressors of the mandible in favor of the elevators established a new rest position at the occlusal vertical dimension. One of the generalizations in physiology that can be demonstrated repeatedly is that the organs of the living mammal function in a state of dynamic balance. In this state, opposing forces that may vary in magnitude from time to time balance each other in establishing the functions of life. The occlusal vertical dimension and the rest position are established in any given patient by a dynamic balance between various factors that tend to close the jaws and those that open them. It is a common observation that in some patients the teeth, when taken out of occlusion by the occlusal reduction of a full crown preparation, will rapidly extrude into occlusion if very accurate temporary crowns are not placed on them. In other patients the teeth that have been taken out of occlusion do not seem to extrude at all. When one is deciding whether to change the occlusal vertical dimension of a patient, he should study the factors that have balanced to produce the vertical dimension and interocclusal distance in that patient. If it seems possible to alter these factors in favor of an increased vertical dimension, then perhaps the bite can be successfully opened. One should always examine the interocclusal distance when he is contemplating increasing the occlusal vertical dimension in a patient. It has been found that increasing the vertical dimension in patients with small interocclusal distance is rarely successful.[23] Increasing the occlusal vertical dimension with fixed restorations or removable appliances may not alter the opposing forces that establish the dimension so that the teeth may intrude into the alveolar process or the condyle-fossa relationship of the temporomandibular joint may be changed. These changes may or may not be accompanied by pain dysfunction syndrome. It has been observed that opening the bite in some patients with temporomandibular joint pain syndrome will relieve the pain.[24] This relief is not uncommonly temporary and in those cases in which it recurs after the teeth have been intruded, the dentist is confronted with a most difficult problem. One should always carefully examine for a pathologic condition in the temporomandibular joint, muscle abnormality, interferences in the slide, balancing interferences, lateral deviations in the slide, and open or heavy centric stops at the patient's occlusal vertical dimension before considering opening a patient's bite.

CENTRIC RELATION CLOSURE ARC AND TERMINAL HINGE POSITION

Zola[25] has demonstrated a shiny facet in a depression in the medial wall of the glenoid fossa of an unspecified number of skulls. He has also demonstrated that the meniscus may be only 0.2 mm thick over the medial pole of the condyle as it is positioned in these depressions. The seating of the right and left condylar medial poles in these depressions will establish a bony support for the mandible in its superior position and establish an axis about which it may rotate. It is reasonable that this anatomic relationship would establish a terminal hinge axis with a kinematic point on the face where this axis emerges from the head. This definite depression in the medial wall of the glenoid fossa cannot be demonstrated on many human skulls; so these findings will not explain the presence of a terminal hinge axis in all patients. McCollum and Stuart[26] reported that the terminal hinge axis has remained constant in a few patients for as long as 9 years. The significance of the terminal hinge axis to jaw registration for occlusal restoration was pointed out by Moulton[27] in 1960.

Beck[28] located the terminal hinge axis on 12 subjects and studied its location relative to the image of the condyle on lateral cephalometric radiographs. Disregarding the complicated distortion of the cephalometric radiograph, one can see from his study that the terminal hinge axis fell within the condyle in seven of his 12 subjects. In the other five subjects it was located posterior to, anterior to, or within the neck of the condylar process. Schallhourn[29] located the terminal hinge axis in 70 dental students and then marked the arbitrary axis point 13 mm anterior to the tragus on a line to the outer canthus of the eye. He found the average discrepancy between these two points to be 1.7 mm. Ninety-seven percent of the arbitrary axis points fell within 5 mm of the hinge axis points. The hinge axis points tended to lie slightly posterior to the arbitrary point. Fox[30] has estimated that cementation of crowns produces occlusal errors of 0.05 to 0.08 mm. He then calculated that an error of 1 mm in locating the terminal hinge axis is acceptable because it will not result in greater occlusal discrepancy than 0.08 mm.

TYPES OF OCCLUSAL FUNCTION

Before one can properly diagnose and plan treatment for the occlusal restoration of a patient, he must know how the patient's teeth occlude during function. There are three general types of occlusal function found in the human dentition. These are balanced occlusion, working-side occlusion (group function), and cuspid-rise or cuspid-protected occlusion. All three are based on the assumption that opposing teeth are in contact in a centric stop position when the jaws are closed in maximum intercuspation position. The type of occlusal function in a specific patient may not be bilateral. It is not uncommon, for example, to find cuspid-protected occlusion on one side and working-side occlusion on the other in young patients.

Balanced occlusion is that relationship of the teeth in which they are in contact on the right and left sides and in the anterior and posterior simultaneously when the jaws are closed within the functional range. In this type of occlusion there is a buccal-to-buccal contact on the working side of the mouth and at least one contact of an upper lingual cusp against a lower buccal cusp on the balancing side. This type of occlusion is considered ideal in complete denture construction because three-point contact provides stability of the denture bases against the alveolar mucosa during occlusal function.

Working-side occlusion is that type of occlusal function in which the cuspids and one or more posterior teeth are in contact, buccal-to-buccal, on the working side but there is no tooth contact on the balancing side. Weinberg[31] has reported that 65% of 100 patients having at least 28 natural teeth had this type of occlusion. Working-side occlusion is found in the Australian aborigines who abrade their teeth excessively throughout life. One explanation for the high incidence of working-side occlusion (no tooth contact on the balancing side) in the human dentition can be found in the data of Conant.[32] In this study a sound-transmission method was used to measure the forces exerted between the teeth in the chewing cycle in an unspecified number of subjects. The relationship of force exerted between the teeth to the amount of filtered and amplified 1-kilohertz sound transmitted from the forehead to the chin was determined on one subject. On the basis of this calibration of the system it was found that when subjects chew a soft bolus of food like chewing gum they exert maximum force between the teeth in the maximum intercuspation position at the top of the chewing cycle. When, however, they are chewing a tough bolus of food like raisins, the teeth move through maximum intercuspation into a balancing relationship on the bolus side and exert maximum closing force in this position. It therefore seems reasonable that the balancing inclines of the teeth would abrade away slightly ahead of the working inclines since more force is applied in this tooth position against tough and abrasive foods. It has been observed that balancing interferences are often associated with temporomandibular joint pain syndrome.[9,33] These interferences are not infrequently found in mouths with missing lower molars and mesial tipping of the more distal molar. They are also found in postorthodontic patients when occlusal adjustment has not been accomplished after the band spaces close up and the teeth tighten up.[34]

Cuspid protected occlusion is that type of occlusal function in which there are even centric stops around the arch in the maximum intercuspation position but any lateral or protrusive movement of the mandible immediately discludes the posterior teeth, with the lower cuspid occluding against the lingual surface of the upper cuspid.

D'Amico[35] pointed out the significance of this type of occlusal function when he noted that ancient California Indian skulls showed abraded cuspids and incisors with an occlusal function resembling that of the aborigine, whereas the modern California Indian (eating a soft diet) has cuspid-protected occlusion. Weinberg[31] reported that only 19% of 100 patients with 28 natural teeth in his study had cuspid-protected occlusion. This type of occlusal function would tend to put very heavy forces on single teeth, the cuspids, in eccentric occlusal positions. It has been noted that in the cat[36,37] the periodontal membranes of the teeth, especially the anterior teeth, are richly innervated with receptors whose primary cell bodies lie in the mesencephalic nucleus of the trigeminal nerve. These receptors are directionally oriented around the tooth roots so that slight displacement of the cuspid inhibits the motor output to the jaw-elevating muscles and stimulates the anterior belly of the digastric muscle. These neurons with specialized receptors, then, constitute the sensory side of a jaw-opening reflex.

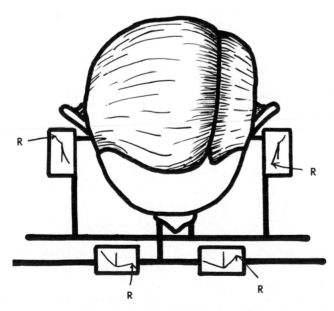

Fig. 16-3. Bennett path and gothic arch tracings of a pantographic tracing. *R*, Extreme right movement of mandible.

This type of proprioceptive mechanism may function in patients with cuspid-protected occlusion to prevent traumatic occlusion and destruction of the cuspid periodontium. There is no agreement today among the men most experienced in occlusal restoration as to whether or not cuspid-protected occlusion is a healthy and desirable occlusal function. Some believe that the lateral forces of occlusion should be distributed to as many teeth as possible,[33] whereas others believe that the cuspids can withstand these forces and the posterior teeth may show premature periodontal deterioration when subjected to the lateral forces of balanced occlusion.[38] Only 16% of the patients in Weinberg's study had balanced occlusion of their natural teeth.

One can best visualize the movement of the mandible relative to the maxilla in both functional and nonfunctional positions by studying a typical pantographic tracing of a patient. Fig. 16-3 diagrammatically demonstrates four of the six tracings of a pantographic recording. The writing styli are not pictured so that the Bennett path and Gothic arch tracings may be viewed without obstruction. It should be noted that the Bennett path tracing tables are fixed to the maxilla and their writing styli are fixed to the mandible. The Gothic arch tracing tables, on the other hand, are fixed to the mandibular face bow and the styli are fixed to the maxilla. The simultaneous locations of the writing styli for a subject in the extreme right lateral position of the mandible are indicated by the letter *R* in Fig. 16-3. A typical pantographic Bennett path tracing is described in Fig. 16-4. It must be remembered that the stylus is lateral to the condyle and so the Bennett tracing does not duplicate the movement of the condyle in any plane in space. The curved line from the centric occlusion point marked "working-condyle path" represents the combination of rotation and lateral shift of the working condyle.

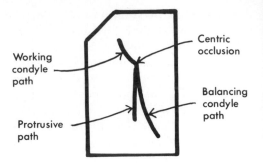

Fig. 16-4. Typical pantographic Bennett path tracing.

The extent of straight lateral displacement of this curve from the centric occlusion point would approximate the actual amount of side shift of the mandible. The angle formed between the "working-condyle path" and the sagittal plane is reported to range between 0 and 35 degrees.[39] An angle of 0 degrees would indicate no lateral shift of the mandible. Several studies[39,40] have reported that all patients examined (76 patients) showed Bennett shift of at least one condyle. The tracing marked "balancing-condyle path" anterior to the centric occlusion point represents the movement of the condyle as it translates down and medially on the articular eminence when the mandible is moved to the opposite lateral position.

The third tracing represents the path of the mandibular stylus when the patient protrudes the jaw straight forward.

A typical pantographic Gothic arch tracing is shown in Fig. 16-5. The apex of the three tracing lines represents centric relation or retruded contact position. The patient's movement from retruded contact to maximum, straight protrusive would produce the tracing so labeled. When the jaw is moved to a right lateral position the tracing would actually move toward the patient's left, as indicated, because the stylus is fixed to the maxilla and the tracing table moves with the mandible. When the jaw is moved to a left lateral position, the tracing would run

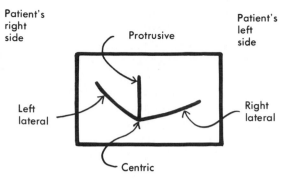

Patient's right side — Protrusive — Patient's left side

Left lateral — Right lateral

Centric

Fig. 16-5. Typical pantographic gothic arch tracing.

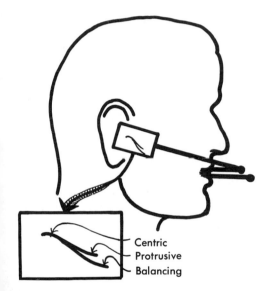

Centric
Protrusive
Balancing

Fig. 16-6. Typical pantographic condyle path tracing.

from the centric occlusion point to the patient's right, as indicated.

A typical pantographic condyle path tracing is shown diagrammatically in Fig. 16-6. The mandibular side arm with its vertical and horizontal writing styli is not shown. It will be noted that the centric relation point is not located at the posterior end of the tracing. The portion of the tracing posterior to the centric point is traced when the jaw is moved laterally to the side of the tracing table. The condyle tracing table is fixed to the maxilla and is

several centimeters lateral to the condyle. The writing stylus is fixed to the mandibular face-bow, and when the condyle rotates, the stylus is moved posterior to its centric relation location. When the patient moves into straight protrusive, the condyle usually does not drop so far inferiorly as it does when the jaw is moved to the opposite lateral position, as indicated. The angle between these paths is known as the Fischer angle. Only a small portion of the protrusive condyle path is traced before the lower anterior teeth have protruded beyond the upper anteriors. The length of the condyle path utilized in functional occlusal positions depends on the amount of horizontal and vertical overlap of the anterior teeth.

There are many variations in pantographic tracings observed in patients, but the examples described demonstrate a fairly common set of tracings. Isaacson[39] has beautifully demonstrated the variability found in the Bennett path tracings in nine patients.

PROPRIOCEPTION IN THE STOMATOGNATHIC SYSTEM

The major receptors that subserve the function of proprioception are the muscle spindles and Golgi tendon organs. The muscle spindles are very complicated structures usually found in the central parts of the muscles.[41] There are two types of muscle fibers within the spindles that do not produce tension when they contract. These fibers have separate motor innervations and function only to alter the firing rate of the primary and secondary endings of the proprioceptive nerves. The muscle spindles, then, have a double motor and double sensory innervation and they provide the central nervous system with information on the instantaneous length and the rate of change of length of the muscle in which they are located. They help ensure that muscle tension will be proportional to stretch, and they allow smooth coordination of phasic (intentional) movement with posture. The Golgi tendon organs are located in the ligaments and tendons of the muscles and are also constantly firing into the central nervous system.[42] The tendon organs have sufficiently low thresholds to tension to play a part in the moment-to-moment control of muscular contraction.

There are several unique features in the proprioceptive mechanism of the stomatognathic system. The cell bodies of the proprioceptive nerves in the muscles that elevate the mandible are found within the central nervous system in the mesencephalic nucleus of the trigeminal nerve.[43,44] One would expect these primary sensory neuron cell bodies to lie in the semilunar ganglion since all the other proprioceptive cell bodies are located outside the central nervous system in the dorsal root ganglia. Secondly, there are very few muscle spindles in the lateral pterygoid muscles and anterior belly of the digastric.[45,46] The typical reciprocal activity of antagonistic muscles has been demonstrated[47] in the mandibular muscles. When the mandibular muscles are freed from their insertion in the cat and are stretched, electrical activity in the antagonistic muscles is inhibited. This type of muscle function is typically attributed to the reciprocal activity of muscle spindles located in the antagonistic muscles. Since there are few muscle spindles in the depressor muscles of the mandible, one must find another explanation for these observations in the stomatognathic system. It has been shown that the capsule of the temporomandibular joint is richly innervated with proprioceptive nerve endings.[48] Griffin[49] has demonstrated recently that the meniscus of the temporomandibular joint is richly innervated by Golgi tendon organs in the area of attachment of the superior belly of the lateral pterygoid muscle. Jerge[36] has demonstrated in the cat that the periodontal membranes of the teeth, especially the anterior teeth, are innervated by complicated nerve receptors whose cell bodies lie in the mesencephalic nucleus of the trigeminal nerve. He has shown that these nerves may innervate single tooth periodontal membranes or two or more adjacent teeth and the adjacent gingival tissue. These receptors in the periodontal membranes are directionally oriented; pressure applied to the teeth is followed by jaw-opening movements. It therefore seems that the organs that need protection from jaw-closing action, the teeth, provide a large part of the sensory side of a jaw-opening reflex. The depressor muscles are protected by the Golgi tendon organs in their attachments and by the receptors in the temporomandibular joint.

It follows, then, that any time a dentist alters or restores the occlusal surface of a tooth having occlusal function, he is dealing directly with the proprioceptive innervation of the muscles. It has been shown[34] that muscle spasms rapidly disappear in the temporal muscles when occlusal interferences have been removed, as evidenced by electromyographic recording from the muscles. In cases where occlusal interferences were corrected with splints, the muscle spasms recurred almost immediately upon removal of the splint. These observations seem to indicate that the proprioceptive nerves from the periodontal membranes, the muscles, ligaments, and joints of the stomatognathic system, are extremely sensitive to the occlusion of the teeth. It also seems evident that an altered proprioceptive input attributable to occlusal interferences will lead to muscle pain and spasm in many patients.

Leff[50] has demonstrated that very slight changes in occlusal position of the teeth greatly alter the maximum closing pressure of the mandibular elevators. He first measured the amount of closure of the subjects' teeth into soft acrylic resin interocclusal records. Then he placed casts of the subjects' arches in the acrylic records and applied pressure until the casts closed down to the same distance as that measured in the mouth. The pressures exerted on the casts were then read from a gage in the system. He found that the average pressure exerted on the teeth with the mandible closing in the maximum intercuspation position (in an unspecified number of subjects) was 110 pounds. When the mandible was shifted just a few millimeters to a lateral position, the maximum pressure exerted dropped to 10 pounds. When the subjects protruded a few millimeters, the pressure measured 55 pounds; when they closed back in the centric relation closure arc toward retruded contact, they could exert only 19 pounds. These data indicate that the proprioceptive receptors of the stomatognathic system are very effective in limiting the contraction of the mandibular elevators so as to protect the structures of the temporomandibular joint in the retruded contact position of the condyle and the teeth when they are occluding on inclines instead of on stable centric stop positions of opposing teeth.

SUMMARY

Many of the complicated and intricate interactions of the structures of the stomatognathic system have been studied and described so that the dentist is now able to measure or approximate its normal function in his treatment of the abnormalities of the mouth and jaws. There is, on the other hand, a large part of stomatognathic function that we do not understand. This void in our knowledge daily faces the dentist in his practice and limits his ability to properly diagnose and plan the treatment of his patients.

The movement space of the mandible, telling us where the patient can move his jaws under various conditions, is understood today and we are able to use some of this information in dental treatment procedures. Posselt has demonstrated that most patients have a centric relation closure arc in which the mandible can rotate about an imaginary axis with the condyles positioned superiorly in the glenoid fossae. In some patients this position is established by the seating of the condyle medial poles into facets in the medial wall of the fossae. The tissues in the posterior of the joint are not firm or stable enough to establish the superoposterior position of the condyle. Most patients can maintain the centric relation closure arc only for the first 2 cm of jaw-opening, at which point the condyles must translate down and forward out of the fossae. The identification of this deflection point in the posterior border movement of a patient's jaw serves as an excellent landmark for determining centric relation in our patients. Most patients with natural teeth, when closing the jaws in the centric relation closure arc, occlude in a retruded contact position and slide up and forward approximately 1 to 2 mm into a maximum intercuspation position. Their mandible moves down and slightly backward from maximum intercuspation to its rest position. In the movement from maximum intercuspation to rest position the condyles translate down and forward approximately 1 mm and rotate a small amount.

The retruded contact position is usually not used in the masticatory cycle, but most patients close back into this position when swallowing and cleansing the mouth. At the top of the masticatory cycle, the teeth first contact in the working-bite relationship, slide up into maximum intercuspation, and then move on into a balancing relationship on the bolus side. More pressure is exerted between the teeth when they have reached the balancing relationship than in the earlier occlusal positions when tough foods are being masticated. This finding may explain the observation that few people have balancing contacts of their natural teeth.

Electromyographic studies have shown that the posterior temporalis muscle is usually showing electrical activity at the clinically determined rest position of the mandible. The muscles that have been examined have revealed a resting range of approximately 11 mm instead of a single rest position of the jaws. The concept that the mandibular muscles are relaxed when the jaw is in its rest position does not seem to be true. Rest position and occlusal vertical dimension both represent a dynamic balance between the opposing forces that close and open the mouth. Many factors such as the addition of a palatal base plate will affect the rest position of the mandible.

When one is considering increasing the occlusal vertical dimension in a patient with temporomandibular joint pain syndrome, one should carefully examine for a pathologic condition of the joint, muscle trismus, interferences or lateral deviation in the slide from retruded contact to maximum intercuspation, balancing-side interferences, and uneven centric stops before opening a patient's bite.

There are three general types of occlusal function for the dentist to consider in his diagnosis and treatment planning. These include balanced occlusion, working-side occlusion, and cuspid-protected occlusion. Any one of these occlusal function patterns may be bilateral or unilateral, and their recognition in a crown and bridge patient is vital to accurate treatment planning.

The proprioceptive mechanism of the stomatognathic system is still poorly understood, but several unique features of the mechanism have been described. There are few muscle spindles in the lateral pterygoids and anterior belly of the diagastric. There is, therefore, a deficiency of muscle spindles in the mandibular depressors, whereas the elevators are richly supplied with spindles. It has been shown, however, that the periodontal membranes of the teeth in animals are well innervated with directionally oriented proprioceptive endings. The attachment of the superior belly of the lateral pterygoid into the joint meniscus and the joint capsule are also richly supplied with Golgi tendon organs. It seems, therefore, that the very organs that must be protected from excessive forces of mandibular elevation are those that house the proprioceptive receptors required to trigger that protection.

SELECTED REFERENCES

1. Posselt, U.: Studies in the mobility of the human mandible, Acta Odont. Scand. **10**:10, 1952.
2. Posselt, U.: Range of movement of the mandible, J.A.D.A. **56**:10, 1958.
3. Beyron, H.: Occlusal relations and mastication in Australian aborigines, Acta Odont. Scand. **22**:597, 1964.
4. Kydd, W. L., and Sander, A.: A study of posterior mandibular movements from intercuspal occlusal position, J. Dent. Res. **40**:419, 1961.
5. Hodge, L. C., Jr.: A study of mandibular movement from centric occlusion to maximum intercuspation, master's thesis, Emory University School of Dentistry, Atlanta, Ga., 1965.
6. Ramfjord, S. P.: Dysfunctional temporomandibular joint and muscle pain, J. Prosthet. Dent. **11**:353, 1961.
7. Cobin, H. P.: The temporomandibular syndrome and centric relation, N.Y. Dent. J. **18**: 393, 1952.
8. Kyes, F. M.: Temporomandibular joint disorders, J.A.D.A. **59**:1137, 1959.
9. Shohet, H.: The treatment of ear, facial, head and other pains associated with pathologic temporomandibular joint, J. Prosthet. Dent. **9**:80, 1959.
10. Hodge, L. C., and Mahan, P. E.: A study of mandibular movement from centric occlusion to maximum intercuspation, J. Prosthet. Dent. **18**:19, 1967.
11. Kabcenell, J. L.: Effect of clinical procedures on mandibular position, J. Prosthet. Dent. **14**:266, 1964.
12. Graf, H., and Zander, H. A.: Tooth contact patterns in mastication, J. Prosthet. Dent. **13**:1055, 1963.
13. Moore, E. E.: Movies and slides demonstrating the chewing of various foods with and without deflective occlusal contacts: chewing and centric—clinical lecture, A.D.A. Annual Session, Dallas, Texas, 1966.
14. Ingervall, B.: Retruded contact position of mandible, a comparison between children and adults, Odontol. Revy **15**:130, 1964.
15. Ingervall, B.: Retruded contact position of mandible in the deciduous dentition, Odontol. Revy **15**:414, 1964.

16. Bennett, N. G.: A contribution to the study of the movements of the mandible, Proc. Roy. Soc. Med. **I**:79, 1908.
17. Nevakari, K.: An analysis of the mandibular movement from rest to occlusal position, Acta Odont. Scand. Suppl. 19, 1956.
18. Garnick, J., and Ramfjord, S. P.: Rest position: an electromyographic and clinical investigation, J. Prosthet. Dent. **12**:895, 1962.
19. Preiskel, H. W.: Some observations on the postural position of the mandible, J. Prosthet. Dent. **15**:625, 1965.
20. Ingervall, B.: Relation between retruded contact, intercuspal, and rest positions of mandible in children with angle class II, division 1 malocclusion, Odontol. Revy **17**:28, 1966.
21. Young, P.: A cephalometric study of the effect of acrylic test palatal piece thickness on the physiologic rest position, J. Philipp. Dent. Assoc. **19**:5, 1966.
22. Vaughn, H. C.: The external pterygoid mechanism, J. Prosthet. Dent. **5**:80, 1955.
23. Moulton, G. H.: Centric occlusion and the freeway space, J. Prosthet. Dent. **7**:209, 1957.
24. Posselt, U.: Physiology of occlusion and rehabilitation, Philadelphia, 1962, F. A. Davis Co.
25. Zola, A.: Morphologic limiting factors in the temporomandibular joint, J. Prosthet. Dent. **13**:732, 1963.
26. McCollum, B. B., and Stuart, C. E.: A research report, South Pasadena, Calif., 1955, Scientific Press.
27. Moulton, G. H.: The importance of centric occlusion in diagnosis and treatment planning, J. Prosthet. Dent. **10**:921, 1960.
28. Beck, H. O.: Clinical evaluation of the arcon concept of articulation, J. Prosthet. Dent. **9**:409, 1959.
29. Schallhorn, R. G.: A study of the arbitrary center of the kinematic center of rotation for face-bow mountings, J. Prosthet. Dent. **7**:162, 1957.
30. Fox, S. S.: The significance of errors in hinge axis location, J.A.D.A. **74**:1268, 1967.
31. Weinberg, L. A.: A cinematic study of centric and eccentric occlusions, J. Prosthet. Dent. **14**:290, 1964.
32. Conant, J. R.: Sound transmission used for studying masticatory force distribution patterns, J. Periodont. **33**:322, 1962.
33. Schuyler, C. H.: Factors contributing to traumatic occlusion, J. Prosthet. Dent. **11**:708, 1961.
34. Jarabak, J. R.: An electromyographic analysis of muscular and temporomandibular joint disturbances due to imbalances in occlusion, Angle Orthodont. **26**:170, 1956.
35. D'Amico, A.: Canine teeth—normal functional relation of the natural teeth of man, S. Calif. Dent. Assoc. J. **26**:6, 1958.
36. Jerge, C. R.: Organization and function of the trigeminal mesencephalic nucleus, J. Neurophysiol. **26**:379, 1963.
37. Kizior, J. E., Cuozzo, J. W., and Bowman, D. C.: Functional and histologic assessment of the sensory innervation of the periodontal ligament of the cat, J. Dent. Res. **47**:59, 1968.
38. Stuart, C. E., and Stallard, H.: Diagnosis and treatment of occlusal relations of the teeth, Texas Dent. J. **75**:430, 1957.
39. Isaacson, D.: A clinical study of the Bennett movement, J. Prosthet. Dent. **8**:641, 1958.
40. Aull, A. E.: Condylar determinants of occlusal patterns, J. Prosthet. Dent. **15**:826, 1965.
41. Matthews, P. B. C.: Muscle spindles and their motor control, Physiol. Rev. **44**:219, 1964.
42. Matthews, B. H. C.: Nerve endings in mammalian muscle, J. Physiol. **78**:1, 1933.
43. Corbin, K. B.: Observations on the peripheral distribution of fibers arising in the mesencephalic nucleus of the fifth cranial nerve, J. Comp. Neurol. **73**:153, 1940.
44. Corbin, K. B., and Harrison, F.: Function of mesencephalic root of fifth cranial nerve, J. Neurophysiol. **3**:423, 1940.
45. Gill, H. I.: Neuromuscular spindles in human lateral pterygoid muscles, J. Anat. **109**:157, 1971.
46. Karlsen, K.: The location of motor end plates and the distribution and histological structure of muscle spindles in jaw muscles of the rat, Acta Odont. Scand. **23**:521, 1965.
47. Kawamura, Y., Funakoshi, M., and Takata, M.: Reciprocal relationships in the brain-stem among afferent impulses from each jaw muscle on the cat, Jap. J. Physiol. **10**:585, 1960.
48. Thilander, B.: Innervation of the temporomandibular joint capsule in man, Trans. Roy. Schools Dent. Stockh. Umea, pp. 9-67, no. 7, 1961.
49. Griffin, C. J.: Inhibition of the linguo-mandibular reflex, part I: Golgi type organs of the pes menisci, Aust. Dent. J. **10**:376, 1965.
50. Leff, A.: Gnathodynamics of four mandibular positions, J. Prosthet. Dent. **16**:844, 1966.

GENERAL REFERENCES

Awazawa, Y.: Electron microscope investigation of the dentin with particular regard to the nature of the area surrounding the odontoblast process, J. Nihon Univ. School Dent. **5**:31, 1962.

Barber, D., and Massler, M.: Permeability of active and arrested carious lesions to dyes and radioactive isotopes, J. Dent. Child. **31**:26-33, 1964.

Beveridge, E. E., and Brown, A. C.: The measurement of human dental intrapulpal pressure and its response to clinical variables, J. Oral Surg. **19**:655, 1965.

Björn, H.: Periodontal viewpoints on crown and

bridge prosthodontics, Sverige Tandlakarforb. Tidn. **58**(12):497-504, 1966.

Bulow, F.: Histochemical and electronmicroscopical aspects of human buccal mucosa, Acta Pathol. Microbiol. Scand. **66**:409-425, 1966.

Croft, L., and Stanley, H. R.: The effect of a chilled water spray on the human pulp during cavity preparation, Oral Surg. **22**:66-71, 1966.

Diamond, R. D., Stanley, H. R., and Swerdlow, H.: Reparative dentin formation resulting from cavity preparation, J. Prosthet. Dent. **16**:1127-1134, 1966.

Eidelman, E., Finn, S. B., and Koulourides, T.: Remineralization of carious dentin treated with calcium hydroxide, J. Dent. Child. **32**:218-225, 1965.

Frank, R. M.: The ultrastructure of the tooth from the point of view of mineralization, demineralization and remineralization, Int. Dent. J. **17**(4):661, 1967.

Held-Wydler, E.: Natural (indirect) pulp capping, J. Dent. Child. **31**:107, 1964.

Henry, P. J., and Mitchel, D. F.: Tissue changes beneath fixed partial dentures, J. Prosthet. Dent. **16**:937-947, 1966.

Jacobs, R. M.: Effect of the mechanism of muscle tonus on mandibular rest position, J. Can. Dent. Assoc. **32**(10):594-598, 1966.

Kawamura, Y., and Majima, T.: Temporomandibular joint's sensory mechanisms controlling activities of jaw muscles, J. Dent. Res. **43**:150, 1964.

Koulourides, T., Cueto, H., and Pigman, W.: Rehardening of softened enamel surfaces of teeth by solutions of calcium phosphates, Nature **189**:226-227, 1961.

Koulourides, T., Feagin, F., and Pigman, W.: Remineralization of dental enamel by saliva in vitro, Ann N.Y. Acad. Sci. **131**(2):685-730, 1965.

Krysiński, Z.: [Individual variability of mastication efficiency], Czas Stomat. **20**(3):299-306, 1967.

Lindén, L., and Brännström, M.: Fluid movements in dentine and pulp, Odontol. Revy **18**:227, 1967.

Löe, H.: Reactions of marginal periodontal tissues to restorative procedures, Int. Dent. J. **18**(4):759, 1968.

Luostarinen, V., and Scheinin, A.: Dynamics of repair in the pulp, Acta Physiol. Scand. **68**:126, 1966.

Marcum, J. S.: The tissue response to different crown marginal depths, J. Kentucky Dent. Assoc. **20**:21-28, 1968.

Mjör, I. A.: Histologic studies of human coronal dentine following the insertion of various materials in experimentally prepared cavities, Arch. Oral Biol. **12**:441, 1967.

Nyborg, H.: Healing processes in the pulp on capping: a morphologic study, Acta Odont. Scand. **13**:9-130, 1955.

Skinner, C. N.: Physiology of the occlusal coordination of natural teeth, complete dentures, and partial dentures, J. Prosthet. Dent. **17**(6):559-565, 1967.

Stanley, H. R., and Swerdlow, H.: An approach to biologic variation in human pulpal studies, J. Prosthet. Dent. **14**:365-371, 1964.

Storey, A. T.: Sensory functions of the temporomandibular joint, J. Can. Dent. Assoc. **34**(6):294-300, 1968.

Van Huysen, G.: The microstructure of normal and sclerosed dentine, J. Prosthet. Dent. **10**:976, 1960.

Weiss, M. B.: Histological effects of silver nitrate on adult pulps, J. Indiana Dent. Assoc. **39**:294-299, 1960.

Wooten, J. W.: Physiology of the temporomandibular joint, Oral Surg. **21**:543-553, 1966.

17

Vertical dimension and masticatory muscle therapy

August J. Kaleta

Problems of facial pain, muscle imbalance, and jaw dysfunction, although treated empirically, may not be resolved satisfactorily without consideration of the underlying neuromuscular function. In many instances, a clinician must make certain diagnostic evaluations that drastically influence his judgment as to what therapeutic procedures may be indicated commensurate with the physiologic profile of a given patient. Although far from complete, basic research has provided a wealth of biologic data that has given the clinician a better understanding of the etiology and the efficacy of certain therapeutic procedures. As the philosopher Frederick Jensen has stated: "What we think we know today shatters the errors and blunders of yesterday and is disregarded tomorrow as worthless. So we go from larger mistakes to smaller mistakes so long as we do not lose courage. This is true of all therapy; no method is final."[1]

The remarks presented on specific neuromuscular activity within the oral apparatus are by no means intended to compete with the basic texts in physiology or neurology. My purpose is to examine some of the current literature pertinent to certain clinical problems and to stimulate future investigation into the subject matter.

VERTICAL DIMENSION

Vertical dimension is a rather abstract clinical concept intended to be used as an index to anterior face height. The term, itself, has been commonly defined as a measurement of the face taken between two arbitrarily selected points (such as the chin and base of the nose) conveniently located above and below the mouth, usually in the midline. Normally, reference marks are placed on the skin surface, but if lateral cephalometric radiographs are used, orthodontic landmarks such as the nasion and gnathion can be identified (Fig. 17-1). The cephalometric technique is an excellent method if comparisons or serial studies are to be made.

The topic of vertical dimension has been the subject of considerable controversy. At first, teeth were given sole credit for establishing the final vertical dimension of the face. It was believed that the gum pads were in approximation at birth and that, as the teeth erupted, the maxilla and mandible were forced apart with a corresponding increase in face height.[2,3]

Brodie[4] was able to demonstrate that at birth the jaws were found to be separated by the tongue, which occupied the entire mouth cavity and extended over the ridges lending support to the lips and

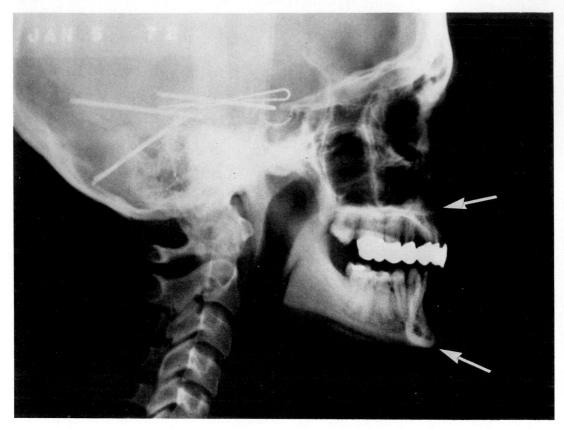

Fig. 17-1. Lateral cephalometric radiograph. *Arrows,* Reference points (nasion and gnathion) used in measurement of vertical dimension.

cheeks. With eruption of the dentition and growth of the jaws, the tongue, maturing at a slower rate, was gradually enclosed by the alveolar processes and the teeth. At no time were these teeth in continuous contact.

Thompson[3] resolved much disagreement when he recognized that there were two separate and distinct measurements possible to evaluate face height, one with the teeth in occlusion (occlusal vertical dimension) and the second with the mandible in its passive postural position (rest vertical dimension). A third quantity, the interocclusal distance (free-way space), represents the gap present between the upper and lower dental arches when the mandible is in its passive postural, or rest, position.

From a developmental standpoint, a distinction should also be made between anterior and posterior face height. Anterior morphologic face height is dependent on the height of the anterior portions of the maxilla and mandible; the length, inclinations, and degree of eruption of the anterior teeth; and the amount of horizontal and vertical overlap present in the incisors. Posterior morphologic face height is dependent on the height of the maxilla, the depth and position of the glenoid fossae relative to the maxillae, the length of the ramus and the condyloid process of the mandible, the degree of

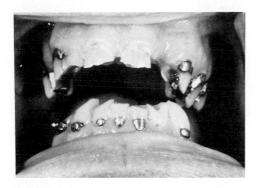

Fig. 17-2. Severe coronal destruction resulting in loss of occlusal vertical dimension. (From Malone, W. F., editor: Electrosurgery in dentistry, American Lecture Series, Springfield, Ill., 1974, Charles C Thomas, Publisher.)

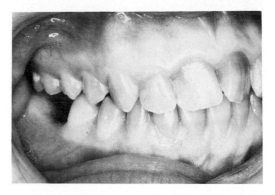

Fig. 17-3. Bite collapse caused by loss of mandibular posterior teeth resulting in decreased occlusal vertical dimension.

eruption of the posterior teeth, and the magnitude of the gonial angle.[5-7]

Occlusal vertical dimension

The magnitude of the occlusal vertical dimension depends on the disposition of bones, teeth, and skeletal muscle. In view of the labile nature of bone, the role of the masticatory muscles in the development of the facial skeleton warrants consideration. It is generally accepted that the form of certain skeletal parts depends, to a significant degree, on the activity of its attached musculature.[9] For example, experimental evidence indicates a definite relationship exists between the development of the temporalis muscle and the ensuing form of the coronoid process. Thus extrinsic muscular factors may serve to augment or perhaps even supersede any intrinsic or genetic factors within the bone itself.[10] Moss[11] associates these extrinsic factors with "functional matrices" in growth determination. Tension that is developed on bone by muscle contraction can be associated with normal cortical recession (involving surface resorption) as well as with outward bone deposition.[12]

The three factors bone, teeth and muscle combine to establish a stable occlusal vertical dimension after the natural growth periods.[13,14] There is cephalometric evidence to indicate, however, that in certain instances there may be a slight increase in morphologic face height during adult life.[15]

The occlusal vertical dimension exists as a functional entity and is amenable to local changes. The measurement can decrease in quantity because of wear or abrasion of the teeth (as in extended bruxism), loss or collapse of the posterior dentition (Figs. 17-2 and 17-3), or inadequately fabricated prostheses. A reduced or inadequate vertical dimension can also exist as an inborn hereditary quality, or it can be associated with lack of growth or an oral habit.[16] Some of the most perplexing problems a restorative dentist is called upon to treat involve adult patients with a class II orthodontic relation possessing an excessive vertical overlap of the anterior teeth. Clinical symptoms associated with this condition include pain, tinnitus, clicking in the temporomandibular joints, tension and fatigue in the facial and masticatory musculature, labial migration of the upper incisors, disruption of normal phonetic patterns, and impingement of the lower incisors on the palatal tissue. In many instances, restorative measures can only be instituted after

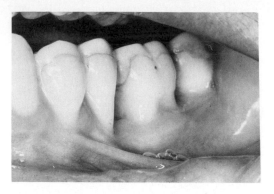

Fig. 17-4. Use of temporary acrylic overlays to restore occlusal vertical dimension and establish satisfactory occlusal plane.

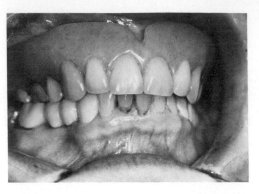

Fig. 17-5. Heat-cured acrylic temporary bridges used to maintain predetermined occlusal vertical dimension and establish posterior arch support.

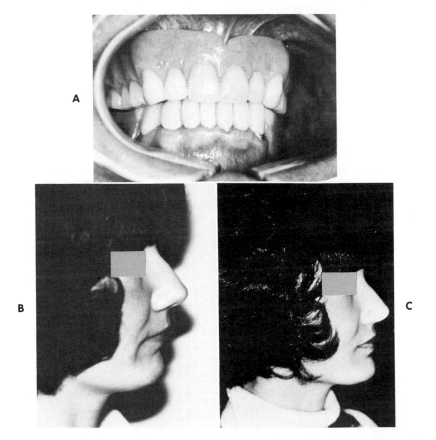

Fig. 17-6. **A,** Transitional partial denture and temporary occlusal splint for patient in Fig. 17-2. Prostheses can be altered until satisfactory occlusal vertical dimension can be established. **B,** Preoperative profile of young adult prior to bite-plane therapy and general prosthodontic dentistry. **C,** Postoperative picture of patient in **B.** Reduced interocclusal relationship is a critical step that must be programmed over a definite period of time. (**A,** From Malone, W. F., editor: Electrosurgery in dentistry, American Lecture Series, Springfield, Ill., 1974, Charles C Thomas, Publisher.)

orthodontic or oral surgical procedures have established a new occlusal relation. Any attempts to increase or reestablish lost occlusal vertical dimension must be exercised with utmost care. Factors taken into account include the patient's age, general health, emotional stability, and condition of the periodontal supporting tissues. Success or failure will often depend on the magnitude of the interocclusal distance. Encroachment or obliteration of the freeway space can place excessive stress on the periodontal tissues and the masticatory musculature, leading to painful, inflamed muscle tissue or acute muscle spasm.

When restorative procedures alone are used in establishing a new occlusal vertical dimension, the use of a temporary prosthesis is most beneficial. Insertion of temporary acrylic crowns, bridges, overlays, or transitional partial dentures allows the dentist to establish a new vertical dimension that could theoretically be modified slightly according to the individual patient's needs (Figs. 17-4 and 17-5). The prosthesis can be worn for extended periods of time to ensure the patient's adaptability to the new vertical height while also providing an adequate functional occlusion (Fig. 17-6). On an experimental basis there is evidence to indicate that deliberate increases in the occlusal vertical dimension may be compensated for by a reorganization of the facial skeleton and its attached musculature. However, this adaptation to extrinsic change is more likely to occur during periods of *growth* rather than *in the mature adult.*[17]

Rest vertical dimension

The rest position of the mandible is usually described as a habitual postural position. The individual is in a comfortable, upright posture, and the condyles are in a neutral, unstrained relation in their respective fossae.[18] It seems paradoxical that rest position, a definite clinical concept, is defined in terms that are not readily subject to clinical observation. Muscle equilibrium or condylar position cannot be determined easily without the use of elaborate equipment. Perhaps a simpler, more practical definition would present rest position as a postural base, from which all masticatory, articulatory, and swallowing movements are initiated and to which the mandible unconsciously returns at the cessation of such activities.[19]

At any moment in time, mandibular posture is determined by the balance existing between the overall tension in the supramandibular musculature in relation to prevailing gravitational forces (Fig. 17-7). Certain investigators maintain that mandibular posture is determined solely by the counterbalanced elastic forces exerted by the masticatory and hyoid musculature on the mandible.[20,21] This hardly seems possible in view of the fact that the mandible falls open when subjects in the sitting position fall asleep or are sufficiently anesthetized. In addition to this, other observations have shown that the mandible falls backward in unconscious subjects in the supine position, that passive opening of the mouth occurs after administration of neuromuscular blocking agents, and that normal mandibular posture is not maintained in patients afflicted with bulbar poliomyelitis in whom the virus has affected the motoneurons of the trigeminal nerve located in the pons.[19] If muscle elasticity were the sole determining factor, mandibular posture would not be affected by varying neurologic activity.

Cephalometric and electromyographic studies have demonstrated conclusively that the rest vertical dimension is by no means immutable.[7,22] It varies with changes in head and neck posture, with phases of the respiratory cycle, with changes in emotional state, with age, and in the presence of pain or psychic tension.[15,23-26] It also changes because of

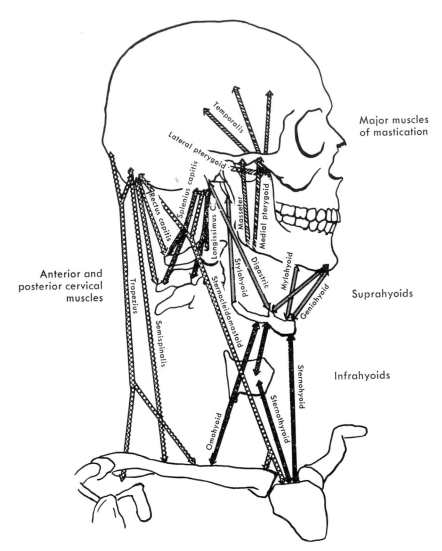

Fig. 17-7. Schematic representation of head and neck (stomatognathic) musculature. *Arrows,* Force vectors establishing craniomandibular balance.

pathologic disturbances such as chronic illness and senile debility.[28]

Since a direct relationship exists between mandibular posture and masticatory muscle activity, it would seem advisable to review some of the pertinent research regarding skeletal muscle.[29]

PROPERTIES OF MASTICATORY MUSCLE

Much of the early research regarding masticatory muscle was performed on cadaver material. Anthropometric methods were used to determine the extent of muscle portions, the direction of muscle resultants, and their moment arms projected in sagittal and transverse planes.[30] Investigators believed that once the origin and insertion of a muscle was known, as well as the fiber direction relative to the joint, the function could be established.[31-33] Unfortunately the fiber anatomy of the masticatory muscles is quite complex. Many are pennate or multipennate in arrangement, complicating fiber analysis. Indeed, the presence of a separate and distinct muscle, the zygomaticomandibularis, is still postulated to exist between the deepest layers of the masseter and the inferior lateral surface of the temporalis.[34,35] Individual fibers may insert into tendons or aponeuroses without extending the entire length of the muscle. Multibellied muscles may include more than one fiber direction.[36] At a given muscle length, certain fibers may be relaxed or even folded while other fibers are taut. The individual muscle may act as a synergist rather than as a single unit.[37] Finally, as muscle contraction produces movement of the mandible, the physiologic activity of the muscle changes as the movement continues.[38] There is electromyographic evidence to indicate that the lateral pterygoid muscle may in fact act as two separate and distinct muscles—one belly active during opening movements, the other during closing movements.[39,40] One therefore cannot speak of muscle fiber activity in the same absolute terms as might be used to describe force vectors.

Striated muscle force is length dependent. The length-tension curve illustrates that with increasing passive stretch of a muscle, increased resting tension is recorded. The total isometric tension consists of two parts—initial (resting) tension and active (developed) tension. Developed tension, produced by active contraction of myofibrils, rises to maximum at an optimal muscle length and then decreases with increasing length. Resting tension rises exponentially as the muscle is stretched. The resting tension at optimal length is usually quite small compared to the active tension.[41] The total magnitude of force production in the complex masticatory muscles will depend not only on the length of the individual fibers, but also on the orientation of fibers, lever arms, and inhibitory feedback from certain mechanoreceptors in the tendons and periodontal ligaments. A clinical measurement such as maximal bite force, then, is a complex function dependent on both anatomic and physiologic factors. This is reflected in the inconsistency of experimental measurements.[42]

Masticatory muscles in a variety of animal species, including man, have been analyzed histochemically.[43-46] Other biochemical and biomechanical studies have indicated the presence of at least three distinct fiber types.[47] Two types have relatively short twitch-contraction times (type FF—fast contracting, fast fatiguing; type FR—fast contracting, fatigue resistant). A third type (type S—slow contracting, fatigue resistant) is extremely resistant to fatigue, an important factor in postural muscles.[46] In these studies the presence of glycogen and adenosine triphosphatase activity is related to the velocity of contraction, whereas the level of oxidative enzymes is more closely related to resistance to fatigue.[48]

MUSCLE TONE AND MANDIBULAR POSTURE

Rest vertical dimension, as a variable quantity, is directly proportional to the total mass of the mandible and its attached soft tissue, relative to prevailing gravitational forces, and is inversely proportional to the aggregate tension (tone) present in the supramandibular musculature. The mass of the mandible can be decreased by extraction of teeth, resorption of basal or alveolar bone, and mandibular alveolectomies. The mass can be increased by bone deposition or insertion of restorative dental prostheses.

As with striated muscle elsewhere in the body, the amount of tension or tone in the masticatory muscles is a resultant of the elasticity provided by the connective tissue components (tendons, fasciae, intramuscular septa), by the contractile protein aggregates, and by the number, size, and frequency of firing of active motor units within specific muscles.[49-51] The motor nerve represents the final common path from the central nervous system. Once the motor unit is activated, membrane depolarization occurs and the ensuing muscle contraction initiates a change in length or an increase in tension within the muscle fibers.

The number of muscle fibers in a motor unit varies from muscle to muscle and within individual muscles. The number of striated muscle fibers that are found in a motor unit vary proportionately with the degree of control necessary in a movement. Experimental evidence indicates there are as few as five muscle fibers per unit in the rectus oculi externus, 100 to 300 fibers per unit in the intrinsic laryngeal muscles, and 600 to 900 fibers per unit in the masseter and the temporalis.[52,54] Although most of the motor units in both the suprahyoid and infrahyoid musculature are believed to be relatively

small, the major masticatory muscles appear to contain a mixture of large and small motor units. The small (phasic) motor units in both groups of muscles are employed mainly in the production of rapid mandibular movements associated with speech and mastication. The larger (tonic) motor units are used primarily in sustained biting and in postural regulation.[30,52]

Under normal circumstances the elastic properties of muscle are invariable. They provide a constant background of static (resting) tension between the origins and insertions. Muscle tone will vary then with changes in activity of the dynamic motor units. The activity is dependent on facilitatory or inhibitory impulses originating within the nervous system. The

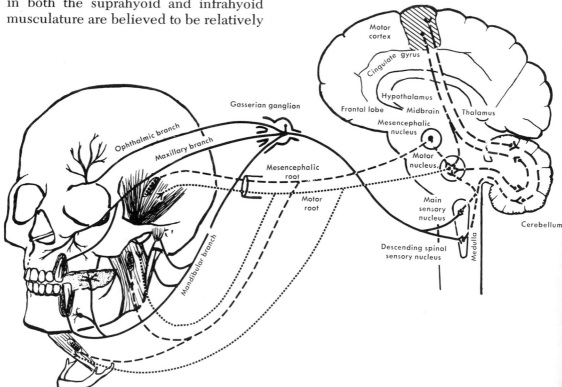

Fig. 17-8. Schematic representation of sensorimotor pathways involved in maintenance of muscle tone and mandibular posture in stomatognathic system.

neurologic influences are provided by both peripheral and central reflex systems[19] (Fig. 17-8).

Peripheral postural reflex systems

Two peripheral control systems are of major importance in maintaining mandibular posture. They include the myotatic reflex, originating from the muscle spindles, and the articular reflexes, originating from the temporomandibular joint mechanoreceptors.

The presence of spindles within the masseter, temporalis, and medial pterygoid has been observed by a number of investigators.[54-56] Freimann[56] notes that there are 160, 217, and 155 spindles located within these respective muscles in man. Karlsen[57] has described the location of spindles within the central portion of the muscle, with the origin and insertion areas being devoid. The presence of

muscle spindles within the lateral pterygoid had long been a debatable point. However, they have now been described in the lateral pterygoid of man, the miniature swine, and the monkey.[57-59]

The muscle spindle has long been regarded as a primary regulator of postural muscle activity. The myotatic postural reflex is provided mainly by afferent discharges from the primary (annulospiral) and secondary (flower-spray) receptor endings related to the nuclear bag and nuclear chain fibers within the spindles (Fig. 17-9). The nuclear bag fibers register instantaneous length and any change in length (phasic activity) occurring among the muscle fibers. The nuclear chain fibers appear to register primarily the instantaneous length (tonic activity) of the muscle. The contractile portions of both the nuclear bag and the nuclear chain fibers are innervated by gamma mo-

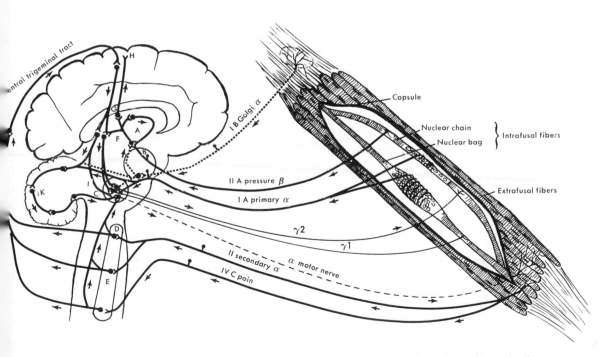

Fig. 17-9. Reflex pathways with specialized sensory nerve endings (muscle spindle apparatus, Golgi tendon organ, mechanoreceptors in muscle fasciae) located within masticatory skeletal muscle. Receptors facilitate or inhibit muscle contraction in effort to maintain physiologic homeostasis.

tor nerves. The nuclei for these fusimotor nerves are located within the trigeminal motor nucleus in the pons. The gamma motor nerves are responsible for regulating the sensitivity of the nuclear bag and chain fibers to stretch (gamma bias).[61] The afferent fibers from the spindle receptors turn rostrally in the mesencephalic tract to reach the main mesencephalic nucleus located within the midbrain. It is here that their cell bodies are located. Reflex collaterals then project caudally to the motor nucleus, relaying on the alpha motor nerves. The system is mainly monosynaptic and facilitatory to neurons innervating the mandibular elevator muscles and polysynaptic and inhibitory to those nerves innervating the mandibular depressors.[62]

With the mandible at rest, the frequency of tonic afferent discharges from the muscle spindles depends upon the degree of passive stretch applied to the muscles by gravitational force acting on the mandible, and upon activity of the static fusimotor neurons that innervate the nuclear-chain intrafusal fibers within the spindles.[19]

Articular postural reflex effects are exerted by afferent discharges from mechanoreceptors within the temporomandibular joint capsule. Low-threshold, slowly adapting (type 1) mechanoreceptors are distributed throughout the fibrous cap-

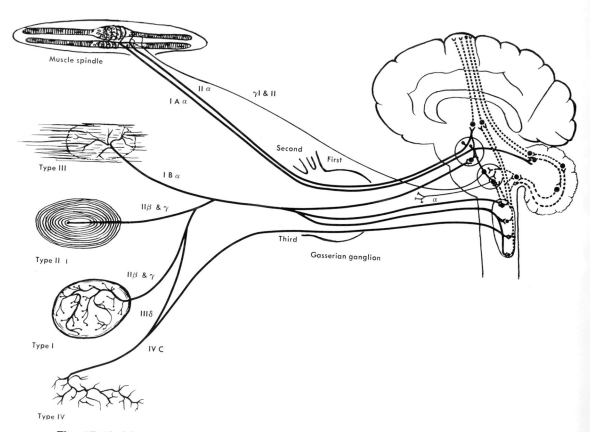

Fig. 17-10. Muscle spindle apparatus and mechanoreceptors located within temporomandibular joint capsules modify muscle tonicity and provide constant proprioceptive feedback.

sule.[64] The threshold of some of these mechanoreceptors is so low that they are continuously stimulated by mechanical stress to parts of the joint capsule even when the mandible is at rest. Like the gravitational stretch applied to the mandibular muscles, this articular stress is also related to head posture and mandibular mass.

The afferent discharges from these mechanoreceptors are transmitted via the articular branches (auriculotemporal, posterior deep temporal, masseteric) of the trigeminal system to the sensory nuclei in the pons and medulla (Fig. 17-10). From here they are relayed to the motoneuron pools of the mandibular musculature.[63] Data accumulated from the study of the reflex systems of other joints suggest that articular mechanoreceptor afferent fibers generally synapse on fusimotor rather than on alpha motoneurons.[65,66]

The present understanding is that low-grade postural motor unit activity encountered in the supramandibular muscles is continually modulated by the interaction (within the motoneuron pools of the individual muscles) of the reflex inputs from the type 1 articular mechanoreceptors with the myotatic reflex system operated through the muscle spindles, against the background influence of a variety of central reflex systems.[19]

Central postural reflex systems

Although the scope of this chapter does not permit a detailed discussion, mention should be made of the central facilitatory and inhibitory control systems that modulate the afferent impulses originating in the specialized sensory nerve endings located within the muscles, joints, ligaments, mucosa, and periodontium of the masticatory apparatus. The central control systems coordinate activity occurring in the mesencephalic, the main sensory, the descending spinal sensory, and the motor nuclei of the trigeminal system maintaining physiologic homeostasis.

The constant sensory input is continually discriminated or modulated by the vestibular, cerebellar, and cervicoarticular projection systems, by the brainstem reticular formation, and by corticobulbar tracts originating in the cerebral cortex.

These projection systems provide the means of effecting voluntary and involuntary phasic changes in mandibualr posture, plus they contribute to the tonic reflex facilitation and inhibition of both the alpha and gamma mandibular motoneurons.[67]

MUSCLE DYSFUNCTION

Trauma, parafunctional habits such as bruxism and tooth-clenching, and occlusal irregularities, if they occur outside the range of normal adaptation of the masticatory apparatus, can lead to pathologic changes within the oral musculature. These changes can range anywhere from localized muscle soreness (myositis) to an acute muscle spasm. Muscle spasm is normally attributed to isolated contraction of certain motor units in response to excessive stimuli from the central nervous system or to an accumulation of abnormal metabolic end-products within the muscle tissue. Electromyographic studies indicate that any local irritating factor or metabolic abnormality of a muscle, such as severe cold, lack of blood flow to the myofibers, or overexertion of an inflamed muscle can elicit pain and other types of sensory impulses that are transmitted from local receptors to the spinal cord, causing reflex muscle contraction. The contraction in turn restimulates the same sensory receptors to increase the intensity of afferent impulses and the subsequent reflex contractions. A positive-feedback system leading to an acute muscle spasm may occur.[68]

Development of spasm in one or more of the masticatory muscles can be attributed to fatigue, overcontraction, or overextension. The spasm itself can lead to symptoms of pain (diffuse, localized, or referred), limitation of mandibular movement, and changes in mandibular position resulting in an apparent functional malocclusion. If the spasm persists and the abnormal jaw relation continues, the teeth may gradually shift to accommodate the new position. Degenerative changes may occur in the temporomandibular joint (arthritis) or in the muscles themselves (contracture). The condition becomes self-perpetuating if the organic changes result in an altered chewing pattern that continually reinforces the original spasm and its concomitant pain.[69]

The key to successful clinical management of muscle dysfunction rests in the correct diagnosis of the primary etiologic factors. In this regard, special emphasis must be placed on the clinical history, occlusal analysis, palpation of the cervical and masticatory musculature, identification of abnormal habits affecting mandibular movements, radiographic examination, and evaluation of psychic or emotional difficulties.

MASTICATORY MUSCLE THERAPY

Clinical treatment of mandibular dysfunction attributable to muscle spasm is directed at the relief of acute pain and the restoration of normal muscle length. The most commonly advocated procedures involve use of occlusal bite plates or splints, intramuscular injections of local anesthetics, drug therapy including tranquilizers or muscle relaxants, external massage, heat or diathermy, psychotherapy, periodontal therapy, occlusal equilibration, or occlusal reconstruction.

At times normal muscle-reflex activity can bring about resolution of an acute spasm. In this regard, reciprocal inhibition of a muscle can sometimes completely relieve a spasm or cramp. If the patient will purposefully contract the antagonistic muscles, the reflex inhibition of the agonist muscles may restore normal tone. In an opposite manner, forced contraction of a spasmodic muscle may cause

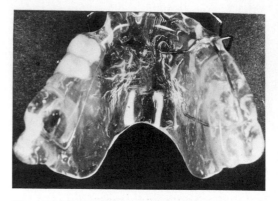

Fig. 17-11. Modified Hawley appliance designed to function as occlusal bite plate providing simultaneous occlusal contact of all posterior teeth. Insertion of plastic teeth in edentulous area can temporarily enhance esthetics.

autogenic inhibition to occur if the Golgi tendon organs are sufficiently stimulated.[70]

Bite plates or occlusal splints are of great value in the treatment of functional muscle disorders. A bite plate eliminates the disturbing effects of occlusal interferences in centric or eccentric jaw excursions. A modified Hawley retainer or Sved appliance can prevent contact of the posterior teeth and still allow functional jaw movements (Fig. 17-11). An acrylic table built up behind the maxillary anterior teeth serves as a stop for the lower incisors. Since it may allow extrusion of the posterior teeth, this type of appliance should not be worn longer than 3 to 6 weeks. If a prolonged period of disengagement is necessary, the use of an occlusal splint is preferred. The splint covers the occlusal surfaces of all the teeth, preventing any untoward movement (Fig. 17-12). The splint should be unobtrusive and comfortable to wear. It should also allow for simultaneous contact of all the opposing teeth.

If effective, muscle hypertonicity and pain will usually disappear within a few weeks. After the elimination of pain, the patient should be instructed to wear the

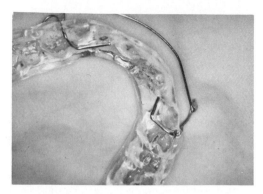

Fig. 17-12. Heat-cured acrylic bite plate. Complete coverage of occlusal and incisal surfaces will prevent further coronal destruction.

bite plate or splint only during those intervals when clenching or grinding is most likely to occur.[71]

For acute muscle spasms the use of ethyl chloride spray may be helpful. The painful area is isolated and the direction in which motion is impaired, registered. Ethyl chloride is then sprayed on the overlying skin. The spray acts as a counterirritant, masking the primary discomfort. The head or mandible is then moved toward the painful site. As movement continues, painful sites in other oral or cervical muscles may be localized. These are then sprayed and the muscle excursions continued. Passive stretching is quite beneficial in restoring normal muscle length.

If this procedure is ineffective, myofacial trigger areas, if present, can be isolated and injected with 1 to 2 ml of lidocaine without vasoconstrictor. The injection is made intraorally or extraorally, whichever is more convenient. During treatment, range-of-motion muscle exercises within painless limits are again instituted. Although these methods may produce only transient symptomatic relief, they have a definite diagnostic value. In addition, when jaw opening is severely limited by myospasm, anesthetic blocking may allow enough man-

dibular movement for impressions to be taken and an occlusal splint fabricated.

Barbiturates, tranquilizers, and muscle relaxants have all been advocated for the treatment of functional muscle disorders. These drugs may provide temporary relief of acute symptoms and a general decrease in muscle tone, a useful adjunct to supportive occlusal therapy. Controlled pharmacologic and clinical studies of these drugs have failed to demonstrate any direct effect on peripheral myospasm when given orally.[71] The drugs appear to be more effective in alleviating symptoms of neurotic tension and anxiety.

External massage and heat and cold therapy are important adjuncts in the treatment of myofacial pain and muscle spasm. Their major purpose is to restore circulation and remove toxic products from the affected muscle tissue. Limitation of jaw motion resulting from any shortening of the masticatory musculature can also be treated by ultrasonic therapy to increase extensibility. Such therapy permits subsequent range-of-motion exercises to restore normal mandibular function.

Treatment of masticatory muscle disorders should be directed toward the removal of any acute symptoms. This is imperative if the underlying primary cause is to be identified and isolated. It is only after this has been accomplished that any irreversible corrective procedures should be contemplated.

REFERENCES

1. Jensen, F.: In Graber, T. M.: Orthodontics: principles and practice, Philadelphia, 1972, W. B. Saunders Co.
2. Thompson, J. R.: The constancy of the position of the mandible and its influence on prosthetic restorations, Illinois Dent. J. **12:**242-247, 1943.
3. Thompson, J. R.: The rest position of the mandible and its significance to dental science, J A.D.A. **33:**151-180, 1946.
4. Brodie, A. G.: On the growth pattern of the human head from the third month to the eighth year of life, Am. J. Anat. **68:**209-261, 1941.
5. Atwood, D. A.: A cephalometric study of the

clinical rest position of the mandible. Part 1: The variability of the clinical rest position following the removal of occlusal contacts, J. Prosthet. Dent. **6**:504-519, 1956.

6. Atwood, D. A.: The variability in the rate of bone loss following the removal of occlusal contacts, J. Prosthet. Dent. **7**:544-552, 1957.

7. Atwood, D. A.: Clinical factors related to variability of the clinical rest position following the removal of occlusal contacts, J. Prosthet. Dent. **8**:698-708, 1958.

8. Atwood, D. A.: A review of the fundamentals on rest position and vertical dimension, Int. Dent. J. **9**:6-19, 1959.

9. Avis, V.: The relation of the temporal muscle to the form of the coronoid process, Am. J. Phys. Anthropol. **17**:99-104, 1959.

10. Felts, W. J.: Transplantation studies on skeletal organogenesis. I: The subcutaneously implanted long bone of the rat and mouse, Am. J. Phys. Anthropol. **17**:204-215, 1959.

11. Moss, M. L.: The primary role of functional matrices in facial growth, Am. J. Orthodont. **55**:566-567, 1969.

12. Hoyte, D. A., and Enlow, D. H.: Wolff's law and the problem of muscle attachment on resorptive surfaces of bone, Am. J. Phys. Anthropol. **24**:205-214, 1966.

13. Kaleta, A. J., Kruzan, W. C., and Grimm, A. F.: Masticatory muscle growth and adaptability: studies utilizing metallic implants, J. Dent. Res. **53**(suppl.):204, 1974 (abstract).

14. Kaleta, A. J., and Malone, W. F.: Masticatory muscle: a preview for the rationale of the centric closure position, Illinois Dent. J. **43**:83-97, 1974.

15. Tallgren, A.: Changes in adult face height due to aging, wear and loss of teeth and prosthetic treatment, Acta Odont. Scand. **15**(suppl. 24):1-122, 1957.

16. Lee, R. L., and Gregory, G. G.: Gaining vertical dimension for the deep bite restorative patient. In Lundeen, H. C., editor: Dent. Clin. North Am. **15**:743-763, 1971.

17. McNamara, J. A.: Neuromuscular and skeletal adaptations to altered orofacial function, doctoral thesis, University of Michigan, Ann Arbor, Michigan, 1972.

18. Academy of Denture Prosthetics: Glossary of prosthodontic terms, J. Prosthet. Dent. **10** (suppl.): Nov.-Dec. 1960.

19. Wyke, B. D.: Neuromuscular mechanisms influencing mandibular posture: a neurologist's review of current concepts, J. Dent. **2**(3):111-120, Feb. 1974.

20. Lynn, A. M., and Yemm, R.: External forces required to move the mandible of relaxed human subjects, Arch. Oral Biol. **16**:1443-1447, 1971.

21. Yemm, R., and Berry, D. C.: Passive control in mandibular rest position, J. Prosthet. Dent. **22**:30-36, 1969.

22. Garnick, J., and Ramfjord, S. P.: Rest position: an electromyographic and clinical investigation, J. Prosthet. Dent. **12**:895-911, 1962.

23. Fish, S. F.: Respiratory associations of the rest position of the mandible, Br. Dent. J. **116**:149-159, 1964.

24. Olsen, E. S.: Radiographic study of variation in the physiologic rest position of the mandible in seventy edentulous individuals, J. Dent. Res. **30**:517, 1951.

25. Preiskel, H. W.: Some observations on the postural position of the mandible, J. Prosthet. Dent. **15**:625-633, 1965.

26. Yemm, R.: A comparison of the electrical activity of masseter and temporal muscles of human subjects during experimental stress, Arch. Oral Biol. **16**:269-273, 1971.

27. Graber, T. M.: Orthodontics: principles and practice, Philadelphia, 1972, W. B. Saunders Co.

28. Sicher, H.: Positions and movements of the mandible, J.A.D.A. **48**:620-625, 1954.

29. Kaleta, A. J.: Histologic and radiographic studies on the masticatory musculature of the miniature pig, master's thesis, University of Illinois Medical Center, Chicago, 1974.

30. Carlsöö, S.: Nervous coordination and mechanical function of the mandibular elevators, Acta Odont. Scand. **10**(suppl. 11):9-126, 1952.

31. Lord, F. P.: Observations on the temporomandibular articulation, Anat. Rec. **7**:355-362, 1913.

32. Lord, F. P.: Movements of the jaw and how they are effected, Int. J. Orthodont. **23**:557-563, 1937.

33. Reigner, H.: Die Physiologie und Pathologie der Kieferbewegungen, Arch. Anat. Physiol. **23**:98-102, 1904.

34. Parsons, F. G.: The joints of mammals compared with those of man, J. Anat. Physiol. (Lond.) **34**:41-68, 1899.

35. Sicher, H., and DuBrul, E. L.: Oral anatomy, ed. 6, St. Louis, 1975, The C. V. Mosby Co.

36. Schuhmacher, G. H.: Funktionelle Morphologie der Kaumuskulatur, Jena, 1961, VEB Gustav Fischer Verlag.

37. Grant, P. G.: Biomechanical analysis of the masticatory apparatus of the rhesus macaque (primates: *Macaca mulatta*), master's thesis, University of California, Berkeley, Calif., 1973.

38. Hiiemae, K.: The structure and function of the jaw muscles in the rat (*Rattus norvegicus* L.), III. The mechanics of the muscles, Zool. J. Linn. Soc. **50**:111-132, 1971.

39. Grant, P. G.: Lateral pterygoid: two muscles? Am. J. Anat. **138**:1-10, 1973.

40. McNamara, J. A.: The independent functions of the two heads of the lateral pterygoid muscle, Am. J. Anat. **138**:197-206, 1973.

41. Ramsey, R. W., and Street, S. F.: The isometric length-tension diagram of isolated skeletal muscle fibers of the frog, J. Cell. Comp. Physiol. **15**:11-34, 1940.
42. Carlsson, G. E.: Bite force and chewing efficiency, Front. Oral Physiol. **1**:265-292, 1974.
43. Baker, G., and Laskin, D.: Histochemical characterization of the muscles of mastication, J. Dent. Res. **48**:97-104, 1969.
44. Masuda, K., Takahashi, S., and Kuriyama, J.: Studies on the fiber types of the guinea pig masticatory muscles, Comp. Biochem. Physiol. **47A**:1171-1184, 1974.
45. Ringquist, M.: Histochemical fiber types and fiber sizes in human masticatory muscles, Scand. J. Dent. Res. **79**:366-368, 1971.
46. Taylor, A., Cody, F. W., and Bosley, M. A.: Histochemical and mechanical properties of the jaw muscles of the cat, Exp. Neurol. **38**:99-109, 1973.
47. Henneman, E., and Olson, D. B.: Relations between structure and function in the design of skeletal muscles, J. Neurophysiol. **28**:581-598, 1965.
48. Burke, R. E., Levine, D. N., Tsairis, P., and Zajac, F. E.: Physiological types and histochemical profiles in motor units of the cat gastrocnemius, J. Physiol. **234**:723-748, 1973.
49. Basmajian, J. V.: Muscles alive: their functions revealed by electromyography, ed. 2, Baltimore, 1967, The Williams & Wilkins Co.
50. Basmajian, J. V.: Electromyography: its structural and neural basis, Int. Rev. Cytol. **21**:129-140, 1967.
51. Granit, R.: The basis of motor control, New York, 1970, Academic Press, Inc.
52. Carlsöö, S.: Motor units and action potentials in masticatory muscles, Acta Morphol. Neerl.-Scand. **2**:13-19, 1958.
53. Carlsöö, S.: An electromyographic study of the activity of certain suprahyoid muscles (mainly the anterior belly of the digastric muscle) and of the reciprocal innervation of the elevator and depressor musculature of the mandible, Acta Anat. **26**:81-93, 1956.
54. Faaborg, A.: Electromyographic investigation of intrinsic laryngeal muscles in humans, Acta Physiol. Scand. **41**(suppl.):140, 1957.
55. Barker, K.: The structure and distribution of muscle receptors. In Symposium on Muscle Receptors, Hong Kong, 1962, Hong Kong University Press.
56. Freimann, R.: Untersuchungen über Zahl und Anordnung der Muskelspindeln in den Kaumuskeln des Menschen, Anat. Anz. **100**:258-264, 1954.
57. Karlsen, K.: The location of motor end plates and the distribution and histological structure of muscle spindles in jaw muscles of the rat, Acta Odont. Scand. **23**:521-547, 1965.
58. Christensen, L. V.: Muscle spindles in the lateral pterygoid muscle of the miniature swine, Arch. Oral Biol. **12**:1203-1204, 1967.
59. Honée, G. L.: An investigation on the presence of muscle spindles in the human lateral pterygoid muscle, Nederl. T. Tandheelk. **73**:43-48, 1966.
60. Karlsen, K.: Muscle spindles in the lateral pterygoid muscle of the monkey *(Macacus irus)*, Arch. Oral Biol. **14**:1111-1112, 1969.
61. Mountcastle, V. B.: Medical physiology, ed. 13, St. Louis, 1974, The C. V. Mosby Co., vol. I.
62. Szentagothai, J.: Anatomical considerations of monosynaptic reflex arcs, J. Neurophysiol. **11**:445-461, 1948.
63. Thilander, B.: Innervation of the temporomandibular joint capsule in man, Trans. Roy Schools Dent. Stockh. Umea 2(7):1-67, 1961.
64. Kawamura, Y.: Recent concepts in the physiology of mastication. In Staple, P. H., editor: Advances in oral biology, New York, 1964, Academic Press, Inc., vol. I.
65. Freeman, M. A. R., and Wyke, B. D.: Articular reflexes at the ankle joint: an electromyographic study of normal and abnormal influences of ankle joint mechanoreceptors upon reflex activity in the leg muscles, Br. J. Surg. **54**:990-1001, 1967.
66. Larson, L. E., and Thilander, B.: Mandibular positioning: the effect of pressure on the joint capsule, Acta Neurol. Scand. **40**:131-143, 1964.
67. Evarts, E. V.: Relation of discharge frequency to conduction velocity in pyramidal tract neurons, J. Neurophysiol. **28**:216-228, 1965.
68. Guyton, A. C.: Textbook of medical physiology, ed. 4, Philadelphia, 1971, W. B. Saunders Co.
69. Laskin, D. M.: Etiology of the pain-dysfunction syndrome, J.A.D.A. **79**:147-153, 1969.
70. Schwartz, L.: Disorders of the TMJ, Philadelphia, 1959, W. B. Saunders Co.
71. Bell, W. H.: Non-surgical management of the pain dysfunction syndrome, J.A.D.A. **79**:161-170, 1969.

18

Occlusal and morphologic considerations in restorative dentistry

Raymond Henneman, David L. Koth, William F. P. Malone, Boleslaw Mazur, Richard N. Pipia, Hosea F. Sawyer, and Stanley D. Tylman

The science of occlusion has undergone an inordinate proliferation of academic information. A search for the "optimum" occlusal (Fig. 18-1) scheme in removable prosthodontics or "ideal" occlusal design for fixed restorations of the natural teeth has sponsored the initiation of concentrated research and longitudinal clinical evaluation studies.

The dentist who conscientiously attempts to keep abreast with this information is overwhelmed with the multiplicity of diverse therapeutic approaches. These conflicting theories of occlusal treatment have disconcerted many dentists.

Why the current emphasis on occlusal therapy? The high-velocity instrumentation and improved accuracy of impression materials have proceeded without the accompanying proportionate academic exposure to the basic principles of occlusion.[1] There is also the tendency of the patient to desire these refined dental procedures in a shorter period of time.

Primarily, classical texts in crown and bridge prosthodontics have been partially effective because of nonspecific discussions of occlusal anatomy of cast restorations and their effect upon supportive structures. Secondly, these texts also presented information concerning the determinants of occlusion, equilibration techniques, and occlusal morphology as if all patients possessed a skeletal neutro-

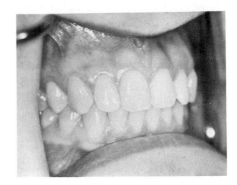

Fig. 18-1. Optimal arch position is conducive to a "normal" occlusal range.

occlusion. These concepts associated with a neutro-occlusion are merely guidelines.[2] When there are disparities in a maxillomandibular relationship, crossbites, and neglected dentitions with a myriad of sequelae, that is, periodontal problems, the dentist still encounters insurmountable restorative problems. However, it is still an undeniable fact that occlusion should be the cornerstone on which clinical dentistry is structured.

TREATMENT VERSUS THEORY

The dental practitioner is unimpressed with general statements, although true, that sound clinical practice is based upon a working knowledge of muscle physiology, anatomy, and supportive tissue pathology. A clinician considers these

420

generalities not applicable to his clinical profile. The rationale of sound treatment must be based upon "identifiable difficulties," that is, questionable abutment, for restorative dentistry. Limitations of treatment, despite the potential of the dentist's ability to restore every tooth in both arches, must be emphasized prior to treatment. Secondarily, the dentist should perform the least amount of dentistry required for a given patient. The primary object of restorative dentistry should be to prevent or intercept as many problems as possible.

There is no panacean approach to treatment that will reduce chair time and alleviate the painful process of deep intellectual activity. Hard-core literature research is a mandate to adequate treatment of the variety of patients the dentist will encounter.

The last two decades have seen many changes in our approach to restorative dentistry. Dentistry has rightfully emphasized comprehensive care for the individual patient rather than merely timely repair procedures. Conversely, mouth rehabilitation can be the restoration of the form and function of the masticatory apparatus to as nearly a normal condition as possible without extensive dentistry. Comprehensive patient care can be accomplished with conservative treatment in many cases. It is apparent that comprehensive total patient care is not synonymous with full mouth rehabilitation, complete crown coverage, or even replacement of all 28 teeth.

Techniques that emphasize one clinical approach for all patients will always appeal to the profession. Unfortunately, there are institutions and study groups that employ practices of this nature because of gifted clinicians who can perform clinical feats because of their innate ability to compensate for obvious deficiencies in one empirically designed therapeutic approach for all patients. It is even more ludicrous when all practi-

tioners with diverse backgrounds and abilities are expected to excel in extensive restorative dentistry with a solitary clinical approach. These introspect theories are appealing because of their oversimplification or singular approach to diverse problems.

DEVELOPMENT OF DENTITION

The human dental occlusion is a composite craniofacial growth, neuromuscular development, and maturation of the dentition. Occlusal function of the adult dentition formally begins as the 6-year molars erupt into contact and intercuspate. The occlusal surface relationship of the 6-year molars aids in the determination of the height of the face. As the anterior teeth erupt, centric closure forces develop. As the deciduous molars are exfoliated, the permanent premolars eventually erupt into occlusion (Fig. 18-2).

As the growth and development of the jaws continue, the mandibular molars tip forward, while the maxillary molar teeth grow downward and backward. The result produces an occlusal curve in the sagittal plane known as the curve of Spee (Fig. 18-3).

As the mandible moves in chewing, the mandibular buccal cusp tips contact the buccal cusps of the maxillary teeth caus-

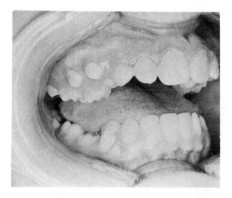

Fig. 18-2. Mixed dentition whose exfoliation schedule endangers a normal arch position for succedaneous teeth.

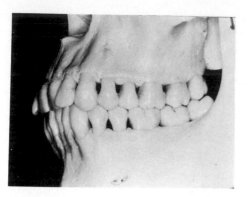

Fig. 18-3. Buccal view of class I malocclusion showing curve of Spee on mandibular arch.

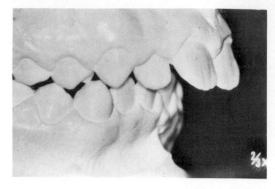

Fig. 18-5. Class II malocclusion relationship is better served with orthodontic treatment. Skeletal disparities, as shown, are an insurmountable restorative problem.

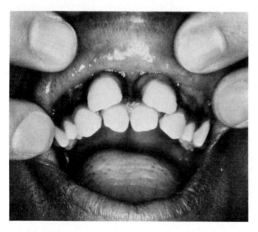

Fig. 18-4. Early diagnosis of insufficient arch length will aid orthodontic treatment and reduce incidence of difficult restorative cases.

ing a buccally inclined maxillary quadrant. The mandibular quadrant assumes a lingual inclination with the exception of the first premolars. This action produces a curve in the frontal plane (perpendicular to the curve of Spee) known as the curve of Wilson. Most of the growth and development takes place during the teen-age period. It is from the tenth year through the sixteenth year of life that occlusal problems should be recognized and reviewed for possible orthodontic and orthopedic treatment. Early recognition

of a disparity between maxillomandibular growth or deviation of the midline will ensure a greater measure of success of orthodontic treatment (Fig. 18-4).

Occlusion adapts and changes throughout the life of the patient. During the second and third decades of life, there is a decrease in both the overbite and overjet relationship of the anterior teeth because of a downward and forward positioning of the mandible.

With all the variables in growth from nutrition, heterogeneous genetic impact, and so forth, a review of the population obviously reveals occlusion exists in a variety of combinations and is as unique as the individual (Fig. 18-5).

MASTICATORY SYSTEM

The masticatory system consists of the dentition, the periodontal structures, supportive bone, the temporomandibular joints, neuromuscular system, the lip-cheek-tongue system, and salivary and vascular systems.

The functions of the masticatory system are the masticatory act, swallowing, and the production of speech sounds. Mastication is of prime importance and can be divided into three stages: incising, chewing, and deglutition.

Incising

During incision, the mandible moves in a protrusive or lateral protrusive position to permit the maxillary and mandibular anterior teeth to shear and penetrate food introduced into the mouth. At the completion of the incisive bite, the food rests on the tongue from where it is directed to the posterior teeth for further tearing and mulling.

Chewing

The chewing movement is multidirectional and cyclic in nature. Because of the rotary nature of the closing movements of the mandible, the interocclusal distance is larger in the anterior part of the mouth than in the posterior at any degree of mouth opening. This notable difference in interocclusal distance is in accordance with the functional demands in incisive chewing.

When the bulk of food has been cut off by incisors, it is torn and partly crushed in the premolar areas, where adequate space can be provided without excessive muscle distention while the mandible is being opened. After the initial chewing strokes have reduced the particle size of the bolus of food, trituration takes place in the molar regions where interocclusal distance remains minimal to conclude the usual chewing cycle.

Repeated efforts to reduce the size of the bolus of food is performed by this stomatognathic system. The minced food and saliva mixture is positioned on the occlusal tables of the lower posterior teeth after each stroke. It is hypothesized that response-related tooth contacts mediate appropriate muscles to contract by means of proprioceptors in the periodontal ligament. The chewing cycle ceases when the bolus of food reaches a consistency suitable for swallowing. There is a decided increase in the occlusal contact of the teeth during heavy mastication. Chewing is a complex neuromuscular activity and the interrelationship

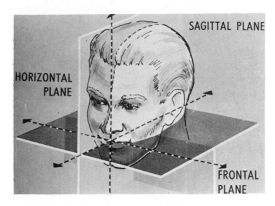

Fig. 18-6. Diagram of facial planes associated with gnathology. (From Guichet, N. F.: Principles of occlusion—a teaching manual, Anaheim, Calif., 1970, Denar Corp.)

between mastication and occlusion is critical.

Deglutition

Swallowing begins as a voluntary muscular act and is completed involuntarily. Several swallows are required to empty the mouth of a given food mass. When swallowing salivary secretions only, the mandible is braced in the intercuspal position to provide proper stabilization. Graphically, mastication can be represented in three planes: the sagittal, the horizontal, and the frontal planes (Fig. 18-6).

REVIEW: DENTAL MORPHOLOGY RELATED TO OCCLUSION

The importance of knowing the anatomic form of all individual permanent teeth and their function in the entire permanent dentition is as basic as learning the alphabet prior to written communication in sentence form.

Knowing the dimensions of each tooth and its height of contour cannot be overlooked or minimized. The mesiodistal dimension of each tooth establishes contact with the adjacent tooth and stabilizes the dental arch. The faciolingual

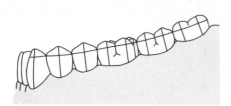

Fig. 18-7. Diagrammatic buccal view of mandibular arch showing curve from canine to terminal molar. This has been named "curve of Spee."

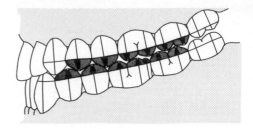

Fig. 18-8. Lateral (working position) excursion of mandible showing premolar and first molar contacts.

contours protect the supportive structures. Lastly, the functioning occlusals have specific contours needed in the preparation of food-particle size for digestion, and the lingual surfaces of the maxillary anteriors are functioning surfaces that play an important role in phonetics as well.

Function

The variable functions of different teeth are a means of dividing the human dentition into the following four classes:

Incisors—cut

Canines—tear or hold

Premolars—reduce particle size

Molars—mill or grind

Each class of teeth is more thoroughly understood in relation to its function by a prior study of its position in each arch. Secondly, the dynamics of both arches functioning together should be understood on the basis of their position and interdigitation according to their occlusal topography.

The functional surface of the mandible or lower arch of teeth is designed in a curvature, anteroposteriorly, commonly referred to as the curve of Spee (Fig. 18-7). The teeth also exhibit a curvature in a mediofacial manner (curve of Wilson), and the entire arch is curved from the distal of the right third molars to the distal of the left third molars, when viewed from the occluding surface (arch form).

The mandibular arch has reciprocating

curves to the maxillary arch, and they function together with efficiency (Fig. 18-8).

One may note that the functioning surface of the maxillary anteriors is the incisal and lingual surfaces as the mandibular teeth cut, moving their incisal surface against the maxillary antagonists. It is interesting to note that the power of the biting force can be or is near maximum as the incisals of both arches contact. This is the farthest point from the temporomandibular joint and considered to be the facial extremity of the arch.

In the maxillary arch, the force of bite is transferred from the facial border of anteriors to the lingual border of the functioning surface in posteriors, with the transition occurring in the premolar area.

In the mandibular arch, however, the force of bite remains in the facial border of the entire arch. Because of the angulated position of the teeth in a faciolingual plane, the forces brought to bear on the respective arches are better distributed along the axis of the teeth, taking full advantage of the radicular anchorage to the bone.[3]

Cusp position

In the construction or rebuilding of any occlusal or functional surface of a tooth or teeth, it is important to establish a satisfactory relationship of the elevations and depressions of each tooth with each other in function. The elevations (cusps) of the

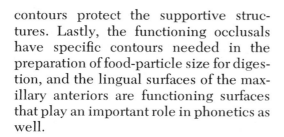

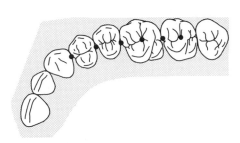

Fig. 18-9. Maxillary arch with illustration *(black circles)* of mandibular stamp-cusp contact in centric occlusal position (type cusp to embrasure).

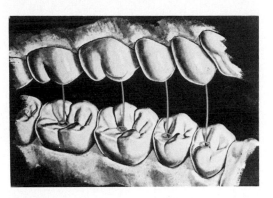

Fig. 18-10. Stamp-cusp placement of lingual cusps of maxillary arch as shown on occlusal table (central groove) of mandibular arch. (Courtesy Dr. Everett V. Payne, Beverly Hills, Calif.)

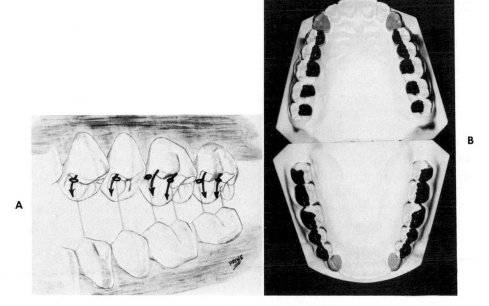

Fig. 18-11. A, Stamp-cusp placement of mandibular buccal cusp shown on maxillary arch. **B,** Diagram of maxillary and mandibular stamp cusps *(in dark)* with "broad areas" that are possible occlusal contact surfaces. *Light areas* on four canines are guarding inclines, and cusps *in white* are gliding or idling cusps. (**A,** Courtesy Dr. Everett V. Payne, Beverly Hills, Calif.)

maxillary arch and the cusps of the mandibular arch that stabilize the power of occlusion are known as stamp or support cusps. They are, as we saw previously, the lingual of the maxillary and the buccal

or facial of the mandibular teeth (Fig. 18-9).

The proper location of these stamp cusps may be seen in the diagram of a proximal view showing that the maxillary

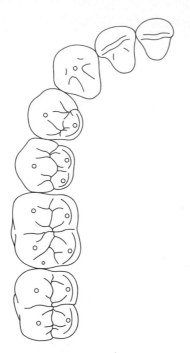

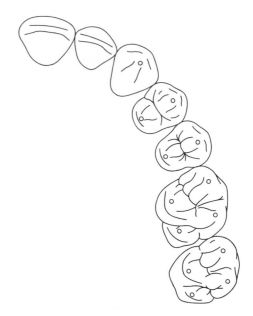

Fig. 18-12. Occlusal arch form of left mandibular quadrant. Circular areas represent placement of cusps: buccal cusps of mandibular arch are stamp cusps, and lingual cusps are called shearing or guiding cusps.

Fig. 18-13. Occlusal arch form of left maxillary quadrant. Circular areas represent placement of cusps: lingual cusps are stamp cusps on maxillary arch, and buccal cusps are shearing or guiding cusps.

is located in the lingual one third of the faciolingual dimension of the tooth, and the mandibular is in the buccal or facial one third. Each of these cuspal (stamp-cusp) elevations will rest in the depressions of its antagonists when the arches are in maximal closure. The location of each of these stamp cusps in a mesiodistal relation will be discussed as we review each of the types of teeth in anatomic detail (Figs. 18-10 and 18-11).

The remaining elevations, called the shearing or guiding cusps (lingual of mandibular and facial of maxillary), will also be located and their position discussed as the mandibular arch changes its position with the maxillary in function (Figs. 18-12 and 18-13).

The depressions in the occlusal topography of each posterior tooth varies and gives each tooth identifiable traits. The

depressions, called fossae, are the uniting of grooves that have the distinct variable properties of width, depth, and extent of curvature. The deepest depressions and culminations of the secondary grooves is known as the central groove. These depths are never contacted by the opposing cuspal elevations. Rather, the walls of these grooves—the triangular, marginal, and secondary ridges—are the holding contacts as the two arches come together in centric occlusion. This is commonly referred to as a fossa, or, in some instances, an embrasure. To obtain maximum stability in occlusion or maximal closure of the arches, it is important that the opposing classes of teeth have their respective stamp or support cusps exhibit some form of tripodism (Fig. 18-14).

Each quadrant in the entire dentition has four classes of teeth present. A de-

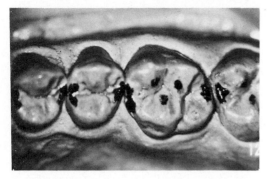

Fig. 18-14. Naturally occurring tripodization of maxillary first molar. This is a rare clinical observance.

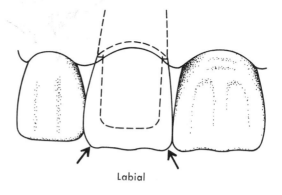

Labial

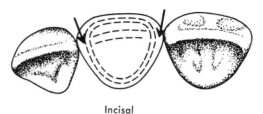

Incisal

Fig. 18-15. Maxillary right central incisor. *Arrows*, Exact positions of mesiolabioincisal and distolabioincisal point angles.

scription of each class and the types within each class as well as their relationship in centric occlusion are now briefly reviewed.

CLASSIFICATION OF TEETH
Incisors

There are eight incisors. Each arch contains four teeth of this class.

Each quadrant has two incisor types— central and lateral. Their names relate to their position to the midsagittal plane.

centrals
maxillary Widest and most prominent horizontal cutting blade and two vertical functional lingual cutting blades at the proximal borders (Fig. 18-15).

mandibular Smallest horizontal cutting blade working as the antagonist to the maxillary central incisor and functioning by cutting or incising food with the maxillary central incisor's horizontal and vertical cutting blades.

laterals
maxillary Smaller replica of the maxillary central incisor.

mandibular Equal in size or slightly larger than the mandibular central incisor; both function in the same manner as the central type of incisor.

Canines

There are four canines. Each arch contains only two teeth in this class; conse-

quently, each quadrant has one and only one type of canine (Fig. 18-16).

Both the maxillary and mandibular canines are single cusped teeth with sloping cutting blades in a mesial and distal direction. The maxillary canine has a functional lingual surface with a prominent lingual ridge joined to a bulbous cingulum. The maxillary canine is positioned labial and distal to the mandibular canine in centric occlusion. In function, the mandibular canine occludes against its maxillary canine antagonist to tear, cut, or hold food. The cuspal elevations of these antagonistic canines contact each other in all excursions of the mandible and are called guarding cusps.

Premolars

There are eight premolars. Each arch contains four teeth of this class.

Each quadrant has two premolar types —first and second. They are numbered in the order that they appear in an anteroposterior position (Fig. 18-17).

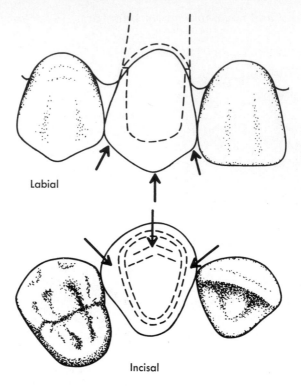

Fig. 18-16. Maxillary right canine. *Arrows,* Placement of three incisal cones.

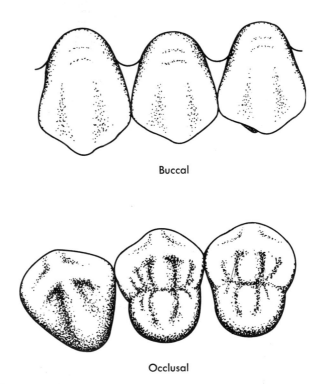

Fig. 18-17. Occlusal and buccal views of maxillary premolars and canine.

It is important to restate at this time that the elevations of these remaining posterior teeth may be described as multicusped (stamp-support or shearing-guiding), with the stamp cusps being the maxillary lingual cusps and the mandibular buccal cusps. The shearing cusps are the buccal cusps of the maxillary teeth and the lingual cusps of the mandibular teeth.

The relation of these cusps to the curve of Spee, as we view the buccal aspect of opposing quadrants, is described as follows, with the mesiodistal positions given in relation to opposing teeth and their height in relation to the curve of Spee and adjoining cuspal elevations.

first premolar

  maxillary A two-cusped tooth whose buccal and lingual elevations border the functional surface. The buccal cusp is slightly larger and resembles the canine from the buccal aspect. The tip of this cusp is on line with the curve of Spee and divides the mesiodistal width of the crown. The lingual cusp is smaller and is visible from the buccal aspect as it divides the mesial cuspal ridge of the buccal cusp in half. It lies slightly above the curve of Spee. The support area of this cusp in centric occlusion is the distal fossa of the mandibular first premolar.

  mandibular A two-cusped tooth with a nonfunctional lingual cusp, much smaller than the buccal cusp, that is usually joined to the buccal cusp by a prominent transverse ridge. The buccal cusp divides the mesiodistal diameter when viewed buccally and has its support area in the mesial fossa of the maxillary first premolar in centric occlusion.

second premolar

  maxillary A two-cusped tooth with both buccal and lingual cusps being approximately equal in size. The lingual cusp has its support area in the distal fossa of

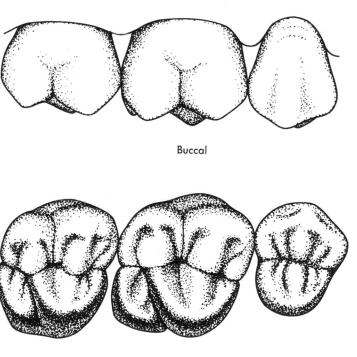

Buccal

Occlusal

Fig. 18-18. Maxillary molars shown from buccal and occlusal views.

the mandibular second premolar. The buccal and lingual cusp height rest on the curve-of-Spee line.

mandibular A two- or three-cusped tooth. The buccal cusp is the largest with the mesiolingual cusp next in size if three cusps are found. The buccal cusp divides the width of the crown, and its support area is the mesial fossa of the maxillary second premolar. The function of the premolars is to reduce food-particle size.

Molars

There are twelve molars. Each arch contains six teeth, with each quadrant having three teeth of this class.

All molars are multicusped teeth and are numbered in progression: first, second, and third moving distally from the previous class, the premolars (Figs. 18-18 and 18-19).

first molars The first molars are the largest occluding or functioning surface used to mill or grind food in preparation for swallowing.

maxillary first A four-cusped tooth, three of which are major in size. The order of cusp size, from largest to smallest is (1) mesiolingual, (2) mesiobuccal, (3) distobuccal, and (4) distolingual (Fig. 18-20). Viewed buccally, the two buccal cusps appear to be of equal length and are on the curvature line. The apex of each of these cusps divides the mesial and distal halves of the crown width. The tip of the mesiobuccal cusp is in line with the mesiobuccal groove of the mandibular first molar. The horizontal plane that would touch the cusp of the maxillary canine and buccal cusps of both premolars would only contact the mesiolingual cusp of the maxillary first molar. The mesiolingual cusp would be visible between

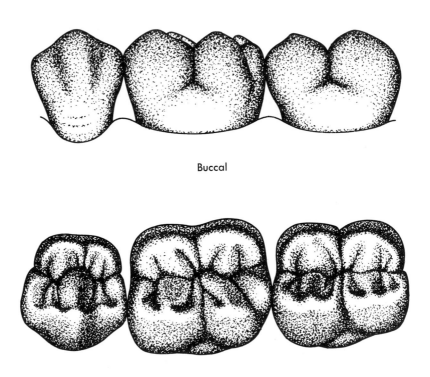

Buccal

Occlusal

Fig. 18-19. Mandibular molars shown from occlusal and buccal views. Note position of proximal contact areas.

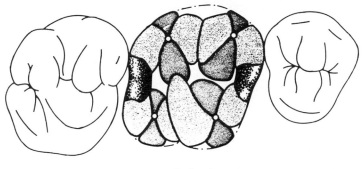

Occlusal

Fig. 18-20. Maxillary first molar cusp tips with illustrated triangular cuspal inclination. Note size of marginal ridges.

the two buccal cusps viewed from the buccal aspect. The support area for the mesiolingual cusp is the central fossa of the mandibular first molar. Viewed occlusally, the two buccal cusps form a facial plane that would be parallel to the midsagittal plane of the skull. The mesiolingual cusp is joined to the distobuccal cusp by an oblique ridge. The major elevation of the mesiobuccal cusp (triangular ridge) projects distolingually into the central fossa.

mandibular first A five-cusped tooth, four of which are major in size and the fifth called the "distal cusp." This tooth is the only posterior tooth whose dimension in a mesiodistal direction is greater than its buccolingual dimension. The mesiobuccal cusp has the support area of the embrasure formed by the maxillary second premolar and the maxillary first molar. It may, however, occlude in the mesial fossa of the maxillary first molar in a dental class II relationship. The distobuccal cusp lies in the central fossa of the maxillary first molar. The distal cusp usually occludes in the distal fossa of the maxillary first molar. An occlusal view may show a wide variety of groove patterns between the triangular ridges of its five cusps. The mesiobuccal cusp and the mesiolingual cusp seem to form a transverse ridge with their respective triangular ridges. The remaining triangular ridges of the other cusps converge toward the center of the central fossa.

maxillary second May be a three- or four-cusped tooth. Usually it is a smaller replica of the maxillary first molar, which may have a complete absence of the distolingual cusp. Viewed buccally and occlusally, it is smaller than the first molar. It occludes with the mandibular second molar in the same manner as did the first molar with its antagonist.

mandibular second A four-cusped tooth with all the cusps about equal in size. The mesiobuccal stamp cusp finds its support area in the occlusal embrasure of the maxillary first and second molar's marginal ridges. The distobuccal cusp lies in the central fossa of the maxillary second molar in centric occlusion.

third molars

maxillary and mandibular thirds These are the most variable types in this class of teeth. Their form usually resembles the first molars in their respective arches and occlude in a similar way.

DETERMINANTS OF OCCLUSION

An understanding of how muscle functions, how occlusal surfaces of the teeth interact, and when other anatomic structures regulate mandibular movements is essential to the restorative dentist.

There are five determinants of occlusion,[4] ranked according to four components:

Posterior components

1. Left temporomandibular joint

2. Right temporomandibular joint

Anterior components

3. Occlusion of teeth

Physiological component

4. Neuromuscular responses, which include chewing, swallowing, and the production of speech sounds

Psychologic component

5. Emotional responses, which include bruxism and eccentric habit patterns

Physiologic aspects of the stomatognathic system are described in more detail in the preceding chapters. It is essential that there be an understanding of the interrelationship of the determinants of occlusion and knowledge of the movements that the mandible is capable of executing in order to have occlusal morphology restored satisfactorily.

POSITIONS OF MANDIBLE

In the median or sagittal plane, there are two basic reference positions—the rest position (the position of the mandible most frequently assumed for the longest periods in the course of a day) and centric occlusion, which is a position of maximum intercuspation of the teeth. Centric occlusion has also been referred to as intercuspal position, acquired centric, and habitual centric. This is the vertical position of the mandible in which the cusps of the maxillary teeth interdigitate with the mandibular teeth. The distance between rest position and centric position is known as the free-way space. An individual with the mandible at rest position is capable of further separation of the maxilla and mandible to accommodate a larger bolus of food. If the individual is requested to close from rest position to centric occlusion, the mandibular teeth will strike close to maximum interdigitation but the initial contact will depend on the posture or skeletal makeup of the individual. See Chapter 17.

Other movements that regulate restora-

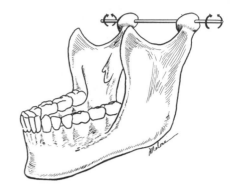

Fig. 18-21. Hinge-axis rotation.

tive procedures are centric relation. This is also called terminal hinge position (Fig. 18-21), centric relation occlusion, and retruded contact position. The average distance between centric occlusion and centric relation is approximately 1 mm. If the mandible is retruded, a hinge movement can be traced by the mandibular incisors from centric relation to a point ¾ inch away on a consistent arch. If there is an attempt to open the jaw beyond ¾ inch, the condyles can translate downward and forward. Using the terminal hinge axis as a premise then becomes questionable if ¾ inch is exceeded because it is not always reproducible with special consideration. Interocclusal recording devices or methods should ordinarily be within the arch of closure to ensure reliability before translation of the condyles. See Chapter 12.

In the vertical plane, masticatory motion is projected in the form of a teardrop. One of the more important aspects of occlusion is the lateral excursive movements of the mandible during function. The mandible is moved to the right side so that the mandibular buccal cusps and the maxillary buccal cusps oppose each other (not necessarily in contact posteriorly); the right side is called the working side or functioning side. Concomitantly, the relationship of the buccal cusp and inclines to the maxillary lingual cusps and inclines on the left side of the arch is called the balancing or non-functioning (idling) side. The converse would be true when the mandible moves to the left.

It is obvious that deviations from the normal occlusal surfaces cause interferences in smooth mandibular excursions. The adaptation of a patient to a change in occlusal scheme because of a restoration with incongruent cusp placement is usually accompanied by deleterious supportive tissue response.

CENTRIC RELATION

It is uncommon to observe patients with centric relation and centric occlusion coincident when one reviews dentitions within a normal range. There is a great deal of evidence illustrating an asymptomatic occlusal pattern of patients who do *not* have centric relation and centric occlusion coinciding. Conversely, orthodontics, prosthodontics, restorative dentistry, and periodontics cannot utilize some arbitrary point as a primary premise or reference point. Obviously, dentists must not only be aware of limitations of the registration of interocclusal records, but develop a standardized method that is reproducible. Whether the patients are treated using a terminal hinge is subject to a variety of clinical factors, such as the complexity of the work.

The terminal hinge axis or centric relation occlusion is used because of the following:

1. Centric relation is reproducible. It can be an unstrained muscular position or a slightly strained ligamentous type of position.
2. Centric relation records would provide a record that would allow smooth retrusive movements regardless of an anterior slide.

Occlusal contact during mastication occurs more commonly in centric occlusion. However, smooth movement from the working intercuspal position toward maximum intercuspation at the midline is essential to a satisfactory masticatory pattern. Most antagonistic tooth contacts that develop horizontal forces are usually considered destructive. Elimination of these undesirable contacts are difficult because of the lack of visibility of the dentist and control of the patient's movements. Clinically, treatment should be to modify the occlusal scheme of the patient to relieve distressed tissues and, one would hope, coordinate the determinants of occlusion so that the patient possesses at least an innocuous occlusal profile.

DEFINITIONS OF OCCLUSION

Simply stated, "Occlusion is the harmonious meeting of the teeth." However, there are more refined definitions, as follows:

pathologic occlusion A pathologic occlusion is one that is in insufficient harmony with the anatomic and physiologic controls of the mandible so that a pathologic condition is precipitated.[4]

physiologic occlusion A physiologic occlusion is one that is in sufficient harmony with the anatomic and physiologic controls of the mandible so as not to produce a pathologic condition with the tissues of the stomatognathic system.[5]

Any discussion of optimum occlusion relates to the occlusal pattern of a given patient. There is no one exact occlusal relationship for all patients, merely a range in normal. Capricious occlusal designs, regardless of how elaborately implemented, may not provide the most favorable stress distribution for each system. Most definitions are merely guidelines.

CLASSIFICATION OF FUNCTIONAL OCCLUSION

There are three main patterns of occlusion: canine-protected occlusion, group-protected (unilateral balance) occlusion, and bilaterally balanced occlusion. This

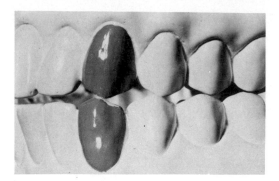

Fig. 18-22. Maxillary and mandibular teeth that contact in a "canine-protected" occlusion during lateral excursions of mandible.

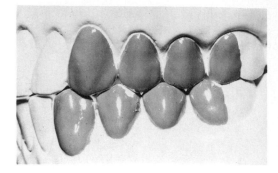

Fig. 18-24. Teeth usually involved in "group-function" occlusion during lateral excursion of mandible.

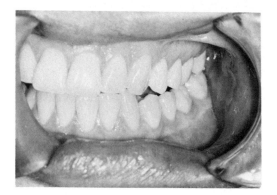

Fig. 18-23. Unilateral balance (group function) in natural dentition.

is not an inflexible listing because a combination of these groupings will be seen daily in dental practice.

Canine protection

Canine protection is associated with the younger patients[6] (17 to 26 years of age) with natural dentition. Bilateral canine protection is commonly observed with Angle's class II static skeletal classification. Micrognathic mandibles and variations in vertical and horizontal overjets of the maxillary anterior teeth characterize class II relationships. This skeletal relationship may be complicated by cross-bite relationships that defy the at-

tainment of optimum arch position without orthodontics prior to restorative procedures (Figs. 18-22 and 18-23).

As these patients move the mandible from centric closure position with the teeth in contact to lateral excursions, the maxillary and mandibular canines immediately disengage the posterior dentition. The canines and incisors permit the maxillary and mandibular molars to contact only upon centric closure position.

Group function

Group function or protection is commonly associated with patients over 30 years of age. Unilateral balance is another synonymous term for group function. Group function refers to the position and intercuspation of the buccal cusps of the mandibular arch meeting the buccal cusps of the maxillary arch during lateral excursions of the mandible (Fig. 18-24). The contacting cuspal ridges of the working side involve the canine, premolars, and occasionally, the mesiobuccal cusp of the maxillary first molar. Balancing-side interferences are noted more frequently in group function than a canine-rise type of occlusal scheme. The canine, however, provides predominance for disengagement of the dentition during function.[7] The need for periodontal therapy would suggest that this type of occlusal scheme be programmed for those patients whose

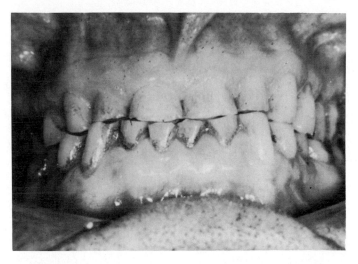

Fig. 18-25. As teeth are abraded, simultaneous loss of vertical dimension is compensated by their passive eruption and their periodontium but not to same dimension that it had in early years. Slightly increased freeway space may be necessarily incorporated in prosthodontics. Bilaterally balanced occlusion is a common observation.

dentition is subjected to secondary traumatic occlusion. If the patient has a naturally occurring group-function occlusal pattern without symptoms or bone loss, restorative work that modifies the occlusion to a canine protection can result in hypermobile canines.[8] A high percentage of restorative work is fabricated with a group-function occlusal scheme in mind and is based upon the dynamic articulation of a patient in a near neutro-occlusal arch position.

Bilateral balanced occlusion

Balanced occlusion in the natural dentition is usually associated with patients past 50 years of age who possess well-developed mandibular musculature. Bilateral balance is the objective in complete denture service and opposing bilaterally free end saddles. A certain segment of our populace with a natural dentition also has a bilaterally balanced occlusion (Fig. 18-25). If the patients move the mandible to the right to exhibit full maxillary and mandibular buccal cusp interdigitation, the left side will show the mandibular buccal cusps striking the lingual inclines of the maxillary teeth. It is more commonly observed on the molars. If these patients are asymptomatic and possess well-defined bone support, the restorative occlusal scheme should mimic the preexisting occlusion of the patients.

Equilibration or occlusal treatment in this group, whether it be at one of the phases before, during, or after restoration, possesses unparalleled pitfalls. This is attributable to the years of attrition, or possibly abrasion, that assisted in developing the unique contact of the teeth during function.

In summary, restorative dental work that will maintain an acceptable degree of biologic tolerance will imitate the previously existing occlusal pattern, rather than adapt a universal scheme of occlusal therapy, such as balanced occlusion for all patients.

EQUILIBRATION

Occlusal equilibration is generally defined as selective inclined plane reduction of teeth in an attempt to develop the harmonious contact of the maxillary and mandibular teeth during all functional and nonfunctional movements. The guidelines for equilibration are based upon clinical symptoms of the patients and radiographic evaluation of bone support.

It is imperative the dentist be familiar with acceptable, organized methods of treatment despite the fact that many patients will present clinical conditions that transcend traditional methods. The risk of any treatment can be reduced by realization of the limitations of any given procedure. Nevertheless, the acknowledgment of limitations should not discourage the clinician, but simply increase the desire to seek information to better serve patients. For example, if there is an inordinate disparity in the patient's skeletal maxillomandibular relationship, equilibration becomes an elusive art with unpredictable results.

Primary occlusal trauma is an indication for occlusal equilibration, for example, if a tooth becomes hypermobile because of a "high" restoration. Another indication is balancing-side prematurities where vertical bone loss is noted radiographically. Cusp modification is usually accomplished initially during the course of periodontal therapy and concomitantly with restorative dentistry for the patient. Normally there is a 6-month hiatus between periodontal therapy and initiation of extensive restorative work.

Methods of equilibration

There are two general methods a dentist can follow when equilibration is indicated. These methods are classified as to the sequence of implementation. One method starts from the centric relation position and proceeds to lateral excursions of the mandible. The second method is initiated with lateral excursions of the mandible and proceeds to refinement of centric relation occlusion.

The first method is more traditional and is usually associated with removable prosthodontics but is applicable to natural dentitions. The sequence is as follows:

1. Centric relation disharmony
2. Nonfunctional prematurities (balancing side)
3. Functional prematurities (working side)
4. Nonfunctional inclines (including eccentric habits)
5. Correct posterior prematurities in protrusive removable prosthodontics

The second method is as follows[9]

1. Correct the incisal relationships during protrusive movements.
2. Review the canine relationship as it moves to centric closure position. The mandibular canine is incisal edge to incisal edge with the maxillary canine. The idling (balancing) side is observed for interferences of stamp cusps of opposing arches. Interferences are more commonly found in the molar areas.
3. The opposite lateral excursion is then checked.
4. Centric closure position is checked in midmost, uppermost, and most distal mandibular position.

The rationale of Stewart's method (second sequence) is regarded as a more pragmatic approach when the dentist is required to locate prematurities in the natural dentition. Dentists are at a distinct disadvantage if they must determine a subtle prematurity with all the teeth in or near maximum intercuspation. The problem is magnified when the patient possesses a subtle difference between maximum intercuspation and the most posterior retruded contact position during centric closure.[10] The method of checking the lateral-protrusive position first and gradually testing occlusal contacts toward centric relation occlusion is considered far more comprehensive and more conducive to programmed refinement of occlusal contacts in the natural dentition.

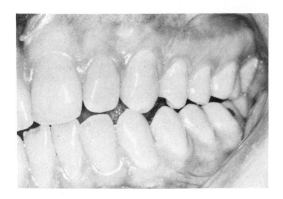

Fig. 18-26. Canine interference during protrusive movement. Equilibration should be cautiously performed.

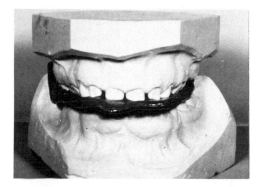

Fig. 18-27. Diagnostic casts with interocclusal record prior to mounting on articulator.

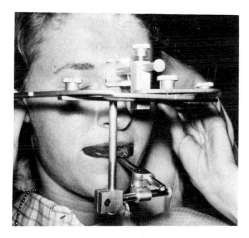

Fig. 18-28. Initial steps in recording maxillomandibular plane of occlusion using Whip-Mix face-bow. (Courtesy Dr. Anda Solarski, Chicago.)

Prerestorative equilibration

Prerestorative equilibration can be one of the most or the least beneficial dental procedures performed for the patient. This depends on the discretion of the dentist (Fig. 18-26). Any beneficial selective inclined plane reduction is preceded by radiographic evaluation and review of the mounted diagnostic casts of the patients (Figs. 18-27 and 18-28). Any therapeutic alteration of an occlusal pattern is tempered by time. Further modification of cusp position or height should be implicitly accomplished with restorative dentistry. Refinement of occlusal therapy is described in Chapter 19.

Occlusal disharmony or prematurities with accompanying periodontal breakdown should be noted by the restorative dentist and left undisturbed. The periodontist is then able to assess the relationship of tooth contact to specific bone loss. Continued occlusal adjustment can then be accomplished in conjunction with restorative procedures.

Equilibration can be accomplished by use of small diamond stones, such as a football-shaped stone or a number 6 or 8 carbide bur. The selection of instruments is usually dictated by the preference of the dentist. The articulator paper employed for marking tooth contacts can vary in color and thickness. Standardization of color and thickness of paper will increase the proficiency of the dentist, such as blue for protrusive position and red for lateral excursion of the mandible.

COMMON SENSE OCCLUSION FOR RESTORATIVE DENTISTRY

There are certain clinical situations that when recognized will assist the dentist during occlusal treatment. These are the more common problems facing dentists in daily practice.

1. *Note the edentulous areas in the oral cavity.* There may be gross discrepancies in the plane of occlusion because of supraeruption or gravita-

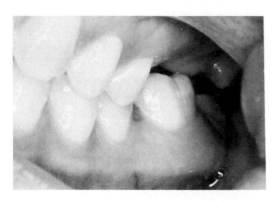

Fig. 18-29. Supraeruption of mandibular first molar attributable to prolonged loss of antagonist.

tion of a tooth lacking an antagonist. The tooth noted to be in poor arch position must be placed in acceptable arch position or removed before any prosthesis is fabricated on the opposing arch (Fig. 18-29).

2. *Evaluation of the mesiolingual cusp of the maxillary first molar.* This centric cusp may be elongated because of placement of undercarved multiple restorations of the mandibular first molar. Restoration of the mandibular arch without attention to the opposing occlusion can trigger an unfavorable intercuspal relationship in a single or multiple casting treatment[11] (Fig. 18-30).

3. *Keep the marginal ridges of proximal teeth congruent.* The marginal

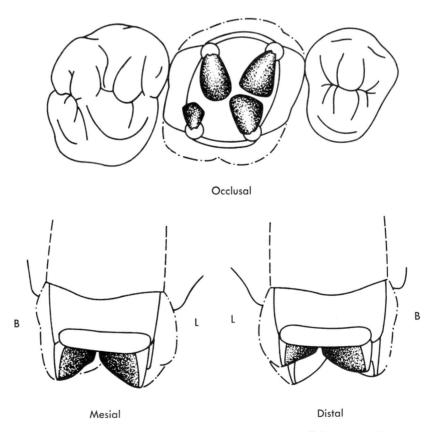

Occlusal

Mesial   Distal

Fig. 18-30. Maxillary molar has primary cusp triangle, the Trigon, consisting of three major cusps. Major cusps are structural with heavy triangular ridges.

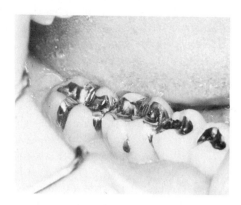

Fig. 18-31. Intracoronal restorations are always preferable when cusp-fossa relationships are within normal range. Every attempt is made to keep proximal marginal ridges even at contact of one tooth to another.

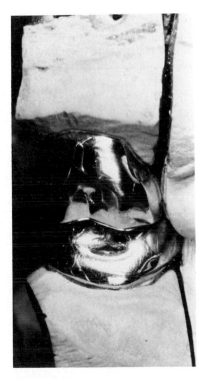

Fig. 18-32. Restoration of terminal molars prior to further restorative procedures. Vertical dimension is preserved in this manner.

ridges of the anticipated restorations should be kept commensurate with the existing dentition if the plane of occlusion is acceptable. If there is contact in a more retruded mandibular position (seen in about 90% of the patients) before maximum intercuspation, the anterior slide should be smooth to reduce the chances of periodontal destruction (Fig. 18-31).

4. *Remove malpositioned third molars.* They are generally poor abutments because of inconsistent root formation and lack of bone support. Poor hygiene is encouraged because of their unpredictable arch position, and they are commonly a cause for malocclusion.

5. *Maintain the occlusal vertical dimension of the patient.* Violation of existing vertical dimension is the most common cause of failure of all restorative dentistry.[12] If quadrant work is anticipated, posterior occlusal stops should be maintained so that the original asymptomatic neuromusculature complex will not be jeopardized by expediency (patient or dentist) to complete treatment of a neglected oral cavity in a matter of weeks. The following are three ways to maintain vertical dimension:

   a. Restore the second molar first as posterior stops, and wait an appropriate period of time for adjustment before further tooth reduction. Conversely, leave the terminal molar untouched to use as an occlusal vertical reference (Fig. 18-32).

   b. Place restorations in alternate quadrants and wait until they feel natural to the patient, such as upper right quadrant followed by the lower left quadrant, lower right quadrant, upper left quadrant, and finally the anterior quadrant, maintaining, if possible, the sanctity of the canines.

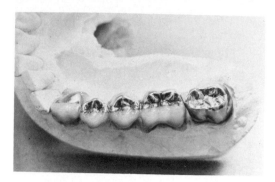

Fig. 18-33. Occlusal view of mandibular porcelain-fused-to-metal restorations. Lingual stamp cusp will contact gold surfaces, facilitating occlusal refinement. (Courtesy Francis W. Summers, Maywood, Ill.)

    c. Formulate an anterior guidance system by establishing the incisal guidance first. Six anterior teeth should *not* be reduced at one time if possible. One canine should be left to provide an occlusal scheme and a morphologic template for the prepared canine.

6. *Use dental materials where they are indicated.* One specific example is the use of complete porcelain coverage for all the restored teeth. Gold occlusal surfaces permit an attrition rate similar to enamel surfaces. Porcelain-to-porcelain occlusal surfaces do *not* afford the latitude for periodic adjustment or the attrition rate necessary during eccentric movements of the mandible. Therefore, complete porcelain occlusal surfaces should be a rare restorative procedure (Fig. 18-33).

A complete and immediate disengagement of the posterior occlusion because of a canine-protected occlusion might allow the use of porcelain-to-porcelain occlusal surfaces. This restorative approach is usually a dictate by the patient for maximum esthetics.

ORGANIZED OCCLUSAL TREATMENT

Because of the advent of high-velocity instrumentation and the increased tooth reduction resulting, a mythical Armageddon looms within each dentist. Specific courses of study should be taken prior to undertaking extensive restorative dentistry. In the early 1950s, the arduous tasks of tooth reduction of an upper canine with a 6000 to 11,000 r.p.m. handpiece intercepted many occlusal disharmonies by restricting the amount of tooth structure prepared. Today there are many excellent texts and courses directed at improving the dentist's knowledge of occlusion. Dawson's text presents an in-depth discussion of occlusion in a comprehensive manner.[13]

One of the more comprehensive approaches to emphasize the principles of articulation is Payne's systematic addition of colored wax (Figs. 18-34 and 18-35). The Payne approach is predicated upon a neutro-occlusion with a unilateral balance in lateral excursions. Thomas has a similar approach, but develops a modified cusp-fossa relationship to place articular stresses along the long axis of the teeth.

Another direction for gaining information concerning occlusion and the finer points of articulation is the use of pantography. This clinical procedure will help the dentist to elucidate the refinement of mandibular movements.

METHODS OF APPROACH TO OCCLUSAL TREATMENT
Gnathology

Gnathology is broadly defined as the study of jaws. There are other connotations that have evolved from this basic definition. Some gnathologists have purposely developed the profile that complex, expensive instrumentation is the most important feature of the gnathologic approach. However, the instrumentation is secondary to the prerestorative evaluation of the patient performed during

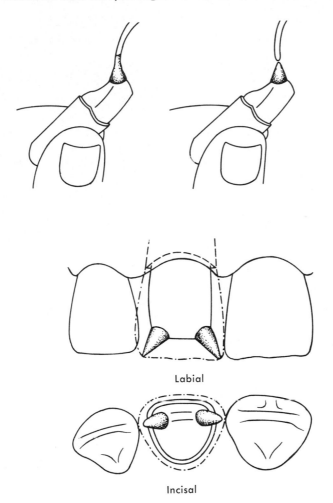

Fig. 18-34. Cone type of wax-up to accentuate placement of incisal edge on maxillary central incisor.

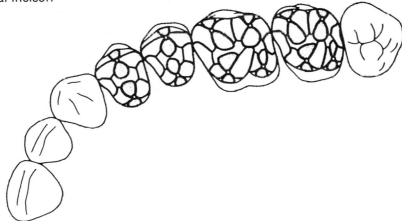

Fig. 18-35. Wax-up of maxillary arch, occlusal view. Note triangular cuspal formation and programmed placement of marginal ridges.

gnathologic analysis. The gnathologic groups usually use the temporomandibular joint as their primary premise or reference area. The science of gnathology is involved with recording the three axes of rotation of the condyle: horizontal, vertical, and sagittal within their respective planes. There is a pragmatic implementation of the occlusal scheme in the form of a mutually protected occlusion, with the anteriors providing protection for the posteriors and vice versa.[14] Determinants of occlusion are coordinated to construct a suitable occlusal plane for the patients. Gnathology possesses, inherently, a greater amount of latitude than do other techniques of oral rehabilitation.

The contributions of the gnathologic groups have been considerable, but all the aids for oral rehabilitations are merely that, if the dentist is the only one who is the recipient of the information. If the instruments or articulators are too expensive or complex, they will never realize their full potential impact upon the dental profession. The laboratory technician who implements the cases by prescription direction of the dentist must be thoroughly familiar with the concepts if they are to be exploited to the benefit of the populace. Extensive restorative dentistry requires many arduous hours interrupted by moments of sheer frustration. A lack of dedication or knowledge by the technician to management of difficult cases can add immeasurably to the discomfort of the patient and frustration of the dentist.

Pankey-Mann-Schuyler

The P.M.S. approach to oral rehabilitation is based upon the intellectual concepts of Monson and Bonwill with a pragmatic reliance upon the influence of incisal guidance.[15,16] The articulators associated with this technique have previously been nonarcon in type, that is, Hanau and Dentatus.

The advantages of the P.M.S. technique are the following:

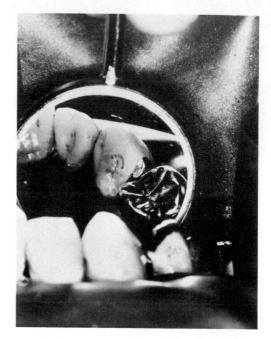

Fig. 18-36. Lingual surface of canine is preserved whenever possible. This disoccluding surface is critical to maintenance of a mutually protected occlusion.

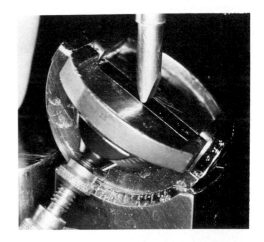

Fig. 18-37. Incisal guidance table set on Hanau Articulator to mimic naturally occurring incisal guidance in natural dentition.

1. The incisal guidance is more reliable because it is closer anatomically to the treated area than to the condyle (Figs. 18-36 and 18-37).
2. Canines are made of unyielding

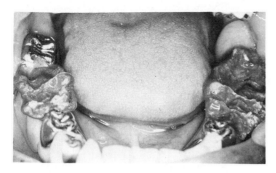

Fig. 18-38. Chew-in technique for gold occlusals on removable partial prosthesis opposing maxillary quadrant restored with onlays.

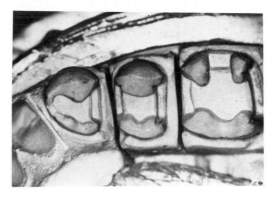

Fig. 18-39. Quadrant of overlay preparations prior to multicolored wax–addition technique.

tissue, which provides a more reliable interocclusal record.

3. There is minimal modification of vertical dimension with the P.M.S. technique because the records are taken at approximately the same occlusal plane of occlusion as the intended occlusal therapy.

4. A functionally generated path technique for less involved cases is also possible (Fig. 18-38). The P.M.S. and Meyer "chew-in" techniques are precursors to this popular restorative technique. Functionally generated path techniques can be very successful in quadrant dentistry or even for total reconstruction where proper anterior guidance has been previously established.

Undergraduate dental education is merely an introduction to these principles. The need for advanced training and education is the responsibility of the dentist to increase his knowledge based upon his initial exposure to these techniques. Chapter 12 describes methods to secure interocclusal records, whereas the refinements of preinsertion and postinsertion equilibration are presented in Chapter 19. Dr. Mahan has shown the interrelationship of basic science information in the sixth edition (Chapters 5, 7, and 12) (see also this edition, Chapter 16), whereas the discussion of vertical dimen-

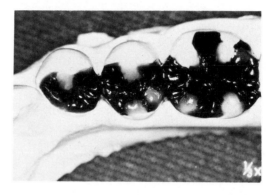

Fig. 18-40. Multicolored wax–addition technique, which facilitates cusp placement during laboratory procedure.

sion in Chapter 17 of the seventh edition emphasizes the importance of neuromuscular balance.

Wax-up methods

There are many courses and methods that have been instituted to enhance the dentist's comprehension of occlusal relationships. One of the more effective teaching methods has been the systematic addition of colored waxes that was introduced by Payne, improved and systematized by Thomas, and refined by Lundeen for undergraduate education (Figs. 18-39 and 18-40). Payne's approach should be mastered first because it is based upon the cuspal interdigitation as noted in Angle's classification of neutro-

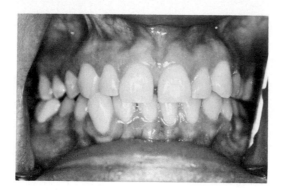

Fig. 18-41. Occlusion at two planes is ideally treated with orthodontic movement.

occlusion. Thomas's wax-up is a similar method, but it has a modified cusp-fossa relationship to place articular stress along the long axis of teeth. These innovations have been particularly useful in diagnostic wax-ups of complex restorative cases. Fabrication of treatment restorations and completion of difficult preparations have also been made easier by these perceptive techniques.

DIFFICULT OCCLUSAL RESTORATIVE CASES

Before the dentist commits himself to altering occlusion, he must be convinced that the clinical conditions present do not prevent or limit the success of the intended modification. The following conditions represent dental problems that, when treated, realize only a limited success rate or at best require an inordinate degree of supervision, that is, perennial 2- to 3-month recall.

1. Occlusion at different levels (Fig. 18-41)
2. Occlusion with excessive vertical overlap
3. Occlusion with horizontal overlap (overjet)
4. Occlusion with a prognathic mandible
5. Occlusion with mobile teeth
6. Occlusion with influence by wear from bruxism
7. Occlusion with an anterior or posterior cross-bite
8. Occlusion with abnormal tongue and swallowing habits
9. Occlusion treated previously
10. Abnormal but functional occlusion of convenience[12]

Additional problem cases are the following:

11. Patients with a history of temporomandibular joint disturbances
12. Young patients who have had a full mouth rehabilitation because of a congenital anomaly, such as amelogenesis imperfecta
13. Patients with a history of mental disturbance or conversion hysteria[17]

In summary, empirical techniques do not indicate the physiologic condition of a patient's occlusion. Failures or limited success rates in restorative dentistry are influenced more by unfounded vertical dimension modifications, uniform occlusions for all cases, and the limitations of restorative procedures than by a particular articulator or method of recording interocclusal positions (Fig. 18-42).

PAIN-DYSFUNCTION SYNDROMES

The influence of occlusion in such cases is somewhat overemphasized, but undeniable. Dentistry has classified patients with this affliction by their physical characteristics, personality traits, and subjective symptoms.[18,19]

1. Seventy to 80% of these patients have accompanying psychologic disturbances. These patients at least have a psychologic predisposition to excessive nocturnal bruxism or clenching, which can cause self-inflicted trauma on a susceptible temporomandibular joint.
2. Symptoms are usually bizarre. There is trismus of maxillomandibular musculature, deviation upon closure, and radiating pain.
3. Most patients with chronic symp-

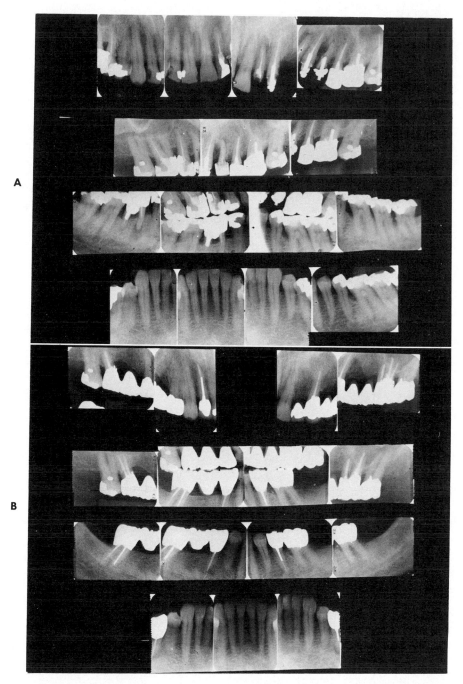

Fig. 18-42. A, Preoperative radiograph of difficult restorative case. **B,** Postoperative radiographs. Prognosis is guarded, at best, with this previously treated occlusion.

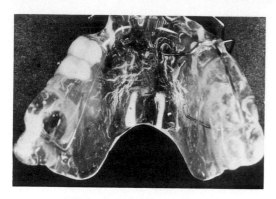

Fig. 18-43. Bite plane with Hawley anterior and ball clasps posteriorly used to alleviate temporomandibular discomfort and assist in determination of acceptable vertical dimension.

toms may experience remissions but rarely cures.

The most effective means of treatment are the following:

1. Bite-plane therapy with programmed equilibration over an extended period of time (Fig. 18-43).
2. Orthodontic treatment for younger patients or patients with adequate bone support.
3. Removal of extruding or supra-erupted teeth that interfere with normal function.
4. Maintenance therapy, which can include muscle relaxants, hydrotherapy, and psychologic consultation.
5. Injections of local anesthetics or anti-inflammatory agents in the case of arthritic conditions demonstrable in laminographic radiographs.

Conservative treatment is far more desirable than drastic therapeutic procedures. A combination of treatment of the above is common. Full mouth rehabilitation should be a rare procedure until the acute symptoms are alleviated. Provisional splinting should precede any permanent alteration of vertical dimension. Most cases of this type are usually classified as long-term, programmed treatment.

SUMMARY

"Normal occlusion" implies not only the centric closure positions, but also the full range of functional movements of the mandible. The importance of occlusion is self-evident; however, the technical aspects of restorative dentistry and the limitations of treatment because of bizarre occlusal relationships have not received sufficient attention in dental research.

The individualistic chewing behavior of the patient must be respected. For a patient who has obviously enjoyed a wide range of freedom during lateral excursions of the mandible, it would be undesirable to develop an occlusion that restricts its movements. The restorative work and its effect upon the delicately balanced equilibrium of the neuromuscular complex is undeniable. Occlusal harmony is well served by conservative restorative dentistry that preserves vertical dimension and helps to maintain the periodontal health of the dentition.

Lastly, there are cases that fail, regardless of the type of treatment instituted by the dentist. Some patients have a propensity to loss of teeth regardless of the most refined interdisciplinary treatment. However, early recognition of clinical symptoms and propitious recall systems may prolong the retention of teeth or advert complete denture service for the majority of patients in this classification.

SELECTED REFERENCES

1. Ingraham, R.: Occlusion and operative dentistry, Dent. Clin. North Am. **13**(3):591-597, 1969.
2. Malone, W. F.: The occlusal epidemic—profile of confusion. Illinois Dent. J. **39**:643-652, Oct. 1970.
3. Henneman, R. F., Vlazny, A. L., and Malone, W. F.: Oral morphology laboratory manual, ed. 2, Chicago, 1975, Loyola University Department of Fixed Prosthodontics.
4. Guichet, N. F.: Principles of occlusion—a teaching manual, Anaheim, Calif., 1970, Denar Corp.
5. Tylman, S. D.: Theory and practice of crown

and fixed partial prosthodontics (bridge), ed. 6, St. Louis, 1970, The C. V. Mosby Co.

6. Scaife, R. R., Jr., and Holt, J. E.: Natural occurrence of cuspid guidance, J. Prosthet. Dent. **22**(2):225-229, Aug. 1969.

7. D'Amico, A.: A study of the comparative functional mammalian masticatory systems, J. South. Calif. State Dent. Assoc. **33**(10-12):450, 504, 546, Nov. 1965.

8. O'Leary, T. J., Shanley, D. B., and Drake, R. B.: Tooth mobility in cuspid protected and group function occlusion, J. Prosthet. Dent. **27**(1): 21-25, 1972.

9. Stuart, C. E.: The methods of approach—determinants of occlusion and occlusal adjustments, Van Nuys, Calif., 1962.

10. Trapozzano, V. R.: Occlusion in relation to prosthodontics, Dent. Clin. North Am., p. 315, March 1957.

11. Lundeen, H. C.: Occlusal morphologic considerations for fixed restorations, Dent. Clin. North Am. **15**(3):649-671, 1971.

12. Brecker, S. C.: Practical oral rehabilitation, J. Prosthet. Dent. **10**(6):1001-1008, 1959.

13. Dawson, P. E.: Evaluation, diagnosis and treatment of occlusal problems, St. Louis, 1974, The C. V. Mosby Co.

14. Thomas, P. K.: Syllabus on full mouth waxing technique in rehabilitation tooth to tooth, cusp fossa concept, Post Graduate Education. University of California, San Francisco Medical Center.

15. Mann, A. W., and Pankey, L. D.: Oral rehabilitation utilizing the Pankey-Mann instrument and a functional bite technique, Dent. Clin. North Am., pp. 215-230, March 1959.

16. Pankey, L. D., Mann, A. W., and Schuyler, C.: Teaching manual for occlusal rehabilitation, ed. 4, Feb. 1967, Pankey-Mann-Schuyler Institute.

17. McElroy, D. L., and Malone, W. F.: Handbook of oral diagnosis and treatment planning, Baltimore, 1969, The Williams & Wilkins Co.

18. Block, L. S.: The prosthodontist and the temporomandibular joint syndrome, J. Dent. Med. **12**:74-78, 1957.

19. Bell, D. H.: Mandibular equilibration: harmony of structure and function. In Boone, M., editor: American Equilibration Society Compendium **8**:276-288, 1968, Indianapolis, Indiana.

GENERAL REFERENCES

Arnold, N. R., and Frumaker, S. C.: Occlusal treatment: preventive and corrective occlusal adjustment, Philadelphia, 1976, Lea & Febiger.

Beyron, H.: Optimal occlusion, Dent. Clin. North Am. **13**:545, 1969.

Fabrick, R.: Occlusion in adolescents, Dent. Clin. North Am. **13**(2):451-459, April 1969.

Granger, E. R.: Practical procedures in oral rehabilitation, Philadelphia, 1962, J. B. Lippincott Co.

Guichet, N. F.: Applied gnathology: why and how, Dent. Clin. North Am. **13**:3, July 1969.

Huffman, R., Regenos, J., and Taylor, R.: Principles of occlusion, Columbus, Ohio, 1969, Huffman & Regenos Press.

Kraus, B. S., Jordan, R. E., and Abrams, L.: Dental anatomy and occlusion, Baltimore, 1969, The Williams & Wilkins Co.

Lucia, V. O.: Modern gnathological concepts, St. Louis, 1961, The C. V. Mosby Co., pp. 25-36.

Mann, A. W., and Pankey, L. D.: Concepts of occlusion: The P. M. philosophy of occlusal rehabilitation, Dent. Clin. North Am., pp. 621-636, Nov. 1963.

McCollum, B. B., and Stuart, C. E.: A research report, South Pasadena, Calif., 1955, Scientific Press.

Moffet, B. C.: The morphogenesis of the temporomandibular joint, Am. J. Orthodont. **52**:401-415, 1966.

Posselt, U.: Physiology of occlusion and rehabilitation, London, 1968, Blackwell Scientific Publications, pp. 65-102.

Ramfjord, S. P., and Ash, M. M.: Occlusion, Philadelphia, 1966, W. B. Saunders Co.

Reider, C. E.: Development of a simplified system for clinical evaluation of occlusal relationships. Part I. Acquisition of information, J. Prosthet. Dent. **33**:264, 1975.

Reynolds, J. M.: Occlusal wear facets, J. Prosthet. Dent. **24**:367, 1970.

Richetts, R. M.: Occlusion—the medium of dentistry, J. Prosthet. Dent. **21**:39, 1969.

Schweitzer, J. M.: Concepts of occlusion: a discussion, Dent. Clin. North Am., pp. 649-671, Nov. 1963.

Shore, N. A.: Occlusal equilibration and temporomandibular dysfunction, Philadelphia, 1959, J. B. Lippincott Co.

Sicher, H., and DuBrul, E. L.: Oral anatomy, ed. 6, St. Louis, 1975, The C. V. Mosby Co.

Stallard, H., and Stuart, C. E.: Concepts of occlusion. What kind of occlusion should recusped teeth be given? Dent. Clin. North Am., pp. 591-606, Nov. 1963.

Stuart, C. E.: Good occlusion for natural teeth, J. Prosthet. Dent. **14**:717, 1964.

Weinberg, L. A.: Radiographic investigation into temporomandibular joint function, J. Prosthet. Dent. **33**:672, 1975.

19

Preinsertion and postinsertion occlusal considerations and equilibration*

J. Marvin Reynolds

The science of occlusion encompasses much more than just the interrelationships of teeth. It involves the total stomatognathic system in health and disease. Occlusion is a physical, neuromuscular, and psychologic phenomenon. An understanding of the interdependence of the teeth, the periodontium, the musculature of the head and neck, and the temporomandibular articulation is needed. It is essential to know the manner in which each is affected in normal and abnormal functions.[1]

There is a mutual relationship between the contact of teeth, the position of the condyles, and the muscular activity associated with the mandible. The teeth control conditioned reflex activities more than innate reflexes. Therefore interferences are probably less damaging during learned functional activities.[1] Tooth contact occurs as a result of some closing action of the mandibular muscles. The occlusal contact results in sensory feedback

to the central nervous system.[2] The information either reinforces or modifies the neural information (engram) that will be responsible for the next analogous activity. Each occlusal contact is the result of neuromuscular activity and each contact releases neuromuscular activity. Thus dentists can modify muscular activity by any dental procedure that alters the occluding surface of a tooth.

DEFINITIONS OF OCCLUSAL TERMINOLOGY

The following terms are used in this chapter. Their definitions are outlined.

arch segments
  incisor segment Part of the dental arch containing the incisor teeth.
  canine segment Part of the dental arch containing the canine, the lateral incisor, and the first premolar.
  posterior segment Part of the dental arch containing the premolars and molars.
bruxofacet Any flat, glossy area on a tooth with well-defined borders that has been caused by empty-mouth tooth-to-tooth rubbing.
deflective occlusal contact Tooth contact that deflects or has the potential to deflect condylar movement; any tooth contact that prevents joint-tooth stabilization of the mandible.
dysfunction State of functional disharmony in which the forces developed during function result either in pathologic changes in the tissues or in some functional disturbances.
functional disturbance Muscular hyperactiv-

---

*I consider myself fortunate to have become acquainted with, and to have studied with, many of the leading dentists in fixed prosthodontics and occlusion. Each has made a major contribution in my professional development, but there is one dentist who has had the most influence on me, especially in making me aware of the importance of occlusion. The example he set instilled in me the importance of professional excellence. Thus I dedicate this chapter to John D. Adams.

ity associated with occlusal disharmonies causing fatigue, myositis, fibritis, or spasm resulting in uncoordinated, evasive, or restricted movement.

interceptive occlusal contact Initial tooth contact that stops or diverts the normal closure of the mandible.

intercuspal position (IP) Occlusal position of maximum intercuspation; focal apex (terminal point) of all mandibular movements with a cranial component; occlusal position that has the most cranial location.

laterotrusive contact Contact occurring on the side of the mandible in laterotrusion (side-shift); synonym: *working contact.*

laterotrusive side Side of the mandible that has moved away from the median plane and is located lateral to intercuspal position; synonym: *working side.*

mediotrusive contact Contact occurring on the side of the mandible in mediotrusion; synonym: *balancing contact, nonworking contact, idling contact.*

mediotrusive side Side of the mandible that has moved toward the median plane and is located medial to intercuspal position; synonym: *balancing side, nonworking side, idling side.*

muscular contact position (MCP) Initial tooth contact position after closure of the mandible from rest by a minimum of muscular effort.

orthofunction State of functional harmony in which the forces developed during function are kept within the adaptive physiologic range and all tissues maintain a state of physical health.

retruded contact position (RCP) Occlusal contact position when the mandible is retruded.

shear cusps Cusps not involved in intercuspal-position contacts; cusps not involved in fossae or marginal ridge contact.

support cusps Cusps that occlude in intercuspal position; cusps that occlude in fossae or on marginal ridges.

symptom-provoking contact Pair of bruxofacets that when pressed together generate an abnormal symptom of which the patient is aware.

CONCEPTS OF OCCLUSION

All the concepts of occlusion might be analyzed in the following manner.[3]

Interarch relationship
1. Intercuspal position at retruded contact position
2. Intercuspal position not at retruded contact position

Excursive tooth guidance
1. Maximum guidance (bilateral balance)
2. Segment guidance (working-side balance or group function)
3. Minimum guidance (posterior disocclusion or canine guidance)

Occlusal morphology
1. Natural anatomy
2. Modified anatomy
3. Flat anatomy

Intertooth relationship
1. Cusp to ridge
2. Cusp to fossa
3. Cusp to embrasure
4. Cusp to plane
5. Plane to plane

This outline permits 24 possible combinations or plans. Is one plan significantly better than another and, if so, under what circumstances? At the present time, it is doubtful that any one plan can be scientifically proved to be better. Many concepts of occlusion are based on the static interrelationship of teeth and on positional relationships of the arches. These concepts should be correlated with the functional state of the temporomandibular articulation.

Joints like the temporomandibular joint permit movement and provide the mechanism to gain a mechanical advantage through the principle of levers. A lever system must have an effective fulcrum present. Joint stabilization is also necessary to ensure reciprocal muscular activity when work is done.

During mastication, the fulcrum may shift to the bolus of food. In fact, this may be associated with the initiation of a new masticatory cycle. However, the teeth should never be the principal fulcrum during empty-mouth closures or contact movements.

The force vectors in the temporomandibular joints tend to swing the condyles up and forward during shortening of the closing muscles and then move the condyles back along the articular eminences. The most effective braced position of the mandible exists when the condyle-disc assembly is uppermost against the articular eminences.[4] Radiographically, this position is determined when the temporomandibular joint spaces are symmetric and equal on both sides. When the temporomandibular joint spaces are asymmetric, either a disc is disarranged, or some of the mandibular muscles are in spasm, or the occlusion of the teeth has deflected the condyle position.

The teeth should permit the condyles to travel to the upper limits in the joint compartments and permit the closing muscles to shorten through a power contraction. This means that the intercuspal position of the teeth must relate to vertical factors of the joints and muscles.[5] The teeth and temporomandibular joints should be considered as one functional unit, sometimes called the articular triad.[6] When the intercuspal position of the teeth is not integrated with a positioning of the joints that is favorable to the musculature, the occlusion is predisposed to causing microtrauma in the joint-muscle system or the tooth-periodontal attachment apparatus or the tooth itself.

Centric relation is defined as the most retruded position of the mandible.[7] This is usually determined intraorally by some type of clinical procedure. If the mandibular position is unrelated to condyle-fossa position, sometimes the condyles will be positioned too far posteriorly and inferiorly when the mandible is retruded. Another misconception about centric relation is that it is a functional position. Border limits do not normally involve functional movements but are end points of intraborder movements. Any intraborder movement should have the privilege of reaching any border position.

It seems that another dimension should be added to centric relation—that of the uppermost and midmost position of the

condyles in the glenoid fossae. When this is done, then intercuspal position (IP) and retruded contact position (RCP) should coincide at a vertical level that is the focal apex of all mandibular cyclic movements with a cranial component. Actually, retruded contact position and intercuspal position are closer together in more individuals than is usually given credit. During any hinge closure, a given point on a mandibular tooth will arc up and forward at an angle of about 45 degrees.[8,9] This means that approximately 1 mm of anterior movement of a tooth will occur with each 1 mm of vertical closure without any bodily change of the condyle relative to the articular eminence. In a situation like this, the linear slide will actually be about 1.4 mm without any forward movement of the condyles.

When a slide from retruded contact position to intercuspal position is observed, the vertical component should be considered along with the forward component. When each component is about equal, the condyles are mainly rotating during the slide (Fig. 19-1). Any bodily

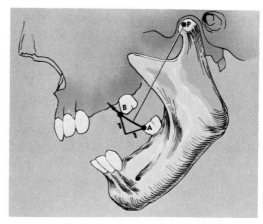

Fig. 19-1. Normal closure of mandible about its axis, *P,* will move cuspal elements of mandibular teeth up and forward along an arc, *AB,* at an angle of about 45 degrees. For each unit of vertical closure, cusp will move forward about same amount without any bodily change of condyle.

displacement of the condyles will be no more than 0.1 to 0.2 mm. When the anterior component of a slide predominates, the condyles are pulled forward (Fig. 19-2). If the vertical component predominates, the closure is probably pivoting around a posterior interfering tooth and the condyles will be deflected down and back (Fig. 19-3).

A slide from retruded contact position to intercuspal position needs to be correlated with three factors: its magnitude, the vertical and anterior components of the slide, and the position of the condyles when the teeth are in intercuspal position.

Empty-mouth excursive tooth guidance is another occlusal consideration. How many teeth are needed in the guidance and where should they be located? Does some form of group guidance have any advantage over minimum guidance?

It is difficult to maintain constant occlusal and condylar relations. There are subtle changes in the occluding surfaces of teeth from attrition, slight alterations in

tooth positions when intertooth forces change, differences in the thickness of the disc, and the gradual decrease in the transjoint distance through remodeling processes associated with normal aging. The type and rate of change are different for each individual.

When the occlusal surfaces of teeth rub on each other, wear occurs.[10] Wear is caused by the nature of the material, the area in contact and the frequency of contact. Group function and bilateral balance not only increase the number of teeth in contact but also increase the range of movement where contact is possible. Either situation will increase the amount of wear of the teeth.

Another factor to consider when there is multitooth guidance is that the wear may be uneven among the teeth. Posterior teeth move shorter distances than do anterior teeth for each degree of lateral rotation. Different materials may be involved. The slower wearing tooth will eventually develop an interceptive or deflective contact.

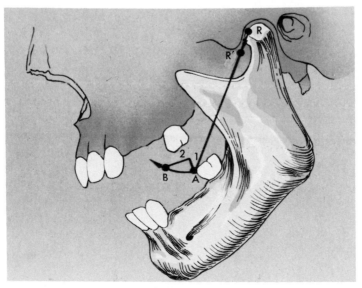

Fig. 19-2. Mandible closes so that cuspal elements of mandibular teeth move along an arc, *AB,* where anterior component predominates. When this occurs, condyle must move down and forward during closure, *R* to *R'.*

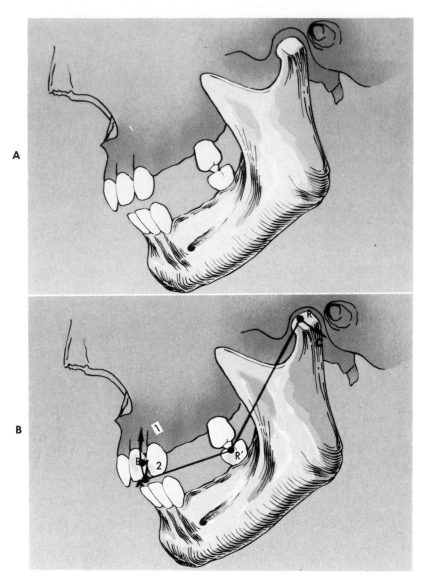

Fig. 19-3. A, Mandible closes on maxillary cusp that is in supraclusion. **B,** As closure continues, axis may shift from condyle, *R,* to upper contact on tooth, *R'.* When vertical component of closure predominates, condyle is probably twisted down and back toward *C.*

When more than one pair of teeth in the posterior segment provide guidance, an interceptive or deflective contact will occur on the most posterior tooth either as a result of uneven wear or with an effective loss of vertical height through the joints. The more distal the contact, the more damaging it may become. Joint height does decrease as degenerative processes associated with aging set in.[6]

The relationship of the articular triad will remain stable for a longer period of time if wear can be minimized. To do this, intercuspal position should be reached as a dead stop without any slide. Only a single pair of teeth should provide

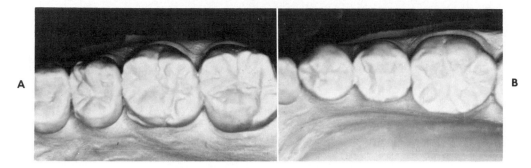

Fig. 19-4. A, Maxillary posterior teeth of caries-free dentition. **B,** Mandibular posterior teeth of caries-free dentition. Note numerous developmental and supplemental grooves creating a variety of spheroid ridges, and the absence of flat planes.

guidance in any excursive movement. The guidance should occur either in the canine or incisor segment, and all guidance should occur just outside the normal cyclic movements used in speech, mastication, and expression.

As long as the mandible is tripoded (both temporomandibular joints and one pair of occluding teeth), joint-tooth stabilization can never be lost. As more and more teeth participate in guidance, more legs are added to the system and the articular triad will eventually be lost. A stable joint-tooth relationship will also be lost. The result will be the creation of a fulcrum on a tooth. The consequence will be a muscle-tooth stabilization of the mandible that will cause an imbalance in muscle activity leading to myospasm.

As teeth develop flat occluding surfaces, wear is accelerated and occlusal stability is reduced. Wear can be reduced and horizontal forces minimized when the area available for contact is small and the potential for contact is kept in the central part of the teeth.

A sectional study of articulated casts from good dentitions shows mainly space between the opposing surfaces of teeth in intercuspal position. The contacts are between spheroid surfaces. The combined area of contact is extremely small and has been estimated to total only about 4 to 5 mm. Each contact is surrounded by

space. The space created by well-developed supplemental and developmental grooves may be very important for a well-organized, stable, stress-free occlusion (Fig. 19-4).

Another aspect of good, unworn dentitions is the reciprocal arrangement of opposing elevations and depressions. Such an arrangement provides escape routes for cusps in excursive movements and the mechanism for developing a definite intercuspal position. There seems to be clinical evidence that the preciseness of the intercuspal position may be just as important as its location, within certain limits.

Everything seems to indicate that nature's own anatomy is the best form for the occlusal surfaces of teeth. It should be maintained or reestablished routinely in our clinical procedures (Fig. 19-5). If we make an error, it should be on the side of more detail, not less. Certainly, flat surfaces should be avoided.

The intertooth location of intercuspal-position contacts should be correlated with a specific type of excursive guidance. From centric relation the mandibular teeth have an anterior component to all excursive movement paths (Fig. 19-6). Therefore lower support cusps need to be occluded more mesially for a balanced articulation than when disocclusion is desired. The reverse is true for upper sup-

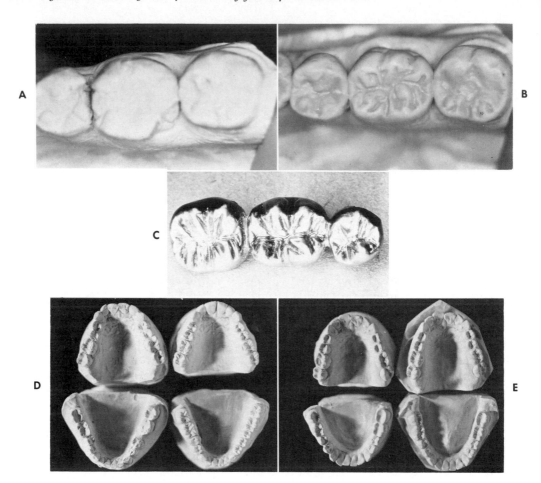

Fig. 19-5. A, Mandibular first molar has fractured lingual cusp and a carious MODB amalgam restoration. Second premolar has a fractured disto-occlusal amalgam restoration. **B,** Finished new restoration of that in **A**. Second premolar has a disto-occlusal amalgam, and first molar has complete veneer crown. **C,** Three-unit mandibular posterior bridge prior to cementation. **D,** Before and after casts where all teeth were restored except mandibular six anteriors. Two maxillary lateral incisors and mandibular left first molar were restored with three-unit bridges. All other restorations were either all metal or ceramometal-veneer crowns. **E,** Before and after casts of dentition where occlusion was altered by selected grinding. Notice that natural occlusal anatomy was recreated in each restorative procedure.

port cusps since maxillary teeth have an apparent posterior component to all excursive paths from retruded position (Fig. 19-6).

Specifically, in a completely balanced articulation (bilateral balance) the lower support cusps need to occlude in intercuspal position on the distal part of the upper teeth. The upper support cusps need to occlude on the mesial part of lower teeth. The molars will have a second cusp occluding in an opposing central fossa that is positioned relative with the other cusps in that arch. From these locations of intercuspal-position contacts, the mesial parts of lower support cusps will slide against the distal cusp slopes of upper teeth in any excursive movement.

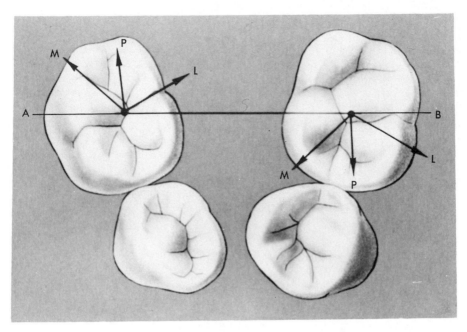

Fig. 19-6. Representation of opposing maxillary and mandibular teeth as they would be positioned in dental arch. Line *AB* represents frontal plane in area of tooth contact in retruded contact position. Lines *L* represent laterotrusive paths of opposing cusps. Lines *M* represent mediotrusive paths and lines *P* protrusive. Notice that from retruded contact position all excursive movements of mandibular teeth have an anterior component and all excursive movements of maxillary teeth have an apparent posterior component.

Distal parts of upper support cusps will slide against mesial cusp slopes of lower teeth (Fig. 19-7, *A*).

For a group-function articulation (unilateral balance), the lower support cusps are positioned to occlude in intercuspal position on upper mesial marginal ridges. From this location, the upper marginal ridges and distal cusp slopes of the upper facial cusps will provide guiding surfaces in any laterotrusive movements. The lingual embrasures will provide space for disocclusion during mediotrusive movements of the lower support cusps (Fig. 19-7, *B*). In this type of guidance, both opposing marginal ridges may have intercuspal-position contacts, but the contact on the distal marginal ridge increases the chance of contact in mediotrusive movements. The upper support cusps are

occluded in intercuspal position on lower distal marginal ridges when cross-tooth laterotrusive guidance is desired; otherwise the upper support cusps are occluded in lower distal fossae. Again, the molars will have a cusp occluded in the opposing central fossa to function in harmony with the other cusps.

In anterior guidance and posterior disclusion, a cusp-to-fossa occlusion in intercuspal position should predominate. This means lower support cusps will occlude on the mesial parts of upper teeth. The facial and lingual embrasures will provide space for disocclusion of the posterior cusps during laterotrusive and mediotrusive movements (Fig. 19-7, *C*). The organization of the placement of the second cusp on molars in the opposing central fossa and the associated ridge and

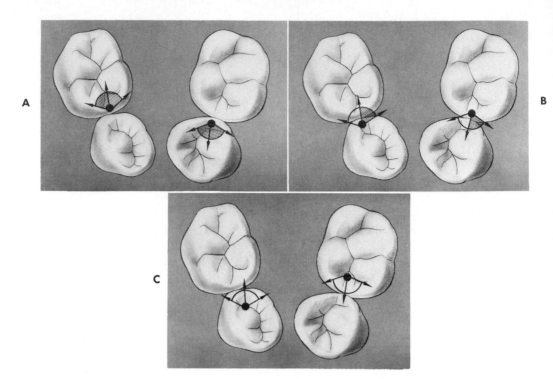

Fig. 19-7. A, Proper location for intercuspal-position contacts when balanced occlusion is desired. Adjacent cuspal inclines *(shaded areas)* provide bulk for excursive tooth contact. **B,** Proper location for intercuspal-position contact when group function is desired. **C,** Proper location for intercuspal-position contacts when disocclusion is desired. Adjacent embrasures will provide space for excursive glide paths.

groove directions must be very precisely organized to assure disocclusion of these cusps in all excursive movements.

An occlusion may seem fine on initial clinical examination or with unmounted casts. The arch form and position of the teeth are satisfactory and the teeth seem to occlude well. However, unless the final closure of the teeth is integrated with a positioning of the joints that is favorable to the musculature, the occlusion may be predisposed to causing dysfunction.

The occlusion should permit joint-tooth stabilization of the mandible without causing splinting or twisting or hyperactivity of the musculature. There should be no need for muscular stabilization of the mandible in intercuspal position or retruded contact position or any other position. Neither should the teeth have the potential to function as a fulcrum in any empty-mouth closures. The condyle-disc assembly must be permitted to function anywhere on the posterior slopes of the articular eminences without deflective or interceptive contacts.

An optimal occlusal plan is one that has the intercuspal position at centric relation, but central relation must include the uppermost and midmost condylar position. There should be minimum excursive guidance, natural anatomy on the tops of teeth, and intercuspal-position contacts occurring between teeth with like names in a predominantly cusp-to-fossa relationship.

AN OPTIMUM OCCLUSAL PLAN

The main features of an occlusal plan that seems to promote a state of orthofunction, remain mechanically stable, feel comfortable, look well, and are listed as follows:

Anterior component

1. The maxillary anterior teeth should overlap the mandibular anterior teeth in intercuspal position.
2. The anterior teeth should contact in the intercuspal position during empty-mouth power closures.
3. The coupled anterior teeth should remain free of contact during normal movements of the mandible associated with speech, mastication, and expression.
4. The length, tilt, and position of the maxillary anterior teeth should form a comfortable seal with the inner side of the lower lip as labiodental sounds are pronounced.

Posterior component

1. All mandibular posterior teeth should close evenly against the maxillary posterior teeth when the condyles are bilaterally seated in their uppermost and midmost articular position.
2. The posterior teeth should contact in intercuspal position at a vertical level that will permit the jaw-closing muscles to shorten through their power contraction.
3. The lingual cusps of the maxillary premolars and distolingual cusps of the maxillary molars should occlude in the distal fossa of the lower teeth respectively.
4. The mesiolingual cusps of the maxillary molars should occlude in the central fossa of the mandibular molars.
5. The facial cusps of mandibular premolars and the mesiofacial cusps of the mandibular molars should occlude in the mesial fossae of the maxillary teeth respectively.

6. The distofacial cusps of the mandibular molars occlude in the central fossae of the maxillary molars.
7. Subsummit surfaces of support cusps contact crests of ridges that surround the opposing occlusal fossae in intercuspal position. The contacts should occur within 1 mm of the cusp tip and within 1 mm of the central groove alignment.
8. The intercuspal position is reached as a dead stop with minimal muscular activity.
9. The horizontal overlap of the shearing cusps should be enough to keep the cheek and tongue free of the tooth-contact area in intercuspal position.

Eccentric component

1. Teeth distal to the genial tubercle should not occlude in any eccentric closure or contact movement.
2. There should be bilateral guidance in the incisor segment in straight protrusion.
3. Laterotrusive guidance should occur on a pair of teeth in the canine segment.
4. The optimal clearance of the posterior teeth is 1 mm in all positions when the anterior teeth are in edge-to-edge contact relationships.
5. The angle of cusp inclines involved in laterotrusive movements becomes progressively steeper from the most posterior tooth to the most anterior tooth (Fig. 19-8).
6. The angle of cusp inclines involved in mediotrusive movements becomes progessively less steep from the most posterior tooth to the most anterior tooth (Fig. 19-8).

Esthetic component of maxillary teeth

1. The incisal edges of the maxillary anterior teeth form a convex downward curve that is similar in outline to that formed by the lower lip in smiling (Fig. 19-9).
2. The facial cusp tips of the maxillary

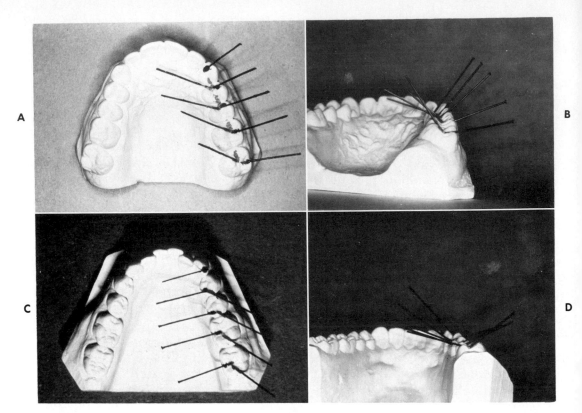

Fig. 19-8. A, and **C,** Plastic rods are attached to cusp inclines of casts from an unworn natural dentition. Rods represent cusp paths of opposing support cusps in laterotrusive and mediotrusive movements. **B** and **D,** Angle of cusp inclines involved in laterotrusive movements get progressively steeper from most posterior tooth to most anterior tooth. Angle of cusp inclines involved in mediotrusive movements get progressively less steep from most posterior tooth to most anterior tooth.

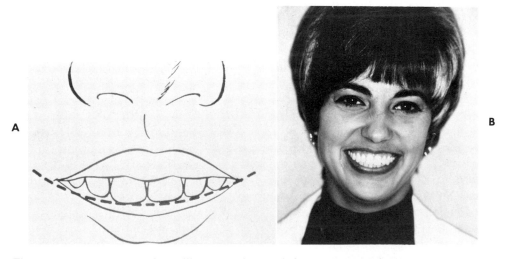

Fig. 19-9. Incisal edges of maxillary anterior teeth form a convex downward curve that tends to follow outline of lower lip in smiling.

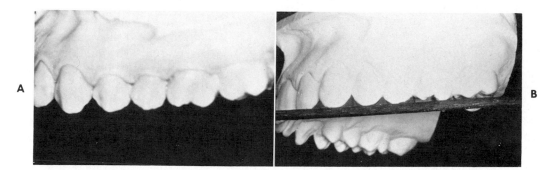

Fig. 19-10. Facial cusp tips of maxillary canine and premolars and first molar fall on same plane. Facial cusp tips of second molar and third molar (when present) are progressively short of this plane.

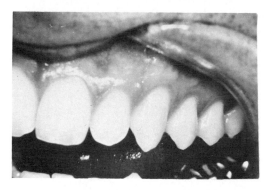

Fig. 19-11. Natural anatomy and arrangement of maxillary anterior teeth form a V-shaped incisal embrasure that gets progressively wider and deeper from central incisors to first premolar. Profiles of facial surfaces of posterior teeth are parallel and similar to those of canines. Geometric shape of incisal embrasures is very important in reestablishing natural esthetics in anterior teeth. Posterior cusp-tip length, its shape, and outline of facial profiles are important in reestablishing proper harmony of these teeth.

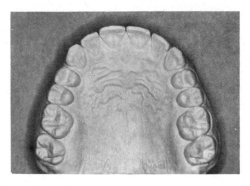

Fig. 19-12. Facial cusp tips of posterior teeth and incisal edges of anterior teeth tend to form a parabolic curve in dentitions that display optimal esthetics and occlusal form.

canine, the premolars, and first molar on each side fall on the same plane. The facial cusp tips of the second and third molars become progressively farther above the plane (Fig. 19-10).

3. The V of the incisal embrasures between maxillary anterior teeth is progressively deeper and wider

from central incisor to first premolar (Fig. 19-11).

4. The arch outline as formed by the incisal edges of anterior teeth and facial cusps of posterior teeth should form a parabolic curve (Fig. 19-12).

Functional component of maxillary teeth

1. The lingual cusp tips of the maxillary first premolars will be short of a plane connecting the facial cusp tips (Fig. 19-13).

2. The lingual cusp tips of the maxillary second premolars will fall on a plane connecting the facial cusp tips (Fig. 19-13).

3. The facial cusp tips of the maxillary

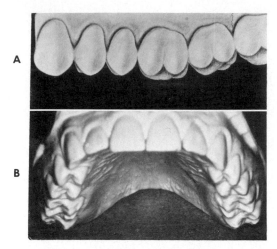

Fig. 19-13. A, Lateral view of posterior teeth displaying optimal cusp length for optimal function. **B,** Occlusal view of natural dentition displaying optimal occlusal plane. On first premolars, lingual cusps are slightly shorter than facial cusps. On second premolars, lingual and facial cusps are about same length. On first molars, lingual cusps are slightly longer than facial cusps. On second molars, lingual cusps are longer than facial cusps. The difference is more than on first molars. Geometric form of occlusal plane represented in **B** and pattern of cusp inclination represented in Fig. 19-8, *b* and *d,* is mechanically correct. This is necessary because mandibular movement is controlled from two centers (left and right temporomandibular joints). During any lateral movement, one condyle moves downward, forward, and inward while the other condyle rotates.

first molars will be short of a plane connecting their mesiolingual cusp tips. The mesiolingual cusp tip is more inferior than any other cusp in the arch (Fig. 19-13).
4. The facial cusp tips of the maxillary second molars will be short of a plane connecting their mesiolingual cusp tips by more than 1 mm. The lingual cusp tips are more superiorly located than the lingual cusps of the first molars (Fig. 19-13).
5. The plane of occlusion is a spiral.

6. The lingual concavities of the maxillary anterior teeth should permit the rotational components of condylar movements to occur without tooth slidings.

This plan organizes the teeth to permit segment function as well as mutual protection. The main load in retruded contact position and intercuspal-position closures is borne by the posterior teeth. The anterior teeth protect the posterior teeth in all eccentric closures. The incisors, canines, and posterior teeth can function independently without interference from the other teeth. Extrusive contact of all teeth occurs just outside the normal jaw movements made during mastication, speech, and expression. The condyles can reach any position in the joint compartment without guidance or interference from the teeth. A joint-tooth stabilization of the mandible is possible in any occluded position.

This plan encourages a stable neuromuscular functional pattern without undue strain or trauma to any of the individual units of the stomatognathic system.

FUNCTIONAL CLASSIFICATION OF OCCLUSION

An ideal occlusal plan is necessary to form a common base line to evaluate all diagnostic and treatment procedures involving occluding surfaces. Most persons deviate in varying degrees from the optimal plan, yet many have perfectly normal functions. Dental patients can be divided into four general categories based on functional responses from the occlusion of their teeth. Two groups can be classified as being in orthofunction and two groups as being in dysfunction.
Orthofunction
Class 1. Patients have ideal or optimal occlusion.
Class 2. Patients have occlusal disharmonies without symptoms or with insignificant symptoms.

Dysfunction

Class 3. Patients have occlusal disharmonies with symptoms that are either mild, transient, or subclinical but are at a level that has some significance.

Class 4. Patients with definite dysfunction symptoms of which the patient is aware.

The number or severity of occlusal disharmonies does not necessarily determine whether a patient has orthofunction or dysfunction. Other factors that influence the functional status include the following:

1. Genetic component
2. Psychologic component
   a. Intelligence
   b. Emotional health
   c. Behavior pattern
3. Physical component
   a. Age
   b. Sex
   c. Occupation
   d. Nutrition
   e. Life style
   f. Resistance
   g. General health

As environmental factors that affect the psychological and physical components change, internal and external stimuli may be altered and a shift back and forth between orthofunction and dysfunction may occur.

SUBJECTIVE PATIENT SIGNS AND SYMPTOMS THAT MAY INDICATE MANDIBULAR DYSFUNCTION

When mandibular dysfunction occurs, it is usually caused by some disturbance of the neuromuscular mechanism that controls mandibular movement. Noxious stimuli will cause an imbalance in muscular function. The causes may be mechanical, emotional, infectious, metabolic, or nutritional. The first two are by far the most frequent causes. Whether mechanical or emotional, or something else, if the trauma is severe enough or long enough, myospasm will develop.[11]

Some head and neck symptoms that result from mandibular dysfunction are the following:

1. Headache
2. Earache
3. Toothache
4. Pain or discomfort anywhere about the head and neck
5. Muscular tiredness or weakness
6. Restricted or inhibited jaw motion
7. Joint noises
8. Bruxism
9. Stuffed-like sensation or fullness in the ears
10. Pressure-like sensations around or behind the eyes
11. Sensitivity during chewing
12. Pulling or drawing sensations along the neck or shoulders
13. Dry mouth
14. Fullness sensation in the throat
15. Certain types of vertigo

Anyone with any of the above symptoms must be suspected of having mandibular dysfunction. Organic disturbances can cause similar signs. Even though the incidence of organic disease is low, such disorders should first be ruled out. Then caries and periodontal causes should be ruled out. After that, occlusion must be the prime suspect.

The first step in making an occlusal evaluation is to start with a six-item questionnaire to quickly screen the patient (Fig. 19-14, *A*). If the questionnaire result is negative, the patient can be considered to have a healthy stomatognathic system.

For each positive-answered question in the screening questionnaire, the following information is obtained[12]:

When were you first aware of the discomfort?

Where is the discomfort located?

What type of discomfort is it?

How often is the discomfort?

Does the discomfort have a pattern?

What makes the discomfort better?

What makes the discomfort worse?

Do you take anything for discomfort?

Does the discomfort interfere with your daily activities?

Significant information is recorded.

The patient is also asked to rank each positive symptom as either mild (1), moderate (2), or severe (3). The number for the ranking is recorded in the column for the occlusal index score. The total score for the six questions is the occlusal index.

The index is used to provide a quick tentative occlusal diagnosis based on subjective symptoms. Statistics are being gathered on the occlusal index score. It seems that an index score that is less than 4 indicates the patient is in orthofunction. A score between 4 and 6 probably indicates either a borderline case of orthofunction or a person with mild dysfunction. An index of 7 or more generally indicates that the patient has definite dysfunction.

When the index reaches 5 or more, further diagnosis is certainly desirable. Regardless of the index score, further occlusal evaluation is suggested when a single question is scaled at a level of 3 unless it can be explained by other existing dental conditions.

OBJECTIVE SIGNS AND SYMPTOMS THAT MAY INDICATE MANDIBULAR DYSFUNCTION

The procedures in an occlusal examination should be aimed at identifying unstable maxillomandibular conditions, finding physical signs of dysfunction, and determination of the degree of functional harmony or disharmony.

The following physical findings often do not provide stable maxillomandibular relations:

1. Poor intercuspal position
2. Lack of anterior guidance
3. Slide from retruded contact position to intercuspal position in which the vertical or horizontal component of the slide predominates

4. Asymmetric slide from retruded contact position to intercuspal position
5. Unilateral contact in retruded contact position
6. Mediotrusive contact of teeth
7. Laterotrusive contact between molars
8. Protrusive contact between molars

The following physical findings indicate some degree of dysfunction in the absence of any organic disorders.

1. Muscular contact position does not equal intercuspal position when a precise intercuspal position exists
2. A maximum interincisal opening that is less than 40 mm
3. Significant deviation of the mandible during opening or closing
4. Restricted or guarded excursive contact movements (less than 8 mm)
5. Pain during mandibular movement
6. Palpation soreness in one or both temporomandibular joints
7. Uncoordinated condyle-disc movement pattern
8. Bruxofacets
9. Accelerated facets of wear
10. Palpation soreness in the muscles that move and stabilize the mandible, head, and neck
11. A scalloped border on the tongue
12. A crease in the cheek mucosa

The more advanced these symptoms are, the higher level of dysfunction present. Trigger areas of pain in muscles and a positive provocation test are usually positive indications of tooth-related dysfunction.

OBJECTIVE CLINICAL EXAMINATION
(Fig. 19-14, *A*)
Intercuspal position

A good intercuspal position is probably one of the most important aspects of a healthy occlusion. The intercuspal position should be a well-defined position (precise). There should be mul-

MEDICAL COLLEGE OF GEORGIA
SCHOOL OF DENTISTRY

Patient's Name_____ Date_____

Screening Questionnaire

			Degree of Discomfort

Yes   No

_____ _____   1. Do you ever have headaches?   _____

_____ _____   2. Do you ever have pain, discomfort, or other sensations (ringing, roaring, stuffiness, etc.) in, in front of or behind the ear?   _____

_____ _____   3. Do you ever have pain, discomfort, or other sensations (tiredness, pulling, weakness, burning, etc.) about the face, eyes, throat, neck or shoulder?   _____

_____ _____   4. Does it ever hurt to chew or does a tooth get in the way when you close your teeth together or is your bite ever uncomfortable?   _____

_____ _____   5. Does it ever hurt to open wide, take a big bite or have any difficulty in opening the mouth wide?   _____

_____ _____   6. Does your jaw ever make noise (popping, cracking, grating, etc.) or does your jaw ever lock? _____

Occlusal Screening Index

Summary_____
_____
_____
_____
_____
_____
_____

A

OCCLUSAL EXAMINATION

1. **INTERCUSPAL POSITION:**

      ___good IP   ___IP=CR   ___IP=MCP   occlusal sounds:

      ___poor IP   ___IP≠CR   ___IP≠MCP   ___dull   ___sliding   ___multiple

2. **RELATIONSHIP OF THE ANTERIOR TEETH IN IP:**

      ___normal contact   ___tissue contact

      ___V. overlap   ___open

      ___H. overlap   ___crossbite

3. **RETRUDED CONTACT POSITION:**

      RCP: Slide from RCP to IP: ___straight   ___right   ___short   ___flat (H)

      ___premolar   ___bilateral   ___left   ___long   ___steep (V)

      ___molar   ___unilateral

4. **OPENING—CLOSING MOVEMENT:**

      ___mm opening   ___painful   ___passive stretch

      TMJ sounds: early   late   continuous

      right   _____   _____   _____   40 mm

      left   _____   _____   _____

      MM ⌊_⌊_⌊_⌊_⌊_⌊_⌊_⌊_⌊_⌊_⌊

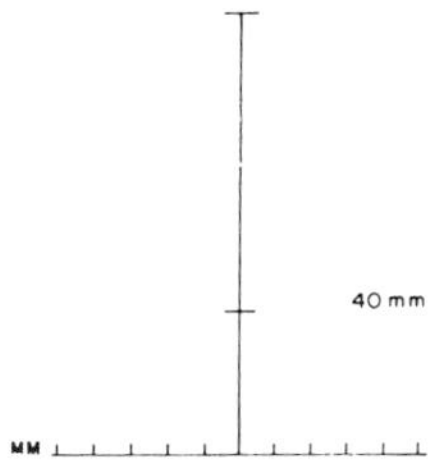

Continued.

Fig. 19-14. A, Front side of occlusal screening and examination chart.

5. **EXCURSIVE GUIDANCE:**

right lateral: _____ no canine segment contact _____ mediotrusive contact

left lateral: _____ no canine segment contact _____ mediotrusive contact

protrusive _____ R _____ L deviation _____ posterior segment contact

6. **BRUXOFACETS:**

R | 1 2 3 4 5 6 7 8 | 9 10 11 12 13 14 15 16 | L   _____ + provocation test

32 31 30 29 28 27 26 25 | 24 23 22 21 20 19 18 17

7. **ORAL—FACIAL PALPATION:**

RIGHT   **LEFT**

R   **DATE**   **DATE**   L

joints
1. lateral to capsule
2. dorsal to capsule

extraoral musculature
3. deep masseter
4. superficial m. — body
           insertion
5. anterior temporal
6. posterior temporal
7. vertex
8. neck — nape
      base
9. sternocleidomastoid — insertion
              body
10. medial pterygoid
11. posterior digastic

intraoral musculature
12. temporalis tendon
13. lateral pterygoid

8. **NOXIOUS ORAL HABITS:**

_____

_____

9. **IMPRESSION:**

_____ dysfunction _____ borderline _____ orthofunction

10. **OTHER PROCEDURES:**

_____ TMJ X-rays _____ drug therapy _____ stabilization splint _____ palliative procedure other: _____

11. **OCCLUSAL TREATMENT PLAN:**

_____

_____

_____

_____

Fig. 19-14, cont'd. B, Back side of occlusal screening and examination chart.

tiple, simultaneous contacts distributed throughout the occlusal scheme. There should be joint-tooth stabilization of the mandible in the intercuspal position. The least acceptable intercuspal position should have at least two pairs of contacting teeth on each side; one in the molar area and one in the canine segment.

A good way to examine the intercuspal position is to check each pair of occluding teeth with a strip of 1 mil Mylar recording tape (other types of Mylar strips or cellophane or wax can be used). Say to the patient: "Close your teeth together normally and hold." Check each pair of teeth with the tape. If the tape holds, there is contact; if the tape pulls, there is no contact. The use of marking ribbon or articulating paper is not so accurate because of the ballistic effect of swinging the mandible closed to obtain the markings. The mandible can be deflected or teeth can move to give a false marking.

When an acceptable intercuspal position exists, check the muscular contact position. Say to the patient: "Tap on your back teeth hard and slow." Listen with a stethoscope under the cheekbone on both sides of the mouth and compare. A single sharp impact sound is heard when MCP = IP. This indicates that the intercuspal position is within the physiologic limits of the patient at this time. In other words, when MCP = IP, the patient has the ability to close the mandible repeatedly into the intercuspal position, which indicates some level of orthofunction. A dull, sliding, or multiple sound is heard when MCP ≠ IP. When this occurs, either a poor intercuspal position exists or some form of functional disturbance is present, or there is muscular bracing of the mandible or the location of intercuspal position is unacceptable.

Relationship of anterior teeth (Fig. 19-14, *A*)

Anterior guidance is probably next in importance to a good intercuspal position. To have anterior guidance, the teeth must make contact in intercuspal position. The nature of the contact can be lighter than that for posterior teeth. This will allow for the slight vertical movement of posterior teeth during a power bite. The amount is about 1 mil (½ mil for each lower and each upper tooth). Disclusion of all posterior teeth should occur within the first ½ mm of movement, or 1 degree of rotation.

The anterior teeth should also exhibit some vertical and horizontal overlap. The question is how much of each? It is difficult to disocclude the posterior teeth when the intercuspal-position contact is near the incisal edge of the maxillary teeth. It is also difficult to maintain stable contacts and smooth guidances when the intercuspal-position contact is below the cingulum. The preferred location is somewhere between these two extremes. The ratio is not known, but clinical experience suggests that the horizontal overlap should be only about one third to one half as much as the vertical overlap. The lingual concavity of the maxillary anterior teeth should be a mirror image of the facial surface of the opposing mandibular tooth.

Examine for intercuspal-position contacts of the teeth in the anterior segment. Say to the patient: "Close your back teeth together and bite hard." Check each pair of teeth with a Mylar tape. At least one pair of teeth should contact each other in each canine segment and one contact on each side of the midline in the incisor segment.

Retruded contact position (Fig. 19-14, *A*)

Examine the relationship of retruded contact position and intercuspal position. When they differ, what is the nature of the slide? Does the slide from retruded contact position to intercuspal position deviate to the left or to the right? Is the initial contact in retruded contact position unilateral or bilateral? Does the contact occur on molars or premolars?

A movement of more than 1 mm is classified as a long slide. How does the vertical component of the slide compare with the horizontal component? A flat slide is one where the horizontal component predominates. A steep slide is one where the vertical component predominates.

Slides that tend to be long or steep or lateral seem to cause more dysfunction than those that are short, flat, and straight. A unilateral contact in retruded contact position seems to be more damaging than bilateral contact and is worse as the initial contact involves teeth farther back in the posterior segment.

Opening-closing pattern (Fig. 19-14, *A*)

Steady the butt end of a millimeter ruler between the maxillary central incisors, and sight along the lateral edge of the ruler. Say to the patient: "Open straight down as wide as you can; then close on your back teeth." Observe the character of the pathway of the mandible as the patient opens and closes. The mandible should not deviate much to either side if the joints and musculature are normal and in orthofunction.

Steady the butt end of the ruler on a lower incisor at the midline to measure the maximum interincisal distance. Say to the patient: "Open your mouth, wider, as wide as you can." An opening of less than 40 mm indicates some form of restricted opening. If the opening can be stretched a few more millimeters, the cause is probably the result of myospasm.

Listen for sounds of the temporomandibular joints. Place a stethoscope over the lateral aspects of each joint as the patient opens and closes. A single sound seems to be more often associated with muscular dysfunction than with continuous noise. The prognosis is better from occlusal therapy if the click (pop) occurs in the early or intermediate phase of the opening. A late click often indicates some form of intrajoint disarrangement. Some type of joint deterioration or degeneration is suspected with continuous noises. Joint noise is often the first sign of dysfunction.

Excursive movements (Fig. 19-14, *B*)

Examine for tooth contacts in left lateral, right lateral, and protrusive movements from intercuspal position to the edge-to-edge positions. Any mediotrusive contact has the potential of causing dysfunction. This is also true to a lesser degree for interferences between any posterior teeth in protrusion. Laterotrusive contact of teeth in the posterior segment may be acceptable so long as no tooth contacts harder than a tooth in the canine segment. Any difficult or restricted movement of the mandible during the preceding phases of the examination should be suspected as a sign of some muscular dysfunction or mechanical blockage. A person should be able to protrude or move laterally from intercuspal position at least 8 mm.

Bruxofacets (Fig. 19-14, B)

The occluding surfaces of teeth are carefully examined for bruxofacets. Suspected areas are brought into contact. Say to the patient: "Bite hard on these teeth without letting your jaw move." Maintain up to 1 minute. Any discomfort or pain experienced is a positive provocation test. A positive response indicates a direct connection between the facet and the symptom and is then referred to as a symptom-provoking contact.

Oral-facial palpation (Fig. 19-14, *B*)

Systematic palpation of the muscles and their tendons is probably one of the best ways to diagnose both subclinical and clinical levels of dysfunction. The muscles are palpated bilaterally and simultaneously with firm but gentle pressure. The main pressure is exerted with the middle finger of each hand. The adjacent fingers may be used for the adjacent area.

Facing the patient, palpate the areas as indicated on the examination chart. A firm thrust of 1 to 2 seconds at each area is used. Watch for the palpebral reflex (blinking of the eyelid) which is a reliable positive response. For each area palpated, ask the patient: "Do you feel any difference between the two sides?" If the response is yes, ask: "'Does it hurt or is it just an increased sensation to pressure? If the response is hurt, ask: "Is it just tender or is it pain?" The positive responses are marked with a (1) if increased pressure, with a (2) if tender, or with a (3) for pain.

Be alert for habit patterns that may play a secondary role in causing dysfunction. Diagnostic casts* are a most helpful aid both in diagnosis and treatment planning. Many of the tooth relationships can be examined better on diagnostic casts. Projected occlusal treatment can be verified.

The composite findings in the questionnaire and clinical examination should make it possible to conclude whether the patient has orthofunctional occlusion, or is on the verge of developing dysfunctional problems or already has dysfunctional sequelae. The class 4 patient will have pain (usually unilateral), muscle tenderness, joint noise, and limited jaw opening.[11,13]

In summary, the clinical findings that tend to indicate mandibular dysfunction are as follows:

1. Sound phenomenon in one or both temporomandibular joints
2. Palpation soreness in the muscles that move and stabilize the mandible
3. Palpation soreness in one or both temporomandibular joints
4. Maximum opening less than 40 mm
5. Pain during mandibular movement
6. Deviation of midline on opening or closing

---

*Casts mounted on an articulator with a face-bow transfer and a centric-relation interocclusal record.

7. Positive provocation test
8. MCP ≠ IP

Oral habits (Fig. 19-14, *B*)

The following occlusal conditions seem to be the prime occlusal causes of mandibular dysfunction:

1. A poor intercuspal position
2. A muscle-tooth stabilization of the mandible in intercuspal position
3. A lack of anterior guidance
4. Unilateral contact in retruded contact position
5. A slide from retruded contact position to intercuspal position that is either asymmetric, long, or steep
6. Any mediotrusive contact
7. Laterotrusive guidance on molars
8. Deflective contact movements to and from the intercuspal position

OCCLUSAL DIAGNOSIS AND TREATMENT PLANNING

The extent and type of occlusal therapy will be dictated by the functional state of the mandibular system, existing dental conditions, what alterations are possible, and the amount of occlusal involvement necessitated by other restorative needs.

A limited fixed prosthodontic involvement is defined as consisting of no more than four restorations and does not include more than 75% of the teeth in any one posterior segment. An extensive fixed prosthodontic involvement is defined as any situation that includes all the occluding teeth in any one posterior segment or consists of at least five posterior restorations that involve three teeth in a posterior segment on one side and two teeth in a posterior segment on the other side.

All patients deserve to have a state of orthofunction. It is only on the basis of jaw function that you can determine whether the patient's occlusal relationships merit perpetuation in the restorative treatment or to what extent modifications should be made in the occlusal scheme.

A patient in orthofunction does not need occlusal therapy, that is, any alteration to his or her occlusal scheme. However, it is important to avoid introducing new occlusal interferences that may precipitate problems as restorative procedures are performed.

1. Typical patient A
   a. Is in orthofunction (class 1 or 2).
   b. Has limited fixed prosthodontic needs.
   c. May or may not have occlusal disharmonies.
   Typical treatment
   a. Maintain a good IP and the interrelationship of IP, MCP, and RCP.
   b. In general, maintain existing eccentric guidances. Guidance may be eliminated on teeth being restored in the posterior segments provided that a new guidance is not created more posteriorly.
   c. Reestablish normal tooth anatomy on the new restorations.
2. Typical patient B
   a. Is in mild dysfunction (Class 3).
   b. Has limited fixed prosthodontic needs.
   c. MCP ≠ IP.
   d. May have a poor IP.
   e. Frequently has mediotrusive contacts.
   f. Frequently has irregular contact movements.
   Typical treatment
   a. Remove symptom-provoking bruxofacets by selective grinding.
   b. Harmonize MCP and IP.
   c. Make the slide from RCP to IP short and even.
   d. Eliminate all mediotrusive contacts.
   e. Provide smooth guidance into and out of IP.
   f. The restorations are fabricated to perpetuate the modified occlusal scheme.
3. Typical patient C
   a. Is in orthofunction (class 2).
   b. Has extensive fixed prosthodontic needs.
   c. Usually has limited occlusal disharmonies—no pattern.

Typical treatment
   a. Maintain existing relations and restore each quadrant separately as with typical patient A
   b. Or create an optimal occlusal scheme (if attainable) by selected grinding.
   c. The restorations are fabricated to maintain and reinforce the new occlusal scheme.
4. Typical patient D
   a. Is in mild dysfunction (class 3)
   b. Has extensive fixed prosthodontic needs.
   c. Usually has a poor IP because of badly broken-down or missing teeth.
   d. Has other types of occlusal disharmonies in varying degrees.
   Typical treatment
   a. Create the framework for an optimal occlusal scheme by selective grinding, orthodontics, and trial (temporary) restorations as required.
   b. The restorations are fabricated to maintain and extend the new occlusal scheme.
5. Typical patient E
   a. Is in severe dysfunction (class 4) with little or no psychologic involvement.
   b. Has extensive or limited fixed prosthodontic needs.
   c. Has symptom-provoking occlusal contacts.
   Typical treatment
   a. The treatment initially should be simple and reversible. A suitable form of palliative therapy is selected. The final occlusal treatment may be extensive, moderate, limited, or none, depending on the type of response to the palliative therapy and other dental needs.
   b. The definitive restorations should be delayed until there is resolution of the significant signs and symptoms of dysfunction.
   c. The restorations are fabricated as with the typical patient B or D.
6. Typical patient F
   a. Is usually in dysfunction (class 3 or 4) with indications of psychologic involvement.
   b. Has limited or extensive fixed prosthodontic needs.

c. Has subjective symptoms that do not match the objective findings.

d. Has pain patterns and muscular-palpation findings that are too uniform and are bilateral in intensity.

Typical treatment

a. Does not change the occlusion.

b. Limits restorative dentistry to just maintaining the existing dentition in a state of good repair.

c. Involves possible referral to appropriate physician.

GUIDELINES FOR OCCLUSAL ADJUSTMENT AND OCCLUSAL THERAPY

When orthodontics is not indicated, occlusal adjustment by selected grinding is often the initial phase of occlusal therapy. The procedure may be limited to just the removal of the symptom-provoking contact or the creation of an optimal occlusal scheme and a different maxillomandibular relationship.

Occlusal therapy is usually performed on patients having some degree of dysfunction. However, treatment procedures necessitated by other existing dental conditions may require some degree of occlusal adjustment on patients in orthofunction.

The purpose of occlusal therapy is to reduce trauma from occlusion and to lower muscular hyperactivity. Regardless of how little or how much change is dictated, the following basic principles should be satisfied:

1. There should be a very precise intercuspal position that will permit joint-tooth stabilization of the mandible.

2. The intercuspal-position contacts should occur within 1 mm of the cusp tips and within 1 mm of the central groove area.

3. Do not reduce or eliminate anterior guidance when the intercuspal position is altered.

4. When intercuspal position and retruded contact position do not coincide, the slide from retruded contact position to intercuspal position should be made symmetric, even, and short.

5. Create contacts in retruded contact position and intercuspal position so that occlusal forces will be directed along the long axis of the teeth.

6. There should be a complete absence of mediotrusive contacts.

7. Establish smooth multidirectional contact movements to and from intercuspal position.

8. Return all occlusal and occluding surfaces to a spheroid form, void of any flat planes.

OCCLUSAL ADJUSTMENT BY SELECTIVE GRINDING

When selective grinding is indicated, the procedure should:

1. Eliminate the interceptive contacts or deflective occlusal contacts, or both.

2. Restore the teeth to contours similar to those of unworn teeth.

3. Eliminate factors that have dysfunction potential.

4. End up with relationships that will be self-sustaining.

The grinding procedure should consist of grooving, spheroiding, and pointing.[14]

Grooving should be the first and basic step of any selective grinding procedure. This is the only way that normal anatomy can be reestablished or maintained. When the interference is located on mesial cusp slopes of upper teeth and distal cusp slopes of lower teeth, the following procedure is followed: Make a groove in the mesial part of the interference on upper teeth and a groove in the distal part of the interference on lower teeth (Fig. 19-15, *B*). Grooves on surfaces involved in laterotrusive movements are made to generally run transversely across the tooth (Fig. 19-15, *A*). Grooves on surfaces involved in mediotrusive movements are made to run obliquely across the tooth (Fig. 19-15, *A*).

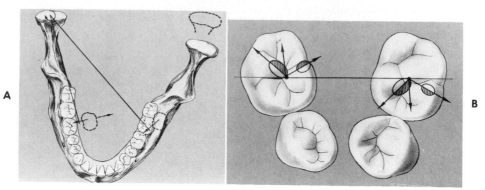

Fig. 19-15. A, During lateral movements of mandible, cuspal elements on laterotrusive side move transversely across opposing occlusal surface while cuspal elements on mediotrusive side move obliquely across opposing occlusal surface. **B,** Occlusal interferences are eliminated by grinding, on distal part of interference on mandibular teeth and on mesial part of interference on maxillary teeth. Transverse depressions (or grooves) are made on laterotrusive inclines, and oblique depressions (or grooves) are made on mediotrusive inclines *(shaded areas).* Diagrams only outline areas of interferences and area of corrections in inner inclines. For each interference on an inner incline, a corresponding interference will exist on an outer incline in opposite arch. The same principles of corrections are used on outer inclines.

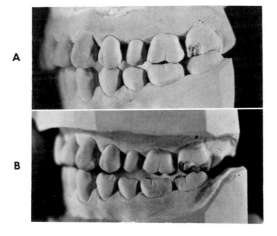

Fig. 19-16. A, Diagnostic casts where laterotrusive interferences occur between central parts of facial cusps in a class II relationship. **B,** Diagnostic casts after an occlusal adjustment by selective grinding. Main part of correction was done on mandibular teeth so that esthetics of maxillary cusps is maintained, yet a reciprocal arrangement of elevations and depressions is established.

When the interference involves the central part of cusps, the following procedure is used: Make two small grooves on each side of the interference on the upper tooth, and then make one large groove in the center of the interference on the lower tooth.

When the interference occurs on unworn areas, always deepen a groove on each side of the ridge that is in premature contact. Then reduce the ridge.

The principle of *spheroiding* is used on the area of the interference not being grooved to either recreate or maintain ridges. The procedure is integrated with the grooving technique to develop a ridge lateral to each groove that is made. A reciprocal arrangement of elevations and depressions is created between the opposing tooth surfaces (Fig. 19-16).

The *pointing* phase consists of reshaping the support cusp tip to a normal form in a location to provide the best position possible for the associated intercuspal-position contact. The cusp tip may be ground to reposition the tip up to 1 mm in any direction. The tip of the cusp is made to migrate toward the opposing central groove alignment and toward mesial parts of upper teeth and distal parts of lower teeth.

The three steps are combined into one smooth operation when carried out clinically.

The method for an occlusal adjustment must be correlated with a specific plan. As outlined, the adjustment procedure is intended to produce a cusp-fossa arrangement of the posterior teeth with intercuspal position at centric relation. Specifically, lower cusps are in upper mesial and central fossae, and upper cusps are in lower distal and central fossae. The interceptive contacts are corrected by reshaping of the surfaces that will come closest to this arrangement. The newly created intercuspal position should be more cranial than the previous intercuspal position. Eccentrically, contact should involve only teeth in the incisor or canine segments. A complete occlusal adjustment of the natural dentition is divided into six steps.

Smile line

The first step of an occlusal adjustment should be aimed at refining the maxillary smile line, which extends from the maxillary first molar on one side around to the first molar on the other side. The incisal edges of the maxillary six anterior teeth should present a smooth-flowing convex-downward curvature, somewhat following the outline of the lower lip during smiling. The facial cusp tips of the first molar, both premolars, and the canine should fall on a straight plane. The cusp tips of these teeth should fall about in the center of each cusp lobe. Make any correction possible by selective grinding.

Retruded contact position

The most difficult part of this phase of occlusal adjustment is mastering a tech-

nique that will consistently and rapidly get the condyles in a functionally seated position. The technique advocated by Dawson[4] works well but takes a lot of training and practice. Any procedure entirely under the control of the dentist is often subject to his own beliefs and perceptions and is more subject to errors.[15]

The technique as advocated by Long[16,16a] permits the patient to position the mandible with little or no assistance from the dentist. A leaf gage made of 10 strips of 0.01-inch acetate is used. The strips are ½ inch wide and 2 inches long and are held together with a rivet at one end.

The leaf gage is placed between the anterior teeth and the patient is asked: "Bite on your back teeth." The minimum number of leaves are used to prevent any tooth contact. Maintain the biting pressure for up to 1 minute. If teeth come into contact, add additional leaves and repeat the procedure. Continue until the relationship stabilizes for 1 minute. The mandible is now ready to start the adjustment procedure. Folds of chamois skin can be substituted for the leaf gage.

Reduce the number of leaves until the first tooth contact is encountered. Place articulating paper between the offending teeth, insert the leaf gage between the anterior teeth and say to the patient: "Bite on your back teeth." Then say to the patient: "Grind your teeth together in a forward and backward motion." The interfering surfaces are ground and the procedure is repeated with one less leaf. One leaf after another is removed until only one remains.

The interceptive contacts in retrusive contact position are eliminated by grooving, spheroiding, and pointing in the following manner:

If the support cusps are not aligned within the desired opposing fossa, corrections are made on the cusp slope or incline to more nearly place the cusp within the fossa. If more correction is needed after the support cusp has been reshaped and realigned the full 1 mm, the fossa is then altered to provide a better seat for the cusp. If the cusp and fossa are in alignment and additional adjustment is needed, either the fossa is deepened or the cusp is shortened—whichever element is least normal or most out of harmony with the other like elements in the arch. Occasionally, cusps and fossae will be so mismatched that a depression will have to be made on a support cusp to serve as a fossa for the opposing support cusp.

As the interceptive contacts in centric relation are ground, aim to eliminate flat surfaces (facets of wear) and reestablish (accentuate) the elements of occlusion. This should result in spheroid ridges. If the occlusal table broadens during the grinding, reshape the outer inclines to bring the width back to normal. The average width of the occlusal table is 5 mm. Continue removing interceptive contacts in centric relation until the slide has been eliminated. Then, evaluate the relationship of the anterior teeth in centric relation.

If the anterior teeth are not in contact, but were prior to the adjustment procedure, continue the adjustment until at least as many anterior teeth are in light contact after adjustment as contacted prior to adjustment.

Lateral excursion

Make a lateral contact movement from intercuspal position to the edge-to-edge position in the canine segment. There should be a single contact between a pair of teeth (usually the canines) in this position. The optimum clearance of the other teeth is 1 mm.

If any posterior teeth interfere or contact in this contact movement, remove the tooth structure as follows:

Laterotrusive side adjustment. If the interference involves a malaligned tooth, remove the tooth structure until that tooth

has been brought back into harmony. Eliminate other interceptive contacts between facets on cusp slopes by making a *transverse depression* in the distal part of the interference on lower teeth and a *transverse depression* in the mesial part of the interference on the upper teeth (Fig. 19-16). All other corrections are usually made on the shear cusps. If the reshaping of the upper shear cusp will detract from the esthetic value of these cusps, corrections are continued on the lower support cusp.

Mediotrusive side adjustment. If the interference involves a malaligned tooth, remove the tooth structure until the tooth has been brought back into harmony. All other corrections are done on support cusps in the following manner: The *mesial* portion of the interceptive contact is eliminated from the *upper tooth* by making a *mesiolingual oblique* groove. The *distal* portion of the interceptive contact is eliminated from the *lower tooth* by making a *distofacial oblique groove* (Fig. 19-16). Repeat the procedure for the opposite lateral excursion.

Protrusive incising position

Test the incisor segment in the edge-to-edge position. There should be bilateral contact in this segment with little or no lateral shift of the mandible. A shift usually means a posterior interference or an asymmetric incisal plane.

If any posterior teeth interfere or contact in the edge-to-edge position, remove the tooth structure from the offending shear cusps until all contact between the posterior teeth has been eliminated. The support cusp is ground on any tooth out of harmony with the occlusal plane.

If the incisor contact is unilateral and correction is desirable, the reshaping is usually made by shortening of the offending maxillary tooth. Do nothing to harm the esthetics or mutilate the teeth. As corrections are made, round over all facets.

Occasionally, an open-bite situation

will not permit edge-to-edge contact of the anterior segments. Establish bilateral contact as far forward as possible.

Round over any facets on teeth in the anterior segment without shortening the clinical crowns.

Make a retrusive contact movement back to the intercuspal position. If the path deviates laterally very much, adjustment is needed to straighten out the path. If a posterior tooth is the cause, correct on shear cusps by grinding either distal slopes of upper teeth or mesial slopes of lower teeth. If an anterior tooth is the cause, correct on the lingual of the upper tooth.

Functional adjustment

If eccentric lateral adjustment is limited to empty-mouth slidings, there may remain interferences that become active only during mastication or bruxism. Strips of chamois skin are used to produce masticatory-like movements. Start with two or three thicknesses of chamois and work down to one thickness. Say to the patient: "Chew the leather bolus on one side." Mark any contacting teeth with articulating paper.

Elimination of the mediotrusive contacts is made to sharpen the cusps and widen the grooves on support cusps without disturbing any intercuspal-position contacts. Laterotrusive contacts are corrected on shear cusps. Anterior contact is corrected by making more of a concavity on the lingual surfaces of the maxillary teeth. Continue the adjustment until no teeth contact when they chew on one thickness of chamois skin.

Repeat the procedure for the opposite side.

Equalization of intercuspal-position contacts

All the teeth that contact in intercuspal position should meet simultaneously without any facial or lingual impact or thrust of the teeth or any skid of the mandible.

With the patient in a reclining position, say to the patient: "Close gently on your back teeth." "Do you feel any teeth that touch harder than any others?" If there is any difference, mark the teeth and adjust until the patient cannot feel any difference. Next, have the patient tap together rapidly on the posterior teeth. Feel each maxillary tooth with the tip of a finger to see if any fremitus can be detected. If so, mark and adjust the involved teeth until no difference in impact can be felt. Check each pair of occluding teeth with a 1 mil Mylar tape to verify the intercuspal-position contacts.

The patient is then seated in the upright position and the above procedures are repeated. This additional step is necessary to make sure that intercuspal position is correlated with jaw-closing movements from this postural position.

The completed adjustment should have light contact between anterior teeth, tight contact between as many posterior teeth as possible, and unrestricted eccentric glide paths of posterior cusps.

In cases of extreme difference between centric relation and intercuspal position, open anterior bites, or other questionable situations, it is most desirable that a cast analysis be performed to ensure that the desired adjustment procedures are reasonable and the aims can be accomplished. Each case must be evaluated on its own merits.

PALLIATIVE PROCEDURES

There are a number of palliative procedures that may be useful in reducing or eliminating dysfunctional symptoms.[1,13,17-19] These procedures are usually used to relieve acute pain and spasm for the class 4 patient. The type of patient in whom palliative procedures are needed fits into a special category and is outside the scope of this chapter.

Some of the more common approaches are listed as follows:

1. Talking with the patient is often

helpful. Explain the nature of the problem and outline how the physical and psychologic components affect muscle response. Show empathy.
2. Soft foods.
3. Good sleeping conditions.
4. A conscious effect to eliminate all clenching and gnashing.
5. Hot and cold packs to acute muscular areas.
6. Jaw exercises.
7. Drugs.
8. Occlusal splints.

Occlusal splints may be useful for typical patient D to check adequate adaptation when a new vertical dimension of occlusion is required or to test new horizontal relations or to evaluate a new scheme of tooth guidance. A splint may be useful for typical patient E to lower muscular hyperactivity before beginning definitive procedures. It is useful to help stabilize the maxillomandibular relationship and should be used anytime there is any question about this relationship. In any case, the splint should be constructed of hard acrylic resin and must fit very accurately and reproduce very precisely the occlusal relations being tested.

POSTINSERTION GOALS

The essential features of the occlusal scheme are established before starting the fixed prosthodontic procedures. Make sure these are maintained when the new restorations are adjusted. The restorations are carefully checked to make sure they fill in any missing links in the occlusal scheme.

Before inserting the new restoration, check the other teeth to see which ones contact in intercuspal position and which ones provide tooth guidance. Insert the restoration and verify the occlusal relations of the other teeth. If they change, then the new restoration needs to be adjusted. In addition, the new restoration should:

1. Maintain a precise intercuspal position.
2. Provide a joint-tooth stabilization of the mandible in intercuspal position and retruded contact position.
3. Not cause unilateral retrusive interferences.
4. Not cause mediotrusive interferences.
5. Not restrict entry into and out of intercuspal position for all eccentric contact movements.
6. Not restrict condylar movement against the articular eminence.

Maintain the occlusal scheme that encourages orthofunction. Remember, occlusal disharmonies do not have to be gross to cause functional disturbances. Low-level, chronic microtrauma will cause dysfunction.

Occlusal management requires a thorough diagnosis based on a complete history and a well-made physical examination of the functional parts. Care must be exercised not to see a disorder where one does not exist or to fail to recognize a disorder that is present. Any change in the occluding surface of a tooth, whether by movement, decay, or restorations has the potential to modify sensory input for muscle response. The ability of the sensory system to detect change is often more acute than our clinical abilities. We must be very careful and precise in our clinical procedures.

SELECTED REFERENCES

1. Schwartz, L., and Chayes, C. M.: Facial pain and mandibular dysfunction, Philadelphia, 1968, W. B. Saunders Co.
2. Beyron, H.: Optimal occlusion, Dent. Clin. North Am. **13:**537, July 1969.
3. Huffman, R. W., Regenos, J. W., and Taylor, R. R.: Principles of occlusion, laboratory and clinical teaching manual, Ohio State University, Columbus, Ohio, 1969, H. & R. Press.
4. Dawson, P. E.: Temporomandibular joint pain-dysfunction problems can be solved, J. Prosthet. Dent. **29:**100-112, 1973.
5. Owens, S. E., Lehr, R. P., and Biggs, N. L.: The functional significance of centric relation as demonstrated by electromyography of the

lateral pterygoid muscles, J. Prosthet. Dent. **33:**5-9, 1975.

6. Moffett, B.: The morphogenesis of the temporomandibular joint, Am. J. Orthodont. **52:** 401-415, 1966.
7. Boucher, C. O., editor: Current clinical dental terminology, St. Louis, 1963, The C. V. Mosby Co.
8. Weinberg, L. A.: Anterior condylar displacement: its diagnosis and treatment, J. Prosthet. Dent. **34:**195-207, 1975.
9. Hodge, L. C., and Mahan, P. E.: A study of mandibular movement from centric occlusion to maximum intercuspation, J. Prosthet. Dent. **18:**19-30, 1967.
10. McAdams, D. B.: Tooth loading and cuspal guidance in canine and group function occlusion, J. Prosthet. Dent. **35:**283-290, 1976.
11. Travel, J.: Temporomandibular joint pain referred from muscles of the head and neck, J. Prosthet. Dent. **10:**745-763, 1960.
12. Wooten, J. W.: Diagnosis of the pain-dysfunction syndrome, J. Prosthet. Dent. **14:**961-966, 1964.
13. Dachi, S. F.: Diagnosis and management of temporomandibular joint dysfunction syndrome, J. Prosthet. Dent. **20:**53-61, 1968.
14. Glickman, I.: Clinical periodontology, ed. 4, Philadelphia, 1972, W. B. Saunders Co.
15. Kantor, M. E., Silverman, S. I., and Garfinkel, L.: Centric-relation recording techniques—a comparative investigation, J. Prosthet. Dent. **28:**593-600, 1972.
16. Long, J. H.: Occlusal adjustment, J. Prosthet. Dent. **30:**706-714, 1973.
16a. Long, J. H.: Locating centric relation with a leaf gauge, J. Prosthet. Dent. **29:**608-610, 1973.
17. Gangarosa, L. P.: Pharmacology of agents used to treat temporomandibular joint problems, J. Prosthet. Dent. **30:**80-86, 1973.
18. Ramfjord, S. P., and Ash, M. M., Jr.: Occlusion, ed. 2, Philadelphia, 1971, W. B. Saunders Co.
19. Wooten, J. W.: Treatment of the pain-dysfunction syndrome, J. Prosthet. Dent. **14:**967-974, 1964.
20. Perry, H. T., Jr.: The symptomology of temporomandibular joint disturbance, J. Prosthet. Dent. **19:**288-298, 1968.

GENERAL REFERENCES

Agnew, R. G.: Differential diagnosis of dental pain, Dent. Clin. North Am., pp. 271-286, March 1963.
Allen, D. L., and McFall, W. T.: An appraisal of temporomandibular joint pain—dysfunction, J. North Carolina Dent. Soc. **51:**11, April 1968.
Alling, C. C., and Burton, H. N.: Differential diagnosis of chronic orofacial pain, J. Prosthet. Dent. **31:**66, Jan. 1974.
Bell, W. E.: Management of masticatory pain. In

Alling, C. C.: Facial pain, Philadelphia, 1968, Lea & Febiger.
Bell, W. E.: Clinical diagnosis of the pain-dysfunction syndrome, J.A.D.A. **79:**154, July 1969.
Bell, W. H.: Nonsurgical management of the pain-dysfunction syndrome, J.A.D.A. **79:**161, July 1969.
Beyron, M. L.: Characteristics of functionally optimal occlusion and principles of occlusal rehabilitation, J.A.D.A. **48:**648, 1954.
DeBoever, J. A.: Functional disturbances of the T.M.J., Oral Science Rev. **2:**106-107, 1973.
Franks, A. S.: Masticatory muscle hyperactivity and temporomandibular joint dysfunction, J. Prosthet. Dent. **15:**1122, 1965.
Freese, A. S.: Temporomandibular joint pain: etiology, symptomatology and diagnosis, J. Prosthet. Dent. **10:**1083-1084, Nov.-Dec. 1960.
Freese, A. S.: The temporomandibular joint and myofacial trigger areas in the dental diagnosis of pain, J.A.D.A. **59:**449, 1959.
Gelb, M., Calderone, J. P., Gross, S. M., and Kantor, M. E.: The role of the dentist and the otolaryngologist in evaluating temporomandibular joint syndromes, J. Prosthet. Dent. **18(5):**497, 1967.
Graf, H., and Zander, H. A.: Tooth contact patterns in mastication, J. Prosthet. Dent. **13:**1055, 1963.
Granger, E. R.: Functional relations of the stomatognathic system, J.A.D.A. **48:**638, 1954.
Greene, C. S., and Laskin, D.: The TMJ pain-dysfunction syndrome: heterogeneity of the patient population, J.A.D.A. **79:**1170, Nov. 1969.
Henny, F. A.: Surgical treatment of the painful temporomandibular joint, J.A.D.A. **79:**171-174, July 1969.
Husted, E.: Surgical management of temporomandibular joint disorders, Dent. Clin. North Am., pp. 601-607, Nov. 1966.
Jagger, R. B.: Diazepam in the treatment of temporomandibular joint syndrome—a double blind study, J. Dent. **2:**37-40, Oct. 1973.
Jankelson, B.: Physiology of human dental occlusion, J.A.D.A. **50:**664, 1955.
Jankelson, B., Hoffman, G. M., and Hendron, J. A., Jr.: The physiology of the stomatognathic system, J.A.D.A. **46:**375, 1953.
Jarabak, J. R.: Electromyographic analysis of muscular and temporomandibular joint disturbances due to imbalances in occlusion, Angle Orthodont. **24:**170, 1956.
Kaplan, R. I.: Concepts of occlusion; gnathology as a basis for a concept of occlusion, Dent. Clin. North Am., pp. 577 and 649, Nov. 1963.
Kraus, H. T.: Muscle function and the temporomandibular joint, J. Prosthet. Dent. **13:**1950, Sept.-Oct. 1963; Dent. Clin. North Am., pp. 553-558, Nov. 1966.
Kornfeld, M.: Mouth rehabilitation—clinical and laboratory procedures, ed. 2, St. Louis, 1974, The C. V. Mosby Co., vol. 2.

Krough-Poulsen, W. G., and Olsson, A.: Occlusal disharmonies and dysfunction of the stomatognathic system, Dent. Clin. North Am., pp. 627-635, Nov. 1966.

Kydd, W. L.: Psychosomatic aspects of temporomandibular joint dysfunction, J.A.D.A. **79:**131, July 1959.

Laskin, D. M.: Etiology of the pain-dysfunction syndrome, J.A.D.A. **79:**148, July 1969.

Laskin, D. M., and Greene, C. S.: Correlation of placebo responses and psychological characteristics in myofascial pain-dysfunction patients, Int. Assoc. Dent. Res. Abst. No. **282:**119, 1970.

Lucia, V. O.: The gnathological concept of articulation, Dent. Clin. North Am., pp. 183-197, March 1962.

Lupton, D. E.: Psychological aspects of temporomandibular joint dysfunction, J.A.D.A. **79:**131, July 1969.

McCall, C. M., Jr., Szmyd, L., and Ritter, R. M.: Personality characteristics in patients with temporomandibular joint symptoms, J.A.D.A. **62:**694, 1961.

Moulton, R. E.: Psychological considerations in the treatment of occlusion, J. Prosthet. Dent. **7:**148, March 1957.

Moulton, R. E.: Emotional factors in non-organic temporomandibular joint pain, Dent. Clin. North Am., pp. 609-619, Nov. 1966.

Moyers, R. E.: An electromyographic analysis of certain muscles involved in temporomandibular movement, Am. J. Orthodont. **36:**481, 1950.

Moyers, R. E.: Some physiologic considerations of centric and other jaw relations, J. Prosthet. Dent. **6:**183, 1956.

Nehlmeyer, C.: Results of a centrally acting muscle relaxant in myogenic inflammatory types of trismus, Oral Surg. **9:**9-11, Sept. 1970.

Perry, H. T.: The symptomology of temporomandibular joint disturbance, J. Prosthet. Dent. **19:**289-293, March 1968.

Perry, H. T., and Harris, S. C.: Role of the neuromuscular system in functional activity of the mandible, J.A.D.A. **48:**665, 1954.

Perry, H. T., Jr.: Muscular changes associated with temporomandibular joint dysfunction, J.A.D.A. **54:**644, 1957.

Posselt, U.: The physiology of occlusion and rehabilitation, Philadelphia, 1962, F. A. Davis Co.

Prentiss, H. J.: A preliminary report upon the temporo-mandibular articulation in the human type, Dent. Cosmos **60:**505, 1918.

Ramfjord, S. P., and Ash, M. M.: Occlusion, Philadelphia, 1971, W. B. Saunders Co.

Ramfjord, S. P.: Bruxism: a clinical and electromyographic study, J.A.D.A. **62:**21, 1961.

Ramfjord, S.: Dysfunctional temporomandibular joint and muscle pain, J. Prosthet. Dent. **11:**353, 1961.

Rees, L. A.: The structure and function of the mandibular joint, Br. Dent. J. **96:**125-133, March 1954.

Ricketts, R. M.: Laminagraphy in the diagnosis of temporomandibular joint disorders, J.A.D.A. **46:**620, June 1953.

Schwartz, L.: Disorders of the temporomandibular joint, Philadelphia, 1959, W. B. Saunders Co.

Schwartz, L. L., and Cobin, H. P.: Symptoms associated with temporomandibular joint, Oral Surg. **10:**399, April 1957.

Schwartz, L.: Conclusions of the temporomandibular joint clinic at Columbia, J. Periodont. **29:**210, July 1958.

Schwartz, L. L.: Ethyl chloride treatment of limited painful mandibular movement, J.A.D.A. **48:**497-507, 1954.

Shore, N. A.: Occlusal equilibration and temporomandibular joint dysfunction, Philadelphia, 1959, J. B. Lippincott Co.

Thompson, J. R.: Temporomandibular disorders: diagnosis and treatment. In Sarnat, B. G.: The temporomandibular joint, Springfield, Ill., 1964, Charles C Thomas, Publisher.

Travell, J.: Temporomandibular joint pain referred from muscles of the head and neck, J. Prosthet. Dent. **10:**745-746, July-Aug. 1960.

Uotila, E., and Kotilainen, R.: Clinical and roentgenologic manifestations of the temporomandibular joint in a dental clinic material, Odontol. Tidskr. **76:**138-145, March 1968.

Updegrave, W.: Evaluation of temporomandibular joint roentgenography, J.A.D.A. **46:**408, April 1953.

Ware, W. H., and Taylor, R. C.: Management of temporomandibular joint disorders, Dent. Clin. North Am., pp. 124-140, March 1968.

Yemm, R.: A comparison of the electrical activity of masseter and temporal muscles of human subjects during experimental stress, Arch. Oral Biol. **16:**269, 1971.

20

Cementing media in restorative dentistry

Gordon J. Christensen

For over 140 years cements resembling those in current usage have been available in dentistry. Weston's Insoluble Cement was introduced in approximately 1880[1] and the Ostermann formula of 1832[2] was the forerunner of the current types of zinc phosphate cement. These cements were similar to certain brands in use today. Weston's cement contained zinc oxide about 81% and aluminum silicate about 19%, and, as today, the liquid was phosphoric acid. In the many years that have passed since the introduction of the zinc phosphate type of cement, significant scientific and technologic advances have been made in nearly all areas of endeavor, and it is inconceivable to the author that dental cements have remained so relatively undeveloped. Nevertheless, there have been some advancements and changes in dental cements over those years and time has allowed the careful clinical evaluation of most of the types of cements.

There are five categories of dental cements in use today for luting inlays, crowns, and bridges to teeth. These are zinc phosphate, zinc polycarboxylate, zinc oxide–eugenol, zinc silicophosphate, and resin. It is apparent that four of these cements contain zinc oxide as one ingredient and that only one cement is significantly different from the others. At this time a new category of cements, glass ionomers, are being introduced. Several

years will be needed to prove their usefulness.

The retention of restorations to teeth has been achieved primarily by mechanical interlocking of pieces of cement into irregularities on the internal surfaces of the fabricated restorations and the cavity preparation surfaces. However, tne polycarboxylate cements have been shown to adhere to calcified tissues by means of a chemical attraction to calcium ions in addition to mechanical interlocking. The introduction of polycarboxylate cements marked the first real change in the mechanism of attachment of cements to teeth since the original development of dental cements. Such true adhesion appears to be desirable because of its potential lessening of microleakage between the tooth and the restoration.

Proportionate use of the various types of cements has been changing considerably in recent years. At the time of this writing the polycarboxylate cements appear to be used to about the same degree or slightly more than zinc phosphate cements. The zinc oxide–eugenol cements are used to a limited degree, and the zinc silicophosphate and resin cements are used only slightly. The degree of use of each type of cement by practitioners is a guide to its popularity and perceived value. During a few years' time, polycarboxylate cements have achieved significant popularity. Despite their popularity, dentists have expressed concern about these cements also.

There are real, unfilled needs in the area of dental cements. Dentists have gone to extensive efforts to make well-fitting cast restorations in an attempt to lessen the cement line exposed to oral fluids. However, clinicians know that the perfect seal of a metal restoration to dental enamel is nearly impossible and that they achieve only a small measure of perfection at the margins. Crown preparations are made to have nearly parallel walls to lessen the chance of dislodging restorations, but dentists do not really know how much retention is needed to resist dislodgment. Stronger, more adhesive, and less soluble or insoluble cements could partially eliminate the currently unfulfilled quest for perfect margins and nearly parallel preparations. In the meantime, dentistry is faced with ever-increasing use of five much less than perfect cements.

This chapter discusses briefly the physical characteristics of the cements as they relate to clinical applications and emphasizes the actual use of each cement in day-to-day fixed prosthodontics.

PROPERTIES OF CEMENTS
Zinc phosphate cement (Fig. 20-1)

The major advantage of zinc phosphate cement is that it has been used for many years. Therefore dentists have become accustomed to its use and know what to expect in most circumstances. These expectations are scientifically and empirically documented,[3,4] and they have guided the development of various concepts about cavity preparations, length of bridges, margin placement, and other factors in fixed prosthodontics.

Zinc phosphate cements in current usage contain zinc oxide and magnesium oxide in the approximate ratio of 9 to 1.[5] The water content is about 33%. The liquid is approximately 50% phosphoric

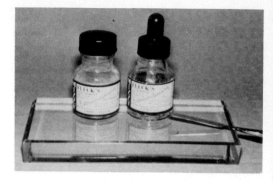

Fig. 20-1. Zinc phosphate cement and its characteristics are well known to dentists and dental assistants. This cement should be mixed slowly on a cool glass slab for optimal incorporation of powder and liquid.

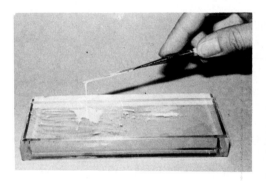

Fig. 20-2. Optimal thickness of zinc phosphate cement mix has been used as a guide when mixing certain other cements. Typical ½- to ¾-inch string of cement following spatula is shown here.

acid buffered by aluminum and sometimes zinc salts. When set, the cement may be described as particles held together by the phosphates. It is commonly known that the more powder and the less phosphates present in a given mix of zinc phosphate cement, the stronger the set cement will be.[6]

With experience, zinc phosphate cement is relatively easy to manipulate. The assistant cools a thick glass slab and incorporates small increments of powder into the cement liquid by mixing powder and liquid together with a wide circular motion on about one half of the glass slab. When the mixture follows the spatula about ½ to ¾ inch from the glass slab, the mixture is ready to be used as a luting medium (Fig. 20-2).

Two major undesirable characteristics are generally attributed to zinc-phosphate cement. The cement appears to have a bad effect on the dental pulp.[7] Nevertheless, recent investigations[8] have indicated that the irritation caused by the cement may be attributable to a "residual film of grinding debris containing bacteria and/or a poor seal between the cement filling and the dentin resulting in leakage of bacteria from the oral cavity to a space between the cement and the cavity walls." This study further states that "zinc phosphate cement per se does not irritate the pulp." Clinicians and patients have observed the immediate pain associated with the cementation of restorations with zinc phosphate cement when anesthesia is not used. However, the real, long-term clinical significance of this alleged pulpal irritation is not well documented. Since zinc phosphate has been used for over 100 years and dentists continue to use it, logic tells one that these dentists do not observe the routine death of pulp or they would discontinue the use of the cement. The elimination of pain on cementation and the overcoming of the uncertainty of undesirable long-term pulpal damage after cementation would be welcomed by the profession. Solubility has been described as a problem with zinc phosphate cement.[9] Certainly a cement that is insoluble in mouth fluids would be very desirable. The dental cements in major use have similar poor solubility characteristics.

Anticariogenic properties would be helpful in a dental cement. Zinc phosphate does not have this characteristic, despite the addition of various fluoride compounds to the cement.

Why has zinc phosphate cement continued in general usage? Its compressive

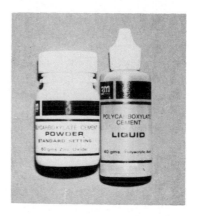

Fig. 20-3. One example of many brands of polycarboxylate cements is 3M Polycarboxylate Cement. The use of one brand over another is related to personal preference more than specific significant differences.

strength ranges from 9,000 to 20,000 p.s.i. with an average value of about 13,000 p.s.i.[10] This wide variation in strength is related to the quantity of powder added to the liquid. The more important characteristic of tensile strength is about 720 p.s.i.[11] However, who knows how much strength is needed? Gilson and Myers[12] have stated that a compressive strength of 8,000 p.s.i. is adequate for retention of cast restorations, but every dentist prepares teeth differently, and, further, there are many types of accepted preparations, each with different retentive characteristics. Zinc phosphate cement has survived despite its described weaknesses. Because of its long-standing use, newer cements are usually compared to it. This chapter will contain some comparisons of zinc phosphate with other cements.

Zinc polycarboxylate cement (Fig. 20-3)

This dental cement has become very popular since its introduction in 1968.[13] This rapid and continued acceptance is evidence of the usefulness of the cement. Numerous research and clinical reports have appeared on the cement, and evidence about its characteristics is now becoming more well known.[14,15] The compressive strength is about one half or more that of zinc phosphate cement, whereas the tensile strength is about the same as zinc phosphate cement. Solubility of carboxylate cements is about the same as that of zinc phosphate, but neither one is adequate. The film thickness of these cements is approximately ±20 μm, which is similar to zinc phosphate.

There are two advantages of this type of cement over zinc phosphate. First, the cement is not irritating to the dental pulp when observed histologically.[16,17] Practitioners have observed this bland nature of the cement clinically. Although the pH of polycarboxylate is similar to that of zinc phosphate cement at the time of cementation,[14] the cement does not cause a pain response when one cements without the use of anesthesia. Second, the cement is the only popular dental material that bonds to tooth structure. Although the actual adhesion of carboxylates to enamel, and in a lesser way to dentin, has

been demonstrated,[13,18] the clinical significance of this bonding has yet to be proved. The forces required to remove inlays cemented with carboxylates were no greater than the forces required for zinc phosphate cement. However, the nature of the breaking of the cement was different. The cement actually adheres to the tooth and the fracture occurs most commonly at the cement-metal junction or within the cement itself. Although the retention of restorations is not increased over zinc phosphate, it is not decreased either, and the seal between the cement and the tooth may decrease future leakage. Further research is required on this subject.

It has been shown[19] that cleaning the surfaces of gold alloys with an airborne abrasive increases the adhesion of polycarboxylate cement to the metal. This appears to have clinical significance and should be considered when using this cement.

Some clinicians have objected to the

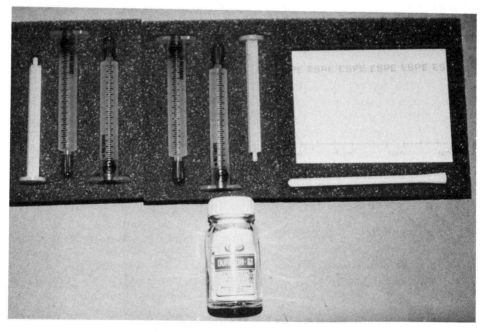

Fig. 20-4. Problem stated by many polycarboxylate cement users has been the relatively uncontrolled thickness of mixed cement. This device introduced by makers of Durelon has allowed easier proportioning of powder and liquid.

thick nature of polycarboxylates as mixed to the manufacturer's specifications. Further, the polycarboxylate liquids became more viscous with time, and it was difficult to determine the actual thickness that could be attributed to the addition of the powder. A measuring device introduced by the manufacturers of Durelon has assisted in controlling the thickness of the mix (Fig. 20-4). The device, resembling a syringe and containing the liquid, allows a more accurate proportioning of powder and liquid for these cements. Mixes that are too thick should be avoided. A correct mix of polycarboxylate cement should resemble the previously described and well-known correct mix of zinc phosphate cements. The cement should follow the cement spatula about ½ to ¾ inch when the spatula is moved upward rapidly. However, mixing the powder and liquid together slowly or mixing on a glass slab is not necessary, since its reaction is very different from the zinc phosphate reaction. The working time with these cements is short—2 to 3 minutes. Therefore the use of these cements is limited to short-span bridges because of working time.

This popular type of cement has been accepted well by practitioners, and if used properly and with care, it has the described advantages. Specific uses are described later.

Zinc oxide–eugenol cement (Fig. 20-5)

Because of the non–pulpal irritating property of these cements, there has been effort exerted to reinforce them sufficiently to allow their use as permanent cements. Polymers have been added[12] and *ortho*-ethoxybenzoic acid (EBA), quartz, and alumina[20] have also been substituted in the mix. The result has been that the strength values for these cements[11] are apparently acceptable for certain cementation tasks. The compressive strength of the reinforced zinc oxide–eugenol cements is in the range of one

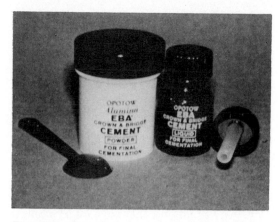

Fig. 20-5. Numerous brands of reinforced zinc oxide–eugenol cements are available. They offer moderate strength and lack of pulpal irritation.

half that of zinc phosphate, whereas the tensile strength is nearly the same as zinc phosphate. Their values are similar to the average values for polycarboxylate cements.

The solubility of the reinforced zinc oxide–eugenol cements has been reported to be in the range of zinc-phosphate cement.[11] However, certain questions concerning the continual leakage of eugenol from the cements have been raised.[21]

The major advantage of reinforced zinc oxide–eugenol cements for final cementation is their palliative effect on the dental pulp. They appear to have no other advantages. Although these cements are not in wide use for permanent cementation, certain practitioners[22] have accepted and supported their routine use.

Zinc silicophosphate cements (Fig. 20-6)

This cement is a combination of silicate and zinc phosphate, and its properties lie in between the expected properties of silicate and zinc phosphate.[23] The advantages of zinc silicophosphate cement appear to be its greater strength and increased translucence when compared to zinc phosphate and its fluoride content,

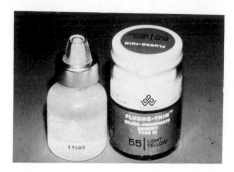

Fig. 20-6. Zinc silicophosphate cement has been useful for very caries-active patients and for those situations where maximum strength characteristics are desirable.

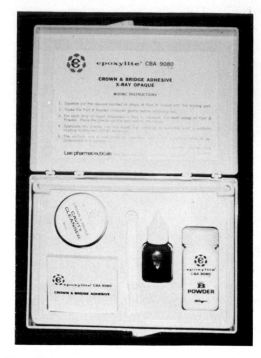

Fig. 20-7. Composite resin cement is very strong, but it has pulp-irritating qualities. Many dentists have used this type of cement to recement old bridges and to cement restorations on endodontically treated teeth.

which provides a potential cariostatic effect.[24] One of the difficulties with the zinc silicophosphate cements has been film thickness. Past forms of this cement have been quite thick and did not allow crowns to seat completely. A new formulation of the cement introduced by S. S. White called "Fluoro-Thin" has a greatly reduced film thickness. Its compressive strength is significantly greater than that of zinc phosphate cement, and it has the potential anticariogenic property afforded by the fluoride content. Further it is available in several hues, which allow better blending of colors under porcelain inlays or jacket crowns. One researcher[25] questions the film thickness of this cement and has stated that its film thickness is excessive. Dentists interested in using the cement should evaluate the film thickness to see if it satisfies their needs. These cements have been reported to have similar solubility to that of zinc phosphate, but this solubility may be advantageous because of the fluoride release and potential cariostatic action. The pulpal reaction to zinc silicophosphate is similar to that of zinc phosphate cement.

The silicophosphate cements appear to be best suited for use in caries-active mouths and under certain ceramic restorations.

Resin cement (Fig. 20-7)

Acrylic resin has had minimal use as a luting material since its introduction for this purpose. However, the composite resins have been suggested for luting. An example is Epoxylite CBA 9080, a crown and bridge adhesive manufactured by Lee Pharmaceuticals. This cement has been reported to have very high strength characteristics when compared with other dental cements.[26] The material is also insoluble in normal mouth fluids. The manufacturer has suggested that the tooth preparation be etched with 50% citric acid before cementing with the resin. Various reports[8,27] on the pulpal irritating potential of these procedures have been published. These reports indicate that a pulpal irritation is produced by the acid-etching or the cement itself, or the bacterial products that form at the cement-tooth interface. Another investigator[25] has questioned the film thickness of this type of cement, stating that it is excessive.

Nevertheless, the high-strength properties and insolubility of this cementing medium make it useful for certain older bridges that lack adequate retention and for cementation of restorations in some cases where the pulp has been removed and endodontics performed.

Other cements

Numerous other cements have been introduced over the years, but few of them have become very popular.

Red and black copper cements are examples. These cements, used to a significant degree in the past, were developed primarily to take advantage of the antibacterial nature of the element contained in them. They have been shown to be excessively irritating to the pulp.

Certain types of *zinc phosphate cement* that are mixed by adding water have been developed. These cements are generally weaker and more soluble than conventional cements.[28]

Cyanoacrylate cements have been developed and used to a limited degree, and some reports have been optimistic[29,30] relative to their retentive properties. However, the ADA Council on Dental Materials and Devices has stated that, "the Council believes that cyanoacrylates, on the basis of current knowledge, cannot be recommended for routine use in dentistry."[31] Practitioners should observe the research literature on these cements and make future judgments about their usefulness.

CLINICAL APPLICATIONS FOR CEMENTS

Each practitioner must decide which cement he desires to use on the basis of available information and past experience. Table 20-1 gives a summary of the information presented in this chapter. The words used to describe the properties of cements are indicative of the numerical values that are available.

CATEGORIES OF CEMENTS FOR APPRAISAL

A careful analysis of Table 20-1 shows that none of the cements is best in all categories. Therefore the use of each one must be based on the needs of practitioners in specific instances. Which cement should be used for the various situations? Suggestions relative to each

Table 20-1. Appraisal of various categories of cements

Cement	Film thickness	Degree of solubility	Pulpal irritation	Compressive strength	Tensile strength	Tooth color matching	Use by U.S. dentists
Zinc phosphate	Good	Moderate	Moderate	Good	Good	Fair	Very common but decreasing
Zinc oxide–eugenol	Good	Moderate plus	None	Fair	Good	Poor	Slight
Zinc polycarboxylate	Good	Moderate	None	Fair	Good	Fair	Very common and increasing rapidly
Zinc silicophosphate	Fair-good	Moderate	Moderate	Good plus	Good plus	Good plus	Very slight
Resin	Fair-poor	None	Moderate plus	Excellent	Excellent	Good	Very slight

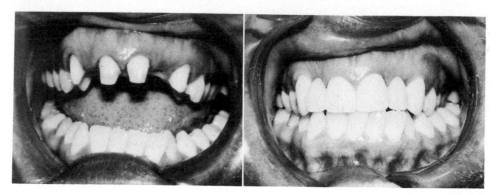

Fig. 20-8. Polycarboxylate cements have gained in popularity significantly over past few years. Additionally, research has supported their use. As a result, one may confidently use polycarboxylate cement to cement routine single-unit restorations or short-span fixed partial dentures, such as the two- or three-unit fixed partial dentures shown here.

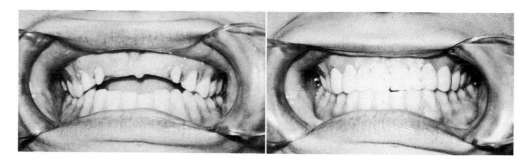

Fig. 20-9. Because zinc phosphate cement provides a long historic perspective by which dentists may observe failure and success and because it has more compressive strength than does polycarboxylate or reinforced zinc oxide–eugenol cement, it is the cement of choice for long-span fixed prostheses or those about which the dentist has concern relative to retention. Such a fixed prosthesis was the one shown here, which replaces two missing central incisors with four small anterior teeth.

cement follow. These recommendations are my opinion based on available research and clinical experience.

For retentive small single-tooth castings on three-unit fixed partial dentures (Fig. 20-8). Polycarboxylate cement is recommended for routine clinical use. Its lack of pulpal irritation, no postoperative sensitivity, and moderate strength values make it acceptable for these situations. Although difficulty has been experienced in the past relative to the proper thickness

for this cement, a new system of proportioning available from Durelon makes proportioning much easier. Zinc phosphate or reinforced zinc oxide–eugenol may certainly be used with assurance for routine cementation also.

For long-span fixed partial dentures (4 units or more) (Fig. 20-9). Polycarboxylate cements have extremely short working times, which makes the seating of long-span bridges difficult. Further, polycarboxylate and reinforced zinc oxide–

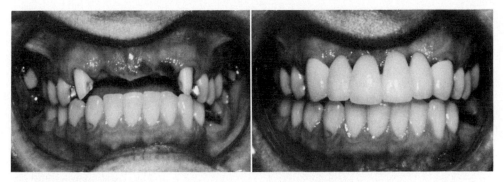

Fig. 20-10. Certain patients have very sensitive teeth, and it is difficult to anesthetize them adequately during treatment. Such teeth are better treated with cements that do not irritate dental pulp. Reinforced zinc oxide–eugenol or *ortho*-ethoxybenzoic acid (EBA) cements are good choices for these patients. Patient shown had very sensitive canine teeth during treatment. However, six-unit fixed prosthesis was not sensitive after it was placed with EBA cement.

eugenol have slightly less strength than zinc phosphate. Therefore zinc phosphate is recommended for long-span fixed dentures.

For very sensitive teeth receiving cast restorations (Fig. 20-10). Reinforced zinc oxide–eugenol or polycarboxylate should be considered. The bland nature of these cements is quite well known clinically and documented in the research literature.

For cast restorations in extremely caries-active mouths (Fig. 20-11). The fluoride content of improved zinc silicophosphate cement, such as Fluoro-Thin, makes it desirable for caries-active mouths. Since film thickness has been reported to be a problem, castings should be relieved internally to allow adequate seating.

For porcelain jacket crowns or porcelain inlays (Fig. 20-12). When color alteration is necessary on such restorations, zinc silicophosphate cement should be considered. Ceramic blend or shaded zinc phosphate cement is also useful in such situations.

For castings that continue to become uncemented (Fig. 20-13). Occasionally cast restorations that have served for many years and have become loose are con-

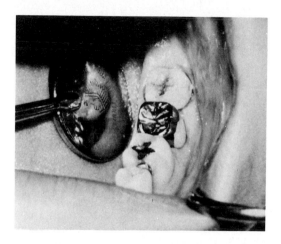

Fig. 20-11. Some mouths are caries active despite all attempts to decrease this activity. Cementation of cast restorations in such mouths with a cement containing silicate (fluoride) may well decrease the possibility of recurrent caries around margins. This onlay was cemented with Fluoro-Thin.

sidered to be salvageable. In such cases a very strong cement is required. The composite resin cement Epoxylite CBA 9080 may be useful. The pulpal irritation of this cement must be considered.

The area of dental cements is changing rapidly. The suggestions that have been

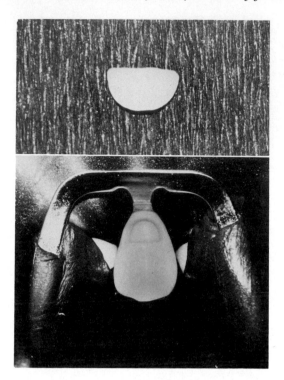

Fig. 20-12. Porcelain jacket crowns or porcelain inlays are less frequently encountered now than in the past. Nevertheless, those dentists who use these restorations need cements that can be varied in color significantly. Such cements are zinc silicophosphate or some types of zinc phosphate.

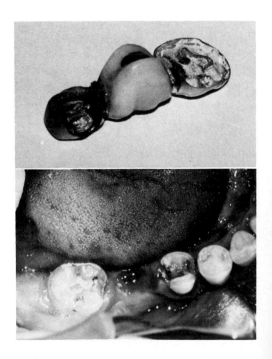

Fig. 20-13. When a fixed prosthesis or crown becomes uncemented, there has often been misjudgment on the part of the practitioner who placed the restoration. When such failure occurs, one is faced with redoing the restoration or attempting to salvage it for a few years. Case shown is an example of this situation. Retainer had come loose from anterior abutment on this three-unit prosthesis. The reason is evident—onlays should not have been used as retainers. Pontic was reshaped correctly, some carious dentin was removed from premolar, deepest portion of preparation was based slightly with calcium hydroxide, and restoration was reseated with Epoxylite 9080 Crown and Bridge adhesive, a composite resin cement. Repaired restoration has served for 3 years at this time.

made are based on information available at the time of this writing. It is expected that information available over the next few years will influence these recommendations. Hopefully, a new category of cement might eliminate the need for the current types of cements.

SELECTED REFERENCES

1. Ward, M. L.: American textbook of operative dentistry, ed. 7, Philadelphia, 1940, Lea & Febiger.
2. Flagg, J. F.: Plastics and plastic filling, ed. 3, Philadelphia, 1890, Sherman & Co.
3. Swartz, M. L., Phillips, R. W., Norman, R. D., and Oldham, D. F.: The strength, hardness and abrasion of dental cements, J.A.D.A. **67**:367-374, 1963.
4. Paffenbarger, G. C.: Dental cements, direct filling resins, composite and adhesive restorative materials: a resume, J. Biomed. Mater. Res. **6**:363-393, 1972.
5. Civjan, S., and Brauer, G. M.: Physical properties of cements based on zinc oxide, hydrogenated resin, o-ethoxybenzoic acid and eugenol, J. Dent. Res. **43**:281, March-April 1964.
6. Paffenbarger, G. C., Sweeney, W. T., and Isaacs, A.: A preliminary report on zinc phosphate cements, J.A.D.A. **20**:1960-1982, 1933.
7. Massler, M.: Effect of filling materials on the pulp, N.Y. J. Dent. **26**:183-198, 1956.
8. Brännström, M., and Nyborg, H.: Bacterial growth and pulpal changes under inlays cemented with zinc phosphate cement and Epoxylite CBA 9080, J. Prosthet. Dent. **31**:556-565, May 1974.
9. Norman, R. D., Swartz, M. L., Phillips, R. W., and Vermani, R. V.: A comparison of the intraoral disintegration of three dental cements, J.A.D.A. **78**:777-782, 1969.
10. Phillips, R. W., Swartz, M. L., and Norman, R. D.: Materials for the practicing dentist, St. Louis, 1969, The C. V. Mosby Co.
11. Phillips, R. W., Swartz, M. L., Norman, R. D., et al.: Zinc oxide and eugenol cements for permanent cementation, J. Prosthet. Dent. **19**:144-150, Feb. 1968.
12. Gilson, T. D., and Meyers, G. E.: Clinical studies of dental cements. IV. A preliminary study of a zinc oxide–eugenol cement for final cementation, J. Dent. Res. **49**:75-78, 1970.
13. Smith, D. C.: A new dental cement, Br. Dent. J. **125**:381-384, Nov. 5, 1968.
14. Phillips, R. W., Swartz, M. L., and Rhodes, B.: An evaluation of carboxylate adhesive cements, J.A.D.A. **81**:1353-1359, Dec. 1970.
15. Powers, J. M., Johnson, Z. G., and Craig, R. G.: Physical and mechanical properties of zinc polyacrylate dental cements, J.A.D.A. **88**:380-383, Feb. 1974.
16. Truelove, E. L., Mitchell, D. F., and Phillips, R. W.: Biologic evaluation of a carboxylate cement, J. Dent. Res. **50**:166, Feb. 1971.
17. el-Kafrawy, A. H., Dickey, D. M., Mitchell, D. F., et al.: Pulp reaction to a polycarboxylate cement in monkeys, J. Dent. Res. **53**:15-19, Jan.-Feb. 1974.
18. Smith, D. C.: A review of zinc polycarboxylate cements, J. Can. Dent. Assoc. **37**:1-8, 1971.
19. Ady, A. B., and Fairhurst, C. W.: Bond strength of two types of cements to gold casting alloys, J. Prosthet. Dent. **29**:217-220, 1973.
20. Brauer, G. M., McLaughlin, R., and Huget, E. F.: Aluminum oxide as a reinforcing agent for zinc oxide–eugenol–o-ethoxybenzoic acid cements, J. Dent. Res. **47**:622-628, 1968.
21. Wilson, A. D., and Batchelor, R. F.: Zinc oxide–eugenol cements: II. Study of erosion and disintegration, J. Dent. Res. **49**:593-598, 1970.
22. Hayes, S. M.: A practical comparison of the three basic types of crown and bridge cements, J. Acad. Gen. Dent. **21**:18-19, Sept.-Oct. 1973,
23. Anderson, J. N., and Paffenbarger, G. C.: Properties of silicophosphate cements, Dent. Progr. **2**:72-75, 1962.
24. Phillips, R. W., Swartz, M. L., Norman, R. D., and Fairhurst, C. W.: Zinc silicophosphate cement: influence of composition on the acid solubility and fluoride content of enamel, J. Prosthet. Dent. **29**:628-631, 1973.
25. Eames, W., Professor of Operative Dentistry, Emory University: Personal communication, Jan. 1975.
26. Lee, H., and Swartz, M. L.: Evaluation of a composite resin crown and bridge luting agent, J. Dent. Res. **51**:756-766, May-June 1972.
27. Ericksen, H. M.: Pulpal response of monkeys to a composite resin cement, J. Dent. Res. **53**:565-570, May-June 1974.
28. Paffenbarger, G. C.: New developments in dental materials: a world-wide survey, Int. Dent. J. **15**:356, Sept. 1965.
29. Bakland, T., and Baum, L.: Cyanoacrylate in the cementation of threaded retentive pins, J. Ga. Dent. Assoc. **47**:13, Summer 1973.
30. Hanson, E. C., and Caputo, A. A.: Cementing mediums and retentive characteristics of dowels, J. Prosthet. Dent. **32**:551-558, Nov. 1975.
31. American Dental Association Council Report: Polymers used in dentistry: Part 1. Cyanoacrylates, J.A.D.A. **89**:1386-1388, Dec. 1974.

21

Coronal-radicular stabilization of endodontically treated teeth for restorative dentistry

Joseph L. Caruso, Joseph C. Morganelli, Hosea F. Sawyer, and Anthony T. Young

Historically, teeth with nonvital pulps have been restored by a subjective system of treatment. Empirical restorative procedures have predominated in the clinical treatment of endodontically treated teeth. Current research and technical advancements have modified the manner in which dentists approach these problems. Comprehensive treatment of patients by multidisciplined specialties has increased the number of retained dentitions and teeth with nonvital pulps.

Plaque-control programs, intermittent restorative materials for caries-control programs, and advanced restorative techniques have increased the longevity of the teeth that were previously extracted. The increased level of the dental education of the populace and school examinations for children have exposed the patient to the potentialities of current dental therapy.

HISTORY

Crowns with dowels were generally used when it was impossible to restore the tooth by means of fillings or other crowns that do not involve the removal of the pulp. If a tooth without a vital pulp is used, every precaution should be taken to ensure periapical tissues that are free of infection.

A root, to be acceptable for this type of crown, must be biologically sound and possess sufficient strength to withstand the forces of mastication. The periodontal structures must also be of adequate amount and distribution to warrant the anticipated restorative procedures.[1]

DOWEL CROWNS

Early dowel crowns were originally designed only for anterior teeth (Fig. 21-1) but currently have been just as successful for posterior teeth. Dowel crowns primarily depend on their retention and resistance to displacement into the root canal. In addition, preparation modifications that permit the final crowns to completely encircle the periphery of the prepared teeth will also increase the resistance to displacement and minimize fracture during function.

Manufactured dowels may be used. Customized dowels may also be made to fit the individual case. The manufactured dowels usually consisted of a pin with a shoulder near the cervical end; from this point the pin is tapered apically. The dowel is extended for several millimeters incisally from the shoulder. For adequate strength, a gold and platinum alloy is commonly employed.

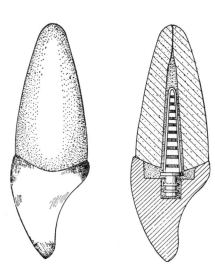

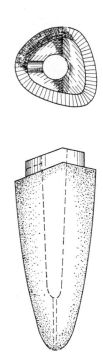

Fig. 21-1. Use of detached type of dowel with all-porcelain crown. Cross sections show relative position of dowel in root and in base of crown. Cement unites tooth, dowel, and crown into one rigid unit (not manufactured today). This former design, connecting the core and dowel with the crown, is currently discouraged.

Fig. 21-2. Coronal-radicular stabilization for a maxillary anterior abutment. Note extent of root preparation with shoulder prior to reception of a dowel.

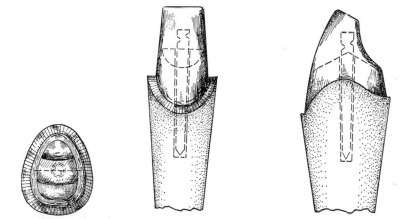

Fig. 21-3. Cast core for porcelain jacket crown encircles plateau portion of preparation and occupies half width of shoulder. Note that some of the coronal portion of tooth is retained whenever possible.

GUIDELINES FOR CORONAL-RADICULAR STABILIZATION[2]

Both anterior and posterior teeth with nonvital pulps are required to have some form of coronal-radicular stabilization. To clarify any misconceptions about post-endodontic treatment, the following guidelines can be followed for restoration of these teeth:

1. The four anterior teeth require cast core and dowel (Figs. 21-2 and 21-3) or a minimum of four pins with a composite[3] buildup of the coronal portion of the tooth.
2. The canines require cast core and dowel unless splinted.
3. Premolar teeth that have lost beyond 50% of their tooth structure usually require that a cast core and dowel be placed.
4. All resected teeth regardless of arch position require a cast core and dowel.
5. Molar teeth that have lost more than 60% of their bulk or are to be considered for an abutment commonly require a cast core and dowel (Fig. 21-4).

Blue Island posts and pins are to be used primarily with premolars and molars after endodontic treatment. Fifty to 60% of their remaining tooth structure must be supportive. Borderline cases between the cast core construction and Blue Island–pin amalgam "buildups" will be at the discretion of the dentist.

These are only guidelines. Imaginative methods will be acceptable provided that a discrete rationale of treatment is provided.[4]

Requirements for traditional core-and-dowel construction

The following traditional methods are considerations:

1. Ideally the length of posts should be equal to, at least, the length of the estimated clinical crown.
2. The post must have an occlusal stop to prevent displacement apically. This is of vital importance since displacement toward the apex commonly results in fracture of the prepared root.
3. Included in this construction should be resistance to rotational forces.
4. Posts, generally speaking, should be of sufficient thickness (minimal size 70) to resist displacement and assist stabilization.

ESTABLISHING RADICULAR SPACE FOR POSTS

The removal of endodontic filling material from the treated root presents a critical step in the final restoration of the

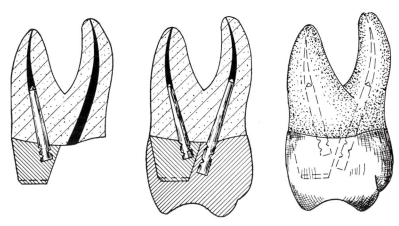

Fig. 21-4. Complete cast crowns for molars are usually fabricated in two parts because of root angulation.

tooth. Perforation of the tooth can result in the loss of the tooth. Great care must be exercised in attempting this procedure, and the safest method of removal should be employed. The two most common types of root-canal filling materials are the following:

1. Semisolid: gutta-percha, chlora-percha, and various pastes
2. Solids: silver points

The first step in treatment of the restoration of endodontic teeth begins with the initial access or approach preparation. Inadvertent excessive removal of tooth structure may result in a weakened tooth. Care must be taken to avoid excessively large pulpal access openings and thinning of the sides of the root canals, especially in the middle third of the root surface. Fig. 21-5 illustrates the stages of removal of the root-canal filling material to the desired length. Fig. 21-5 also illustrates the development of the length and width of the canal necessary for stabilization.

Specific techniques for removal of root-canal filling

Semisolid
Step 1. Heat a Luks plugger in a flame and insert it momentarily into the filler. This procedure should cause the filler to congeal around the plugger. This is repeated until sufficient depth is achieved.

Step 2. Through the use of endodontic reamers and files, the canal is enlarged to provide adequate post room (size 70-80). If the root canal treatment is old, this technique will have obvious limitations. The use of chemicals such as chloroform to soften and facilitate arduous removal of an old filling is helpful. Pezzo reamers, which engage this material, could also be employed.

Solid. The use of silver points to fill anterior canals usually implies the use of a

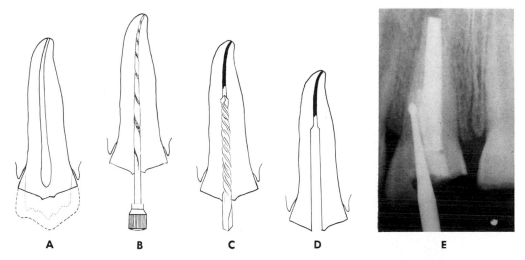

A   **B**   **C**   **D**   **E**

Fig. 21-5. A, Diagram of tooth with loss of tooth structure and internal anatomy of canal system. **B,** Entire length of canal with file in place. Note once again that final shape and size of post room will in part depend on size of file that was used in final preparation. **C,** With increasing diameter of files, internal shape of post core system is achieved. Apical third of canal is endodontic seal. **D,** Internal shape of canal system. Metal post core should correspond as closely as possible both in diameter and length to prepared post room. **E,** In this case tooth can be lost because of hasty preparation for dowel space. Use of rotary instruments in pulpal canal should be a rare occurrence. Hand instruments are more appropriate. This is particularly true in younger patients.

twist-off techique that seals the apex from 2 to 4 mm depending on the tooth.

If any other solid material is used to fill the canal, it is meticulously removed to supply space for the post. If removal becomes impossible, a cervical collar is prepared around the entire circumference of the treated tooth. It can be splinted to a proximating tooth or made part of a splinted prosthesis if post preparation is impossible or particularly hazardous.

Clinical judgment must be employed to weigh the possibility of perforation against traditional "ideals" of coronal-radicular stabilization; that is, length may have to be sacrificed or modified for safety.

Anterior core-and-dowel construction— direct method

Anterior teeth requiring endodontics with a subsequent full-coverage restoration require coronal-radicular stabilization. Fig. 21-6 demonstrates the most common form of coronal-radicular stabilization for single-rooted teeth. However, it is not necessary to completely eliminate all coronal tooth structure. Soundly supported tooth structure can be used to

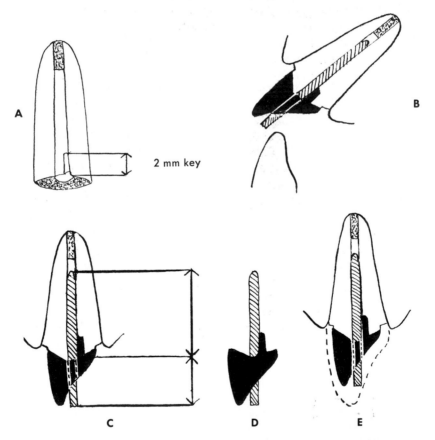

Fig. 21-6. A, Two-millimeter key is usually placed at greatest circumferential width of coronal portion of tooth. **B,** Post is seated and checked for adequate length while coronal portion is developed to resemble a crown preparation. **C,** Radicular post in this illustration is sufficiently long in comparison to length of anticipated crown. **D,** Complete core and dowel to be cemented to prepared root. **E,** Labial surface of coronal portion of dowel should anticipate sufficient clearance for an esthetic veneer.

the advantage of the dentist and patient (Fig. 21-3).

It is conceivable that if the tooth is not involved by caries or large restorations, the placement of a dowel would be sufficient for a tooth not in a strategic occlusal position. A conventional restoration can then be placed over the dowel access opening.

Tooth preparation. It is recommended that, after removal of the root-canal filling necessary for dowel space, the tooth be prepared for the final restoration. This means that the tooth must be fully prepared, with the possible exception of the labial or buccal beveled gingival shoulder for a porcelain-fused-to-metal crown.

Adequately prepared teeth with nonvital pulps will help to avoid overcontouring the completed restoration. The core and dowel should be near completion before cementation. Reduction of cast metal is not only arduous, but the vibration from the air rotor can seriously affect final cementation.

A slot or key in the pulp chamber can be used to achieve further stabilization of the core and dowel. Not only is resistance to rotation essential to the success of the final restoration, but the root preparation should also provide a stop to prevent any apical displacement of the core and dowel.[5]

The root preparation can vary in shape by the tooth size and position; but a funnel-shaped preparation placed 2 to 3 mm into the chamber of root is acceptable. Close adaptation of the casting to this area implies no undercuts.

Fabrication of core and dowel. A dowel of proper size is selected and determined in part by the size of the files and reamers used during endodontic therapy. The dowel should not bind at the apical end. It has been suggested that a dowel one full size smaller than the prepared root-canal diameter is more appropriate and aids the post's insertion. Some dentists

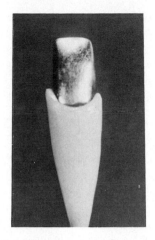

Fig. 21-7. Labial view of core and dowel seated on prepared endodontically treated tooth. Final restoration will be a complete porcelain crown.

are convinced that the length of the dowel within the canal is the critical criterion for the dentist.[6]

Many types of preformed dowels are presently at the disposal of the dentist.[4,7,8] Ordinarily a metal post is placed and held in the prepared root canal after the canal has been lightly lubricated, and wax or plastic is applied to secure it to place. The coronal portion of the core is developed (Fig. 21-7).

Fig. 21-6 illustrates the sequence necessary for the traditional core-and-dowel fabrication for a maxillary incisor.

POSTERIOR TEETH
Pin-retained core

Posterior teeth can present a difficult restorative problem. Access to the canals, divergent canals, diminutive canals, and obliterated canals result in a complicated operative procedure. In posterior teeth where sufficient coronal tooth structure remains, the use of pin-retained amalgams or composites for cores are usually adequate.

The first step is to remove the desired amount of root-canal filling. The removal of the filling material from the largest canal, usually the distal root in lower teeth or the lingual root in maxillary teeth, is accomplished in the same manner as outlined on p. 491. If insufficient tooth structure remains, cast cores are necessary, as shown in Fig. 21-4.

Preparation of tooth structure

If sufficient posterior tooth structure remains, one can create an additional retention into the dentin, using the traditional cavity design as retention in addition to the pins. A screw post of proper size and length (Blue Island) is fitted into the canal. The post should be free of the opposing occlusion, it should not bind excessively, and minimal force should be used to put the post into place. Additional pins can be used to augment the procedure. Until now the discussion has been limited to direct methods of coronal-radicular stabilization, which are used more in anterior teeth. A greater percentage of dentists prefer an indirect method for the posterior teeth.

Cast core restoration—indirect method

In patients who require a complete buildup for tooth structure, the conventional direct method is rarely feasible (Fig. 21-8). In those cases that do require a complete buildup of coronal portions of

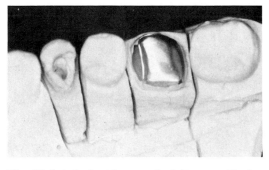

Fig. 21-8. Interlocking casting for mandibular molar on die stone. Indirect method was used for constructing posterior core and dowel prior to complete crown placement.

teeth, an indirect approach is the ideal alternative.

The following are materials used for this impression procedure:
1. Rubber base
2. Polyether

The material of choice depends on the dentist. In this chapter the emphasis will be on the rubber-base impression technique.

Tooth preparation
1. After endodontic therapy, the dentist must evaluate the case in question. Bulk reduction is the initial step. While attempting to visualize an ideal preparation, the dentist anticipates final placement of the margins and functional occlusal positions during preparation.
2. Evaluate the remaining tooth structure. Sharp edges and corners should be rounded to reduce the risk of fracture.
3. Prepare post room. It is advisable to prepare for sufficient length and width. Post position is prepared by use of increasing diameter endodontic files or Pezzo reamers (Fig. 21-5). The diameter of the post position is in part dictated by the diameter of the final endodontic filling. For example, in anterior teeth, where the diameters of the canals are larger, the post core will be larger.
4. One important consideration in the preparation of the internal anatomy of the canal is that anatomically the canal is rarely cylindric, and this point is extremely important to visualize during the preparation of the post system. When one uses files in this stage of the preparation, a rubber stop is needed to indicate the correct length of the post core.
5. To avoid perforation of the canal, the following methods are used:
   1. Use diagnostic radiographs.
   2. Establish the ideal length with the initial file.

3. Check and record measurement with a radiograph.
4. Proceed with increasing diameter of files at this established length with a rubber stop.

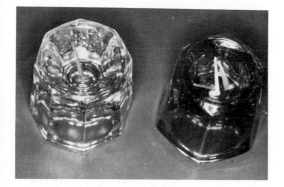

Fig. 21-9. These plastic rods are measured to conform to length of post. They are color coded to be placed in correct canal before impression material is injected.

Impressions

1. It is an important requirement to duplicate the anatomy of the preparation to receive a casting that will adapt to the preparation with maximum retention.
2. Isolate the quadrant and lubricate the internal canal, using a pledget of cotton with solid or liquid petrolatum. This will help minimize the tearing of the impression material.
3. A plastic rod (Fig. 21-9) is adapted to the entire length. This rod is coated with adhesive and dipped in the impression material.
4. Inject the material into the canal and allow material to flow from the canal; insert the plastic rod with the pumping action.
5. Place impression tray into the mouth and hold for 15 minutes. This technique requires a syringe and the heavy-body polysulfide system. See

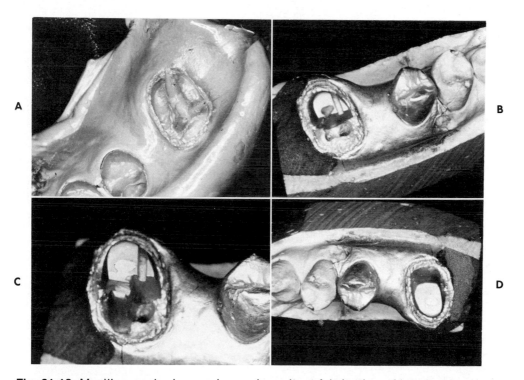

Fig. 21-10. Maxillary molar impression and resultant fabrication of interlocking core and dowel.

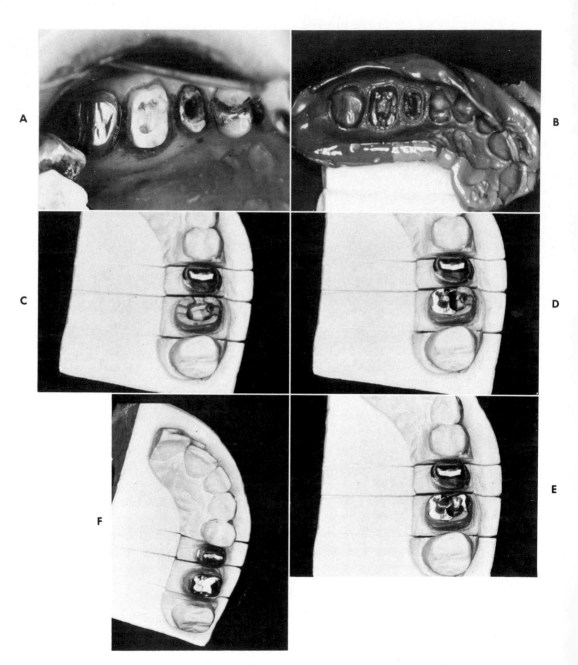

Fig. 21-11. Series of indirect procedures used to construct cores and dowels before final placement of restoration.

Fig. 21-10 for a maxillary molar impression and the resultant fabrication of an interlocking core and dowel.

Preparation for dies

1. The impression is rinsed with water and dried thoroughly.
2. Pour immediately, using vacuum spatulation with a measured portion of stone to water. A die stone is necessary.

Waxing

Conventional waxing techniques are used in order to have a well-adapted casting. A plastic post is needed to add stability to the wax pattern (the post core area). Spruing and casting follow the same direction as any conventional cast restoration.

Casting

Upper molars often receive three separate castings fitting the canals because of the divergence of the maxillary canals.[9] Fig. 21-11 illustrates the complete series of indirect procedures used to construct posterior cores and dowels prior to placement of the final restorations for a complex case.

GENERAL OUTLINE FOR RESTORATION OF ENDODONTICALLY TREATED TEETH[10]

I. *General information.*
   A. Eliminate soft tissue interfering with access to root surface and anticipate a method of temporization.
   B. Decide on the material and method to replace the lost coronal portion of the tooth.
      1. Post- and pin-retained amalgams, composite buildups (foundations).
         a. Blue Island posts.
         b. Anchor-threaded posts.
         c. Serrated stainless posts.
      2. Dowel-retained cast cores.
         a. Anchor systems.
         b. Para post system.
         c. Endo posts.

   C. Use radiographs to monitor the apical seal.
II. *Dowel-retained cast cores (anterior).*
   A. Decide the method of construction.
      1. Direct.
      2. Indirect.
   B. Select materials (manufacturer's) kit.
      1. Anchor system (direct only).
      2. Para post.
      3. Endo post.
III. *Para post.*
   A. Mated twist drills with posts (dowels) 0.036 = 0.070.
      1. Stainless (for foundations) dowels.
      2. Gold (for cast cores) dowel or semiprecious metals.
      3. Plastic (for impression taking) endowels.
      4. Aluminum (used in conjunction with polycrown temporary).
      5. Aluminum pins, plastic pins, precious metal pins, 0.7 mm twist drill.
      6. Jigs (used for drilling pinhole retention).
   B. Technique for cast core.
      1. Prepare root face (eliminate spikes of enamel and bevel angle of canal opening).
      2. Hand ream canal to desired depth of dowel length.
      3. Follow with smallest twist drill and use slow rotation and a light touch.
      4. Continue with succeeding sizes until shavings are no longer endodontic material. Take radiograph with dowel in canal.
      5. With jig corresponding to last-used twist drill in canal, drill pinhole with 0.7 mm drill for torque-preventing pin.
      6. Core-pattern development

depends on whether direct or indirect method of construction is used.
   a. Metal rod corresponding to last-used twist drill and 0.7 mm Ortho pin are used in direct wax-up (Duralay)
   b. Plastic rod corresponding to last-used twist drill and plastic pin are used when developing stone model through indirect-impression method.
7. Develop pattern to look like the appropriate tooth preparation.
8. Cast pattern, pickle, and sandblast.
   a. Eliminate bubbles, which can appear at junction of dowel and core.
9. Polish and cement with phosphate cement, holding core firmly on root face until cement is set.
C. Temporization is developed after step 5.
   1. Relined polycrown, ion crown with acrylic.
   2. Aluminum dowel and aluminum pin.

IV. *Endo post.*
   A. Mated, supposedly, reamers and dowels.
      1. Gold tapered rods.
      2. Plastic endowels.
      3. Base-metal (nonmated) rods.
   B. Technique for cast core.
      1. Prepare root face and cut index ⅛ inch deep into canal.
      2. Hand-ream canal to desired dowel length.
      3. Core-pattern development depends on whether direct or indirect method of construction is used. Check Step 6 above.
      4. Remaining steps as above.
   C. Temporization.

1. Adapt base-metal rod to desired taper by using sandpaper discs.
2. Score portion of base-metal rod extending out of canal.
3. Place polycrown filled with acrylic over base-metal rod.
4. Remove polycrown that will contain rod.
5. Examine and contour to finishing line of root face or to free margin of the soft tissue.

V. *Anchor system.*
   A. Mated and threaded (4 sizes).
      1. Twist drill (blunt-nose drill).
      2. Tap for threading.
      3. Root-facer.
      4. Screwdriver.
      5. Knotched ready-made core and dowel.
      6. Threaded retention posts (notched).
   B. Technique of the one-appointment core-dowel development.
      1. Hand-ream canal to desired length.
      2. Prepare root surface.
      3. Determine canal diameter and match with twist drill.
      4. Follow with removal of remaining side-wall endodontic filling with selected twist drill.
      5. Countersink canal opening with root-facer.
      6. Thread canal with tap by increment of 1 turn forward, ½ turn backward until apical seal is reached.
      7. Shorten dowel to length of canal preparation with Joe Dandy disc, taking care to maintain threads.
      8. Test dowel length by screwing core dowel in canal. Make radiograph. Unscrew dowel and mix cement.
      9. Dip dowel in cement and screw into place with screwdriver.

10. Shape core to desired preparation.
VI. *Dowel-retained cast core (posterior).*
    A. Single-rooted teeth same as anterior.
    B. Two-rooted teeth (bicuspid).
        1. 0.036 para post system.
        2. Hand-parallel dowel holes with 0.036 twist drill to depth of 3 mm.
    C. Three-rooted teeth.
        1. Double-keyed cores.
        2. Indirect method preferred.
    D. Decision on whether dowel-retained cast cores versus pin and dowel–retained composite or amalgam is based on accessibility to area involved and amount of coronal portion of tooth remaining.
VII. *Copings for overdentures.*
    A. Self-retained.
    B. Dowel retained (3 mm).
    C. Lingual shelf.
IX. *Principle of post support (retention).*
    A. Minimum post length should equal restored crown length or engage two thirds of natural root.
    B. Cylindric posts are more retentive than similarly sized tapered posts.
    C. Wrought gold alloy posts are two to four times stronger than cast gold alloy posts of equal diameter.
    D. Serrated posts are 30% to 40% more retentive than are smooth posts.

SUMMARY

This chapter represented a preview of methods for coronal-radicular stabilization for anterior, posterior, maxillary, and mandibular teeth with nonvital pulps. Direct and indirect methods have been described and illustrated.

Methods of core and dowel fabrication have become somewhat easier, but the methods and the materials used are more complex. Continued research will render coronal-radicular stabilization a more routine procedure enhancing the use of endodontically treated teeth in complex restorative dentistry.

SELECTED REFERENCES

1. Tylman, S. D.: Theory and practice of crown and fixed partial prosthodontics (bridge), ed. 6, St. Louis, 1969, The C. V. Mosby Co., p. 580.
2. Malone, W. F., and Smulson, M.: Coronal-radicular stabilization, Loyola University Medical Center dental clinical manual, Maywood, Ill., 1972, Loyola University, p. 7.
3. Newburg, R. E., and Pameijer, C. H.: Retentive properties of post and core systems, J. Prosthet. Dent. **36:**636, 1976.
4. Kahn, H., Fishman, I., and Malone, W. F.: A simplified method for constructing a core following endodontic treatment, J. Prosthet. Dent. **37:**32, 1977.
5. Weine, F. S.: Endodontic therapy, St. Louis, 1972, The C. V. Mosby Co.
6. Grossman, L. I.: Endodontic practice, ed. 5, Philadelphia, 1960, Lea & Febiger.
7. Weine, F. S., Kahn, H., Wax, A. H., and Taylor, G. N.: The use of standardized tapered plastic pins in post and core fabrication, J. Prosthet. Dent. **29:**542, 1973.
8. Gerstein, H., and Evanson, L.: Precision posts or dowels, Illinois Dent. J. **32:**70-73, 1963.
9. Schilder, H.: Filling root canals in three dimensions, Dent. Clin. North Am. **11:**723, 1967.
10. Dinga, P.: Outline of treatment for pulpless teeth, Loyola University Medical Center dental clinical manual, Maywood, Ill., 1972, Loyola University.

GENERAL REFERENCES

Abraham, G. C., and Baum, L.: Intentional implantation of pins into the dental pulp, J. South Carolina Dent. Assoc. **40:**914-920, Oct. 1972.
Baum, L., and Contino, R. M.: Ten years of experience with cast pin restorations, Dent. Clin. North Am. **14**(1):81-91, Jan. 1970.
Bruggers, H., and Coughlin, J. W.: The parallel pin in everyday practice, J. Louisiana Dent. Assoc. **28:**14-18, Winter 1970.
Caputo, A. A., Standlee, J. P., and Collard, E. W.: The mechanics of load transfer by retentive pins, J. Prosthet. Dent. **29:**442-449, April 1973.
Cross, W. G.: A modification of an horizontal non-parallel screw splint, Br. Dent. J. **130:**442-444, 1971.
Duperon, D. F., and Kasloff, Z.: The effects of three types of pins on the tensile strength of dental amalgam, J. Can. Dent. Assoc. **2:**111-119, 1973.
Duperon, D. F., and Kasloff, Z.: The effects of three

types of pins on compressive strength of dental amalgam, J. Can. Dent. Assoc. **11**:422-428, 1971.

Fusilier, C. N.: Cross-pinning for added retention, J. Prosthet. Dent. **31**(4):397-402, April 1974.

Chan, K.-C., and Svare, C. W.: Comparison of the dentinal crazing ability of retention pins and machinist's taps, J. Dent. Res. **52**:178, Jan.-Feb. 1973.

Chan, K.-C., Svare, C. W., and Williams, B. H.: A report of the dentinal crazing producing rate between TMS pins and machinist's taps, Iowa Dent. J. **29**:30-31, Oct. 1973.

Khowassah, M. A., and Denehy, G. E.: A qualitative study of the interface between different dental amalgams and retentive pins, J. Prosthet. Dent. **30**(3):289-294, Sept. 1973.

Lugassy, A. A., Moffa, J. P., and Hozumi, Y.: Influence of pins upon some physical properties of composite resins, J. Prosthet. Dent. **28**(6):613-619, Dec. 1972.

Mattos, F. M., Jr.: A new self-threading pin, J. Prosthet. Dent. **29**(1):81-83, Jan. 1973.

McPhee, E. R.: Pin-retained composite resin cores for posterior teeth, J. Prosthet. Dent. **31**(5):566-569, May 1974.

Moffa, J. P., Going, R. E., and Gettleman, L.: Silver pins: their influence on the strength and adaptation of amalgam, J. Prosthet. Dent. **28**:491, Nov. 1972.

Mondelli, J., and Fonterrada Vieira, D.: The strength of class II amalgam restorations with and without pins, J. Prosthet. Dent. **28**(2):179-188, Aug. 1972.

Nealon, F. H., and Sheakley, H. G.: An extraoral pin technique, J. Prosthodont. Dent. **22**(6):638-646, 1969.

Perez, E. R., Schoeneck, A. G., and Yanahara, M. H.: The adaptation of noncemented pins, J. Prosthet. Dent. **26**(6):631-639, Dec. 1971.

Pherson, J. L.: A simplified root dowel technique, J. South Carolina Dent. Assoc. **39**:115-119, Feb. 1971.

Pruden, W. H., II.: Full coverage, partial coverage, and the role of pins, J. Prosthet. Dent. **26**(3):302-306, Sept. 1971.

Rakow, B., and Light, E. I.: Cyanoacrylates in pin retention, J. Prosthet. Dent. **30**(3):311-314, Sept. 1973.

Shillingburg, H. T., Jr., Fisher, D. W., and Dewhirst, R. B.: Restoration of endodontically treated posterior teeth, J. Prosthet. Dent. **24**(4):401-409, Oct. 1970.

Standlee, J. P., Caputo, A. A., and Collard, E. W.: Retentive pin installation stress, Dent. Pract. Dent. Rec. **21**(12):417-422, Aug. 1971.

Tautin, F. S., and Miller, G. E.: Nonparallel pin splinting for mobile teeth, J. Prosthet. Dent. **29**(1):67-71, Jan. 1973.

Waldman, P. M.: Endodontic pins in vented gold post for rehabilitation cases, Dent. Dig. **77**:638-643, Nov. 1971.

Wenckebach, G. B.: Pin retention with carboxylate cement, J. Prosthet. Dent. **31**(2):190-193, Feb. 1974.

Winstanley, R. B.: Pin-retained amalgam restorations, Oral Health **62**:16-21, Jan. 1972.

22

Precision attachments: an overview

Raoul H. Boitel

A chapter on precision attachments is necessarily but a choice from, and a summary of, the whole subject. The technology of attachments has developed at such a pace that from a very few T-shaped attachments and bar attachments from the years 1915 to 1935 there are now some 120 models of the most diversified designs, ready-made or laboratory fashioned. Most of them are placed intracoronally, and some of them extracoronally, but both serve one and the same purpose—to retain and to attach a removable bridge or partial denture on natural teeth, vital or nonvital.

Another group, often called attachments, actually should be named "stressbreaker joints," although they sometimes are also attachments, if and when they give retention to a prosthetic appliance. Such stressbreakers act as connectors between a rigid and a movable (resilient) system.

It is particularly in Switzerland, known as the country of watchmakers and fine mechanics, that the inventions of new attachments blossomed, not always to the benefit of dentist and patient using them thereafter. Many such models have ceased to exist; they have become part of the history of malcontent in patients and dentists. The choice that is intended to be presented in this chapter is a group of appliances that either have passed the test of many years in the mouth and, what is most important to dentist and technician, are easy to repair or replace; or they

are constructions that by their mechanics promise lasting results. There have been indeed devices that were easy to mount, practical in their use, but very difficult to repair after some breakage or damage from metal fatigue. The ingeniousness of an invention does not always make it practical.

The fathers of the precision attachment were all in the United States of America, and are Bennet, Brown, Bryant, Chayes, Condit, Fossume, Golobin, Kelly, Mc-Collum, Morgan, Peeso, Roach, Sörensen, Supplée (Fig. 22-1) and others who may have escaped my European eye, whereas the Swiss development in the field of attachments picked up momentum before, during, and after the Second World War with Steiger, Müller, Biaggi, and Conod as the forerunners. On the other hand, I am aware of the fact that there must be many useful attachments that are not mentioned in this text except in the classification. To know them all and to know their use would be more than one man's experience in writing this text.

DEFINITIONS

Precision attachments have been conceived as retainers of removable bridgework and partial dentures. Some serve as retainers for full dentures (overdentures) where few abutments remain. The main purpose of each precision attachment, besides retention, is its concealment within or under a restoration, as the es-

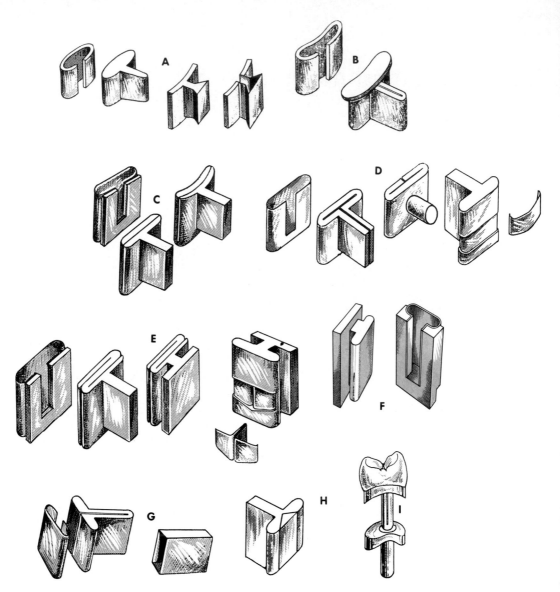

Fig. 22-1. Assortment of old attachments. **A,** Two early attachments made entirely by hand. **B,** Morgan attachment. **C,** Brown-Sörensen attachment. **D,** Early and later forms of Chayes attachment. **E,** Early forms of Stern attachment. **F,** Newer Stern attachment. **G,** McCollum attachment. **H,** Golobin attachment. **I,** Peeso attachment.

thetically better alternative to a visible clasp retainer.

A precision attachment always consists of two functional units, although each functional unit may consist of several parts too. One functional part is the primary part, incorporated into the abut-ment construction, and the other is the secondary part, built into the removable appliance, bridge, partial denture, or full denture. The other designations "male" and "female," "patrix" and "matrix," have caused considerable confusion, since they describe the *shape* of the body

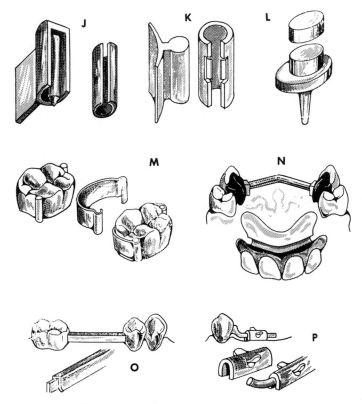

Fig. 22-1, cont'd. J, Condit attachment. **K,** Supplée attachment. **L,** Kelly attachment. **M,** Bryant attachment. **N,** Fossume bar. **O,** Bennett blade. **P,** Gilmore attachment.

of the part in question rather than its *function*. "Male" in a T-shaped attachment belongs to the removable part, whereas "male" in a stud or telescope crown is the primary, fixed part. Thus, in using the sexual terms "male" and "female," "patrix" and "matrix," one designates by male the embraced, enveloped part and by female, the embracing, enveloping part, irrespective of whether it be primary or secondary, fixed or removable.

The main property and purpose of a precision attachment is retention, which is the resistance to removal. Usually, the two functional parts of the attachment are congruent and separable in one direction only. Their contacting walls exert a certain frictional retention. The friction of

rigid walls against each other will cause, with each insertion or removal, a certain amount of wear, which in turn diminishes the frictional retention.

Such attachments, with no adjustable frictional elements, are used exclusively as stress-breaking links or as paralleling devices for nonparallel abutments in fixed bridgework. Additional retention by friction is supplied by various frictional elements. Two of which are as follows:

1. Split attachments with a **T** shape. The split is always in the secondary part, which is easier to repair. The split is always placed vertically, in some attachments with the opening laterally and in others gingivally.
2. Springs in the form of spring wires placed in channels longitudinally in

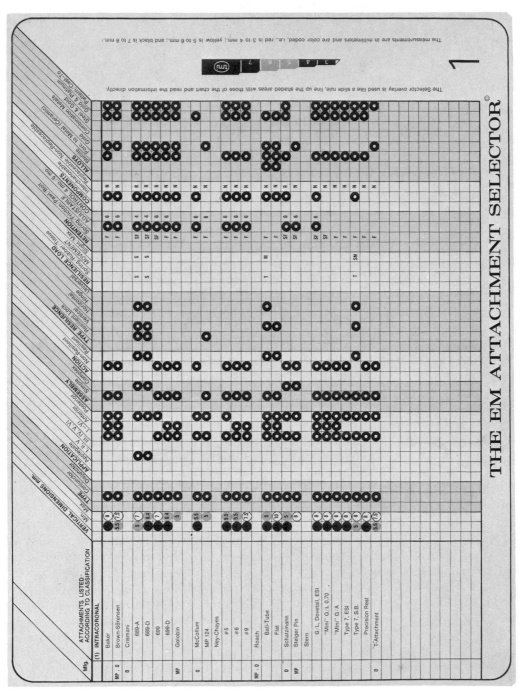

Fig. 22-2. EM Attachment Selector consists of five sheets and gives information on most attachments available today. Measurements are color coded, not shown in black-and-white reproduction. (Courtesy Bell International, Inc., San Mateo, Calif.)

the secondary part, causing friction against the walls of the primary part (channel-shoulder-pin attachments, telescopes). Circular springs as in certain stud attachments (Gerber), lamellated crowns gripping stud cylinders (Baer, Dalla Bona), coil springs in snap-button attachments (Crismani, Schatzmann).

The force necessary to separate an attachment should be between 5 and 12 lb (2.3 and 5.4 kg) of traction. The more attachments there are in a given case, the less is the friction that must be incorporated into the individual attachment. It is an art to combine the proper designs of attachments over a partial dentition so that the removal and insertion will be easy to the patient and at the same time retentive.

The art of precision-attachment dentistry requires special abilities from dentist and technician. Both should be fond of fine mechanics and must be able to cope with every facet of this dimension of precision. Such knowledge alone is a shield against failure caused by overestimation of the mechanical properties of an attachment, faulty indication for a given case, and helplessness in case of damage or wear. Precision attachments are the field of the doers, not the talkers.

CLASSIFICATION AND TYPES

In 1971, 126 attachments were listed and classified by Mensor in his EM Attachment Selector (Fig. 22-2). This selector consists of five charts giving specifications as to type, vertical dimension (minimal and maximal), whether it is for anterior or posterior teeth, whether the assembly is simple or complex, whether the function is rigid or resilient, type of resilience, size of movement, and type of retention. It shows if the attachment is interchangeable or replaceable and finally what type of material and alloy it is made of. Thus the EM Attachment Selector is a useful guide in the forest of attachments.

The attachments mentioned in the EM Attachment Selector are listed below. Certain manufacturers' numbers have been changed, and some 30 new attachments that appeared on the market since publication of the EM Attachment Selector are shown on the list. It is still possible that some newer attachments escaped my notice.

Intracoronal attachments*

Ancra MP	126a
	126b
Baker Attachment	
Beyeler Dovetail	21.03.2
	21.03.3
	21.03.7
	21.08.0
Boos Cylindrical Attachment	
Brown-Sörensen Attachment	
C & L Attachment	
Crismani Dovetail	22.02.4,6,8
Crismani Resilient	61.02.4,6,8
Cylindrical CM	21.02.7
	22.01.2
	22.01.5
Deck Klemmfederattachment	
Flécher Screwed-on Attachment	

---

*Abbreviations:

CM: Cendres & Métaux, S. A., Biel, Switzerland
MP: Métaux Précieux, S. A., Neuchâtel, Switzerland
UGDO: Usine Génévoise de Dégrossissage d'Or, Geneva, Switzerland

Numbers:
Numbers like 121.01.2 are the list numbers of CM.

Terms:
Extracoronal attachment: An attachment built outside abutment crown, into edentulous space.
Intracoronal attachment: An attachment that is built into structure of tooth crown.
Pawl connectors: Built-in frictional element by horizontal snaplock.
Screw units: Two parts, held together by a screw, to connect primary and secondary parts of a fixed-removable appliance.
Stabilizers: Cross-arch stabilization of partial dentures that replace teeth unilaterally. They are usually built into the secondary part of attachments.
Telescope studs: Attachments only used with devitalized teeth. The primary part is soldered to the root cap; the secondary one is concealed within the crown or denture.

Golobin Attachment
I.C. Attachment
Interlock, CM   121.01.2
McCollum Attachment CM   22.03.2
MP 124
Ney-Chayes Attachment   5,6,7
Roach Cylinder-Tube
Roach Flat
Roach Transversal   124.02.5
Roach Resilient   64.01.5
Schatzmann Snap Attachment   22.06.5
                                                            22.07.5

Schröder Attachment
Spang Stabilex   23.01.5
Steiger CSP Attachment
Stern G/L
    G/L Dovetail
    G/L ESI (expansion slot)
    Micro-G/L
    Type 7
    Type 7 Stressbreaker (with ESI)
    T-Attachment
    Precision Rest
Telescopic Crowns
Westin Attachment

Extracoronal attachments

ASC 52 Sphere Supermicro
            Hemisphere Mono
            S-Protect Normal
            H-Protect UGDO
Bival Attachment UGDO
BMB Hinge MP, UGDO
Cuénoud Hinge CM   81.02.5
CM Resilient   76.01.2,5,8
Conex Spang   23.02.5
Crismani   72.02.4
                                                            73.02.4
Dalbo (Dalla Bona) Resilient   63.01.2,5
                                                            63.02.2,5
Dalbo Fix   74.01.5
                                                            74.02.5
Dalbo Hinge (no spring)   83.01
Denon Hinge 90°
Gaerny Hinge MP
Egert MP Telescope
F.M. Hinge
Gerber Hinge   91.01.2
Gerber Hinge Block   92.01.2
Hader Hinge AD MP
Hinge Lock
Hofer Hinge Screw
Huser Conda CM   77.01.5
Inoue Hinge

Inoue Hinge Bolt
Korte Gelenkanker UGDO
Mays Attachment
PR (Pini-Romagnoli) Hinge MP
Pintil
Roach ball   64.01.5
                                                            64.02.5
Sandri Hinge
Stabilex   23.08.5
    Guglielmetti   22.08.5
Steiger Axial Rotation Joint   71.01.5
Steiger Rotation Joint   125.01.5
Stern Gerbert Bolt
Strini Hinge

Telescope studs (push-button attachments)

Ancrofix MP
Anderes MP
Baer & Fäh Cylinder   31.06.2
    Step Cylinder   32.06.2
Battesti Rigid   31.03.2
    Resilient   41.03.2
    Resilient   43.03.2
Biaggi Resilient   43.01.5
Ceka Anchor
Conod   31.01.2,5,8
Dalbo (Dalla Bona) Ball   43.02.8
    Cylinder   31.02.8
    Buffer   44.02.9
    Cylinder Resilient   41.02.8
Egert standard, small
Gerber Resilient Cylinder   32.02.5,8
    Resilient Buffer   42.02.5,8
Gmür   31.04.2,5
Huser Snap Lock   23.04.2,5
Introfix MP
Rotherman Eccentric   32.01.5
    Eccentric Resilient   41.01.5
Sandri MP   B,C,F,G
                                                            1,2,3
                                                            11R,11,12R,12
Schatzmann Snaprox   31.01.5
                                                            31.01.8
                                                            33.02.5
                                                            33.02.8
Spang Bolt Lock   123.03.2
Schneider   32.05.8
Zest Anchor

Bar attachments

Ackermann MP
Andrews Anterior Mini
            Anterior Regular
            Posterior Mini
            Posterior Regular

Baker Bar

CM Bar Round	55.01.5
CM Bar Flat	56.01.5
Dolder Bar Attachment	51.01.5
	51.01.2
Dolder Bar Joint	53.01.2
	53.01.5

Gilmore Bar

Steiger Bar Attachment

Truss Bar

Auxiliary attachments

Screw units

Hruska	34.01.2
	34.02.5
Schubiger Block	33.01.5,8
	33.02.5,8

Screws, pins:
  Bertolini Isodrome
  CM 0.7mm Elasticor for pins
  MP 0.7mm Elastwire for pins
  Introfix MP
Screws with or without housing
  in different sizes
  Hruska screw with tapered anchor
von Weissenfluh shell pins

Pawl connectors

ASC Spring Rests 52, MP	
Gaussen Retainer	102.04.2
Hannes Anker	
Ipsoclip Guglielmetti	102.02.2
	102.03.2
Mini-Pressomatic Rectangular, MP	
Pressomatic Round, MP	
Spang Pushlock	121.03.2
	122.03.2
	123.03.2
Teach E-Z	

Bolts
  B.S. Leaf Spring Bolt
  Ogi Bolt, MP
  Stern-Gerbert

Stabilizers

ASC 52 Anchor, UGDO	
Ancorvis	
BMB Lock, MP	
CM Lock	111.01.2,5
Huser Hook	123.02.2
Snaprox Schatzmann	121.02.2
Williams Hook	

Interlocks

Beyeler Interlock	
CM Interlock	111.01.2
	121.01.2

Double "H" Alder

Sellek Rod & Tube

Stern Micro-G/L 0.7

Latches

Huser Latch	131.01.5

Rests
  Durallium Precision Rest
  McKay Mortice
  Stern Precision Rest
  Vitallium EF Rest
  Wilkinson Precision Rest
  Williams N.C. Rest

GENERAL INDICATIONS FOR ATTACHMENT WORK

The indications for attachment work are governed by various factors that are listed below and are followed each with the question the practitioner should ask himself when he checks the indication for therapy for his patient.

Motivation of patient for oral hygiene and health

Q.: Will the patient be able, by motivation and ability, to clean and preserve the dental work and his oral health, and will the expense for the patient be a good investment for a long period of time?

Economic possibilities of patient

Q.: Is the treatment I mean to propose to the patient within his means, or should I propose a simpler solution so as not to make him feel badly when he must say, "Doctor, I cannot afford this, give me the second best solution."

Health of dental organ and hereditary disposition

Q.: What is the prognosis of the remaining abutments after therapy? Will they be strong enough to warrant the prosthetic appliance I have planned? Is the patient one of the rare ones in whom hereditary factors will destroy the periodontium whatever measures we take and however conscientious the patient is in his preventive measures?

Intellect and practical disposition

Q.: Can the patient understand why we are not just extracting everything and making dentures "to have everything over with," and is the patient manually gifted enough to understand the mechanics and functioning of the appliance he will get? Is he like the professor of nuclear physics who, after trying to remove and insert his attachment bridge without success, paid his bill and sent the denture back with the lapidary sentence: Unusable and useless!

Type of life and surroundings of patient

Q.: Is the patient basically staying in his residential area or is he a migrant, a traveler, an adventurer, a missionary who spends most of his time in a surrounding where specialized dental care is unavailable? For the latter category, attachment work is a risk unless such patients are given a spare appliance. Generally, people who have to stay away from civilization for longer periods of time are better off with simple clasp dentures with a solid framework.

Functional limits of individual attachment or stressbreaker

A part of such indications is given in the EM Attachment Selector (Fig. 22-2)

where one can find, for example, the height an attachment must have in order to be used. Also, the type of frictional retention that may determine its use is shown.

Q.: Is the attachment in question short, long enough, strong enough to warrant its use? Will the freedom of movement in a stressbreaker be adequate to the function of the prosthesis? Will it damage the abutments or not? Will the attachment wear slowly or quickly, and how may we prevent rapid wear? If wear or breakage occurs, is it easy to replace or repair? Who can repair it besides me?

TECHNICAL INDICATIONS
Rigid anchorage

Rigid anchorage of a removable bridge or prosthesis means that the appliance is as rigidly fixed as a cemented bridge and functions the same way. Such removable bridgework could indeed, in most cases, be replaced by fixed bridgework, if only teeth would have to be replaced. However, one will find in many cases loss of bone and soft tissue from trauma, from clefts, from loss of teeth, and from tumor surgery. Such cases can only be solved by removable appliances, because of the extensive tissue-contacting surfaces which require frequent cleaning.

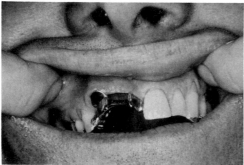 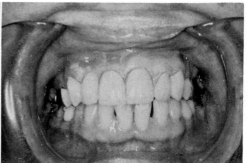

Fig. 22-3. Removable anterior prosthesis. *Fixed part,* Four abutment castings with bar attachment. *Removable part,* Matrix of bar attachment with acrylic replacement of lost bone and gingival tissue invisible to the eye.

Removable instead of fixed bridgework is also desirable if the abutments of a bridge do not have an identical prognostic value. If one anticipates the loss of a distal bridge abutment to happen before the loss of the mesial abutment or abutments, the bridge with a precision attachment on the mesial abutment may become part of a free-end saddle partial denture later. The attachment, mesial abutment, and occlusal gold surfaces could be reused in the denture.

Another indication for removable bridgework is the cross-arch splinting of two lateral bridges. A palatal or lingual bar or a palatal plate may provide this splinting. Finally, I have found that fixed bridgework collects a certain amount of plaque, which is difficult for the patient to remove. Particularly when periodontal disease threatens to endanger the prognosis of a bridge, a removable prosthesis will enable the patient to clean more meticulously around the abutments for better plaque control.

Fig. 22-3 shows a removable anterior prosthesis in a case where only a serious sacrifice of esthetics would allow a fixed appliance. Bone and soft tissue have been lost in a car accident and must be replaced. A fixed bridge for such cases necessitates the use of excessively long teeth, which are placed too far palatally. The result is the well-known "flat look" of the face caused by a retracted lip. The Steiger bar attachment in this case helps to stabilize the arch in the anterior region. Two or three abutments on each side should provide the splinting effect. The patient is able to thoroughly clean around all abutment teeth and along the gingival margin of the bar. A sound retention, consisting of (1) the shape of the bar and (2) the frictional pins visible in the wall of the secondary attachment, guarantees a rigid seat of the bridge. Such a bridge resists any tipping when the patient incises with his anterior teeth.

Fig. 22-4 is an example of cross-arch

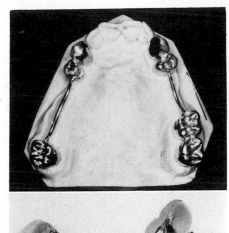
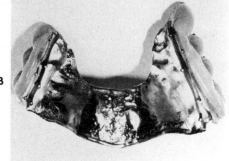

Fig. 22-4. Example of cross-arch splinting of two removable bar attachment bridges by palatal bar (plate). Note frictional pins along the trough.

splinting, solved with two bar attachments laterally and a removable appliance with a palatal plate.

Stress-broken anchorage

Every split-body T attachment (Fig. 22-5) is in fact a stress-broken attachment because it can move very slightly, because of the tiny slit in the body of the secondary part. With wear increasing, this movement becomes more apparent. Such split-body, T-shaped attachments have been used for free-end saddle partial dentures as long as they have been available to the profession. Many such partial dentures turn up in dental offices with badly worn, sometimes broken attachments. Wear and tear depend on tissue resilience underneath the free-end saddle or saddles and, in turn, on the

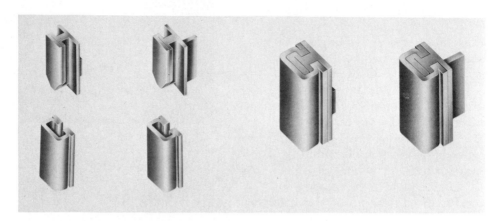

Fig. 22-5. T type of attachment, called McCollum attachment. Split in male part provides frictional retention when activated.

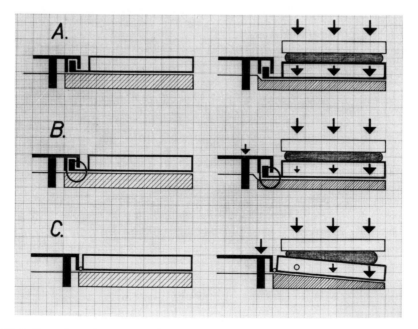

Fig. 22-6. Function of stressbreaker joints. **A,** Unrestrained stressbreaker. Masticatory stress is transmitted to saddle area as it is transmitted to teeth. **B,** Spring restricts full transmission of stresses to saddle tissue mesially; distally there is no restriction. **C,** Principle of hinge. No stress is transmitted to tissue adjacent to hinge, all of it is received by distalmost abutment. The farther distal the force is applied, the more stress is transmitted to the tissue.

tissue resorption, faulty occlusion, and insufficient tissue-bearing surface.

Such excessive and often rapid wear has led inventors to study other solutions that would place the broken stress from the attachment into a separate stress-breaker. The function of such stress-breakers is shown in Fig. 22-6.

The controversy around stressbreakers. Ever since stressbreakers became part of prosthetic dentistry, there has been a controversy as to their usefulness and desirability. Whereas dentists in Switzerland, where most stressbreakers were developed, claimed that stress-breaking was necessary in order to avoid torque and leverage upon the abutment teeth of a free-end saddle denture, the partisans of rigid anchorage, mainly found in the United States, claimed that stress-breaking was not only unnecessary, but even damaging. The rigid attachment, they say, would not cause any damage to the abutments because of the bodily and torque-free movement of abutments.

Both schools have shown success and failure alike. As in so many controversies, an actual scientific proof was never shown by either side in favor of success or failure. Good judgment and, above all, a nontraumatizing occlusion, a healthy periodontium and a patient motivated for strict home care help both sides increase their rate of success and decrease the number of failures. In prosthetic work, there is a long chain of steps to be observed, starting with the prognostic evaluation of a case and periodontal preparation including surgery, splinting, and motivation for home care. Then follows the choice of design, the method of recording jaw relations, the accuracy and knowledge of the dental technician, and finally the knowledge of the chewing habits and of the parafunctional habits of the patient —the response of the particular patient to the dentist's attempts at motivation for prophylaxis. It seems reasonable to assume that if these goals are approached, they will weigh more in the scale of success against failure than the detail of whether one should use a stressbreaker or not for a free-end saddle denture.

There is a particular aspect that should be considered. For several patients, two dentures were made, one rigid, one stress-broken. Asked for their preference, they said without hesitation: "The stress-broken one." The patient's comfort is sometimes a very strong argument!

If a rule of thumb has to be given for such a decision, one might say that a healthy, resistant periodontium usually does not require stress-broken dentures whereas periodontally susceptible or damaged abutments will call for all measures of caution such as splinting teeth into group units and blocks, and stress-breaking the tissue-supported parts of partial dentures. A long saddle may be rigidly attached, but a short one resiliently, since torque upon the abutment decreases with the increase of saddle length.

Requirements of dentist and technician. Abilities no book or chart or selector can provide are experience, the talent to work with small things, and the love of precision with all the difficulties involved in such work. A dentist who wishes to use precision attachments should have a basic understanding of fine mechanics. A good technician is a great help to the dentist, but he is not the whole answer. The dentist must familiarize himself with the mounting procedures after recording, he should practice delicate soldering, he should practice judging the strength and purpose of this or that attachment to assess its limits. He should be able to cut a bar attachment on the parallelometer and wax up a patrix over it. Also, he should be able to cope with any repair or replacements that occur in daily practice. Such repairs often require a good dose of sound improvisation. One should learn how to thread a screw or make a bolt, maybe even how to use a small lathe.

If a dentist is not prepared to do such things himself, he would be well advised to keep away from precision attachments and to concentrate on clasps and do them well!

CONTRAINDICATIONS FOR ALL TYPES OF ATTACHMENTS

Attachment work involves an economic problem. There is a very small number of patients for whom this problem does not exist, and there is no patient who does not expect to have an adequate return against his investment. This return consists of the service, particularly the duration of service restorative work is giving. Should it fail early, the patient will hardly blame himself for the failure. Instead, he will blame the dentist, and with him the dental profession for having failed him.

It is therefore contraindicated to do any expensive rehabilitation work to a patient who has not proved his motivation for home care to his dentist. This is not the place to elaborate upon the duties of the dentist and his auxiliaries respective to patient education and motivation, but there are certain rules that must be followed when doing this kind of prosthetic work:

1. Show the patient the disease in his mouth.
2. Remove the disease by proper cleaning and periodontal therapy.
3. Teach the patient how to keep that oral health.
4. Check the patient periodically if he has learned his lesson and is willing and able to follow it.
5. Then only decide on the modus of rehabilitation.
6. If in view of clinical findings and patient motivation the prognosis is good and favorable, all doors of therapy are open, including precision-attachment work.
7. If clinical findings are unfavorable or the patient is unmotivatable, do your duty as a medical man: Remove

pain, make the necessary extractions, and content yourself and the patient with simple partial or full dentures. This simple alternative may ultimately motivate some patients to do more for their oral health. Crown-and-bridgework, generally speaking, should have a prognosis of 20 years plus. Unfortunately, statistics belie such an estimate and the average life-span is much shorter.

So when and if attachment work is considered for a patient, the question should always be asked: "Will the patient receive adequate return for his investment?" If a patient himself, against the advice of the dentist, insists on work of

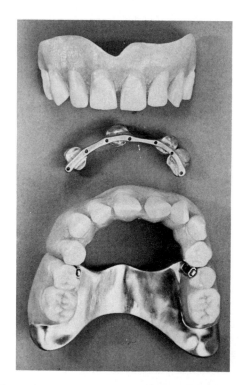

Fig. 22-7. Case with four anterior devitalized abutment roots, joined together with cast post bases and a bar attachment. First bicuspid to first bicuspid is rigidly attached. Distally, twin axial rotation joints hold a palatal plate with four lateral teeth, on resilient tissue.

short duration, prognostically he should be made to sign a declaration to that effect. EXAMPLE: A patient, an industrial manager, appears for consultation. On the basis of clinical and radiologic findings the advice is: Rehabilitation of mandibular teeth with a precision-attachment partial, in the upper arch; extraction of four remaining, damaged incisors; full denture. The patient explains that he will be pensioned in 3 years and that until then he must be certain that his teeth are well retained to give him the necessary personal security as a manager. After his retirement, this would not matter anymore. The four abutments were periodontally treated, fitted with a splint of a bar attachment (Fig. 22-7), and the denture was thus firmly retained. The patient signed a declaration that he was aware of the risk that these retainers would perhaps not last too long because of short roots. Using minutious care, the patient wore that denture for a full 12 years until shortly before he died.

Another contraindication for attachment work is the situation whereby a person lives and stays in a country with underdeveloped dentistry. Whether natives or residents from abroad, such people should have simple robust clasp partials, easily repairable when damaged.

Rather than writing contraindications for each type of attachment here, this chapter gives the specific indication field for each of the attachments mentioned. Certain disadvantages are also shown here.

INDICATION FOR DIFFERENT ATTACHMENTS
Intracoronal attachments without activation

Activation means the frictional or retentive elements that compensate for wear between the primary and secondary parts of the attachment (frictional pins, coil springs). Such a simple attachment is shown in Fig. 22-8. There are others with

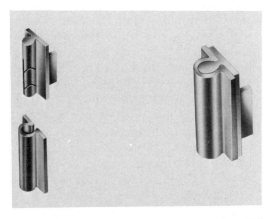

Fig. 22-8. Nonfrictional attachment, the CM (Cendres & Métaux) connector, used for nonparallel abutments in bridgework.

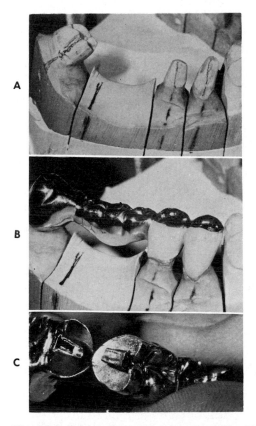

Fig. 22-9. Dovetail rest in a fixed bridge. This rest can be cut into intracoronal part of abutment.

a dovetail cross section. Such attachments are never used in removable work, but for fixed bridgework in order to parallelize the insertion when nonparallel abutments are present. Such attachments could be called "precision rest." The same effect may be obtained with a laboratory-made dovetail rest cut into the abutment crown or overlay and a corresponding casting in one piece with the pontic. This procedure avoids two solderings (Fig. 22-9).

Such attachments may be placed for a possible enlarging of a bridge at a later date. Since the CM cylindrical attachment is very slender, it is well suited for anterior teeth, where space is usually limited. Let us assume a front bridge cuspid to cuspid is made, with three or four abutments. Prognostically, one would expect that the premolars will be the next teeth to go; thus an attachment is placed into the distal side of each cuspid crown and will come into use the moment one or both lateral bridges is made.

Frictional intracoronal attachments

These are the most conventional attachments used in the U.S.: Stern, Ney-Chayes, Brown-Sörensen, McCollum and Baker. Fig. 22-10 shows a stern attachment. The primary part is incorporated into the abutment casting, and the split secondary part into the removable appliance. Wear is compensated for by widening of the split with special, fine wedges, calibrated to the desired degree of friction and wear. Such attachments are usually obtainable in current crown-and-bridge gold alloys or in ceramic golds for the porcelain-to-gold technique.

A special type of this kind of attachment is shown in Fig. 22-11. In addition to the frictional retentions by the split male, this attachment includes a small cam that snaps into place when the attachment male has become completely seated (Fig. 22-11).

Indication. Removable bridges and tooth-supported partials.

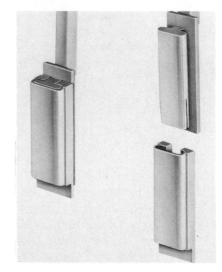

Fig. 22-10. Stern attachment with slit placed gingivally in male part. Strong frame of male and female prevents distortion during soldering.

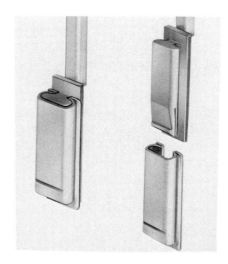

Fig. 22-11. Stern attachment (Models G/L and Micro-G/L) with a snap built in.

Advantages. Available in all countries with developed dentistry; relatively easy to repair.

Disadvantages. Small contacting surfaces, hence relatively rapid wear; friction incorporated into the same body,

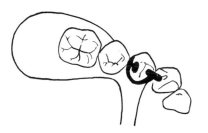

Fig. 22-12. Two attachments in a row for reenforcement and stronger retention.

which gives form retention; unusable on short teeth.

Note that no recommendation was given for using such attachments as retainers of free-end saddle partial dentures. This reservation is caused by the excessive wear of such relatively slender attachments. The resilience movements of the denture upon the saddle or saddles, particularly if rebasing of the saddles

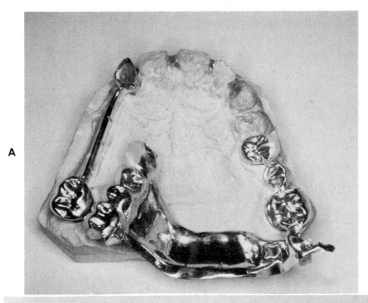

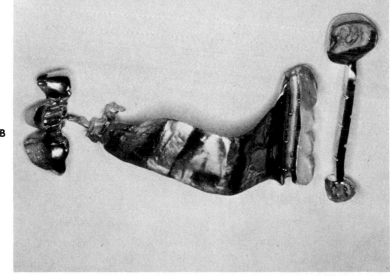

Fig. 22-13. Stabilizer built lingually around abutment crown to amortize lateral stresses upon attachment. **A,** Occlusal view. **B,** Tissue-bearing surfaces.

comes late or is forgotten, cause the denture or saddle to rotate around the attachment. The larger the resilience or the resorption of the tissue under the saddle, the more pronounced this movement will be. Inevitably, such an attachment will wear rapidly and will eventually break in the split part of the male. Wear does not attack the male only, and often one can observe that by replacing the T attachment alone, the attachment does not fit as a new one would. The box has worn too. No replacement is possible here except by destruction of the abutment construction.

Where such heavy wear is anticipated, the following are limited possibilities to reduce it:

1. Two attachments are combined in the same long axis but at right angles with their boxes (Fig. 22-12). This second attachment may be one of the so-called stabilizers (see p. 515).
2. The attachment may be combined with a stabilizer clasp arm placed on the lingual side of the abutment tooth. Such a stabilizer should rest on a shoulder (Fig. 22-13).

Intracoronal attachments with frictional or spring retention

A proved representative of this family is shown in Fig. 22-14. It is a dovetail-shaped attachment with a snap bolt in the male part. The bolt, with a steel coil spring behind it, is held by a threaded ring. The bolt head snaps into the semi-

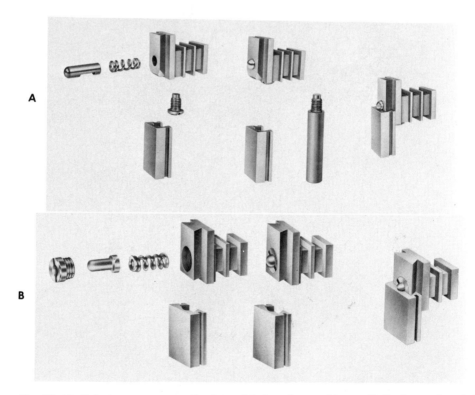

Fig. 22-14. Schatzmann snap attachment in two forms. *Above,* Bolt of snap is retained by screw from gingival surface. Screw prevents bolt from escaping in direction of spring pressure. Large screw is used only for curing saddles in acrylic resin. It is thus retained in the plaster. *Below,* Bolt is retained by frontal screw.

spheric hollow in the female when the attachment is in assembled position. All parts except the female are interchangeable. The Crismani attachment uses a U-shaped wire as a snapper instead of the bolt in the Schatzmann attachment.

Indication. The same as the split-T attachments; removable bridges and tooth-supported partials.

Advantages. No breakage of the male when wearing; easy replacement of parts.

Disadvantages. Dosage of pressure is delicate and must be adjusted according to the number of attachments used in the case.

Extracoronal attachments

Many times, there is no space to place an attachment intracoronally. It then can be placed extracoronally. There are three groups:

1. Rigid, extracoronal attachments, with patrix soldered to the abutment
   Examples: Spang Stabilex
                   Spang Conex
2. Resilient, extracoronal attachment

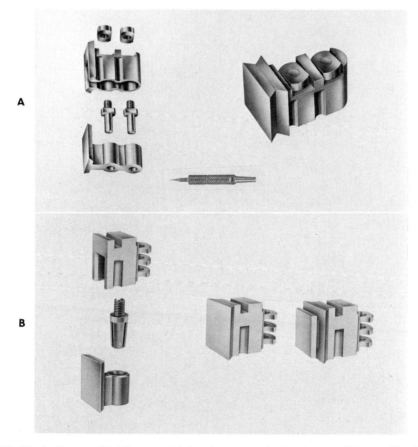

Fig. 22-15. A, Spang Stabilex, a rigid extracoronal attachment. Two split pins are retained in housing by two nuts and are replaceable. They provide frictional retention and can be activated with a little key (below), which is given to patient. This attachment is used for removable bridgework or rigidly attached partial dentures. **B,** Spang Conex is a simpler version of Stabilex, since it has only one split pin, which is conic and a little less retentive. Indication: removable bridgework.

with patrix soldered to the abutment

Examples: Crismani Resilience Joint

Dalbo Resilience Joint

3. Stressbreakers that are interposed between the removable part of a rigid attachment and the resilient part of a denture

Examples: Steiger Axial Rotation and Rotation Joints

Gaerny Hinge

Cuénoud Hinge

Gerber Hinge

4. Bar attachments

Spang Stabilex and Conex. Fig. 22-15 shows the Spang Stabilex and Conex attachments. The primary part, soldered to the distal abutment adjacent to the free-end saddle, is a bar with a double tube, over which fits the secondary part containing two cross-split cylinders as the frictional element. These split pins are activated with a special key, which even the patient can use and with which the pins may also be unscrewed and replaced when necessary. A simpler version is the Spang Conex, with one tube only and a conic cross-split pin as the frictional ele-

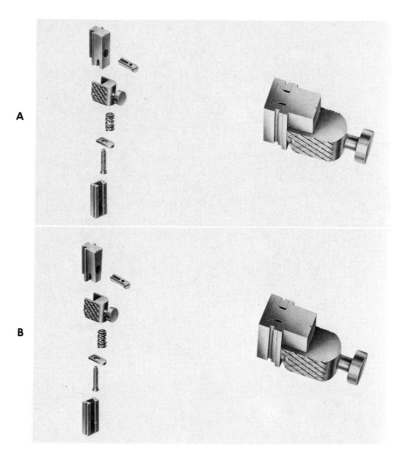

Fig. 22-16. A, Crismani resilience joint with rectangular patrix for unilateral free-end saddles or bilateral ones, which function independently. Return spring brings saddle back into rest position after resilience movement. **B,** Crismani resilience joint with tapered patrix. May be used as attachment for removable bridge and later as resilience joint in bilateral free-end saddle case. Crismani resilience joints are available in two sizes.

ment. The indication for both are removable bridges, partial dentures, and particularly rigidly attached free-end saddles. Rigid attachment of a free-end saddle is particularly indicated when the saddle is long and the tissue is firm. Then the resilience movement under pressure of mastication does not exceed the physiologic movement of the abutment tooth or teeth. In such cases, it is always wise to splint several (a minimum of two strong) abutments together to a group abutment. Also, in unilateral cases, cross-arch splinting with a lingual or palatal bar or plate helps to stabilize the saddle.

Crismani resilience joint. There are two models, one for unilateral free-end saddles and one for bilateral free-end saddles (Fig. 22-16). The matrix is the same as for the rigid Crismani attachment, which is used for removable bridgework. Thus, with the same matrix, it is possible to use (1) the rigid attachment, (2) the unilateral resilience joint, and (3) the bilateral resilience joint. This means that an abutment may serve as a bridge abutment for a certain length of time. If a distal abutment of such a bridge is lost, the mesial abutment can be reused as an abutment for a partial denture, rigid or resilient. Different sizes may be adapted to different abutment heights. Simple mandrels are used to parallelize the Crismani matrices. The housing of the resilience joints with its button retention is cured into the acrylic of the saddle or saddles. All parts except the female of the attachment are interchangeable and replaceable. The whole attachment comes in different sizes, widths, and alloys.

Dalla Bona resilience joint. This is also a combined attachment-resilience joint. The patrix, a rectangular body with a T profile, is soldered to the end-standing abutment, singly or as a group. On its gingival end, there is a ball. Over this T-and-ball body fits a housing that slides along the patrix and ball in a vertical direction. This movement is stopped by a spring interposed between ball and top of the housing. The friction is adjustable by slots in the gingival end of the housing. The slight compression of the blades formed by the slots activates this frictional retention. The retentions and the ring on the back of the housing are de-

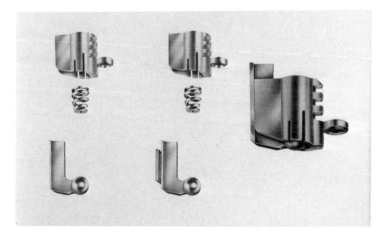

Fig. 22-17. Dalbo (Dalla Bona) resilience joint. Beam with spheric anchor is soldered to distalmost abutment adjacent to saddle. Return spring is self-retained within housing. Slits in housing serve to activate frictional retention. Dalbo joint is used for unilateral saddles or for independently functioning bilateral saddles. Two models each in two sizes are available.

signed to hold the acrylic of the saddle. One can easily replace the steel spring if it breaks from fatigue, by pulling it out of the housing with a hook probe and pushing the new one in until it touches the roof of the housing (Fig. 22-17). This spring must be periodically checked, since breakages from metal fatigue occur and the housing needs to be cleaned too.

Indication. One model is designed for unilateral saddles or independently working bilateral saddles. Another model is used for bilateral saddle cases, where the saddles are joined by a bar across the arch. In such cases, the patrices must be aligned on the same axis, which means that the saddles should be of even length, for example, from cuspid to cuspid. In long-term planning one can first use these attachments as simple slide attachments by blocking the housing with acrylic and using it as a rigid retainer. If at a later date a distal abutment tooth fails and has to be removed, the attachment can be converted into a resilience joint. The idea of the spring in the housing is to return the saddle to its rest position after termination of the resilience movement.

There is still another, newer model (Fig. 22-18) of the Dalbo joint, which has a short housing without spring, where the roof of the housing rests directly on the ball of the patrix. This attachment has only one freedom of movement, the hinge rotation, and is very useful because it is not prone to damage and repairs.

Steiger axial rotation joint and Steiger rotation joint. The original idea of Steiger was to create a stable stressbreaker with axial and rotation freedoms of movement. The male is a flattened cylinder with a screwhole of 1 mm (Fig. 22-19). The female is a tube, congruent to the male, with an oval window on one of the flat sides. The 1 mm screw joins the two and the soldering base is used to solder the male to the framework of the saddle, to a lingual bar, or to a palatal plate. The joint in its fabricated form has only one freedom, that of vertical translation. Fig. 22-20 shows the function of a saddle relative to the resilience joint. If the load on the saddle is distributed, the movement is purely translatory. If there is a mesial or a distal load, the translatory movement is combined with a rotational one. The untouched joint however allows only vertical movement. Thus small reliefs must

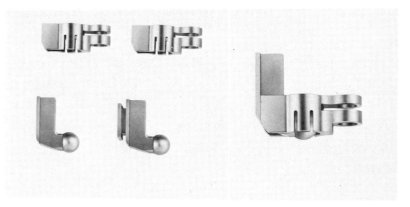

Fig. 22-18. Dalbo rotation joint. This model functions without a spring and is in effect a hinge joint. It makes only a rotation around the ball anchor. It is used as an attachment for bridges or as a joint for free-end saddle denture, unilateral or independently working bilateral case.

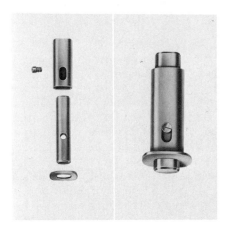

Fig. 22-19. Axial rotation joint (Steiger). *On left, bottom to top,* soldering ring, to be given inclination of gingival tissue before soldering; male; female with oval window and fixation screw, which is screwed into male through oval window. *On right,* Assembled joint. It is used as a resilient connecting link between attachments and saddle denture. Only to be used in bilateral saddle dentures.

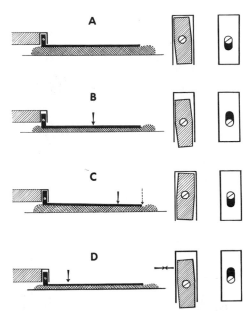

Fig. 22-20. Function of axial rotation joint. **A,** Rest position. **B,** Force applied to middle of denture. **C,** Force applied to distal side of denture. **D,** Force applied to mesial side of denture. Reliefs on male, enlarged in middle column, are of course exaggerated to show location of reliefs. In right column, position of screw (in male) within oval window (in female) is demonstrated.

be made on the joint. Experience over the years has produced the following two facts (Fig. 22-21):

1. Any reliefs made before insertion of a denture by the operator are liable to be excessive and to make the joint too movable. Therefore the patient receives the denture without reliefs. Even after 1 week of use, the reliefs show from pure wear and function. These reliefs are accurate because function has caused them.

2. The oval window on the matrix of the AxRo joint is usually too large for the resilience that one would desire the denture to have. Often, such excessive freedom damages, with the mesial border of the saddle, the gingival papilla distal to the last abutment. Therefore, to reduce the amount of resilience, the AxRo is replaced by the Ro-Joint.

Steiger rotation joint. The Ro-Joint (Fig. 22-22) was originally designed to act

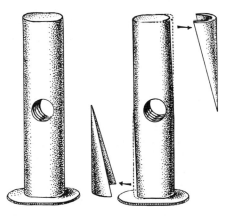

Fig. 22-21. Reliefs on male of AxRo Joint. These reliefs are very slight and will form by themselves when joints are in action and under stress.

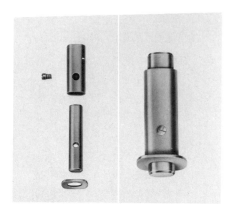

Fig. 22-22. Rotation joint (Steiger). Rotation joint has same components as AxRo Joint, except that oval window is replaced by round one and therefore no axial movement of translation is possible. Is used in unilateral cases, on other side of arch, as a stabilizer, or, in bilateral free-end saddle cases, as a hinge joint. Naturally, a new Ro-Joint has not even the freedom of a hinge movement. It should be worn rigid for a while; then reliefs that are formed by themselves should be retouched slightly to increase hinge movement.

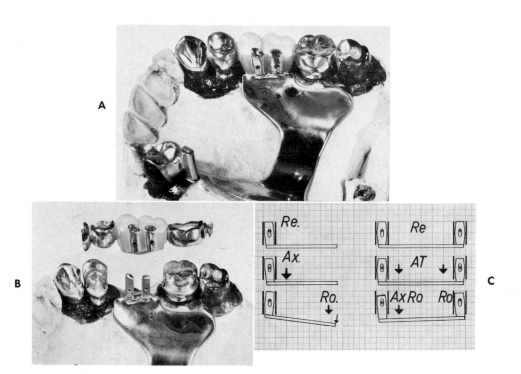

Fig. 22-23. A, Unilateral free-end saddle case. Block of two abutments on patient's right side hold an AxRo Joint. On patient's left side there is a removable bridge, attached by two channel-shoulder-pin (CSP) attachments on bicuspid and first molar. In between, the two pontics are visible, and within them appear two Ro-Joints as stabilizers for contralateral AxRo Joint. **B,** Removable bridge is removed, and CSP patrices, the Ro-Joint males, are separated from CSP matrices, the AxRo females. To disassemble joints, screws would have to be removed. This is only done sporadically when denture is cleaned in laboratory, otherwise they remain assembled. **C,** Function is shown in two planes: on left in sagittal plane; on right in transversal plane. *AT,* Axial translation in a transverse view; *Ax,* axial translation movement; *AxRo,* axial rotation; *Re,* rest position; *Ro,* rotation.

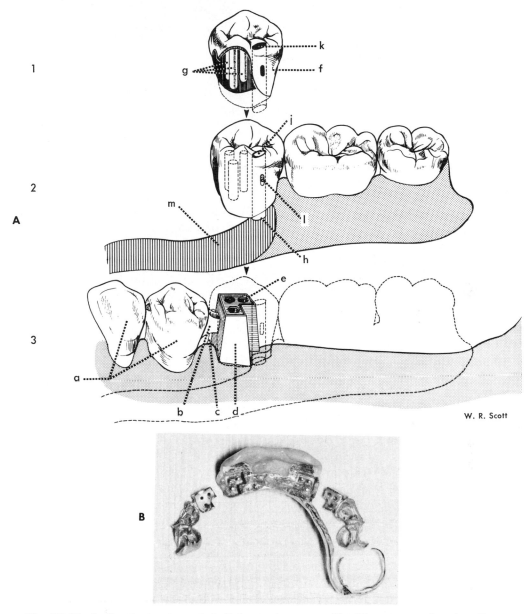

Fig. 22-24. A, Scott attachment. *1,* Telescopic crown *(f)* with cutaway showing three internal parallel iridioplatinum pins *(g)* and an axial rotation joint (see p. 520) placed into recess of connector *(k). 2,* Male of AxRo Joint is soldered at *h* to lingual bar *(m).* It is visible only at occlusal opening *(j)* and near the limiting screw *(l). 3,* Double abutments *(a)* soldered together with external connector *(d).* Connector pinholes *(e)* and an angular recess for placing the AxRo Joint. Telescope crown fits over it accurately. FUNCTION: Retainer with stressbreaker for resilient dentures. **B,** Scott attachments seen from tissue side on replacement of anterior teeth. Soldered twin abutments and external attachments, this time without combination with AxRo Joint, because it is a rigid attachment. Clasp arm is an additional stabilizer against leverage.

as a compensating joint to an AxRo in unilateral saddle cases. AxRo and Ro-joints can only be used in pairs across an arch. They are used either in bilateral free-end saddles, or in unilateral saddle cases with an AxRo on the saddle side and with a Ro-Joint on the tooth-bearing side of the denture. Thus the Ro-Joint acts as a compensating joint to the resilience movement of the saddle side, and as a stabilizer across the arch (Fig. 22-23). As we have commented before, the AxRo with its oval window allows, in many cases, for too much resilience. The Ro-joint has a round window and therefore no axial movement at all. This round window can be enlarged in an axial direction for as little as desirable. If the AxRo allows for 2 mm resilience movement, the case may ask for only 1 or 0.5 of a millimeter. In fact, the Ro-Joint might serve as a pure hinge joint if left in its original state. In such cases however, reliefs should be made as in Fig. 22-19 to allow this rotational movement to take place.

Mounting of AxRo and Ro joints is made on the parallelometer with a special mandrel for parallelizing. Note that the soldering base should be soldered at the angle of the tissue inclination underneath it.

W. R. Scott has combined the AxRo with a pin attachment of his own design (Fig. 22-24).

The bar attachments are described on p. 554.

Scott external precision attachment. The Scott external precision attachment (Fig. 22-24) is used for fixed and removable prostheses. It is connected to double abutments by a horizontal arm, and its position allows for normal contouring and embrasure space. It is a telescopic crown with tapered walls and a recess to house a stressbreaker if so desired. The numerous tapered walls increase the retention. Additional frictional retention is given by the parallel pins. The male of the attachment is available in burn-out plastic.

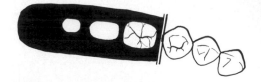

Fig. 22-25. Function of hinge (see also Fig. 22-6). When free-end saddle is attached to hinge, masticatory stresses near hinge are fully transmitted to abutment(s) next to saddle area. The farther away from the hinge that the forces are applied to the saddle, the more they are transmitted to underlying tissue. Therefore masticatory surface of such a saddle should decrease toward distal side, and teeth distalmost only serve to prevent antagonists from erupting.

The attachment, combined with an axial rotation joint, functions as a stable retainer with a stressbreaker for tissue-bearing dentures. The limiting screw of the axial rotation joint ties the attachment to the denture, and the patient removes them as a unit (Fig. 22-24). The attachment can also be used as a rigid connector for tooth-bearing dentures.

Hinges. A hinge functions as described in Fig. 22-25. Pressure on the tooth adjacent to the distal abutment in a free-end saddle will be transmitted almost completely to that abutment, whereas the distalmost tooth of the saddle will transmit the force almost totally to the resilient tissue. One should consider these facts when building the saddle and mounting the teeth. The saddle itself should be extended as distally as possible to get as much tissue-contacting surface as possible. When mounting the teeth, the width of the occlusal table should diminish toward the distal (Fig. 22-25). If a tooth has to be set near the distal margin of the acrylic saddle, because it must retain the antagonist from growing out, this denture tooth should only have a point contact with its antagonist.

Gaerny hinge. Hinges in general are stressbreakers interposed between attachment and the resilient saddle part of a denture. The Gaerny hinge (Fig. 22-26) is a strong construction that is relatively resistant to wear because of the large contacting surfaces between the two parts and because of the shape that locks the two parts in closed position. It represents a cylinder hinge combined with a vertical beam for reenforcement against lateral stresses. It comes in two lengths, 11 and 8 mm, and may be shortened from the top if the teeth are shorter. Shortening does of course weaken the hinge, since it reduces the contacting surface. When and if the tissue under the saddle of the denture is resorbed, this is signaled to the patient

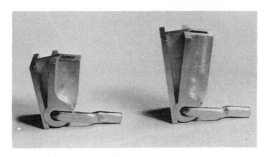

Fig. 22-26. Gaerny hinge consists of three components that are assembled by axis with lever. Hinges should always work independently on each saddle. Axis may be used on both sides, left and right, and is concealed within acrylic resin of saddle, on lingual (palatal) side.

and dentist by a slight opening of the hinge joint in rest position. It is the signal for rebasing. The hinge is always used independently from the other side. It is not advisable to connect the two hinges in a bilateral case, even if they are accurately aligned.

Gerber hinge. The Gerber hinge (Fig. 22-27) can be used singly in unilateral saddles as well as in bilateral saddles, where it is possible to couple them by aligning them vertically and horizontally. In general, the joints should operate individually and independently in bilateral saddle dentures. Only in cases of extreme stress should they be aligned horizontally and connected by a lingual or cross-arch bar. In the latter case they cannot function unless very accurately aligned on the same rotation axis. The soldering plate of the patrix is soldered to an attachment or clasp framework, and the matrix has a retention loop for the saddle acrylic. The linch pin, or axis screw, can be tightened if the hinge shows some wear. The washer serves to limit the rotation movement and may be used for both sides of the arch.

Cuénoud hinge. This type of hinge (Fig. 22-28) is at the same time an attachment, in principle similar to the Dalbo hinge. Its vertical housing forms, together

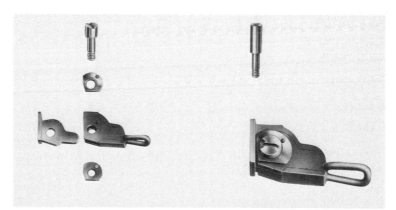

Fig. 22-27. Gerber hinge has four components. Sleeve is shown twice, once from inside and once from outside. It can be turned around to fit left and right side. *On right,* Hinge is assembled; above it, the screw used for mounting joint in acrylic resin.

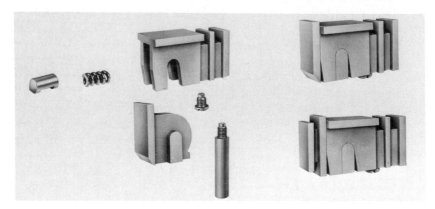

Fig. 22-28. Cuénoud hinge is attachment with hinge joint combined. Housing snaps onto patrix with a coil-spring snapper stud. On assembled hinge are shown reliefs that limit hinge movement.

with the patrix, large contacting surfaces resistant to wear. A snapper with a spring, held in place by a gingival screw, ensures the retention of the attachment. The freedom of hinge movement is given by the two wedge-shaped reliefs on the matrix. This hinge is moderate in height (4.6 mm). It is used in free-end saddles working independently, that is, in unilateral cases.

Screwed-on bridgework. In the chapter on planning bridgework and other restorative dentistry it was said that abutments that have different prognostic value could be used. A three-rooted molar with divergent roots has a longer prospective life-span as an abutment than does a one-rooted third molar with a beet-shaped root. An endodontically treated root is a bigger risk than is a healthy vital tooth. Yet patients confront dentists with their own individual cases, with a certain number of usable teeth as bridge abutments, each of which has to be evaluated as to its prognostic value and its bearing capacity for the restorative piece that the dentist intends to incorporate. Root length, root curvatures, quality of surrounding bone and periodontal tissues, position of the root in the damaged

arch, and size of spacing to be covered are factors influencing this prognostic value. A rigid, one-piece bridge over all abutments does not leave any alternative at a later date. This is where the fixed-removable bridge, screwed onto its abutments or onto groups of abutments, renders invaluable service. If any of the supporting teeth or roots fail, the bridge can be unscrewed and removed from the mouth. The failing abutment may be treated if it is destroyed by secondary caries or affected by endodontic problems. It can be extracted (if it is not an end-standing abutment), and with a small addition on the bridge, the latter may be reincorporated with practically no change or expense to the patient. Even if end-standing abutments fail, a total bridge in many cases can absorb the stresses upon a cantilever end, where the loss has occurred. A temporary bridge for the patient will also allow for attachment work to be performed on the bridge, to replace a loss by a partial denture.

Such fixed removable bridgework has another advantage. It has the same qualities as a fixed bridge but can be thoroughly cleaned by the dentist at chosen intervals. Thus one of the big dis-

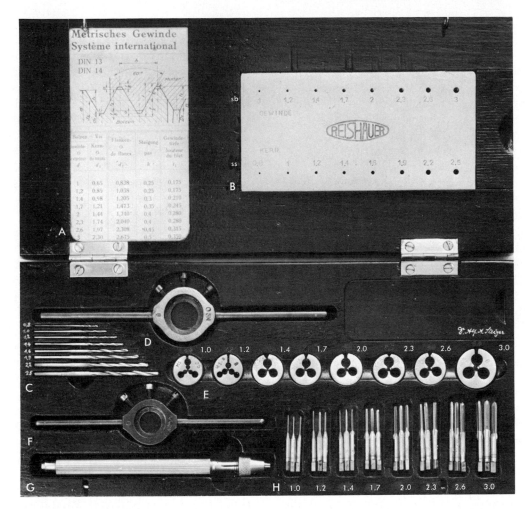

Fig. 22-29. Threading instruments. **A,** Metric thread, international system. **B,** Gages: *sb,* thread from 1 to 3 mm; *ss,* core from 0.8 to 2.5 mm. **C,** Drills. **D** and **F,** Holder for threaders. **E,** Threaders. **G,** Holder for screwtaps. **H,** Taps from 1 to 3 mm.

advantages of the fixed bridge is eliminated.

The placement of the screws is not problematic. A single point must be kept in mind: The screw must have a direction so as to make it easily accessible for a screwdriver in the mouth. Since we try to keep it visually hidden, the logical location is mesiopalatally in the upper, and mesiolingually in the lower arch. As the technician usually cannot visualize the handling of the bridge in the mouth, the dentist should indicate his wishes as to

the exact position and direction of the screws.

Screws are available with or without a sleeve. For dentists and technicians who are unfamiliar with cutting screw threads, the sleeve of a screw is cast into the matrix of the telescopic construction. The head of the screw should be at right angles and flush with the surface of the crown wall. Its minimum diameter should be 1.5 mm. The head of the screw may or may not be conic. The foot of the screw must reach into a shallow dip in the surface of the matrix of the telescope. Measure the thickness of the gold wall before fixing the position of the screw because the dip may form a perforation! Instead of a sleeve melted into the wax pattern of the patrix, the screw thread may be cut into the wall of the casting. With a spiral drill of the diameter of the inner thread the screwhole is drilled, always with oil (castor oil or eucalyptus oil). Spiral drills are brittle, and the critical moment in boring with them is when the inner wall is perforated. This is the time when they are liable to break if lubrication is insufficient and pressure excessive. Each size of screwthreaders (Fig. 22-29) has three subsizes. Progressively, each is used until the screw fits not too tightly and not too loosely.

Construction of a retentive screw. A screw without a conic head can be made without a lathe, just by use of platinum-gold wire or platinum wire and screw taps. The wire of proper size is fastened into a holder. The holder is held in a vise. Then the screw tap is placed by hand at right angles to the wire, of which the end is rounded. With the spreading screw or the two tightening screws, the size of the screw can be very slightly increased or decreased. The slit in the head of the screw is made with a handsaw and a blade of proper width.

For anteriors, the Schubiger block is an excellent screw unit; for posteriors, screws with sleeves of any make will do.

Fig. 22-29 shows a set of threading instruments of the international metric threading system for special dental purposes, sizes 1 to 3 mm. A few preliminary considerations may serve for better understanding of the properties of the threading instruments. Ignorance of these facts leads to immediate damage of the instruments and also of the work at hand, from which a broken screw tap must be removed. A definite tolerance is observed by the manufacturer in order to have screw taps and screw plates corresponding with each other. These tools are made of the best alloyed tool steel or of "heavy duty" high-speed steel. The latter instruments have the advantage of better quality and durability for dental purposes. Since the screw taps may be used in the mouth and may thus come into contact with saliva, chromium-plated instruments are useful. By the process of chromium plating, the instruments get surface hardened. The cutting angle of a screw tap (Fig. 22-30) is widely responsible for the proper pitch and neatness of the thread and for the amount necessary to cut it. Because screw taps and plates are cutting tools, their cutting angles will also have to differ when the dentist cuts different materials (Fig. 22-30). Thus angles between 0 and 2 degrees are used for hard steel; hard castings; steels of average strength; angles of 8 to 20 degrees for iron, soft steel, tough latten, and magnesium alloys; angles of 20 to 40 degrees for copper, aluminum, electrum, and other light-metal alloys. Gold and its alloys belong in the category of light metals, and therefore the threading tools have cutting angles of 20 to 40 degrees.

The choice of the size of the core-boring is the most important factor in a rational threading operation. Most fractures of screw taps are caused by excessively small core-borings. Therefore the manufacturer indicates the sizes of drills for each size of thread (Fig. 22-29). The cutting speed does not matter in hand-threading, whereas for lathe-threading, a certain speed in meters per minute is prescribed. On the other hand, lathe-threading eliminates the danger of misdirection, whereas in hand-threading, misdirection of the screw-tap during the operation may lead to breakage. Finally, it is important to use a proper lubricant, the same as that for milling. This again depends on the material to be threaded. For steel and iron, oils like rape oil, lard oil, whale oil, boring oil, sulfurated mineral oils, and hog fat are preferably used. For gold, euca-

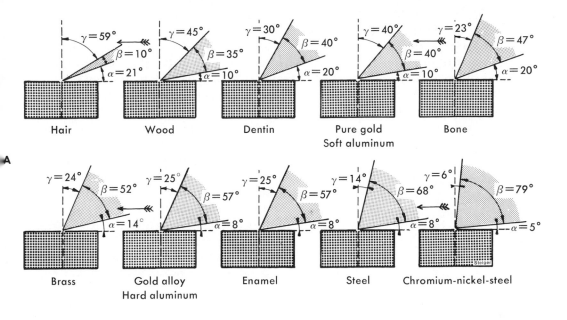

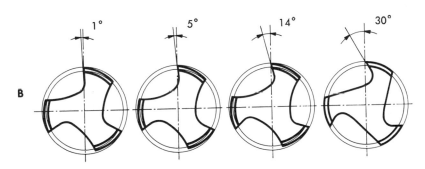

Fig. 22-30. A, Angles of incidence, α, and cutting angles, β, necessary for cutting instruments used on different materials. The softer the material, the larger is α and the smaller is β. The harder the material, the smaller is α and the larger is β. **B,** Principles shown in **A** apply to the cutting edges of threading plates: Almost rectangular cutting edge for steel at 30-degree inclination in order to thread soft metals like aluminum or latten.

lyptus oil is used with good results. It can be used without harm to the patient for work in the mouth.

Procedure of threading. One marks the location of the screwhole on the metal by tracing a cross. The intersection is marked with a tool called the "center." Thus the drill (Fig. 22-31) cannot "walk away" but is guided in the depression left by the center. According to Fig. 22-30, *B*, a bore of 1 mm is required for a thread diameter of 1.2 mm. The 1 mm drill, well lubricated, is pressed against the metal with the proper direction. Intermittently it is removed and reinserted in order to control the operation. The danger of breakage, apart from misdirection of the instrument, starts at the point of perforation.

Because the surface of the dental work pieces are irregular, the blades of the drill, on perforating the material, may cease to cut at different times, and the resulting torque may lead to breakage. Therefore the pressure must be considerably decreased as soon as the perforation

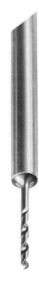

Fig. 22-31. Spiral drill used on dentin or gold. Note cutting head at end of instrument with rooflike inclination. This requires a starting hold made with a center, or on tooth, with very small round bur.

is imminent. Just ahead of the perforation a slight protuberance is noticeable on the surface of the metal. A screwhole that does not perforate the material is done with less risk. After completion of the bore, the screwtap of 1.2 mm in diameter is fastened in the holder. For each size there are three taps marked 1, 2, and 3. Work is started with tap 1, well lubricated. The tip of the tap is without thread, so that it may be inserted into the boring in proper axial alignment. It is turned clockwise with caution and, after a few turns, turned back and cleaned. Again it is lubricated and reinserted for a few more turns. As soon as the thread is finished in its full length, taps 2 and then 3 are used.

To make a screw, a piece of wire 1.2 mm in diameter and rounded at the end is immobilized in a vise, mandrel, or bench chuck. The 1.2 mm screw plate is fastened in the plateholder (Fig. 22-32). Held at right angles to the wire, it is screwed onto the wire with appropriate lubrication. For proper correlation between the diameter of the screwhole and the screw, screw plates may be adjusted with the screws outside on the plateholder. By tightening of the two lateral screws, the plate is compressed and the screw becomes slightly thinner. Tighten-

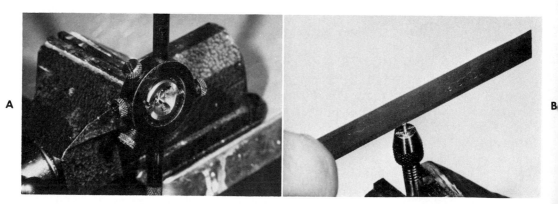

Fig. 22-32. A, Threading plate with holder on wire in process of screw-threading. **B,** Screw is attached in holder held in vise. Screw slit is cut with fine saw.

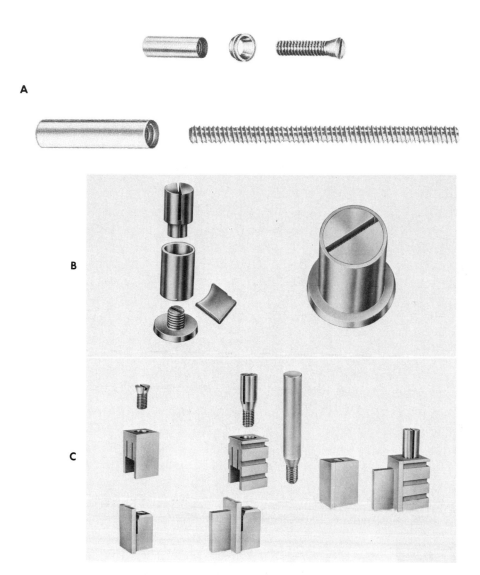

Fig. 22-33. A, Ready-made screw with sleeve. *Above,* With conical head; *below,* piece of screw to be cut off in appropriate length, and the screw slit must be cut for each screw, with a slit file. **B,** Schubiger block, a screw base to be soldered to a post cap on a devitalized root, a sleeve to be built into a crown. This sleeve can be cut to size and inclination of crown surface. Screw nut with screw slit holds the two parts together. Schubiger block is used in fixed-removable bridgework, in crowns, or in making a bar removable. Contratorsion plate is a soldering accessory. **C,** Flécher screwed attachment, used for fixed-removable bridgework or bar attachments. Large screw is a mounting screw only.

ing of the central screw pries the plate apart and makes the screw slightly larger. Thus the fit of the screw in the screwhole can be adjusted to minimum tolerance.

One side of the screw plate has a conic opening, which is to receive the tip of the wire to be threaded. The first thread fillets of the plate are very shallow; they serve to grip the end of the wire and to feed the wire into the deeper fillets, which cut the thread to proper depth. Proper thickness of the thread must be tried in the beginning, so that adjust-

ments may be made on the screw plate if necessary. If the screw is tight, compress the plate by the lateral screws; if it is too loose, pry it apart with the central screw. If the screw is to receive a head, conic or cylindric, a tube with a bore corresponding to the outer diameter of the screw is placed over one end of the screw and soldered at the top. The top is then flattened or rounded, and with a jigsaw for metal, the slit is cut. If the head of the screw must be countersunk in the workpiece, the entrance of the nut thread is milled

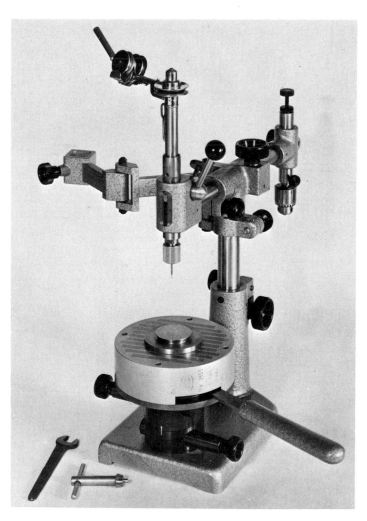

Fig. 22-34. Parallelometer Bachmann, by Cendres & Métaux. Component parts are explained in Fig. 22-50.

out cylindrically or conically. The proper fit of the screwhead is given on the lathe, when the proper amount is turned off with the turning steel.

With some training and enthusiasm and proper care, all sizes of screws of the international system may easily be made —a versatility that is a great help in the planning and construction of fixed removable bridgework. For those unable to perform such work, ready-made screws with corresponding threaded tubes are available in the industry of dental products (Fig. 22-33).

MOUNTING OF INTRACORONAL AND EXTRACORONAL ATTACHMENTS

The mounting of attachments requires adequate equipment, which is usually recommended by the manufacturer. The most important accessory is the surveyor or parallelometer (Fig. 22-34).

On study models, a common direction of insertion should be established. To plan this axis of insertion on models is a must, because it will influence cavity and crown preparation. Sufficient space must be allotted to the attachment boxes if intracoronal retainers are expected to be used. The space available will determine the size and length of the attachment used.

With special holders provided by the manufacturers, the attachment boxes are placed into the waxed-up abutment crowns or overlays, on the parallelometer (Fig. 22-35). Before the wax patterns are invested, the boxes should be withdrawn. They should be soldered in after the castings are completed and not cast to it. The placement of the box for soldering must again be done on the parallelometer because there is practically no tolerance for parallelism between attachments. Once the primary parts are soldered, the position of the secondary part is determined, and the latter may be soldered to the bridge body or the framework of the partial denture.

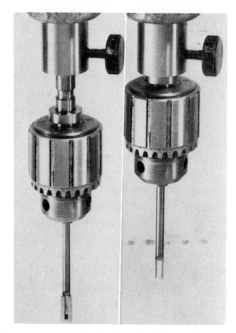

Fig. 22-35. Holder for female T-attachments in parallelometer. Thus several attachments may be parallelized exactly.

Manufacturers usually provide a detailed set of instructions. Also, they provide courses for technicians wishing to familiarize themselves with the use of these construction elements. To follow their advice is to avoid failure.

OPERATIONS PREVIOUS AND BASIC TO MOUNTING ATTACHMENTS
Impressions

Impressions may be conventionally taken with copper band–compound or copper band–rubber base materials, or— after soft-tissue management with threads (Gingipak, Racord, Pascord, etc.) or by electrosurgery—with elastomer or hydrocolloid impressions that may include all preparations at one time. Of all impression methods, the copper-band compound method, first for almost half a century, has become the least accurate and is about to become obsolete. Some practitioners will prefer elastomers (silicones, polyethylene, polysulfide rubber) because they can be metal plated. Others will prefer the ease and accuracy of hydrocolloids and plaster dies. There are a few rules to be observed when root posts with cast bases on devitalized roots are planned. The posthole should be bored with a calibrated drill corresponding to the conicity of the used post. A post should always consist of a wrought wire, not of a cast alloy, because posts made from wrought wires are many times stronger than cast posts. To remove a cast post at a later date is difficult to impossible. To remove a drawn post is easy with the proper instruments. The preparation of the root is started with the posthole. At the head of the stump, a small inlay preparation is made (1) for retentive purposes and (2) to envelop the post by sufficient casting. Posts should be conic 2 to 3 degrees. Parallel posts must have escape channels for the cement, otherwise they cannot be properly cemented. For copper-band impressions, the posts must have a serration at the oral end to retain compound or rubber-base materials. For hydrocolloid impressions, they should be fitted with a little "roof" cut out from a sheet of acrylic (Fig. 22-36). The post is heated, sunk into the acrylic, and chilled.

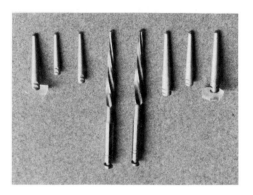

Fig. 22-36. Root posts of iridioplatinum in two sizes and two lengths for each size. For each size there is a drill of same conicity and size. On each side of posts depicted, a post is fitted with "cap" for retention in impression material.

Removal of old posts

Unfortunately, our best efforts in dentistry cannot claim to last a lifetime except in exceptions. Such exceptions mean very lucky patients and dentists. Therefore a young dentist should think about difficulties arising from his own work after 20 to 30 years, a period that lies easily within his professional life expectancy. The older dentist, who may expect many of his pieces of work to survive him, should think of the next professional man who eventually will have to remove his patient's bridges when they will have served their purpose for a period of years. One of these considerations is the placing of posts into root canals. The removal of a post made from wrought wire is very easy with the proper instrumentation.

The post crown is cut at the stem of the post, just underneath the crown, preferably from the lingual side, with a fissure bur. The dentist is then faced with a root surface and a post flush with it; so he uses the Pivotex, the Clavulex, or the Thomas instrument (Fig. 22-37).

First, a trepan bur (circular saw) of proper size is used to cut around the post into the root inlay, or into the dentin or the cement around the post, whatever the situation will be. The depth of bore will be about 1.5 mm. Then the same-size threading instrument is used to cut a thread into the protruding head of the post. It is advisable to oil the threader with mineral oil before use. With at least two, or better three threads cut, the threader is unscrewed, and then in sequence the steel and the rubber ring are inserted. The lever instrument is applied, with the rubber ring pressing against the tooth and the steel ring against the upper lever (Fig. 22-37, *B*). With a finger on the head of the threader, the lever is screwed tight until the post pops out, attached to the threader. A cast post cannot be removed in this way because it will tear off right underneath the threaded part when leverage is applied. Such posts have to be

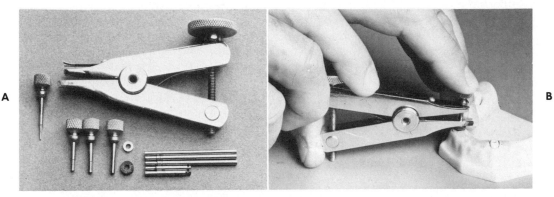

A

B

Fig. 22-37. A, Thomas post extractor with its components. With a trepan bur, post to be removed is circumcised. Same-size threader cuts three or four threads into post. Extractor pushes down upon metal ring, rubber ring, and root and pushes up against threader. **B,** Operation of removing post. Screw down extractor and hold finger over threader to prevent it from popping out.

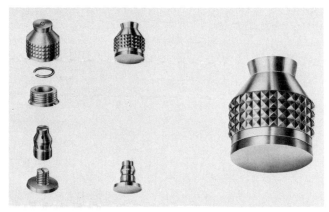

Fig. 22-38. Gerber retention cylinder, RZ. *On left,* Base for components, core, cylinder screw, spring, and housing. *Middle bottom,* Base and screw assembled (screw in with a drop of acrylic resin). Serrations in surface of cylinder housing increase retention in acrylic resin.

drilled out completely. Everybody who has tried this once knows what is involved in such a procedure: loss of root material, possible perforation, and despair over the time involved.

TELESCOPE STUDS (PUSH-BUTTON ATTACHMENTS)

Telescope studs, as attachments, are also known under the name of cylindric friction-grip anchors. This category applies only to devitalized root stumps without crowns. The use of modern endodontia along with a sound judgment of where its use has a good chance of success may save many a healthy and strong root as an abutment for a bridge or a partial denture, or as the last tooth-supported retention for a full denture (overdenture). A glimpse into the classification shows that studs have become widely used; inventions in this field never seem to stop. Their greatest advantage is the replaceability of their parts.

Rigid attachments

Gerber retention cylinder. Fig. 22-38 shows a Gerber RC (retention cylinder). The five component parts are the base, screw, retention core, inner cylinder, and spring. The base is soldered to the root cap of the abutment. In the center of the base is a sturdy screw, which practically never breaks. Upon that screw fits a core, the retention core, which is screwed on along with a little bit of self-curing acrylic. The excess acrylic comes out through a little venthole. To remove this core, should it become necessary, slightly heat the core by contact with a hot instrument, and then easily unscrew it. At this stage, the parts still remain in the mouth. Over that core fits the removable unit—the cylinder that is polymerized into a bridge tooth, a partial, or a full denture. The cylinder contains an inner cylinder that holds the split-ring spring. Inner cylinder and snap spring may be easily replaced in no time at all by use of a special screwdriver provided by the manufacturer. The snap retention results from pushing the split-ring spring over the bulge of the retention core. This ring spring is held in place by the inner cylin-

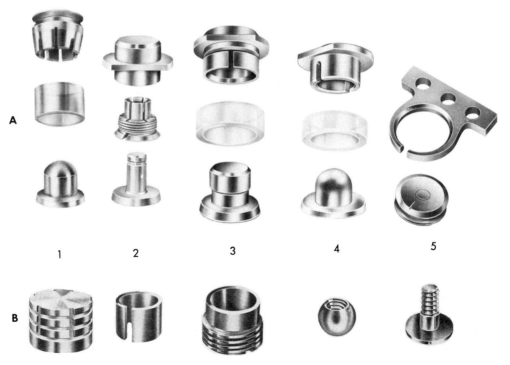

Fig. 22-39. A, *1,* Dalla Bona cylindrical anchor; *2,* Schneider anchor; *3,* Baer-Fäh anchor; *4,* Baer-Fäh anchor, short model; *5,* Rothermann eccentric anchor (horizontal). **B,** Sandri ball anchor. Its component parts are shown as they are assembled. Frictional sleeve is retained in this model by screw. In another model, it is retained by a square spring that snaps into a circular channel in housing. Sandri anchors are popular because of their small vertical dimension.

der. Studs of this type are rigid when assembled. Fig. 22-39 shows some other models of this type:

Dalla Bona cylindrical anchor. The housing is split six times and is slightly conic. A plastic sleeve slips over it to keep the acrylic away from the elastic part. The housing and its sleeve are incorporated into crown or denture, and the base is soldered to the root cap. The dentist can activate the housing by prying slightly apart the segments between the slits. A similar anchor exists with a ball base.

Schneider anchor. It is a solid anchor with a threaded bushing fitting into the housing, which is replaceable without repair of the denture or crown by unscrewing. Frictional adjustment is possible. The anchor is relatively large in height.

Baer-Fäh anchors. No. 4 is only 2 mm high, a size that is often very useful. The friction is obtained by activation of the split housing enveloped by the plastic sleeve. Only the sleeve is replaceable.

Rothermann Eccentric. The Rothermann eccentric anchor is particularly popular for its small height of only 1.7 mm. In its first model, it showed frequent breakages because the clasp part was of wrought wire, soldered to the perforated base. The new model depicted is made of one-piece wrought alloy fashioned into shape and so promises less repairs. Repairs are more difficult than with the cylindric housings.

Resilient anchors

Telescope studs as described above are rigid attachments. Some of them are available as resilient anchors. Fig. 22-40 gives a few examples of such resilient anchors. We recognize the same component parts as in the rigid design. In addition, there is a plastic spacing ring, which is used only for mounting. The spacing ring holds the housing slightly away from the surface of the soldering base. Thus a resilience way of 0.4 mm is created. It is often argued that this resilience way will have disappeared after a few months. This is mostly correct. On the other hand, the difference in resilience in different tissue areas will have been overcome by that time, and the denture will have "settled." Here again, the discussion is still open as to what anchor to choose for

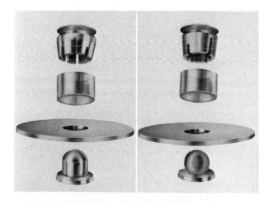

Fig. 22-40. Two Dalla Bona resilient anchors. *On left,* With cylindric core; *on right,* with ball core on soldering base. Plastic ring is space holder during mounting procedure. Its thickness determines maximum resilience movement.

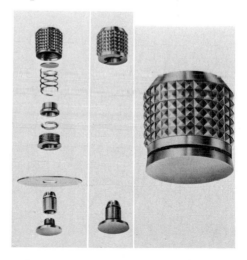

Fig. 22-41. Gerber cylindrical buffer. Also a resilient anchor. Core, screw, small spring, sleeve, return spring, plate, and cylinder are replaceable.

an overdenture, a rigid or a resilient one. A few examples for resilient anchors are the Gerber Retention Buffer, Battesti Resilient Anchor, Dalla Bona Buffer Anchor, Sandri Resilient Anchor, and Rothermann Eccentric Resilient Anchor (Fig. 22-41).

Mounting of telescopic studs

Each model requires a small amount of special equipment for mounting, which is provided by the manufacturers. The axis of insertion must be established on the parallelometer just as for the other attachments. The soldering base is placed upon the root cap with a special holder from the parallelometer, fastened with burn-out plastic or sticky wax, invested with an auxiliary holder, and soldered.

Experience has shown that the root caps should not be tapered toward the occlusal (Fig. 22-42) because this invites tissue proliferation and inflammation. Instead, the root cap should imitate the base of a crown with an inverted taper. Tissue proliferations should be cut away by electrosurgery and left to heal with a periodontal pack.

Such studs must sometimes absorb quite sizable forces. In acrylic dentures, breakages and fissures are often observed to occur from the torque of a stud cylinder within the acrylic plate. To avoid such breakages, the denture plates are reenforced with a metal base designed to translate those forces to a larger surface of the plate. At the site of the studs, this base consists of small "grips," cast rings that envelop the stud cylinder but leave a small space for acrylic between grip and cylinder (Fig. 22-43). Formerly, these grips were soldered to the cylinders, but then replacement of a cylinder was a large operation because the base had to be severed from the cylinder. Such a destroyed grip had to be recast and resoldered, thus necessitating also a reprocessing of the acrylic part. With the present method, one simply uncovers the cylinder with a bur and then heats the cylinder with a hot instrument and pushes it out of the grip. There is an auxiliary holder, which makes this heating process easy. To remount the new cylin-

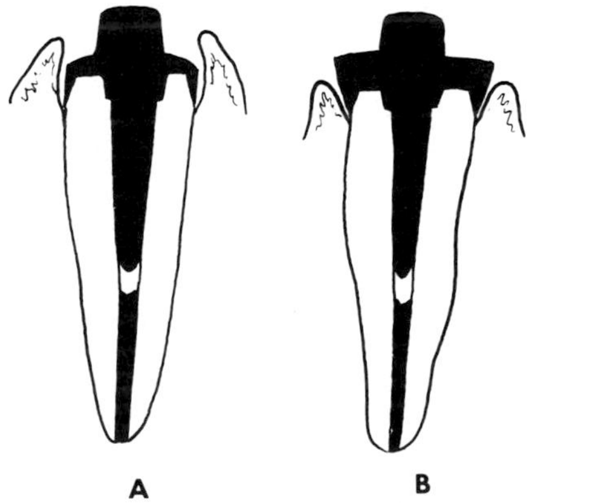

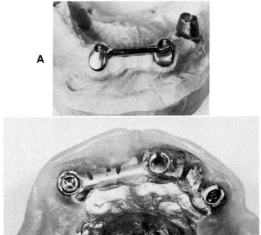

Fig. 22-42. A, Wrong shape of cast root base, rounded shape; tissue grows over it and proliferates. **B,** Correct shape simulates neck of tooth crown.

Fig. 22-43. Two post bases with studs. In the back a crown stump receiving a telescope crown. Two bases are joined by a bar attachment. **A,** Construction cast. **B,** Overdenture.

der, it is placed upon the core in the mouth, the denture is inserted over it, and with a drop of self-curing acrylic, the space between cylinder and grip is filled and the defect is closed. For the root caps, only ready-made posts of a durable and resistant platinum-iridium-gold alloy with a taper of 2 to 3 degrees are used. Cast posts are entirely insufficient because they are too weak.

Overdenture

Telescopic studs are the ideal anchors for overdentures. An overdenture is a full denture that is supported by one or several roots (Fig. 22-44). Its purpose is to provide the patient with a few remaining supports by his natural roots, to compensate for sometimes missing retention of poor alveolar crests and to give the patient a period of adaptation after making him lose most of his natural teeth and giving him the strange feeling of a set of teeth on a plate. To many patients, the mere feeling that a denture snaps into place, instead of just staying on the palate by air pressure, gives them a security that helps them to make the best of a regrettable situation. To make the abutments of an overdenture last, the patient must be taught meticulous care to clean the studs and root caps. Plaque under a denture may considerably shorten the lifetime of such abutments. Overdentures may also be supported by a Dolder bar joint (see p. 563), which is a retainer allowing for resilience and a rotational movement of the denture.

Nonretentive supports such as *A* to *C* in Fig. 22-44 may be used where the alveolar crests and saliva texture provides sufficient retention. Such nonretentive supports will probably last longer than rigid or stress-broken, retentive anchors, but they provide little or no retention.

Laboratory-made precision attachments

In Europe, laboratory-made attachments became known during the First World War, when ready-made attachments from the United States were unobtainable. At the time, for a dentist to make his own attachments was quite a feat, since casting methods were still in a rudimentary stage. One of the great pioneers in laboratory-made attachments was Alfred Steiger, who, by his ingeniousness and careful planning, created a class of attachments unparalleled in durability and variability. His inventions,

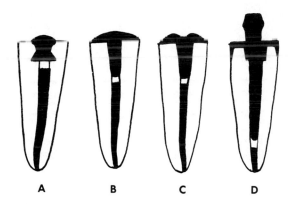

Fig. 22-44. Overdenture bases. **A,** Root with root canal filling and amalgam obturation, simplest version. **B,** Fully cast base, convex at surface. **C,** Same, but with a central depression in convexity; congruent part in denture centers itself into depression. **D,** Long prefabricated post with cast base and stud base soldered to it. Large choice in studs, rigid or resilient, has been partially shown previously.

with slight modifications have survived into our modern times and still count in among the best retainers we have.

Channel-shoulder-pin attachment (Steiger)

The channel-shoulder-pin attachment (CSP) is a laboratory-made attachment and may be adapted to all conceivable crowns, overlays, inlays, porcelain-to-gold crowns, and vital or nonvital teeth. If properly constructed, the CSP is so resistant to wear and tear that it may claim to survive the tooth or the patient! A variation to the CSP attachment is the Steiger bar attachment, an extracoronal attachment, described on p. 520. Both these attachments consist of three elements as the name suggests: The channels, elements that guide the matrix onto the patrix into its seat; the shoulder, a supporting element receiving and transmitting shearing forces or axial stresses;

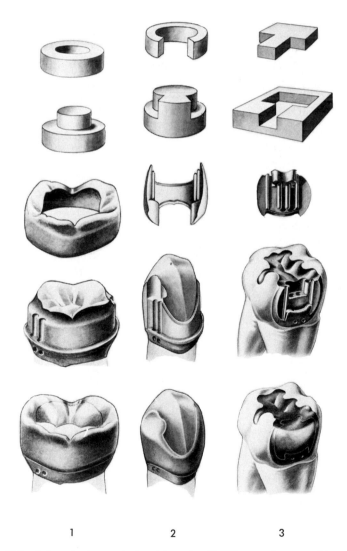

1   2   3

Fig. 22-45. Principle of channel-shoulder-pin (CSP) attachment. Shapes: *left,* ring shape; *middle,* horseshoe shape; *right,* T shape. (From Steiger, A. A., and Boitel, R. H.: Precision work for partial dentures, Zurich, 1959, Berichthaus, Buchdruckerei.)

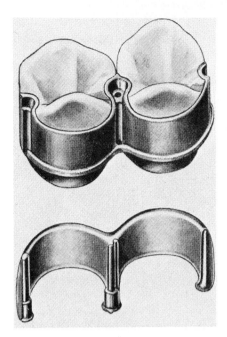

Fig. 22-46. Horseshoe type of CSP attachment as used for porcelain-to-gold techniques. Note dovetail anchorage between abutments, also cast sleeve, into which frictional pins are soldered. (From Steiger, A. A., and Boitel, R. H.: Precision work for partial dentures, Zurich, 1959, Berichthaus, Buchdruckerei.)

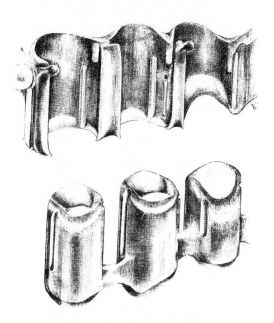

Fig. 22-47. Horseshoe type of attachments as shown by Gaerny. He connects the individual attachment crowns almost at their base and closes interdental space to prevent contamination with food and debris.

and last the pins, which provide the frictional element. They oppose a reasonable measure of resistance to the separation of the matrix and the patrix. Naturally, the proper design of the attachment body is paramount for success. Faulty design has led, in dental practice, to most of the failures observed. Since there is no limit to the possibilities of design, they are subdivided into three main groups. A rule is established for all of them: The design must be such that the matrix (without the frictional pins) must not be displaceable except in the direction of removal and insertion. Even if strong lateral forces or torque are applied, there should not be the slightest movement between patrix and matrix.

Fig. 22-45 shows the three basic designs of the CSP attachment: cylinder, horseshoe, and T. The most resistant de-

sign is the cylinder in all its variations. It applies to full crowns, three-quarter crowns, overlays, and post crowns.

The horseshoe design applies mainly to porcelain-to-gold crowns without occlusal gold surfaces (Fig. 22-46). A modification of the horseshoe design has been adopted by Gaerny for his CIS attachments* (removable closure of the interdental space) (Fig. 22-47). Such horseshoe type of attachments must be made very strong in order to avoid "opening" of the attachment on the open end, by torque. Also, a dovetail junction of continuous attachments (Fig. 22-48) or deep channels on single abutment attachments must keep proper retention.

The T design has been all but abandoned, because it is the weakest of all. It may be used on an end-standing abutment tooth as a supplementary attach-

---

*Gaerny, A.: Removable closure of the interdental space, Quintessenz, Berlin, 1972.

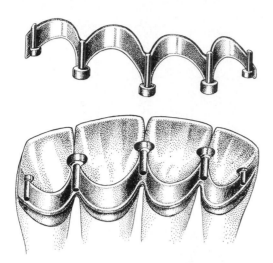

Fig. 22-48. Continuous clasp type of CSP attachment. Not in use very frequently since it unnecessarily thickens area that may be critical for proper speech sounds. In a splint, endstanding attachments may often be preferable.

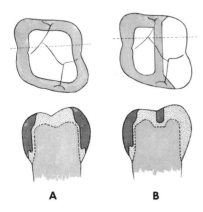

A   B

Fig. 22-49. A, Ring type of cylindric CSP attachment from above and from side in cross section. **B,** Modified cylinder attachment, leaving buccal surface untouched.

ment, for example, on the mesial of a single second-molar bridge abutment. It is just as easy, though, to cut a modified cylinder attachment (Fig. 22-49).

Materials necessary for CSP attachments

Parallelometer. The name "parallelometer" is not descriptive or correct for this

sort of instrument, since "meter" would imply a measuring device, which it is only partly. It should be defined as a multipurpose parallelizing machine because it combines the following devices in one instrument:

1. Isodrome—a drilling and milling machine, driven by a laboratory motor with flexible driving axle or Doriot type of attachment.
2. Pantostat—a lever with two parallel hinge joints, conventionally called a surveyor in prosthetics.
3. Pin-seating device—device for the parallelism of frictional pins in CSP attachments or for the parallelism of stress-breaker joints of resilient partial dentures; the only part that would deserve the name "meter" is a millimeter scale indicating the boring depth of the drill press.

Parts of Cendres & Métaux parallelometer (Fig. 22-50)

BASE WITH ADJUSTABLE WORKING TABLE. Loosening of knob *b* allows the table to be turned around a perpendicular axis. Loosening of knob *b* allows any oblique position desired for surveying clasp work or establishing the correct axis of insertion for precision work. With both lines at the front of the table in alignment, the table is horizontal, that is, perpendicular to the boring and working axis of the instruments. Lever *c,* inserted into the opening on the side of the table, serves to activate a magnet inside the table. In the forward position of the lever, the magnet is active, and in backward position, inactive. The magnet serves to immobilize a model with a special steel disc incorporated in its base, on the working table. With lever *c* held firmly and both knobs loosened, the table can be brought into any oblique position without rotation by a knob that moves backward and forward.

VERTICAL BEAM WITH RACK. The vertical beam supports all the working parts of the instrument with the exception of the table and serves to raise and lower the hori-

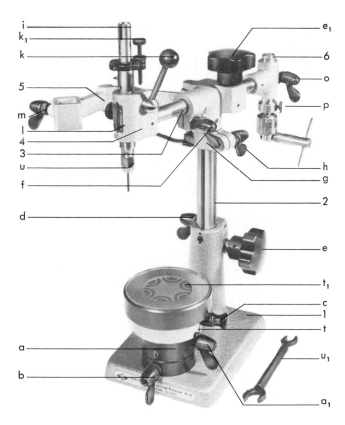

Fig. 22-50. Parallelometer Bachmann, Cendres & Métaux. *1,* Base of instrument; *2,* vertical beam; *3,* horizontal beam; *4,* working head with slip joint for laboratory motor; *5,* Pantostat; *6,* pin-seating device. *a, a₁,* and *b,* Knobs for table adjustments; *c,* magnet lever; *d,* fixation screw for vertical movement; *e,* knob for vertical movement; *e₁,* knob for horizontal movement; *f,* scale for measuring boring depth; *g,* joint for rotation of horizontal beam on vertical beam; *h,* fixation screw; *i,* slip-joint connection; *k,* lever for vertical movement of drillhead; *k₁,* limiting screw for depth of bore; *m,* fixation screw for Pantostat; *n,* inner cylinder of pin-sealing device; *o,* fixation screw for pin-seating device; *p,* fixation screw of outer cylinder against inner cylinder; *q,* adjusting screw for accurate height adjustment; *t,* working table; *t₁,* magnet; *u,* chuck for screw drills; *u₁,* wrench for chuck.

zontal beam that is attached to its top. Knob *e* moves the beam up and down; knob *d* is the fixation screw against this movement. The cogwheel, which drives the vertical beam, is concealed in the base shaft.

HORIZONTAL BEAM. The horizontal beam serves to move the working instruments in a horizontal plane. The knob for horizontal movement is *el.* A cog-

wheel allows a linear displacement, which is arrested by a fixation screw *f.* The joint *g* allows a rotation of the horizontal beam around a vertical axis in order to place the different working parts into working position over the table. Fixation screw *h* arrests the rotational movement.

DRILL HEAD. The drill head serves to drive drills, milling and cutting instru-

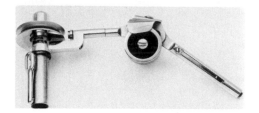

Fig. 22-51. Slip-joint adapter for laboratory motor.

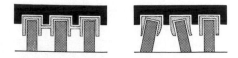

Fig. 22-52. *Left,* Parallel abutment preparation, primary crowns and secondary attachments. *Right,* Unparallel abutment preparation, parallelized crowns, and secondary attachments.

ments. The top *i* is a slip-joint connection for the laboratory motor. Certain laboratory motors require a slip-joint adapter (Fig. 22- 51) by S. S. White or KAVO drill head chucks for different-sized drill shafts to fit into the drill head, which is tightened by a screw wrench. Lever *k* serves to move the bur, drill, or milling instrument in a vertical direction, and scale 1 indicates the boring depth in millimeters.

PANTOSTAT. The pantostat, pantograph arm (surveyor), with two toggle joints, moves horizontally. Its free end carries a holder of square cross section for a pencil or any rod suited to the purpose. The square shape allows the fixation of different-sized instruments, which need not be round in cross section. Fixation of the instrument is obtained by screw *m*. If desired, the pin-seating device 6 may be fastened in the pantostat arm.

PIN-SEATING DEVICE. The pin seater serves to seat the frictional pins of the CSP attachments into the waxed-up restorations (see p. 540). The rod is removable from its shaft by loosening of the fixation screw *o*. The lower end of the pin seater carries an adjustable chuck for shafts of different sizes. In this chuck the pin holder or the joint holder or the holder for precision attachments of the T type is fastened. The pin seater consists of an outer cylinder held by a shaft 6 and an inner piston *n*, which may be lowered by manual traction into the exact desired position. Since the piston is retained by a spring, it must be fastened into the de-

sired position by fixation of screw *p*. Adjustment screw *q* serves to lower the fixed piston a small distance. Loosening of fixation screw *p* causes the release of the spring inside the cylinder, and the piston retracts into the cylinder.

Working axis on parallelometer. Each study model must be examined for the establishment of a common axis of insertion and removal of the planned removable appliance. For single bridge abutments, not soldered into groups, this working axis must *approximately* determine the axis of abutment preparation. For group abutments, it must nearly coincide with the axis of preparation. This makes it clear that this working axis should be determined on a study model *before* the cutting of the teeth. Where there is doubt about the axis, tentative abutment preparations on the study models may be very worthwhile. At the same time, one should decide which of the abutments shall be soldered into splinted groups. Single abutments or groups of abutments between them need not be completely parallel, if there is sufficient space for parallel-cut or parallel-adapted attachments (Fig. 22-52).

MOUNTING OF AXIS. The study model (or later, the master model) is placed upon the parallelometer table. The axis rod is fastened into the chuck of the pin seater or of the drill head, whichever seems more convenient. The nipple is lowered into proximity with the center of the model. The table is now moved into an oblique position that places the model at

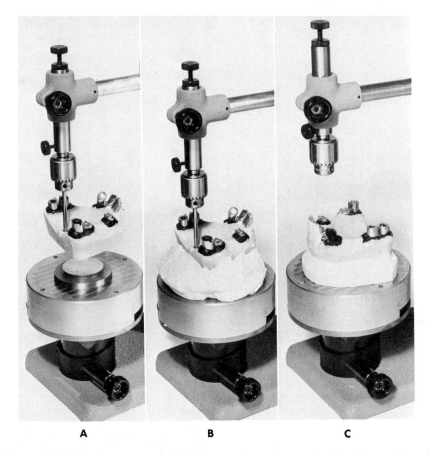

A   **B**   **C**

Fig. 22-53. Placing of master model in correct working axis. **A,** Axis rod has been cemented in desired position and is fixed into pin-seating device of parallelometer, above working table, where a magnetic disc has been placed. **B,** Plaster has been poured onto disc and table, and model was lowered into plaster. **C,** Master model has a base that is perpendicular to working axis.

a desired angle that will constitute the working axis of the model (Fig. 22-53). The area below the nipple in the plaster of the model is hollowed out to a depth corresponding to the length of the nipple. Dental cement is brought into the cavity and the nipple of the axis is lowered into the cement. When the cement has set, the horizontal beam of the parallelometer is raised; thus the model is suspended in midair. The parallelometer table is adjusted to horizontal position and a plaster base containing a steel disc for the magnet is poured under the model. Thus, with the table in horizontal position, the working axis will be established permanently and the axis rod may be removed from its nipple (Fig. 22-54).

Cutting instruments for gold. Straight or helicoid cutters are used for cutting gold on a parallelometer. Fig. 22-55 shows an excellent representative of this type, the Gaerny cutters. They are left rotating, right cutting, and minimally conic to compensate for the torque deformation. Optimal milling speed is 3,000 rpm. The cutters should work without vibration. For small channels, the round end cutters are used (Fig. 22-56).

Lubrication is obtained by equal parts

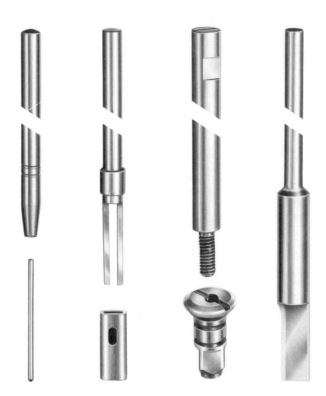

Fig. 22-54. Small accessories to parallelometer. *Left to right,* Pin seater and pin, holder for axial rotation joint, female or T-attachment female, axis rod with base carving knife for parallelizing wax crown walls in CSP attachment work.

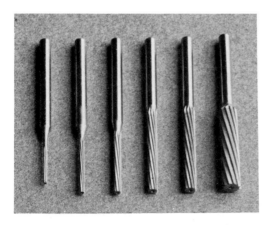

Fig. 22-55. Gaerny cutters for cutting CSP attachments, left-turning and right-cutting.

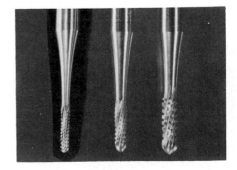

Fig. 22-56. Round-end burs to cut and clean channels in cast patrix and to cut occlusal chamfer in CSP attachments.

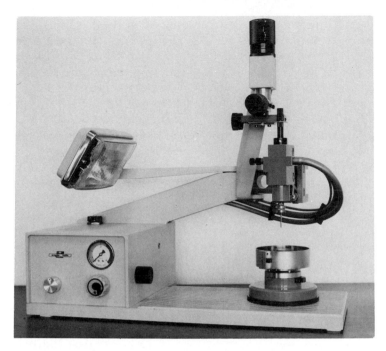

Fig. 22-57. Cutting machine "Fresatore 3 D N 1" Artiglio (Parma, Italy). This is a turbine cutter with lamp.

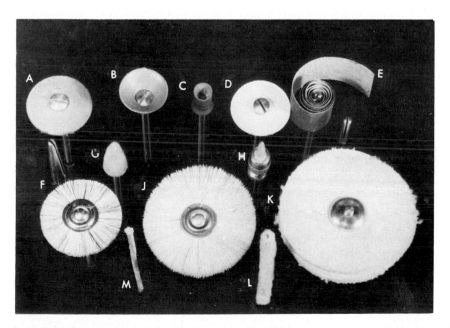

Fig. 22-58. Polishing materials. **A,** Burlew disc. **B,** Rubber cup. **C,** Small rubber cup. **D,** Felt disc. **E,** Split mandrel with abrasive paper strip. **F,** Split mandrel. **G,** Felt cone. **H,** Wood cone. **I,** Wheel brush, hard. **J,** Wheel brush, soft. **K,** Leather wheel. **L,** Pipe cleaner. **M,** Piece of string.

of eucalyptus oil and mineral oil. Cutting should always be done under lubrication. Some technicians use the conventional number of revolutions per minute to cut on the parallelometer; others have started to cut with a turbine cutter (Fig. 22-57) at high speed. For boring holes (pinholes in shoulders), the best instrument is the Spirec drill (by Müller, Biel, Switzerland) or spiral drill by Seitz & Haag (Giessen, West Germany). For tooth preparations it can also be used for pinholes in pinledge techniques. Its boring depth may be limited by a silver sleeve that is pushed over the drill. On the parallelometer, the boring depth may be read on the millimeter scale of the drill press.

Polishing materials. The most frequently used polishing instruments are shown in Fig. 22-58. The art of polishing is a personal matter with every technician. The difficulty in CSP attachment work is not to create undercuts in the patrix by overpolishing. Well-milled surfaces need little polishing.

Measuring instruments. Calipers are used to measure the thickness of a material (Fig. 22-59). The measured distance is enlarged 10 times on the scale so that 0.1 mm can be read as 1 mm. In attach-ment work, it is often very important for one to be able to measure the thickness of a crown when positioning a ready-made attachment or when milling the patrix of a CSP attachment. The *wire gage* for wires of 0.52 to 0.9 mm is useful in measuring all kinds of pins, wires, and posts.

Steps to make a channel-shoulder-pin attachment

1. Establish, on a study model, the tentative axis of insertion of a bridge or partial denture, and fix this axis bodily with the parallelometer (Fig. 22-53) by tilting the table. When fixed, place the table in a horizontal position, and make a plaster base under the model. Make rough preparations on the study model.

2. Prepare abutments on the patient, take impressions, make master model, and cast the base to the model the same way as under step 1 with the study model. The master model should have removable dies.

3. Wax up crowns that will serve as attachment retainers. Transfer crowns by luting them to a post or tripod in the parallelometer and pouring a new base for each of them.

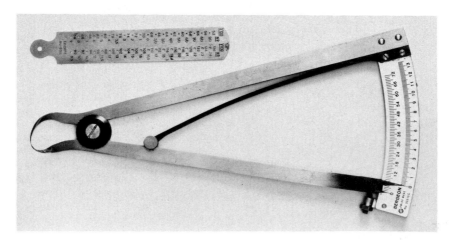

Fig. 22-59. Wire gage from 0.52 to 0.96 mm diameter, 0.02 mm apart. Calipers for measuring gold thickness in crowns and attachments.

4. Cut the parallel walls of the attachment with a wax knife fixed in the Pantostat (Fig. 22-60). Sink the pins at desired locations into the wax walls (steel pins), and lute a wax shoulder over the pins (Fig. 22-61).

5. Invest and cast the patrix, pull out steel pins, if necessary, and remove them with hydrochloric acid.

6. Use cutters to parallelize the attachment walls, and use round-end fissure burs to clean the channels (Fig. 22-62).

7. Fashion an occlusal chamfer with a

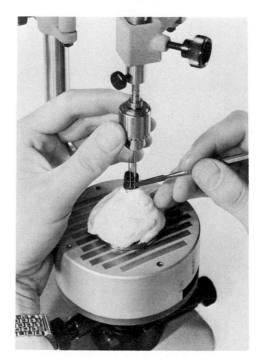

Fig. 22-61. Seating pins into wax patrix with pin-seating device on parallelometer.

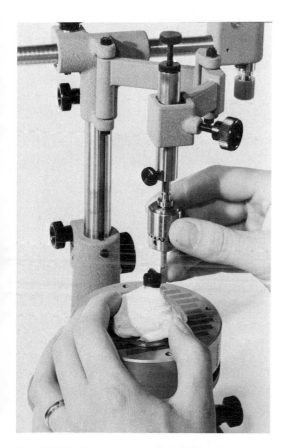

Fig. 22-60. Carving parallel CSP attachment walls on parallelometer. Crown has been transferred from master model to individual model, later used as cutting model.

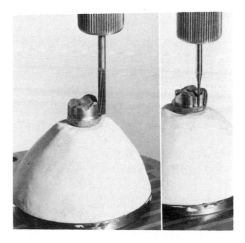

Fig. 22-62. Cast patrix on cutting model. *Left,* Cutting parallel walls. *Right,* Cleaning channels left by steel pins, getting proper depth of channels.

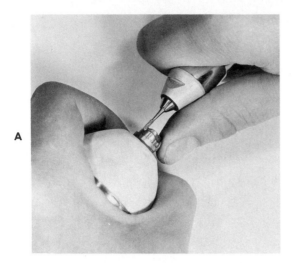

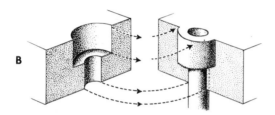

Fig. 22-63. A, Cutting occlusal chamfer on CSP patrix with round-end fissure bur. **B,** Diagram of occlusal chamfer on CSP patrix.

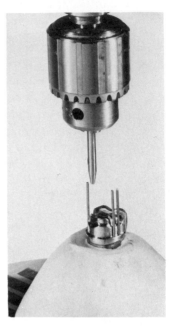

Fig. 22-64. Seating pins into finished patrix before matrix of CSP attachment is waxed.

heavier round-end fissure bur (Fig. 22-63). This chamfer will give more thickness and strength to the occlusal part of the matrix as will be seen later.

8. Polish delicately without creating undercuts.
9. Seat new steel pins into the finished patrix (Fig. 22-64).
10. Wax up the patrix (for this, the die should be intermittently replaced into the master model to check contact and occlusion). Duralay plastic may be used. The advantage is that the pins may be temporarily removed to check and grind in the occlusion (Fig. 22-65).
11. Sprue and invest patrix with pins (Fig. 22-66).

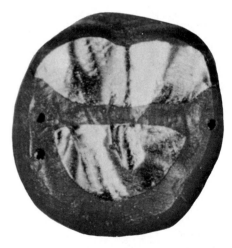

Fig. 22-65. Finished wax-up of matrix with pins removed.

12. Cast patrix, remove steel pins, and make necessary adjustments (stripping, oxidizing for friction marks).
13. Insert platinum-gold pins, fasten them with sticky wax, and invest and solder the pins (Fig. 22-67).

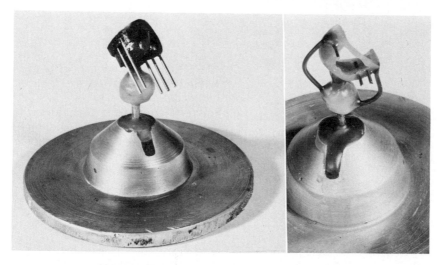

Fig. 22-66. Sprued matrix ready for investing.

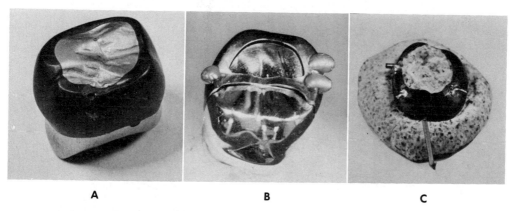

A	B	C

Fig. 22-67. A, Cast and oxidized matrix on finished patrix. **B,** Matrix not quite completely inserted to show limits, with platinum-gold pins waxed into place. **C,** Matrix on soldering investment with pins ready for soldering.

14. Polish and finish, and solder the attachment to the bridge body or partial denture framework.

Fig. 22-68 shows a cross section of the patrix, matrix, channels, and pins. Fig. 22-69 shows with two removable bridges a few possibilities offered by the CSP system. The model was made to demonstrate different attachments rather than to show the indication for removable bridgework. In such a case, it is very likely that a fixed bridgework would be indicated.

Bar attachment

Although the Steiger Bar Attachment belongs to the category of extracoronal attachments, its description is placed here, since it is many times used in conjunction with the CSP attachments and is also laboratory made. The bar attachment is designed to splint two or more single or group abutments to a unit that retains a partial denture and forms a line or, still better, a plane of support (Fig. 22-70). Its precursors were the Gilmore bar and the Bennet blade (see p. 503). The Gilmore

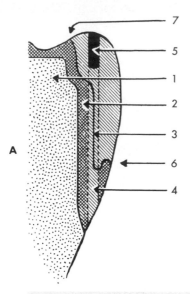

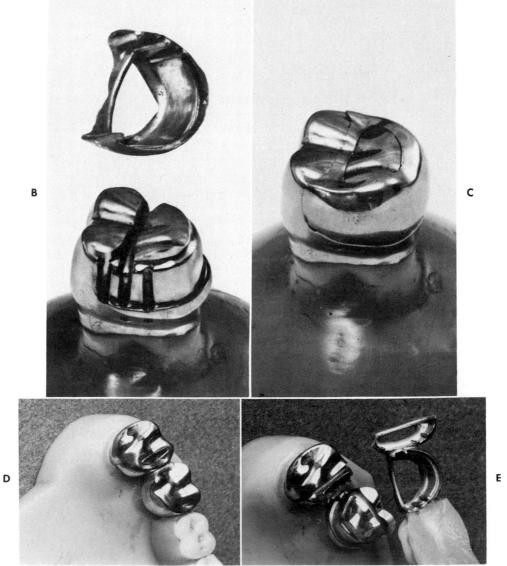

Fig. 22-68. A, Cross section of patrix and matrix assembled. *1,* Tooth; *2,* patrix; *3,* surface of patrix with shoulder; *4,* frictional pin; *5,* soldered part of pin; *6,* bevel of shoulder; *7,* matrix with thick part created by chamfer in patrix. **B,** Modified cylinder design CSP attachment, disassembled. **C,** Same crown assembled, not quite together, to show outline. **D,** Modified cylinder design CSP attachment on construction model, disassembled. **E,** Assembled on construction model.

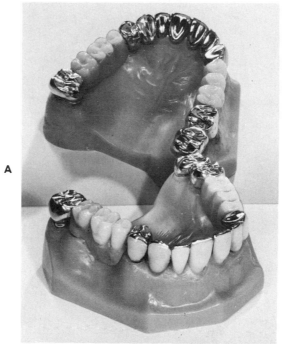

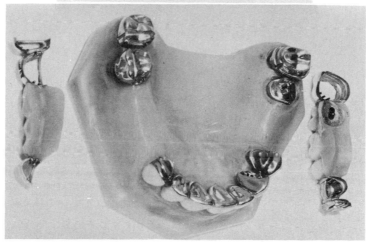

Fig. 22-69. A, Model for various types of CSP attachments. Such a case would be unlikely to be solved with attachments, as fixed bridgework is mostly indicated, but it shows the different adaptations of CSP system. **B,** With bridges removed, design of various CSP attachments becomes visible. When assembled, nothing distinguishes surface from fixed bridgework.

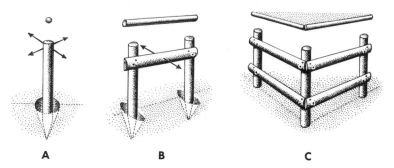

Fig. 22-70. Principle of splinting with bar attachments. **A,** One can easily remove a single fence post from earth by moving it in every direction. **B,** Two fence posts joined together by crossbar are easily movable only in one direction, *arrow*. **C,** Three fence posts, forming a triangle, are all but impossible to remove without particular force; they support a plane.

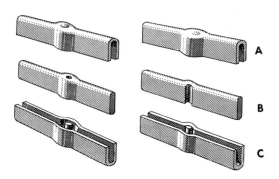

Fig. 22-71. A, Matrix from above. *On left,* With frictional pins in center of bar; *on right,* in one side of matrix. **B,** Two bars with central or lateral channels. **C,** Matrix from below, showing position of frictional pins.

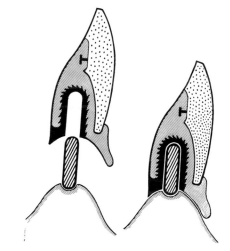

Fig. 22-72. Cross section through bar attachment replacing anterior teeth and lost bone tissue.

bar was a simple, strong gold wire soldered to two abutments across an edentulous space. The wire followed more or less the contour of the alveolar crest, and the partial denture was fastened to it by two or more elastic clamps.

The Steiger Bar Attachment is a cast and fashioned gold bar, flat and upright, following the alveolar crest but with a more or less even occlusal level. The bar is rounded on its edges and parallel on its sides (Fig. 22-71). Since it is laboratory made, it has to be waxed up, cast, and cut

parallel the same way as the CSP attachments. The removable secondary part is also a cast piece and fits like an inverted U over the primary bar on its whole length (Fig. 22-72). On the outside, it carries retentions for the denture part of the appliance. One obtains such retentions by working the outer surface of the matrix with a jeweler's prick (Fig. 22-73). This type of attachment stays very clean

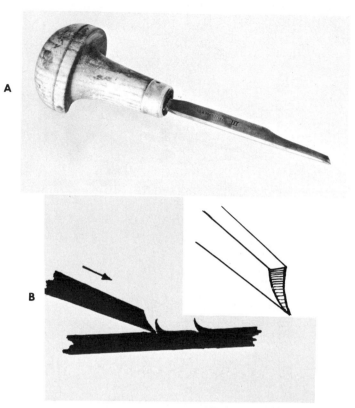

Fig. 22-73. A, Jeweler's prick with handle. **B,** *Inset,* point of jeweler's prick; *in black,* operation of lifting retentions in the gold.

because there are no hollow spaces as we find them under the Gilmore and Dolder bars. Bar and prosthesis are flush with each other on the tissue side. They just touch the gingiva on the whole surface. Frictional pins are placed at chosen intervals on the whole length of the bar (Fig. 22-74). Half their diameter lies in the bar, and the other half in the housing.

The most frequent and ideal application of the Steiger Bar Attachment is in dashboard-accident cases, where anterior teeth and, with them, gingival and bone tissue are missing. A fixed bridge creates the well-known "flat look," because only teeth and no surrounding tissue has been replaced. Such tissue is replaced by a chosen amount of acrylic, so that the lip is sufficiently supported and the teeth are

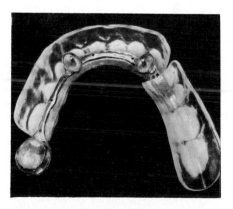

Fig. 22-74. Bar attachment on lower case with three remaining sound teeth, two nonvital, one vital. Bar-supported part is rigidly attached; mucosa-supported part, the saddle, is joined by hinge. The same case was worn for 27 years when last checked, hinge was changed five times, and teeth were newly mounted twice.

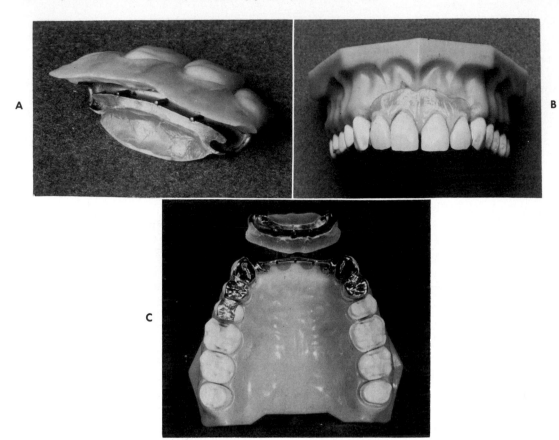

Fig. 22-75. Bar attachment replacing anterior teeth. Pins set into matrix wall are protected from injury.

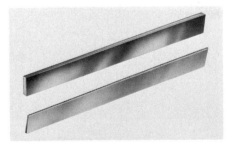

Fig. 22-76. CM (Cendres & Métaux) bar. This bar must be cut to proper shape. Sheet of copper is cut out to follow contour of gingival crest, on model. Then it is laid upon gold bar, and outline is scratched into surface. Then gold bar is milled to proper outline. Matrix is cast same way as in CSP bar.

set in a correct anteroposterior position (Fig. 22-75).

Not everybody has the facilities to make laboratory-made attachments. It is the parallel cutting of the bar part of the attachment that requires special education of the technician. To avoid the cutting process, ready-made bar units have been created. Thus the *CM (Cendres & Métaux) bar* (Fig. 22-76) is simply a sheet of a gold alloy, 1.8 mm in thickness, with a thinner copper sheet. The latter serves to cut out the outline of the bar, according to the alveolar line. The cutout auxiliary sheet is then laid upon the precious-metal sheet to allow the dentist to mark the out-

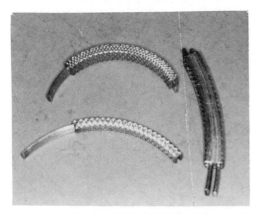

Fig. 22-77. Three of 52 configurations available with Andrews bar system. Single-bar rider is used for anterior applications whereas double bar is used for posterior replacements. The austenitic alloy of the sleeve is die-formed, with a textured surface pressed into outer surface for retention. Each bar has a series of small grooves along its linear surface that provides retention of components while providing a release for sleeves.

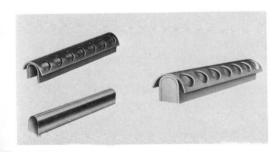

Fig. 22-78. Dolder bar attachment. Rigid attachment, soldered to abutments in order to span edentulous areas, cannot be made to follow outline of gingival crest. Matrix has perforated cover soldered to it as retention for acrylic overdentures.

line there and cut out the exact length and form of the bar.

Another, very useful bar is the *Andrews bar* (Fig. 22-77), made of nonprecious metal. It comes in curved segments, with four types of curvatures and different lengths. Since it is stronger than gold and more resistant to wear, its volume can be kept small. For the posterior region, twin

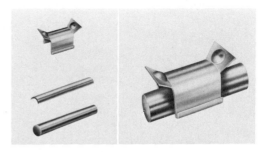

Fig. 22-79. Ackermann bar attachment. Round stiff wire, which can be bent. Individual riders support denture. Inspired from Gilmore bar.

bars may be used to increase retention and friction. Within certain limits, this bar can also be ground to follow the alveolar crest. The bar is soldered to the abutments adjacent to the edentulous space by means of a solder lock. Another ready-made bar is the *Dolder Bar Attachment.* It is available in segments from which the bar can be cut off. The bar has a quadrangular cross section, and the matrix is a U-shaped elastic retainer that can be activated. Perforated flaps retain it in the acrylic of the denture (Fig. 22-78). The bar can only be used as a straight piece because any bending would compromise its parallelism. Also the mounted bar leaves spaces underneath it because it does not follow the irregularities of the alveolar crest.

The *Ackermann Bar* is round and can be bent, and its retainers are short riders similar to the Gilmore Attachment (Fig. 22-79). A variation of the bar attachment is the Dolder Bar Joint (Fig. 22-80). It has an ovoid cross section in the bar and matrix and serves to support full dentures (overdentures) on two or more abutments. Because the ovoid cross section allows a movement of the denture upon the bar, the bar joint acts as a stress-breaker between abutments and denture. If, upon mounting the matrix, one uses the space holder (Fig. 22-80), the denture will, in function, be able to make a resil-

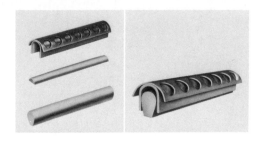

Fig. 22-80. Resilient Dolder bar joint. Bar has ovoid cross section. Housing can be squeezed to snap over bar upon insertion of denture. Housing has same retention as Dolder bar attachment. Half-round wire seen at middle left is interposed between bar and housing upon mounting before curing. This wire is removed after acrylic resin is cured, and denture becomes resilient.

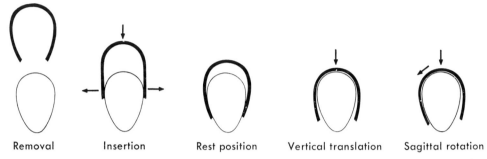

Removal   Insertion   Rest position   Vertical translation   Sagittal rotation

Fig. 22-81. Function of Dolder bar joint. (From Steiger, A. A., and Boitel, R. H.: Precision work for partial dentures, Zurich, 1959, Berichthaus, Buchdruckerei.)

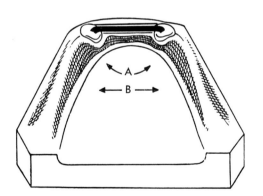

Fig. 22-82. A, Bar joint arrests any movement in transversal plane. **B,** Rotation through sagittal axis is prevented. (From Steiger, A. A., and Boitel, R. H.: Precision work for partial dentures, Zurich, 1959, Berichthaus, Buchdruckerei.)

ient and a rotational movement. Practice shows, however, that this resilient mounting lasts for only a short time, then the denture is down on the bar, and only a rotational movement is left, with the likelihood of a disturbed occlusion (Figs. 22-81 and 22-82). A few variations to the standard application are given in Fig. 22-83.

The root caps supporting the Dolder Bar Joint should be fashioned the same way as root caps with studs (see pp. 535 and 538) to avoid inflammation and proliferation of the gingival tissue around them.

Telescopic crowns

Telescopic crowns are laboratory-made double crowns, with the primary crown cemented to the abutment tooth and the secondary crown soldered to the removable bridge or partial denture (Fig.

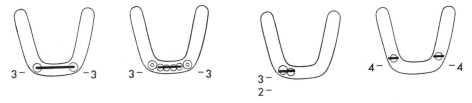

Fig. 22-83. A few examples for mounting bar joint. (From Steiger, A. A., and Boitel, R. H.: Precision work for partial dentures, Zurich, 1959, Berichthaus, Buchdruckerei.)

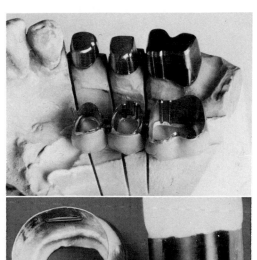

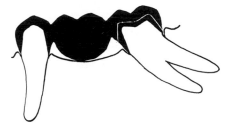

Fig. 22-85. Case of nonparallel abutments. It is very difficult to prepare such abutments parallel without endangering either pulp or retention. Primary thimble can be aligned on outside with second abutment, and fixed bridge can be cemented over thimble. This would be a cemented telescopic crown.

Fig. 22-84. Telescopic crown. **A,** Primary cemented part is a thimble with near-parallel, slightly tapering walls. If no frictional element is included, walls should be as parallel as possible. In a slightly tapering thimble and secondary crown, frictional pins can increase frictional retention. **B,** Klemmfederattachment (Hans Deck). Another method of providing additional retention for a telescopic crown, by horizontal snap-wire.

22-84). Parallelism between abutment preparations must be approximated, though a slight discrepancy may be corrected in the cutting of the primary crowns. This principle may be used also in fixed bridgework, where the frequent case of convergent abutment teeth in a mandibular lateral bridge may pose a difficult problem to the practitioner (Fig. 22-85). The danger of pulp exposure on a tipped tooth prepared to receive a crown is well known. With a primary crown cemented into place, the fixed bridgework may be easily cemented without previous parallelisation of the abutment preparations.

Likewise, removable prosthetic work may be retained by telescopic crowns. If the walls of the contacting crown surfaces are near parallel, this parallelism is a sound retention for a long time. However, such parallel crowns are difficult to separate. In other words, the patient often has difficulty removing his appliance. Therefore a certain conicity (2 to 4 degrees) is preferable. Conic crowns however are nonretentive; so elastic elements must be incorporated into them. Such elastic retentive elements are the pins of the CSP attachment (p. 540), which can be incorporated into the crowns. Slight activation of these pins restores the frictional retention lost by wear.

Another means of retention of telescopic crowns is the spring attachment (Deck Klemmfederattachment, Fig. 22-84, *B*). Such springs are incorporated into the inside wall of the removable crown and upon insertion snap over a slight notch on the cemented crown.

PLANNING

With careful planning, one can anticipate in a large percentage of cases the progressive loss of tooth elements over a long period of time and the preplanned measures that one must then take to compensate for the loss.

Where bridge and partial denture work has become necessary, a process of destruction is in progress. The goal of reconstruction in such a mouth is to arrest (or at least slow down) further destruction and to restore function and esthetics to the highest possible degree. Before reconstruction, many measures may become necessary: functional analysis of the occlusion, endodontia, surgical periodontia, and finally proper temporary replacements that do not jeopardize the preceding measures.

Every arbitrary classification of model cases is incomplete, and if an attempt is made here to present a few typical situations presenting themselves for our inspection, such schematic designs cannot embrace all the problems at hand. Still, it is valuable for the practitioner to analyze his case for statics and dynamics to distinguish between a fully tooth-supported reconstruction, leverage zones, and mucosa-supported areas (Fig. 22-86).

Cases with abutment-supported areas throughout the dental arch (case 1) and small leverage zones are usually solved by fixed bridgework. Anterior leverage

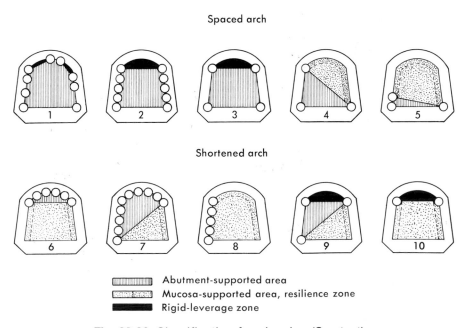

Spaced arch

Shortened arch

Abutment-supported area
Mucosa-supported area, resilience zone
Rigid-leverage zone

Fig. 22-86. Classification for planning (See text).

zones (cases 2, 3, 9, and 10) usually include loss of soft tissue from extractions, surgical operations, or accidents. Replacement of such anterior zones must usually occur by removable appliances that not only replace the teeth, but also place the teeth in their proper position and include acrylic coverage of the soft-tissue area that has been lost. Such cases are ideal for bar attachments (see p. 554).

Wherever mucosa-supported areas present themselves, there will inevitably be a difference of opinion between those who see the solution in a rigid attachment of the removable denture and those who prefer to break the stress between abutments and mucosa-supported denture. Since both schools of thought are in a position to show consistent results, it would be unnecessary to discriminate either method. Let the good man judge for himself. My personal opinion is that maxillary cases may be solved with either method, rigid or stress-broken, provided that a sufficient palatal area is used as a support. The resilience of a maxillary appliance is then minimal. For mandibular free-end saddle cases, the bearing surface is small, resilience is in many cases quite pronounced, and the lateral stability is unsafe, particularly if the ridges are flat and the insertion of movable tissue is adjacent to the crest of the ridge. In such cases, resilient partial dentures may prove less damaging to the abutments. Where there are long, firm mandibular saddles, rigid attachment may also give good results.

There is a difference if the opposing arch to a free-end saddle denture consists of natural teeth or a full denture. A patient who is used to masticating on natural teeth and who is fitted with a unilateral free-end saddle denture will use more masticating force than does the patient with the full denture and should therefore have a stressbreaker. A frequent case is unilateral loss of mandibular or maxillary molars. In such cases, the free-end saddle denture carries a hinge to break the stress (see pp. 523 and 555).

Classification for planning

For examples of denture planning note Fig. 22-86 and consider cases 1 to 4 for the spaced arch and cases 5 to 9 for the shortened arch; 10 is an overdenture case.

Case 1. With healthy abutments, this is the classic case for fixed bridgework. Unfortunately, such ideal circumstances are the exception. Usually, there are good abutments along with weaker ones. If one tries to visualize what the patient's mouth may look like after 5, 10, or 15 years, one may find that certain destructive processes then still may have progressed, even if this process has been slowed down by proper care and adequate dental work. It is then that attachments may be built into a case, to be ready later, when weaker abutments are lost. Fig. 22-87 shows an extreme case of planning. Each abutment could, if necessity arises, be eliminated because the bar is screwed on and the prosthesis is a tertiary stage.

Case 2. The edentulous front is nowadays a frequent car-accident situation (dashboard collision of face). If the teeth are lost, the shrinkage of the supporting tissue, bone, and soft tissue does not offer a good restorative chance to fixed prosthodontics. The teeth of a fixed bridge would have to be built too long, and a typical "flat look" is the unesthetic result of such attempts with a fixed bridgework. This is the classic case for the bar attachment. With such a replacement, it is possible to get excellent esthetic and functional results, along with a situation that allows minutious cleaning of abutments and tissues (Fig. 22-88).

Case 3. Molars and cuspids remain. Provided that the teeth make good and vital abutments, the solution can be the single or combined use of two molar full crowns, two three-quarter crowns, or porcelain-to-gold crowns for the cuspids, and stabilization of the four abutments by bar

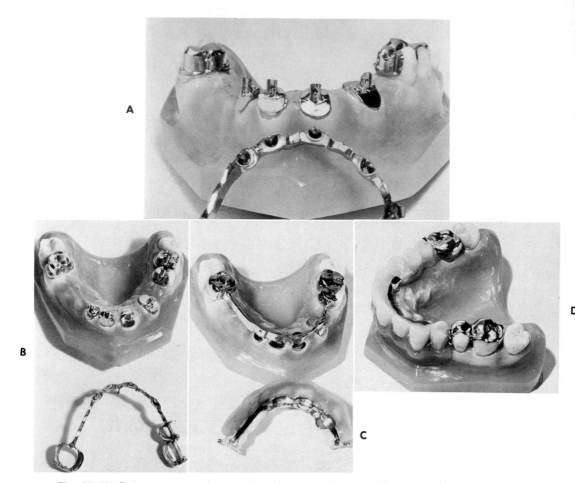

Fig. 22-87. Primary, secondary, and tertiary attachments. Upper partial denture where provision has been made to fix framework on individual abutment teeth in such a manner that loss of any individual abutment will not appreciably affect usefulness of appliance. (Courtesy Dr. Oskar Staehelin, Winterthur, Switzerland.)

attachments. If the abutments are non-vital, the design of the bar attachments remains the same, except that no crowns need be built up (Fig. 22-89). Cast root caps with posts replace the crowns. A full denture, an overdenture, covers the tooth-borne cemented appliance, and the anchorage is rigid. With two good cuspids and two doubtful molar abutments, the cuspids would be joined by a bar attachment and the two molars would get CSP attachments or telescopic crowns. Instead of the bar attachment, it would be possi-

ble to use a Dolder bar, since after the loss of the two molars this would make a resilient overdenture (Fig. 22-90).

Cases 4 and 5. The combination of splinting of the twin abutment, telescopic crowns on all abutments, and a full coverage of palate will give many years of service and optimal retention of the denture. This case can also be solved by CSP attachments and stressbreaker joints (Fig. 22-91).

Case 6. This is the classic case of bilateral free-end saddle extension for max-

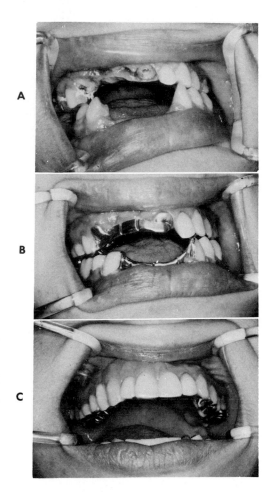

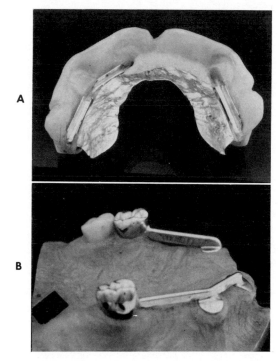

Fig. 22-89. Dolder bar attachments splinting two vital and three nonvital abutments. Prosthesis with partial palatal plate. Since prosthesis is fully tooth supported, metal of plate could actually terminate right behind bar and cast bases. Need for mucosal support is minimal.

Fig. 22-88. Missing and broken front teeth after car accident. **A,** Situation before rehabilitation. **B,** Bar attachments cemented into mouth along with lateral rehabilitation. **C,** Prosthesis in place.

illary and mandibular reconstruction. A splint for the six anteriors will give a good stable basis to a partial denture. The splint may consist of three-quarter crowns, porcelain-to-gold crowns, post crowns on nonvital teeth, crowns on end-standing abutments or added cantilever elements on each side, distal to the cuspids with CSP attachments, or "stabilized" T attachments incorporated as retainers. By "stabilized" one should

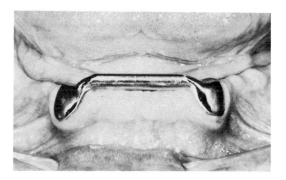

Fig. 22-90. Dolder bar joint on two cuspid roots. Overdenture will rest on this bar (see p. 557), which should be positioned at right angles to sagittal midline of dental arc.

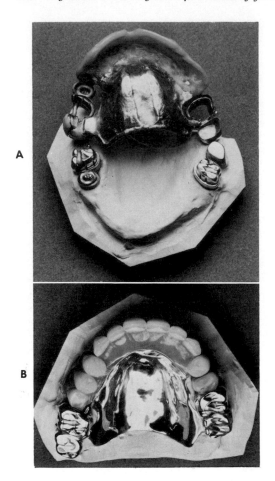

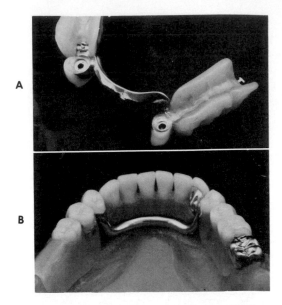

Fig. 22-92. Mandibular unilateral free-end saddle with a hinge joint with stud abutments (nonvital). Posterior abutment possesses a precision attachment of the T type.

Fig. 22-91. Several CSP attachments and two AxRo Joints hold an "almost full denture" in place. Patient was a beautiful woman of about 40 years of age. At 55 she was a candidate for complete denture service.

understand that each attachment is reenforced by an invisible cast clasp arm (see p. 520). The mucosa-supported denture may be soldered directly to the attachments, or two Steiger AxRo Joints may be used to break the stress. If the anterior abutments are nonvital, root caps with posts are built over the roots, and a bar is soldered over the caps, thus splinting them (Fig. 22-7).

Case 7. In unilateral mandibular free-end saddle extension, depending on the periodontal condition of the abutments, splinting of groups of abutments may or

may not be necessary. Even in healthy periodontal conditions, at least two stable abutments could be splinted to form a solid base for the saddle. If three or more stable abutments are splinted, again, a cantilever element is permissible. This is advantageous for esthetics and for the protection of the distal gingival papilla of the distalmost abutment. The saddle is joined to the attachment with a hinge (Fig. 22-92).

To avoid damage to a maxillary tooth–supported denture by group contact and lateral stresses, one should build up the occlusion with cuspid and anterior tooth protection. The saddle is extended far palatally, terminating in a knife-edge. Thus the surface resisting lateral stresses is increased, and, by the knife-edge, the patient hardly feels the border line between saddle and tissue (Fig. 22-93). An alternate treatment, shown in Fig. 22-94, can be used when the posterior teeth have been removed.

Case 8. In the case of the unilateral free-end saddle, with abutments on one side

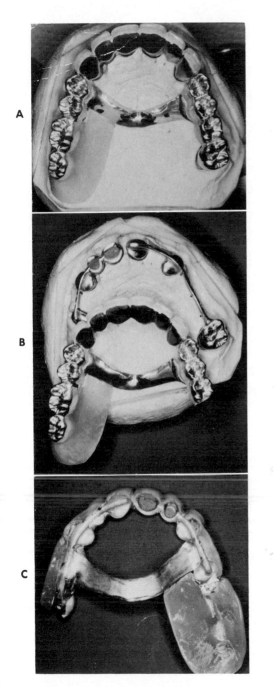

Fig. 22-93. Nonvital anterior abutments joined by a bar attachment. Edentulous area covered by a metal plate.

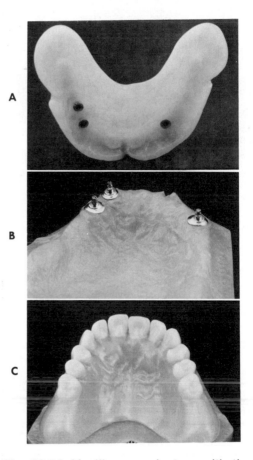

Fig. 22-94. Maxillary overdenture with three abutments left. On three root caps, post bases are fitted with Gerber retention cylinders. Under masticatory stress in molar region, denture will move around axis formed by two distalmost abutments. These retention cylinders should remain retentive; that is, the snap spring should be inserted to give push-button effect. Cuspid abutment on right side (where twin abutments are) should be nonretentive, so as not to receive pulling forces through rotation.

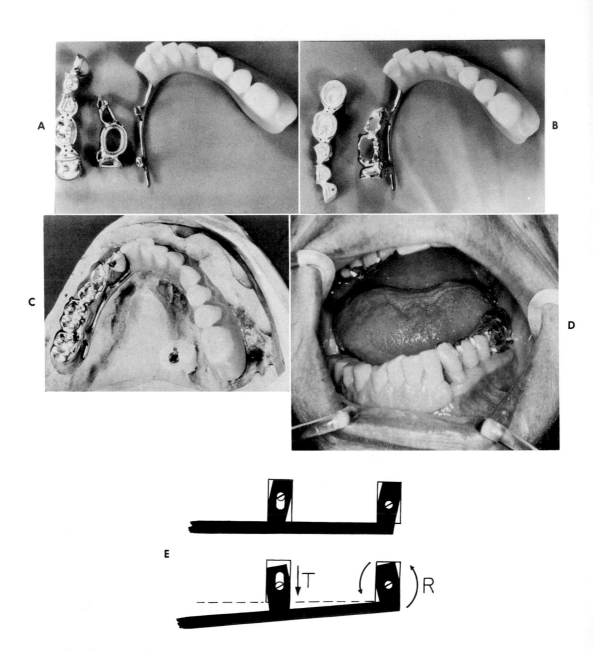

Fig. 22-95. A, Unilateral free-end saddle case with CSP attachments and cross arch splinted by a bar, worn for 26 years (patient died). Two stressbreakers: Anterior is Steiger AxRo Joint; posterior is Steiger Ro-Joint. **B,** Assembled denture and splint. **C,** Case on model, assembled. **D,** Denture inserted in patient's mouth. **E,** Function of stressbreakers. *T,* Translatory movement; *R,* rotatory movement.

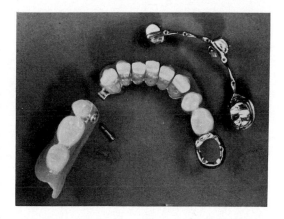

Fig. 22-96. Mandibular free-end saddle extension joined by hinge stressbreaker, on three abutments splinted together by Steiger bar attachment.

of the median line only, splinting of all remaining abutments has proved very useful (Fig. 22-95, *A* to *C*). CSP attachments are also arranged as a secondary splint on at least three abutments (variation: telescopic crowns). The stress-breaking connection with the mucosa-supported part of the denture consists of one Steiger Ro-Joint distally and one Steiger AxRo Joint mesially. The mechanics of this arrangement are shown in Fig. 22-95, *E*. The joints are soldered to a lingual bar or palatal plate that connects with the saddle part of the denture. This case is also classic, because with a straight line of support only, a rigid attachment of the denture would result in a lingual tipping of the abutments when stresses are applied to the saddle side. Loosening of the abutments when rigidly attached to the denture is inevitable. With the AxRo joints the transmission of impulses from the denture to the abutments is considerably lessened.

Case 9. In the case of the unilateral mandibular free-end saddle, three abutments are left and stabilization is obtained by bar-splinting (Fig. 22-96). The free-end saddle extension is joined by a hinge stress-breaker (Fig. 22-92). With healthy abutments and proper patient's care to keep the tissues healthy, such dentures may last 10 and more years, with the maximum being in my experience 18 years so far.

Case 10. Two remaining abutments (cuspids) call for an overdenture. Abutments will preferably be devitalized and covered by stud attachments (Fig. 22-44). They may or may not be splinted and stabilized by a Dolder bar (Fig. 22-90).

SUMMARY

This chapter is an overview of precision attachments fabricated today. About 180 are listed and classified. General, individual, and technical indications are given for the different groups of attachments and some individual models. Some of the difficulties and problems are discussed and show certain contraindications. Mounting of attachments and their repair is only summarily described because an accurate description would exceed the desired volume of this presentation. Each manufacturer gives out specific instructions and accessories for the mounting and replacing process of the whole or of parts of the attachment. Much space is given to laboratory-made attachments as they seem to be of the most resistant types to wear and tear. The CSP (channel-shoulder-pin) attachment and the bar attachments particularly fit this description. These attachments, properly designed and made, outlive the teeth to which they are fixed or the patient who wears them. Ready-made attachments, particularly telescope studs, have replaceable parts and, with proper service, are also durable constructions. Planning of precision attachment work is very important, along with the knowledge of the special indication and limits of each attachment. Also, the mechanics of movement in removable bridgework, partial denture work, and overdenture work must be known by the practitioner, or else he will face frequent breakages, loosening of abutments, and short time of service for his rehabilitations. Precision attachment work is expensive and delicate. In return, it should give the patient long-lasting service.

GENERAL REFERENCES

Boitel, R. H.: A new bar attachment for removable bridges and partial dentures, Trans. Am. Dent. Soc. Europe, 1954.

Cendres & Métaux, S. A.: Attachments and components for prosthetic dentistry, Biel (Bienne), Switzerland, 1974.

Dolder, E.: Die Steg-Prothetik als neue Möglichkeit im gelichteten Lückenbiss, Zahnaerztl. Rundsch. **76:**349, 1967.

Dolder, E.: Steg-Prothetik, Heidelberg, West Germany, 1966, Dr. Alfred Hüthig Verlag GmbH.

Fédération des travailleurs de la métallurgie: Manuel du tourneur, Paris, 1948, La Bibliothèque Française.

Gaerny, A.: Removable closure of the interdental space, Quintessenz, Berlin and Chicago, 1972.

Mensor, M.: The E. M. attachment selector, San Mateo, Calif., 1972, Bell International, Inc.

Preiskel, H. W.: Precision attachments in dentistry, ed. 2, London, 1973, Henry Kimpton, Ltd.

Steiger, A. A., and Boitel, R. H.: Precision work for partial dentures, Zurich, 1959, Berichthaus, Buchdruckerei.

Stern Company, Technical bulletin, 1957.

23

Tooth-supported prostheses (overdentures)

Robert J. Crum

The overdenture is a complete or removable partial denture fabricated over retained teeth that may or may not be modified (Fig. 23-1). It has also been called the tooth-supported denture, overlay denture, telescope denture, and hybrid prosthesis.

The clinical procedures involved with the overdenture technique are simple, and they use a broad spectrum of dentistry. The procedures involve endodontics, periodontics, crown and fixed partial prosthodontics, and removable prosthodontics.

The use of the overdenture is based on the premise that there are distinct advantages to the retention of a *few* natural teeth and real disadvantages to the extraction of *all* teeth. The extraction of all teeth results in a more rapid loss of alveolar bone, complete loss of the sensory input from the receptors in the periodontal ligament, and a transfer of all occlusal forces from the teeth to the residual alveolar ridge.

PREVENTIVE PROSTHODONTICS

The current emphasis on preventive dentistry reflects the importance that is

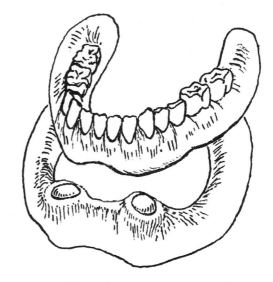

Fig. 23-1. Mandibular overdenture using two reduced canines for support.

placed on procedures that prevent or delay problems in the function of the masticatory system. Prosthodontics plays a role in prevention. Preventive prosthodontics implies the application of procedures that return the masticatory system to good function. The establishment of good integrated oral function has a beneficial effect in that it also acts to lengthen the functional life of all the components of the masticatory system.

The use of sound principles of crown and fixed partial prosthodontics is also

I wish to thank Dr. Lewis L. Landsman for the endodontic treatment of the overdenture patients. Educational materials reproduced through the courtesy of the Dental Service, Veterans Administration Hospital, Hines, Illinois.

569

preventive prosthodontics, since it prevents or delays future prosthodontic problems. The restoration of function through the use of crown and fixed prosthodontics acts to preserve the natural teeth with the periodontal tissues and alveolar bone.

Preventive prosthodontics can still be practiced when the teeth are no longer suitable to support a fixed or removable prosthesis. An overdenture can be considered as an alternative to the extraction of all natural teeth. The use of the overdenture prevents future prosthodontic problems by preserving teeth, their sensory input, and the alveolar bone around these teeth.

The use of the overdenture is one method of reducing the ravages of alveolar bone resorption. The resorption of the alveolar ridge is probably one of the most disabling of all oral conditions. The reason is that it is chronic, progressive, cumulative, and irreversible.[1]

Preventive prosthodontics recognizes the importance of the retention of one or more natural teeth, particularly in the mandible. It is often possible to retain at least two teeth in many patients who are faced with the loss of all teeth. After the loss of all natural teeth, there are not many options left open to the patient. The dentist must present alternatives to the extraction of all teeth—one alternative may be the retention of one or more teeth for an overdenture.

RATIONALE FOR OVERDENTURE
Tooth support for occlusal forces

The roots of the teeth offer the best available support for occlusal forces. Miller[2] stated that the maxillae and mandible were designed to house the teeth—they were not designed to support dentures.

The problems associated with the conventional complete denture supported by the alveolar ridge are evident to every dentist. It is obvious that the alveolar ridge does not offer support for occlusal

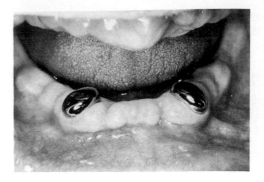

Fig. 23-2. Devitalized reduced mandibular canines with gold copings.

forces, since it is not so adequate as the roots of the teeth.

The overdenture utilizes retained teeth as its primary support. The teeth are reduced to improve the crown-root ratio and to reduce the horizontal torque. Occlusal forces, transmitted along the long axis of the teeth, appear to be the most compatible with the health of the periodontal ligament.

Alveolar bone preservation

It has been shown in a recent study that the retention of teeth for overdentures acted to preserve the alveolar bone.[3] Alveolar bone loss in patients with mandibular overdentures was compared to that of patients with conventional mandibular dentures during a 5-year study. The methods of the study involved the use of comparative cephalometric radiographs and serial study casts. The mandibular canines were retained for the patients with overdentures (Fig. 23-2), and all natural teeth were extracted for the patients with conventional dentures. The investigators found that there was 10 times more bone loss in the patients with conventional dentures than in the patients with overdentures. They observed that the patients with conventional dentures had a loss of 5.2 mm (mean) in the vertical height of the alveolar bone in the anterior part of the

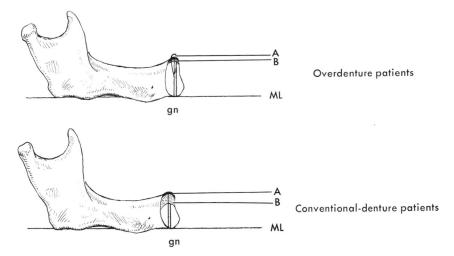

Fig. 23-3. Method of measurement of anterior height of mandibular alveolar processes at **A,** prior to extraction, and **B,** after 5 years of denture wear.

mandible, whereas the loss in the patients with overdentures amounted to only 0.5 mm (Fig. 23-3). It was also noted that the alveolar bone between the canines in the overdenture patients was preserved. It is therefore advantageous to retain mandibular canines since the anterior mandibular ridge is most susceptible to resorption. The anterior portion of the maxillary ridge is not so susceptible to resorption when opposed by a complete mandibular denture.[3] However, the anterior maxillary ridge does show more resorption when opposed by natural dentition.

Tallgren[4,5] has shown that with conventional complete dentures, resorption in the anterior height of the mandible was four times greater than that which occurred in the anterior part of the maxillae. She found that the total linear vertical resorption of the anterior maxillary and mandibular processes during the 7-year period was 8.3 mm (mean)—the mandibular process showed a loss of 6.6 mm whereas the maxillary process showed a loss of 1.7 mm of alveolar bone. Atwood[1] found in one subject that the vertical

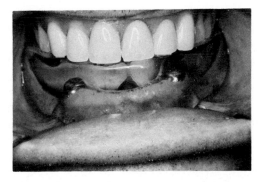

Fig. 23-4. Clear acrylic base over two gold copings with occlusal loading. Alveolar ridge tissues exhibit minimal blanching, since canines protect alveolar ridges.

bone loss of the anterior part of the maxillae was 3 mm whereas the loss in the anterior part of the mandible was 14.5 mm over a period of 19 years. From these studies it is apparent that alveolar bone resorption in the anterior part of the mandible occurs at a very rapid rate after the extraction of all natural teeth.

The use of teeth to support an overdenture has both a biologic and a protective effect on the alveolar bone. The

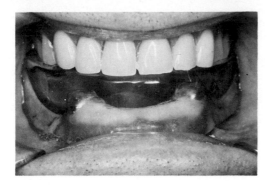

Fig. 23-5. Clear acrylic base relieved in areas of canines. Blanching of alveolar ridge tissues occurs since canines do not protect alveolar ridges from occlusal forces.

very presence of the teeth in the alveolar bone exerts a positive physiologic influence on the preservation of the bone.

It can also be shown that the teeth under an overdenture have a protective effect on the alveolar ridge. This can be demonstrated by placement of a clear acrylic baseplate (Fig. 23-4) over two reduced mandibular canines with occlusal loading.* Here the two canines assume the major portion of the load and the alveolar ridge is protected. Notice that there is minimal blanching of the tissues upon occlusal loading. In the other photograph (Fig. 23-5), the clear acrylic has been relieved so that the mandibular canines do *not* support the baseplate. One can see that the mucosa between the canines and distal to the canines exhibits blanching as a result of the occlusal loading. It is apparent here that the use of the teeth under an overdenture acts to protect the ridge tissues from overloading.

Preservation of sensory input from periodontal receptors

Proprioception and perception. The preservation of the sensory input from the periodontal ligament receptors is one of

---

*Personal communication, 1977, Dr. Vincent Urbanek, School of Dentistry, Medical College of Georgia, Augusta, Ga.

the major objectives in the use of the overdenture. The sensory input from the periodontal ligament receptors contains information regarding the direction and size of the occlusal forces. It has been stated that the periodontal receptors are mainly responsible for the ability of the mandible to close directly into intercuspal position without interferences.[6] The sensory input of the periodontal ligament receptors contributes to the process of proprioceptive sensibility.

Masticatory function is dependent on the integration of sensory input from all the component parts of the system—periodontal ligament, muscles of mastication, temporomandibular joints, epithelial surfaces of the mouth, and tongue. This sensory input originates in sensory nerve endings called receptors. The sum total of the integrated sensory input from these receptors supplies information about the position and movements of the mandible, and this information is called proprioception.

The extraction of all teeth results in the complete loss of all proproceptive input from the periodontal ligament receptors. The use of the overdenture preserves a portion of this proprioceptive input. The proprioceptors of the periodontal ligament are one of the major determinants of masticatory function. The periodontal ligament receptors offer more discrete discriminatory input than could ever be obtained from the oral mucosa.

Most proprioceptive signals from the periodontal ligament are of the subconscious reflex type. Perception therefore differs from proprioception in that perception is the conscious mental registration of a sensory stimulus. Some deliberate conscious mandibular movements may result in some proprioceptive signals being raised to the higher brain levels, and they are then received as perception. Two recent reviews list much of the literature on proprioception and perception.[7,8]

Sensitivity of anterior teeth. The anterior teeth exhibit more acute sensitivity than do posterior teeth, and it is important that they be retained for use with an overdenture where possible.

Numerous studies have shown that the anterior teeth have more sensitivity. It has been observed that a patient's ability to localize a mechanically stimulated tooth was almost 100% in anterior teeth, whereas it was less in posterior teeth.[9,10] Other investigators have observed that the structures in the anterior part of the mouth, particularly the anterior teeth, mucosa, and tongue tip were acutely sensitive.[11-14] This may be related to the findings of Kawamura[14] that there is a greater concentration of sensory receptors in the anterior part of the mouth.

Manly et al.[15] noted that the mean minimal threshold for detection of load on the incisal surface of an anterior tooth (natural dentition) in an axial direction was about 1 gm, whereas the minimal threshold for the occlusal surface of the first molar was 8 to 10 gm. They also determined the mean minimal threshold of detection of load to the occlusal surface of the first premolar in eight wearers of complete dentures. They found that five denture patients were insensitive to a load of 125 gm, two reacted to 83 gm, and one to 56 gm.

These studies show that the anterior teeth give more discrete sensory input. They should be used for the support of an overdenture where possible.

Canine sensory input. Several researchers have found in animal studies that the canine was more sensitive than other teeth. It has been shown that the canines in cats were the most sensitive of all oral structures.[16] Others have also studied decerebrated cats and noted that the neurons for the canines were the most densely distributed[17] and that the canines had more neurons than any other teeth.[18] These studies cannot be done in humans, but they indicate that the canine may

possibly have a greater sensitivity and signal the importance of retaining canines for overdentures where possible.

Directional sensitivity. Directional sensitivity is a term that indicates that the sensory input from the periodontal ligament contains information about the direction of the loading forces.

There are specific sensory nerve endings for various directions of force, such as a lingual force or a buccal force.[14] It has been noted that specific sites in the bulbar and spinal trigeminal nuclei respond to pressure on a tooth from a specific direction.[19] Others have also reported that the teeth were directionally sensitive.[18,20,21]

This quality of directional sensitivity means that the periodontal ligament receptors have a functional individuality.[14] It also signals the neuromuscular importance of the relationship existing between the tooth and its periodontal ligament. Jerge[21] said that the activity of specific muscles or parts of muscles attached to the mandible is directed by specific receptors of specific teeth. The proprioceptive mechanism of directional sensitivity is probably the most important aspect of the sensory input of the periodontal ligament receptors.

Teeth should be retained for use with overdentures to preserve the directional sensitivity of the periodontal receptors. This is based on the assumption that some lateral occlusal forces are transmitted to the supporting teeth by the overdenture.

Perception of nonvital teeth. Studies have shown that human vital and nonvital teeth exhibit equal perceptive responses to occlusal loads.[22,23] The majority of natural teeth selected for use with overdentures are devitalized and treated endodontically.

Dimensional perception. Dimensional perception is the conscious discrimination of different thicknesses of objects between the occlusal surfaces of the teeth. Manly et al.[15] found that the sensitivity of texture judgment of patients with natural dentitions was better than that of patients with complete dentures. They also believed that the sensory input from very small food particles might be of auditory or vibratory origin. This finding of better dimensional perception in patients with natural dentition underscores the importance of preserving the teeth with the periodontal sensory input.

Relationship of periodontal receptors to masticatory muscles. The justification for retaining teeth for an overdenture is supported by research that shows a close relationship between the sensory input of the periodontal ligament receptors and muscle activity. Nerve cells from the periodontal receptors have been found along with those from masticatory muscle spindles in the mesencephalic nucleus.[20] The mesencephalic nucleus is known to have a proprioceptive function. Jerge[21] and Kawamura[14] suggest that the periodontal receptors are involved with cyclic jaw movements during mastication. This facet of sensory input from the periodontal receptors underscores the importance of natural tooth preservation.

Sensory input of teeth with reduced alveolar bone support. A majority of the teeth selected for use with overdentures exhibit a loss of alveolar bone support. This loss of bone support also results in a decrease in the total amount of periodontal ligament attachment around the teeth. This may lead one to question whether a tooth with reduced alveolar bone support has equal sensory input. The perception of occlusal forces in an axial direction was compared in two groups of patients—one with reduced alveolar bone support and the other with normal bone support.[24] This study showed that there was little difference in the perception of occlusal forces between the two groups.

Perception in older individuals. The level of oral perception decreases as age increases.[25,26] The rationale for the reten-

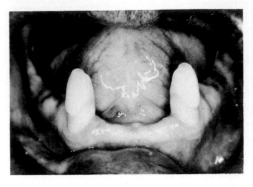

Fig. 23-6. Clinical view of overdenture patient prior to endodontics and reduction of teeth.

tion of teeth for overdentures is based on the preservation of every possible sensory input, particularly in older individuals where the level of sensory capability may be decreasing.

INDICATIONS

The overdentures are not proposed as substitutes for fixed or removable partial dentures.

Overdentures should be considered for every patient where the extraction of all natural teeth is being contemplated. The use of the overdenture is always considered as an alternative to the extraction of all teeth. These teeth may be involved with periodontal disease or caries to such an extent as to render them unsuitable for use with a fixed or removable prosthesis. However, it is often possible to retain one or more of these teeth for the support of an overdenture (Fig. 23-6). Such cases present esthetic problems in replacement with fixed or removable prostheses. The reduction of the clinical crowns of these teeth and periodontal treatment results in more stable teeth with improved crown-root-ratio.

Overdentures are indicated particularly in the mandibular arch where the loss of alveolar bone is more rapid. However, they are indicated for maxillary use where the edentulous maxillae are opposed by natural dentition.

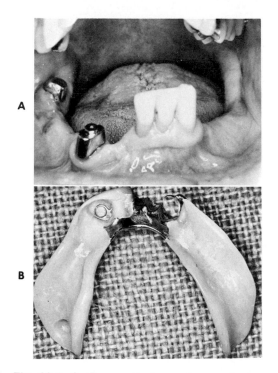

Fig. 23-7. A, Traumatic loss of several mandibular teeth and alveolar ridge—restored with a gold coping on a reduced hemisected second molar. Rothermann attachment was used on right canine. **B,** Distal extension base of partial denture fabricated over hemisected molar in **A.**

Overdentures are indicated for use in patients where there has been a severe loss of alveolar bone in areas of previous extractions. One can project that there will be similar loss of bone in the areas of new extractions. The retention of teeth to support overdentures in these patients will act to preserve the remaining alveolar bone.

Overdentures may be indicated for use in cases involving posttraumatic or postsurgical prostheses. There is usually an urgent need to retain teeth for denture retention and support in these patients. The retention of a single tooth will often mean success or failure to these cases. In the case shown in Fig. 23-7, *A*, there was a traumatic loss of alveolar bone on the right side of the mandible, and it was im-

portant to preserve as many of the natural teeth as possible. The lower right second molar was hemisected after endodontics and a gold coping placed on the reduced portion. The distal extension base of the partial denture uses the reduced hemisected molar for support as an overdenture (Fig. 23-7, *B*). A Rothermann attachment was placed on the right canine.

The retention of teeth for an overdenture should be considered in congenital abnormalities such as cleft palate. The success or failure of a prosthesis will often hinge on the retention of one or two unfavorable teeth. Prior to the extraction of any tooth in a cleft palate or postsurgical case, the proposal to retain the teeth for an overdenture prosthesis should always be considered.

Overdentures are indicated in patients where there may be special considerations. This may involve the use of maxillary overdentures in patients with severe "gag" reflexes. Here, it is often possible to use a maxillary overdenture with a reduced palatal coverage. It may be desirable to use a stud or bar attachment to enhance retention of the denture.

When planning a partial denture, it is often advantageous to retain a molar that may be unacceptable for use as a partial-denture abutment. The reduction of the clinical crown improves the crown-root ratio and makes it suitable for the support of a distal extension base of a partial denture (Fig. 23-8). It is not always necessary to devitalize molars in these situations. There may be situations where a molar may exhibit excellent stability and there are one or two anterior teeth not suitable for partial dentures. The molar may be clasped as in a conventional partial denture and the anterior teeth reduced for an overdenture (Fig. 23-9).

Maxillary overdentures are indicated as a means of correcting prognathic occlusions, and they have been used for this purpose for many years. These class III occlusions may not be amenable to sur-

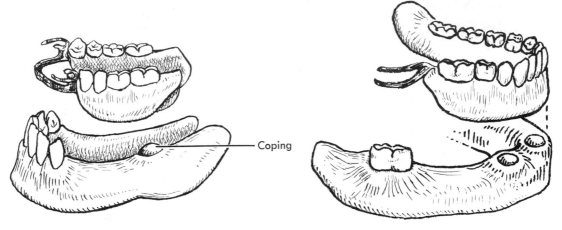

Fig. 23-8. Distal extension base of partial denture that uses a reduced molar for support.

Fig. 23-9. Overdenture with clasp on molar.

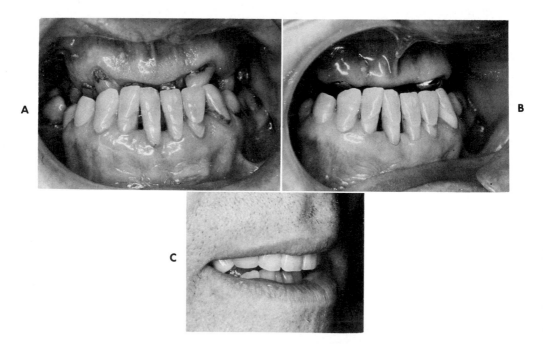

Fig. 23-10. A, Clinical view of prognathic relationship prior to treatment. **B,** Prognathic relationship shown in **A** corrected by maxillary overdenture with copings on canines. **C,** Prognathic relationship shown in **A** and **B** corrected with maxillary overdenture.

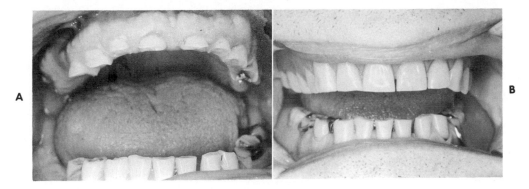

Fig. 23-11. A, Clinical view of severely abraded maxillary teeth. **B,** Maxillary overdenture fabricated over abraded teeth in **A.**

gical correction or orthodontics, and the use of the overdenture results in esthetic and functional improvement (Fig. 23-10). In this case, the maxillary canines were retained and an overdenture was fabricated to correct the occlusion and improve the esthetics. In cases of acromegaly, the class III jaw relation can be rendered functional and esthetic by the use of the maxillary overdenture.[27]

Overdentures are sometimes indicated to improve function and esthetics in badly abraded teeth (Fig. 23-11, A). These stable abraded teeth required minimal modification without endodontics. The maxillary overdenture was fabricated over these abraded teeth (Fig. 23-11, B). This patient has worn the maxillary overdenture for 4 years with a good functional and esthetic result. The labial flange may be reduced in height if desired.

CONTRAINDICATIONS

Overdentures are contraindicated where the remaining teeth can be restored with fixed or removable partial dentures.

Overdentures are contraindicated where the patient cannot achieve good preventive plaque control. This failure of plaque control can be attributed to many factors such as poor patient motivation and physical and psychologic problems.

They are also contraindicated where the endodontic and periodontal treatment cannot be performed satisfactorily.

ADVANTAGES

Preservation of alveolar bone. The overdenture preserves alveolar bone by permitting the stress of occlusal loads to be partly sustained by the retained teeth. It was mentioned previously that research has shown that the use of the overdenture acts to preserve the alveolar bone. The presence of a reduced tooth with a healthy gingiva has a biologic effect on the alveolar bone. The reduced tooth takes part of the occlusal load, and it thus has a protective action on the alveolar ridge. The teeth act as a stressbreaker for the occlusal forces.

Improvement of crown-root ratio. The elimination of the unfavorable crown-root ratio by the reduction of the height of the crown results in a much better prognosis for the retained tooth and its surrounding alveolar bone.

Preservation of proprioception. One of the major advantages of the use of the overdenture is that it preserves the sensory input from the supporting teeth. The sensory input from the periodontal ligament receptors is a major determinant in masticatory function.

Increased stability, retention, and better function. The retained teeth provide a definite tooth support for the overdenture. This results in better stability for the denture. The retention of the supporting teeth also results in bone preservation, and this leads to better denture function. Horizontal occlusal forces are tolerated better because of the presence of the reduced teeth and the preserved alveolar bone.

Psychologic advantages. Acceptance of overdentures by patients is excellent. Many patients associate the complete loss of teeth with aging and senility. The retention of one or two teeth for an overdenture results in a real psychologic stimulus for the patient. They do not consider themselves as edentulous. This increased patient satisfaction results in better patient motivation and is responsible for the rapid adaptation to the use of the overdenture.

Easy placement of denture teeth. The retention of teeth for an overdenture facilitates the proper placement of the artificial tooth.

Less postinsertion problems. The totality of all of the advantages results in less postinsertion problems.

DISADVANTAGES

The main disadvantage of the overdenture is that the clinical procedures consume more time and result in higher expenses.

TREATMENT PLANNING—CRITERIA FOR RETAINING TEETH

Ideally, *teeth should be selected where resorption is most likely to occur.* The greatest amount of alveolar bone resorption after extraction of all natural teeth occurs in the anterior part of the mandible. Therefore the selection of mandibular canines or first premolars should be considered. It has been shown that the lower canine is usually the last tooth to be lost in the natural dentition.[28] However, any tooth will contribute to the support of an overdenture. Occa-

sionally a single lower incisor has been used.

The anterior part of the maxillary ridge is also subject to great resorption potential when it is opposed by natural mandibular teeth. Here, the retention of maxillary canines for a maxillary overdenture would act to preserve the alveolar bone in this area.

Acceptable periodontal prognosis. The tooth to be retained must be amenable to periodontal treatment. The periodontal treatment must result in adequate zones of attached gingiva, normal sulcus depth, and acceptable tissue contour. Teeth should have at least 5 mm of alveolar bone support.[29] Slight mobility prior to periodontal treatment is acceptable. It has been my observation that mobile teeth become firm after reduction of the crown and periodontal treatment. This has also been the observations of others.[30,31]

Acceptable endodontic prognosis. Most teeth being considered for use with overdentures must be capable of being treated endodontically. However, there are cases in older individuals where the pulp chambers and root canals are obliterated, and these would not require endodontic treatment (Fig. 23-11, *A*).

Location and number of teeth. The ideal situation would be to retain at least four teeth situated in an arch to give broad support. For example, such a case would utilize both canines and second molars in the same arch. Such a situation is rarely found. Occasionally, it may be feasible to select more than four teeth. The use of three teeth—two canines and a molar—can also give good support for an overdenture.

The majority of overdentures involve the use of both canines in an arch. The author has found that about 80% of overdenture cases use the canines. The selection of mandibular canines also meets the previous criteria in that they are located in an area of rapid bone loss po-

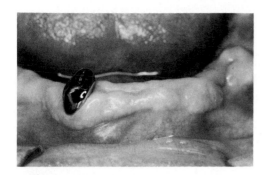

Fig. 23-12. Clinical view of one canine used for support of overdenture.

tential. The canines also occupy an important place in the arch.

There are cases (Fig. 23-12) where only one tooth in an arch will be suitable for retention. These single teeth contribute to better stability and function of the overdenture.

Adjacent teeth in the anterior part of the maxillae or mandible may be retained. Splinting of reduced adjacent teeth is generally not indicated since each reduced tooth usually has adequate stability. Splinting of adjacent teeth may also create an unmanageable oral hygiene problem for the overdenture patient. There are also instances where a molar may be hemisected, and the remaining root used to support the overdenture (Fig. 23-7).

TREATMENT
Preliminary procedures

After selection of the teeth to be retained according to the above criteria, some preliminary procedures need to be performed.

The initial treatment consists of removal of calculus deposits along with oral hygiene instructions to the patient. The importance of plaque control is stressed and reinforced at each treatment visit. The patient must be aware of the need for daily routine plaque removal and be cognizant of the relationship between dental plaque and periodontal disease and caries.

Most of the teeth retained for overdentures require endodontic treatment. Gutta-percha is the preferred choice for the root-canal filling. Most cases will also require some periodontal treatment—the type will depend on the pocket depth, the amount of inflammation, and calculus deposits. *The best long-term results are obtained by completion of the periodontal treatment before one proceeds to the next step of treatment.* This means that the periodontal tissues must be returned to a healthy state with a sulcus of normal depth and attached gingiva.

Overdenture procedures

The teeth are reduced from 1 to 2 mm above the level of the gingival margin. The reduction of the clinical crown results in a more favorable crown-root ratio and gives more room for the placement of the artificial tooth. Crown-root ratios of 1:1 that exist prior to treatment are often changed to a ratio of 1:5 after treatment. If the reduced dentin surface is sound, amalgam restorations are then placed in the top portion of the root canal (Fig. 23-13). The reduced dentin surface and amalgam restoration are polished with sandpaper discs, rubber wheels and tin oxide powder (Fig. 23-14). The polished tooth surface facilitates the removal of plaque (Fig. 23-15).

The overdenture may be fabricated over these reduced teeth on an *interim basis* to determine if the patient will maintain oral hygiene and to see if the patient will need more retention in the overdenture. If the oral hygiene is poor and good patterns of plaque removal cannot be established, it is useless to proceed to coping fabrication. However, when oral hygiene is good, copings or attachments may then be fabricated. This modality of treatment is based on the fact that a gold coping under an overdenture will not prevent caries in the presence of poor oral hygiene.

When the patient expresses a desire for

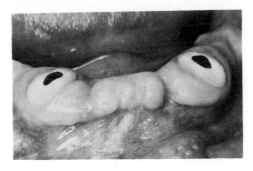

Fig. 23-13. Reduced devitalized canines with amalgam restorations in top portion of canals.

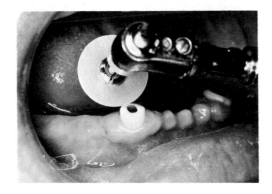

Fig. 23-14. Dentin surface and amalgam restorations are polished.

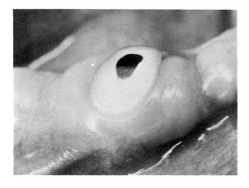

Fig. 23-15. Polished surface of dentin and amalgam restoration.

more retention after wearing the interim overdenture for a period of 6 months to 1 year, stud attachments or bar attachments may be incorporated with gold copings. If the patient states that retention has been adequate with this interim overdenture, then gold copings alone will suffice. One can reline the denture in the area of the reduced teeth only by using autopolymerizing acrylic resin.

The polished dentin surfaces of the reduced teeth with amalgam restorations may remain caries free *provided* that there is a *vigorous program of plaque removal and frequent fluoride treatments.* Since there is an increased risk of caries in these exposed dentin surfaces, it is recommended that these patients be seen on a 3-month recall to have their oral hygiene and caries checked. I have some patients in this category who are caries free at the 5-year level. As stated before, this mode of treatment may be considered as an interim treatment to determine if the patient will cooperate with the oral hygiene program. Lord and Teel[32] have also reported minimal caries occurrence in the polished dentin surfaces of reduced teeth under overdentures.

Shannon* believes that daily self-application of stannous fluorides to these dentin surfaces will provide chemical protection along with a vigorous program of oral hygiene. It is necessary to reinforce the importance of plaque removal, particularly after the reduction of the crowns of the teeth. Most patients find that tooth-brushing around these reduced teeth is difficult, and they need personalized instruction. The use of disclosing solutions aids in the establishment of good oral hygiene procedures.

Gold copings may be fabricated (Fig. 23-16) after good oral hygiene patterns have become established and wherever

---

*Personal communication from Dr. Ira L. Shannon, Director, Oral Disease Research Laboratory, Veterans Administration Hospital, Houston, Texas.

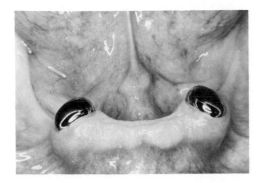

Fig. 23-16. Gold copings on mandibular canines.

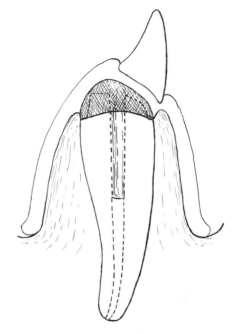

Fig. 23-18. Proximal view of preparation for gold coping. There is more tooth reduction toward labial surface.

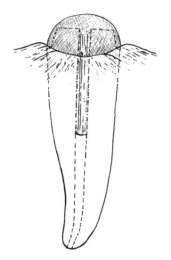

Fig. 23-17. Labial view of preparation of tooth for gold coping.

there is inadequate tooth structure to give support to the overdenture. A preparation is made with slightly tapered axial walls that end in a slight chamfer just below the crest of the gingival margin (Fig. 23-17). A root-canal post is always used to ensure adequate retention in endodontically treated teeth. In vital teeth, pins may be used to add retention to the coping. The gold coping should be rounded with less bulk toward the labial surface (Fig. 23-18). This allows more room for the placement of the artificial tooth. The gold coping should be no more than 2 mm in height above the gingival crest.

Different coping designs have been used for overdentures. These consist of (1) the rounded short coping design with a height of 2 mm above the gingival crest (Fig. 23-16), (2) the tapered coping about 4.5 mm in height,[2,33] (3) the rounded coping with a lingual ledge,[34] and (4) the tapered coping with an occlusal bearing in the denture.[35]

A recent study compared five different coping designs for the transfer of forces from the denture base to the reduced tooth and the alveolar bone.[36] The short coping design displayed the least amount of stress of any of the five designs studied. It also had the least cross-arch effect on the opposite abutment. This design also appeared to transmit its load primarily along the long axis of the tooth except for the posteriorly directed loads. This study indicates that the short rounded coping provided a more optimal stress situation for the reduced tooth under an overdenture.

After cementation of the gold copings, the impressions and jaw relation records are taken in the conventional manner. The use of nonanatomic acrylic teeth is recommended along with a 0-degree incisal guidance. It is often necessary to hollow-grind the artificial tooth which is placed over the retained natural tooth (Fig. 23-18). The teeth are arranged and the wax denture is examined for esthetics and accuracy of records. The overdenture is finished and pressure-indicator paste is placed in the overdenture in the area of the reduced teeth. The acrylic is relieved in the area of the gingival margin inside the overdenture to prevent denture pressure on this gingival tissue. Undercut areas often exist on the labial surface of upper and lower canines. The denture must also be relieved in these areas to facilitate the insertion of the denture. The dentures should then be remounted on an adjustable articulator and selective grinding and mill-in accomplished prior to insertion.

IMMEDIATE OVERDENTURES

The overdenture procedure can also be adapted for use as an immediate overdenture. This technique differs from the conventional immediate denture in that selected teeth are reduced in height and retained as support for the overdenture. The sequence of treatment for the immediate overdenture does have some differences from the conventional immediate denture.

The posterior teeth are extracted first and the alveolar ridges are allowed to heal. Endodontic treatment is then accomplished on the teeth to be retained. Periodontal treatment can also be done

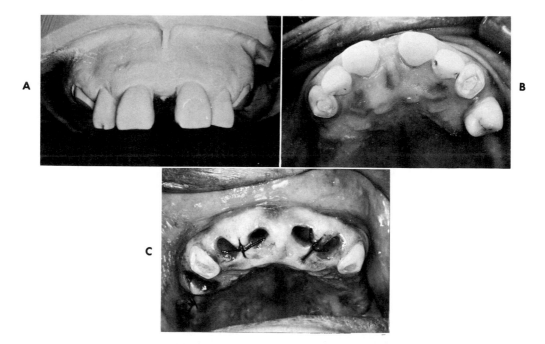

Fig. 23-19. A, Canines to be retained for immediate overdenture are reduced on cast to simulate later reduction in mouth. **B,** Just prior to immediate overdenture insertion, canines to be retained are reduced similar to that done on cast in **A** and amalgam restorations placed in top portion of canals. **C,** Reduced teeth immediately after extraction of other anterior teeth; same patient as in **A** and **B.**

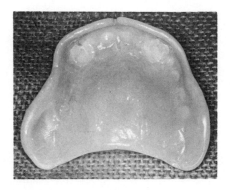

Fig. 23-20. Autopolymerizing acrylic resin is placed in area of reduced canines only for reline of immediate overdenture.

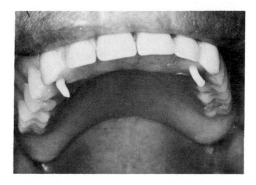

Fig. 23-21. Excess acrylic resin from vent holes prepared for immediate overdenture relining.

around the retained teeth, along with oral hygiene instructions and plaque control.

Final impressions are taken and the master casts are mounted on an adjustable articulator with interocclusal records. The teeth that are to be retained for the overdenture are reduced on the cast (Fig. 23-19, *A*) similar to the manner in which they will later be reduced in the mouth. The anterior teeth, which will be extracted later, are removed from the cast and replaced with artificial teeth as in the usual immediate-denture technique. The remaining artificial teeth are arranged and the occlusal scheme is perfected. The dentures are then processed and finished.

At the appointment for the insertion of the dentures, the teeth to be retained are reduced in height (Fig. 23-19, *B*) similar to that done on the master cast. The top portion of the canal should be sealed with amalgam. The teeth to be extracted are then removed (Fig. 23-19, *C*) and the overdenture is inserted. The acrylic resin should be relieved in the area of the gingival margin area of the retained teeth. Pressure-indicator paste should be used at the time of insertion to ensure that the denture is tissue borne.

On an early subsequent visit, the denture should be relined in the area of the retained teeth only (Fig. 23-20). The acrylic resin should be relieved in the area of the retained teeth and a small vent-hole placed in the center of this area. This allows the acrylic to escape (Fig. 23-21). Autopolymerizing acrylic resin is added and the denture reseated into the mouth. Any excess acrylic should be removed and the area polished.

If desired, gold copings may be placed at a later date after healing has occurred. The placement of gold copings will require a relining procedure in the area of the gold copings. As in all overdenture procedures, good oral hygiene is mandatory.

FOLLOW-UP PROCEDURES
Oral hygiene and fluoride use

Good oral hygiene is mandatory for the success of the overdenture. Poor oral hygiene will result in failure because of caries and periodontal disease. The reduced tooth will continue to serve as stable support for the overdenture as long as there is a vigorous program for plaque removal and frequent applications of fluoride. As stated previously, the placement of gold copings with overdentures will not prevent caries in the presence of poor oral hygiene. Caries in this situation often occurs gingival to the coping.

Patients should be recalled at 3-month intervals to follow up on the patient's oral hygiene and to check on the occurrence of caries and periodontal disease.

Regular fluoride applications should be done on the retained teeth. The use of fluoride is discussed in Chapters 2 and 6.

The occlusal relationship of the teeth should be checked on the recall visits to determine if there has been any change. When occlusal discrepancies are noted, they should be corrected. Slight changes may be corrected by remounting and selective grinding. When occlusal changes are too great to be corrected in this manner, a relining of the denture may be indicated.

Relining procedures

In relining of overdentures, it is necessary to first relieve all the undercut areas on the inside of the denture. It is important that the acrylic in the area of reduced tooth not be relieved entirely so that the vertical stop can be preserved. A small venthole should be made through the denture in the central area of the reduced teeth. This is to allow an escape vent for the relining impression material.

Silicone impression material is recommended for the relining impression. The impression material is placed in the denture and the denture seated with enough force to reestablish the original relationship that existed between the reduced tooth and the denture. If the overdenture has only two teeth for support, the denture with impression material should be seated firmly on these teeth without pressure on the edentulous parts of the denture. The mandible is then guided to light centric relation contact with the opposing dentition.The overdenture reline is then flasked and processed according to the usual relining procedures. Prior to insertion of the relined overdenture, one should do a remount procedure and a selective grinding and milling-in.

PROBLEMS
Fracture of overdenture

The weakest part of the overdenture is the acrylic resin in the area of the sup-

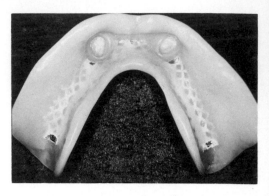

Fig. 23-22. Mandibular overdenture that has been reinforced with Vitallium meshwork.

porting teeth. It is important to make the acrylic base in mandibular overdentures slightly thicker in the area of the supporting teeth. This will usually give the overdenture sufficient strength in most cases. It is also important that acrylic teeth be used in these areas of the reduced teeth.

Occasionally, a patient will fracture the denture during mastication even though there is thicker acrylic in these areas. The overdenture may be reinforced by the placement of a metal meshwork inside the denture (Fig. 23-22).

Poor oral hygiene

The useful life of an overdenture will be severely shortened by poor oral hygiene. Poor oral hygiene will result in the occurrence of caries and periodontal disease. Patients should receive personal instruction regarding their plaque removal and this should be accomplished on a regular follow-up basis.

Inadequate abutment reduction

It is important that the teeth supporting an overdenture be reduced to 1 to 2 mm above the gingival crest. Failure to reduce the teeth sufficiently will result in unfavorable crown-root ratios. It was pointed out previously that the longer copings exert more stress and horizontal force on the root and its supporting alveolar bone and that the short coping presents the least stress.[36]

Coping retention

Short root-canal posts are used to give additional retention to the short copings in endodontically treated teeth. Pins may be used to give added retention in vital teeth with partially obliterated root canals.

ATTACHMENTS

Attachments may be used whenever there is a need for more retention in the overdenture. Attachments and their use are described in detail in Chapter 22. The attachments that are used in conjunction with overdentures are classified as stud attachments and bar attachments.

OVERDENTURE FUTURE

The use of the overdenture is representative of the current trend in preventive prosthodontics. Innovative procedures are currently being tried to gain simple retention with simplified techniques. One of these innovations involves small magnets on the top of gold copings and the placement of the corresponding magnet in the overdenture as currently being used by Vraney.*

Research is also proceeding on methods to preserve alveolar bone. Some investigators are devitalizing teeth, reducing them below the height of the alveolar bone, and closing a surgical flap over them.[37] Other researchers are using vital tooth retention by simply reducing the vital tooth below the crest of the alveolar bone without endodontics and closing the surgical flap.[38]

Overdentures will continue to be used as a method of preserving alveolar bone and the sensory input of the teeth. Research will provide the basis for improved methodology and progress.

SUMMARY

The overdenture provides a modality of treatment that is simple in technique and conservative in purpose. It is based on the premise that the best support for occlusal forces is the roots of the teeth.

SELECTED REFERENCES

1. Atwood, D. A.: Reduction of residual ridges: a major disease entity, J. Prosthet. Dent. **26**:266-279, 1971.
2. Miller, P. A.: Complete dentures supported by natural teeth, J. Prosthet. Dent. **8**:924-928, 1958.
3. Crum, R. J., and Rooney, G. E.: Comparative alveolar bone loss in patients with mandibular overdentures, J. Prosthet. Dent. (to be published).
4. Tallgren, A.: Positional changes of complete dentures—a 7-year longitudinal study, Acta Odont. Scand. **27**:539-561, 1969.
5. Tallgren, A.: The effect of denture wearing on facial morphology, Acta Odont. Scand. **25**:563-592, 1967.
6. Posselt, U.: The physiology of occlusion and rehabilitation, 2 ed., Philadelphia, 1968, F. A. Davis Co.
7. Anderson, D. J., Hannam, A. G., and Matthews, B.: Sensory mechanisms in mammalian teeth and their supporting structures, Physiol. Rev. **50**:171-195, 1970.
8. Crum, R. J., and Loiselle, R. J.: Oral perception and proprioception: a review of the literature and its significance to prosthodontics, J. Prosthet. Dent. **28**:215-230, 1972.
9. Loewenstein, W. R., and Rathkamp, R.: A study of the proprioceptive sensibility of the tooth, J. Dent. Res. **34**:287-294, 1955.
10. Nishiyama, T., Funakoshi, M., and Kawamura, Y.: A study of sensitivity of the human tooth, J. Dent. Res. **46**(suppl.):136, 1967.
11. Grossman, R. C.: Oral sensory threshold determination methods, J. Dent. Res. **43**:833, 1964.
12. Grossman, R. C.: Sensory innervation of the oral mucosae: a review, J. S. Calif. State Dent. Assoc. **32**:128, 1964.
13. Grossman, R. C., Hattis, B. F., and Ringel, R. L.: Oral tactile experience, Arch. Oral Biol. **10**:691-705, 1965.
14. Kawamura, Y.: Recent concepts of the physiology of mastication. In Staple, P. H., editor: Advances in oral biology, New York, 1964, Academic Press, Inc., vol. 1, pp. 77-109.
15. Manly, R. S., Pfaffman, C., Lathrop, D. D., and

---

*Personal communication from Dr. R. E. Vraney, Resident in Prosthodontics, Veterans Administration Hospital, Hines, Illinois.

Keyser, J.: Oral sensory thresholds of persons with natural and artificial dentitions, J. Dent. Res. **31**:305-312, 1952.

16. Corbin, K. B., and Harrison, F.: Function of the mesencephalic root of the fifth cranial nerve, J. Neurophysiol. **3**:423-435, 1940.

17. Kawamura, Y., and Nishiyama, T.: Projection of dental afferent impulses to the trigeminal nuclei of the cat, Jpn. J. Physiol. **16**:584-597, 1966.

18. Kruger, L., and Michel, F.: A single neuron analysis of buccal cavity representation in the sensory trigeminal complex of the cat, Arch. Oral Biol. **7**:491-503, 1962.

19. Kubota, R., and Kawamura, Y.: Quoted in Staple, P. H., editor: Advances in oral biology, New York, 1964, Academic Press, Inc., pp. 93.

20. Jerge, C. R.: Organization and function of the trigeminal mesencephalic nucleus, J. Neurophysiol. **26**:379-392, 1963.

21. Jerge, C. R.: Comments on the innervation of the teeth, Dent. Clin. North Am., pp. 117-127, March 1965.

22. Adler, P.: Sensibility of teeth to loads applied in different directions, J. Dent. Res. **26**:279-289, 1947.

23. Stewart, D.: Some aspects of the innervation of the teeth, Proc. Roy. Soc. Med. **20**:1675-1686, 1927.

24. Edel, A., and Wills, D. J.: Effects of reduced alveolar support on the sensibility of the incisors of humans to axial pressure, J. Dent. Res. **52** (suppl.):946 (abstr.), Sept.-Oct. 1973

25. Litvak, H., Silverman, S. I., and Garfinkel, M. H.: Oral stereognosis in dentulous and edentulous subjects, J. Prosthet. Dent. **25**:139-151, 1971.

26. MacDonald, E. T., and Aungst, L. F.: Apparent independence of oral sensory functions and articulatory proficiency. In Bosma, J. F., editor: Second symposium on oral sensation and perception, Bethesda, Md., Springfield, Ill., 1970, Charles C Thomas, Publisher, pp. 391-397.

27. Nemeth, Z.: The full denture onlay in a case of acromegaly, Dent. Dig. **52**:546-548, 1946.

28. Arpad, T.: [The distribution of the last 1-4 teeth in the oral cavity], Fogorv. Szemle **63**(6):180-186, June 1970.

29. Zamikoff, I. I.: Overdentures—theory and technique, J.A.D.A. **86**:853-857, 1973.

30. Brewer, A., and Fenton, A. H.: The overdenture, Dent. Clin. North. Am. **17**:723-746, Oct. 1973.

31. Morrow, R. M., Feldman, E. E., Rudd, T. D., and Trovillion, H. M.: Tooth supported complete dentures: an approach to preventive prosthodontics, J. Prosthet. Dent. **21**:513-522, 1969.

32. Lord, J. L., and Teel, S.: The overdenture: patient selection, use of copings, and follow-up evaluation, J. Prosthet. Dent. **32**:41-51, 1974.

33. Yalisove, I. L.: Crown and sleeve-coping retainers for removable partial prosthesis, J. Prosthet. Dent. **16**:1069-1085, 1966.

34. Malone, W. F., Gerhard, R. J., Ensing, H., and Morganelli, J.: Imaginative prosthodontics, J. Acad. Gen. Dent. **18**:21-25, June 1970.

35. Morrow, R. M., Powell, J. M., Jameson, W. S., Jewson, L. G., and Rudd, K. D.: Tooth-supported complete dentures: description and clinical evaluation of a simplified technique, J. Prosthet. Dent. **22**:414-424, Oct. 1969.

36. Warren, A. B., and Caputo, A. A.: Load transfer to alveolar bone as influenced by abutment designs for tooth-supported dentures, J. Prosthet. Dent. **33**:137-148, Feb. 1975.

37. Levin, M. P., Getter, L., Cutwright, D. E., and Bhaskar, S. N.: Intentional submucosal submergence of non-vital roots, J. Oral Surg. **32**:834-839, Nov. 1974.

38. Johnson, D. L., Kelly, J. F., Flinton, R. J., and Cornell, M. T.: Histologic evaluation of vital root retention, J. Oral Surg. **32**:829-833, Nov. 1974.

GENERAL REFERENCES

Brewer, A. A., and Morrow, R. M.: Overdentures, St. Louis, 1975, The C. V. Mosby Co.

Brill, N.: Adaptation and the hybrid-prosthesis, J. Prosthet. Dent. **5**:811, Nov. 1955.

Cozza, V. J.: A simple technique for tooth supported complete dentures, J. Colo. Dent. Assoc. **48**:28, 1970.

Crum, R. J., Loiselle, R. J., and Hayes, C. K.: The stud attachment overlay denture and proprioception, J.A.D.A. **82**:583-586, 1971.

Dodge, C. A.: Prevention of complete denture problems by use of "overdentures," J. Prosthet. Dent. **30**:403-411, 1973.

Loiselle, R. J., Crum, R. J., Rooney, G. E., Jr., and Stuever, C. M.: The physiologic basis for the overlay denture, J. Prosthet. Dent. **28**:4-12, 1972.

Lord, J. L., and Teel, S.: The overdenture, Dent. Clin. North Am. **13**:871, Oct. 1969.

Perel, M. L.: Telescope dentures, J. Prosthet. Dent. **29**:151-156, Feb. 1973.

Schweitzer, J. M., Schweitzer, R. D., and Schweitzer, J.: The telescoped complete denture: a research report at the clinical level, J. Prosthet. Dent. **26**:357-372, 1971.

24

Machine-milled copings in periodontal-prosthodontic rehabilitation

Daniel Frederickson and Joachim Nordt

INTRODUCTION AND THEORY

Machine-milled copings make possible a wide range of prosthetic restorations for the periodontally crippled dentition. These copings (Fig. 24-1) are the primary castings in a versatile double-casting technique. The secondary casting (Fig. 24-2) is a telescoped removable prosthesis that is retained by frictional forces generated between machine-smooth metal surfaces (Fig. 24-3). This system provides many of the biomechanical advantages of a fixed prosthesis while giving the patient and dentist access for preventive care, further treatment, or repair.

This is not a new concept. *The American Textbook of Prosthetic Dentistry* (1896) contains a description and illustration (Fig. 24-4) of a technique for removable bridgework!

Removable bridges are devices which are so attached that they may be removed by the operator for the purpose of repair or to gain access to abutments which may possibly require therapeutic aid; again, as a means of bridging spaces to which, owing to the position of the abutments, it would be impracticable to properly adapt fixed bridges. Others are designed and attached so that the patient may remove them for hygienic considerations.

Although the double-casting concept is not new, recent technologic advances have made the method more precise. The development of a device called a Ko-

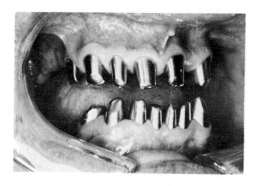

Fig. 24-1. Machine-milled copings are primary castings of versatile double-casting technique for periodontal prosthetic rehabilitation.

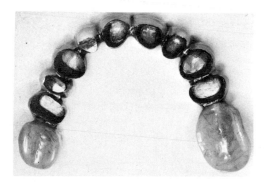

Fig. 24-2. Secondary casting is removable telescope periodontal prosthesis.

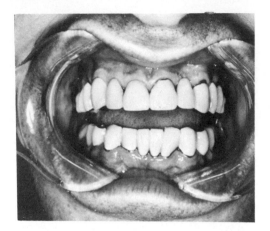

Fig. 24-3. Maxillary and mandibular distal-extension removable partial dentures retained by machine-smooth metal surfaces.

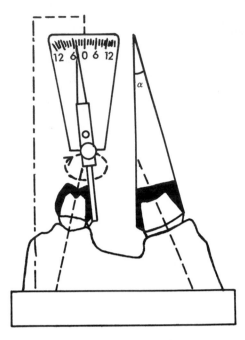

Fig. 24-5. Konometer makes it possible to accurately prepare tapered wax copings.

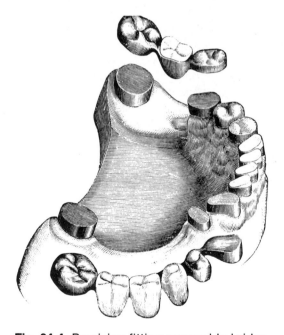

Fig. 24-4. Precision-fitting removable bridgework about 1886.

nometer* and others makes it possible to accurately prepare copings in wax (Fig. 24-5).

A precision milling machine† refines the axial surface of the coping after it is cast (Figs. 24-6 and 24-7). The telescope retainers are produced from wax patterns adapted directly to the machine-milled coping. The final prosthesis is a rigid, precision-telescope removable partial denture.

Körber,[3] a recognized expert in this method, has mathematically described and illustrated the frictional/retention relationship between the coping and the telescoped retainer (Fig. 24-8). Frictional stress may be reduced on weaker abutments by an increase of the angle of taper. Conversely, greater frictional retention is gained by a decrease of the angle. The most favorable angle for coping contour and retention is 6 degrees. As tapers approach parallel, they are often so retentive that the force of removal exceeds the bonding strength of commonly used luting agents (cements) causing the copings to be pulled off the abutment teeth. Copings with tapers greater than 6 degrees

---

*Gerhard Hug, GmbH, 87 Freiburg-Umkirch im Kirchenürstle, West Germany.
†Sistema Artiglio, Strada Naviglia 4, 43100 Parma, Italy.

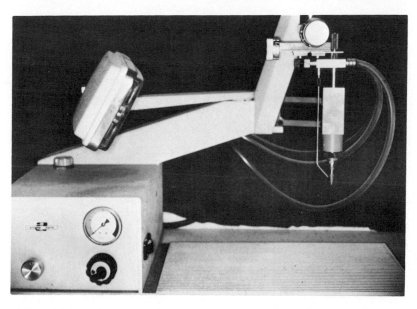

Fig. 24-6. Italian-made Fresatore 3D air turbine milling machine.

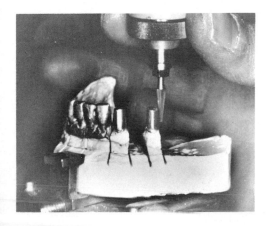

Fig. 24-7. Machine milling the primary casting with a pantographic, air-driven handpiece and finishing bur at 5,000 rpm.

become too bulky at the free gingival margin causing hygiene and esthetic problems.

Depending on abutment distribution retainers may be joined by rigid pontic connectors as in typical fixed bridgework (Fig. 24-9), or lingual bars, palatal straps, and aprons as in removable partial denture construction (Figs. 24-10 to 24-12).

Rarely does the retainer-coping complex have stress-breaking features of some attachments.

The precise fit of the telescope retainers joined by rigid major connectors allows the individual abutments to function together as though they were joined by some type of connector bar. It is this author's experience that healthy abutments can act in this manner as positive retainers and vertical stabilizers without periodontal damage (Fig. 24-13).

CLINICAL CONSIDERATIONS

The patient with moderate to severe periodontitis challenges the dentist who attempts to restore dental form and function with the remaining healthy teeth. The periodontal cripple usually has a history of poor oral hygiene; unpredictable pulpal disease; mobile, nonparallel teeth in malocclusion; root sensitivity, dental caries, and failing restorations. They often have completely edentulous quadrants and long edentulous spaces bounded by abutments of unequal strength. They may also suffer from developmental defects of the jaws and teeth

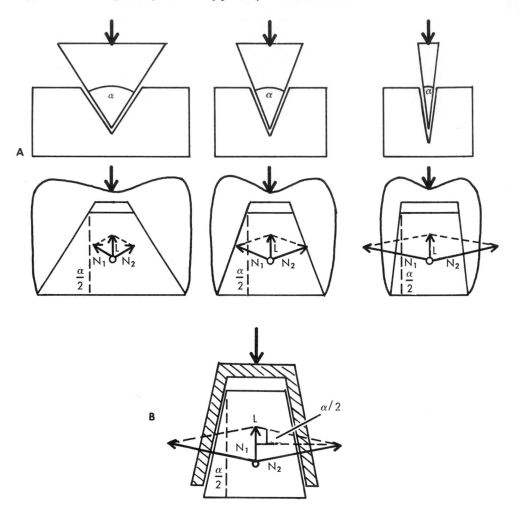

Fig. 24-8. The smaller the angle, the greater the retention.

such as mandibular prognathism, maxillary protrusion, dentinogenesis imperfecta, and other forms of ectodermal dysplasia. Low pain thresholds and difficult attitudes frequently complicate treatment. Fixed crown and bridge procedures are seldom indicated as solutions for such severe conditions.

An alternative treatment approach is the machined coping–telescope removable partial denture system. This periodontal prosthesis is designed so that refabrication is not necessary if one abutment is removed because of failure or because the prosthesis is inadvertently damaged.

Essential to the success of treatment in any periodontal prosthetic rehabilitation is a thorough dental examination and history. Two sets of diagnostic casts are required, with one set mounted on a semiadjustable or completely adjustable articulator so that occlusal patterns may be evaluated. The following items are also recorded: periodontal probe measurements, mucogingival and bony de-

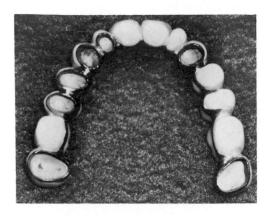

Fig. 24-9. Telescoped retainers joined by pontics as major connectors. Removable ceramometal periodontal prosthesis.

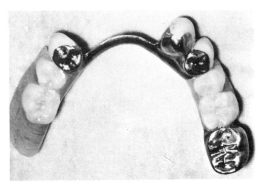

Fig. 24-10. Rigid, lingual bar connecting telescope retainers in unilateral distal-extension removable partial denture case.

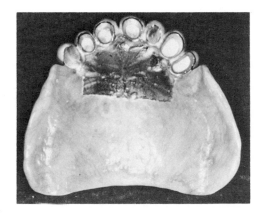

Fig. 24-11. Palatal apron as major connector in flangeless-telescope complete overdenture.

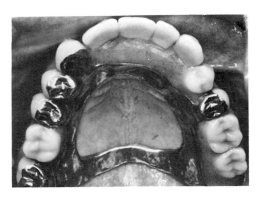

Fig. 24-12. Maxillary-telescope partial denture using an isolated premolar for cross-arch stabilization.

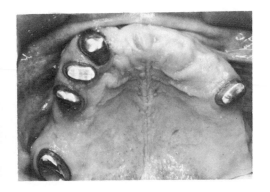

Fig. 24-13. Isolated abutments connected by rigid, precise superstructure act as both vertical and horizontal stabilizers without stressbreakers.

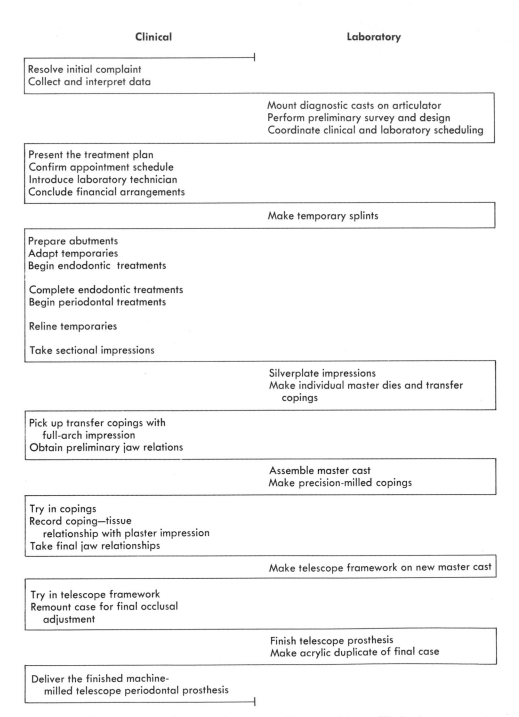

Fig. 24-14. Typical treatment plan for completing precision-milled telescope periodontal prosthesis.

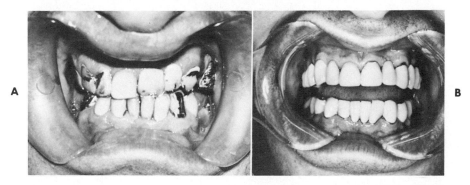

Fig. 24-15. A, This 35-year-old male has multiple missing teeth, moderate periodontitis, and failing dental restorations. Treatment consisted of minor tooth movement, endodontics, and periodontics. Hyperactive gag reflex and low pain threshold are controlled with intravenous premedication. **B,** Finished telescope periodontal prosthesis is retained by frictional resistance between machine-smooth metal surfaces. No luting agent (cement) is required.

fects, missing or impacted teeth, existing restorations, and tooth vitality, mobility, and shade. Radiographs and photographs necessary for diagnosis and or reference are taken.

The patient's personal habits, attitudes, general health, and pain tolerance must be obtained and evaluated. A firm commitment to treatment is made by the patient, including an awareness of his or her financial obligation.

An experienced laboratory technician must be consulted. This should include a discussion of restorative design and the coordination of clinical treatment with laboratory schedules. It is advisable for the technician to meet the patient and observe directly his tooth position and form, esthetics, and patterns of speech.

From this information a diagnostic summary and treatment plan (Fig. 24-14) is derived and used for the case presentation and scheduling. There may also be consultations with specialists who may participate in the patient's treatment. Several case reports are illustrated in Figs. 24-15 to 24-31.

These cases demonstrate that periodontal prosthetic rehabilitations are complex and time consuming. Many chairside hours and much laboratory time must be spent in patient interviews, appliance design, planning, and construction. Evidence of progress along the way is an important psychologic factor for both patient and dentist (Fig. 24-20, *C*). Therefore, it is very important that durable esthetic temporaries be made. It is also necessary to allow adequate time to plan a workable schedule for yourself, your patient, the laboratory technician, and any specialist who may be called upon for consultation and treatment. Thorough pain control is an absolute must in the early stages of mouth preparation. Methods ranging from local to general anesthesia may be used.

CLINICAL AND LABORATORY PROCEDURES

Silver-plated dies, reinforced with acrylic resin, provide the accuracy and durability necessary for machine-milling procedures (Fig. 24-21). Epoxy dies are currently being used successfully. The dies are made from sectional rubber-base impressions. To produce the milling model, vacuum-adapted plastic copings

Text continued on p. 598.

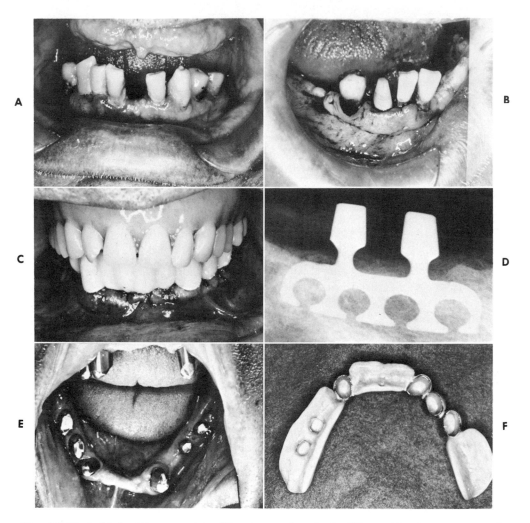

Fig. 24-16. A, Male, 61 years old, with advanced periodontitis and broken upper and lower dentures. Good bone support is present around canines and premolars. **B,** First surgery includes abutment preparation and evaluation, removal of nonrestorable teeth and initial periodontal surgery. **C,** Temporary splint in place after initial surgery. **D,** At second surgery a double-post blade implant is placed. **E,** Precision copings cemented on natural teeth and double-post endosteal implant. **F,** Telescope removable partial denture ready for insertion.

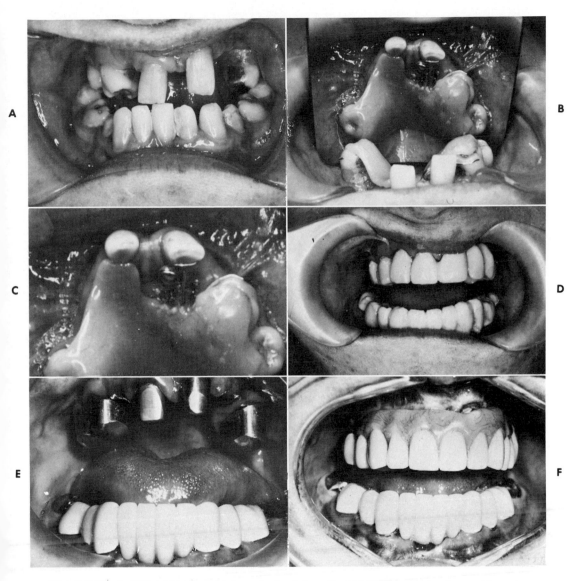

Fig. 24-17. A, This 19-year-old female had Apert's syndrome and advanced periodontitis. Also present are malformed and congenitally missing teeth with gross malocclusion. **B,** Removable orthodontic appliance used prior to telescopic preparation to secure a more favorable arch position. **C,** Treatment included a LaForêt III osteotomy, periodontal surgery, and minor tooth movement. **D,** Tooth preparation and placement of acrylic temporaries preceded definitive periodontal surgery. **E,** Precision-milled copings and fixed bridgework are cemented. **F,** Finished telescope over denture in place.

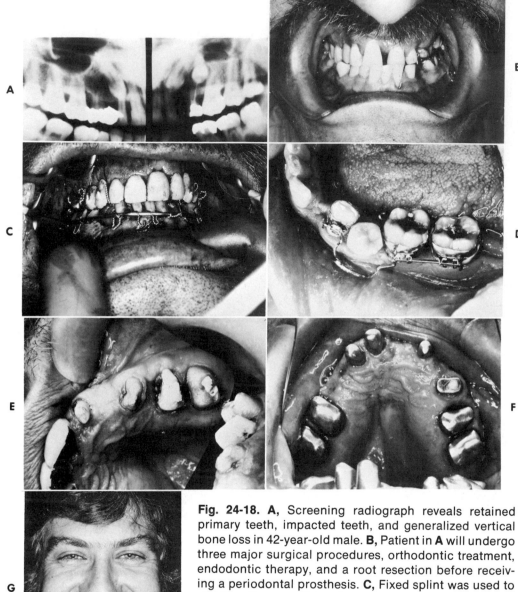

Fig. 24-18. A, Screening radiograph reveals retained primary teeth, impacted teeth, and generalized vertical bone loss in 42-year-old male. **B,** Patient in **A** will undergo three major surgical procedures, orthodontic treatment, endodontic therapy, and a root resection before receiving a periodontal prosthesis. **C,** Fixed splint was used to stabilize the mandible after an oblique osteotomy was performed. **D,** Adult orthodontics to correct cross-bite. Edgewise appliance was also used to stabilize mandible after osteotomy. **E,** Healing root resection on upper first molar mesiobuccal root. **F,** Precision-milled copings in place after surgical removal of impacted canines, root resection, endodontic treatment, and definitive periodontal surgery and mandibular osteotomy. **G,** Telescope removable partial dentures in place. Concluding 21 months of treatment.

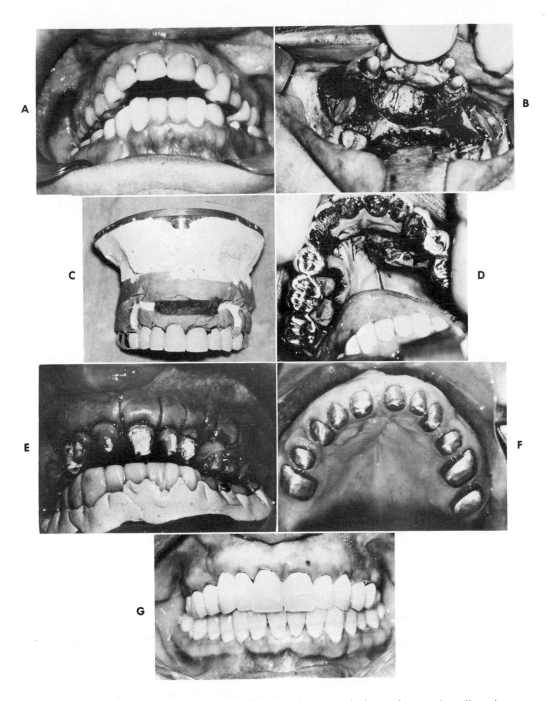

Fig. 24-19. A, Female, 29 years old, with dentinogenesis imperfecta, class II malocclusion with a severe open bite, and generalized moderate periodontitis. **B,** Initial surgery included removal of first premolars and a maxillary osteotomy. **C,** Premaxillary segment was stabilized with an esthetic fixed splint made on a sectioned, articulated cast. **D,** Fixed splint was cemented on anterior teeth first and then on posterior teeth. **E,** Definitive periodontal surgery was performed 4 months after maxillary osteotomy. **F,** Placement of precision-milled copings 8 months after osteotomy and 4 months after periodontal surgery. **G,** Finished maxillary telescope ceramometal periodontal prosthesis. Lower arch was restored with individual ceramometal crowns.

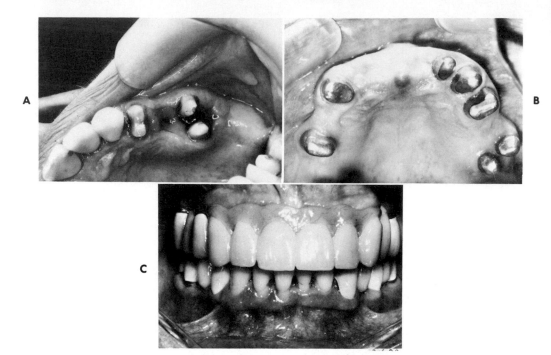

Fig. 24-20. A, Molar trisection resulted in removal of distobuccal root in a 50-year-old female with advanced periodontal disease. **B,** Precision-milled copings cemented. Only the trisected molar was treated endodontically. Removable telescope bridgework allows use of abutment teeth not otherwise suitable for fixed bridgework. **C,** This ceramometal telescope prosthesis with an acrylic veneer replaces extensive bone and tooth loss from advanced periodontal disease in a 50-year-old woman.

are made for each silver-plated die (Fig. 24-22). Duralay acrylic* is added to provide bulk and retention form. The copings are carefully fitted on their respective abutment teeth (Fig. 24-23). Do not impinge or entrap any gingival tissue. If this happens, the relationship of the coping in the pickup impression will be distorted.

Retention locks are cut in the coping and a coating of rubber-base adhesive is added. Rubber-base impression material is then injected around each coping, and the complete arch tray is seated so that a uniform thickness of impression material surrounds each abutment tooth.

*Reliance Dental Manufacturing Co., Chicago.

The final impression should cure 10 minutes in the mouth. Upon removal, inspect for impression material inside the coping. Occasionally, a slight amount is present and can be removed with a sharp scalpel or scissors (Fig. 24-24). If large amounts are present, it probably means that the coping came loose in the impression and the procedure must be repeated. Another excellent material for picking up transfer copings is impression plaster.

Assuming that no distortion has occurred in the final impression, the individual silver-plated dies are sticky waxed into their respective copings (Fig. 24-25). A suitable separating medium is applied and the base is poured in improved stone (Fig. 24-26).

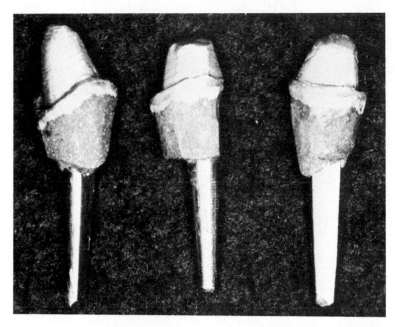

Fig. 24-21. Precision milling requires use of strong master dies like the acrylic reinforced silver-plated ones shown here or epoxy dies.

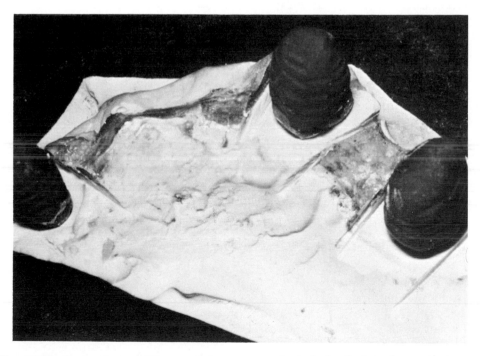

Fig. 24-22. To produce milling model, vacuum-adapted plastic transfer copings are made for each silver-plated die.

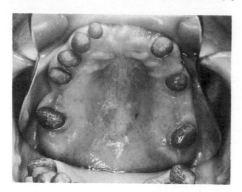

Fig. 24-23. Duralay acrylic resin is added to provide bulk and retention form. Copings are carefully fitted on their respective abutment teeth.

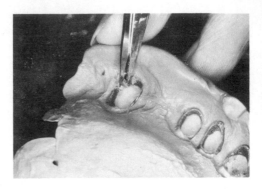

Fig. 24-24. Slight excesses of impression material may be removed with a sharp scissors or scalpel, but large amounts probably mean that coping moved during impression and that pick-up impression must be done over.

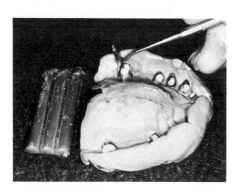

Fig. 24-25. Individual silver-plated dies are tapered and sticky-waxed to their respective copings.

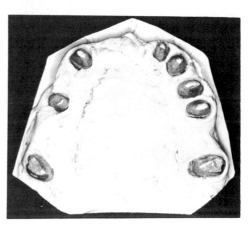

Fig. 24-26. Base of milling model is poured-in stone over well-tapered and lubricated dies.

Waxing, casting, and milling the coping

The machine used for preliminary surveying, final surveying, waxing, and final milling is the Fresatore 3D turbine (Fig. 24-6). Its pantographic motion provides well-balanced three-dimensional movements. It is exceptionally maneuverable, while producing multiple copings with constant taper relationship. The coping should be as thin as possible, so that the case will not be too bulky. Minimum thickness for cast gold is about 0.2 mm. In order to achieve this, plastic copings are adapted to the silver-plated dies, which give some security against wax-pattern distortion. The plastic coping is cut 1 mm short of the margin and placed back on a lubricated die. The margins are then waxed and a sufficient amount of wax is added to the plastic coping. The waxed coping is placed back onto the master model and reduced with a carving tool of proper taper (Fig. 24-27). These cutting blades vary from 4 to 10 degrees. Their usage depends on the inclination of the abutment and the number and health

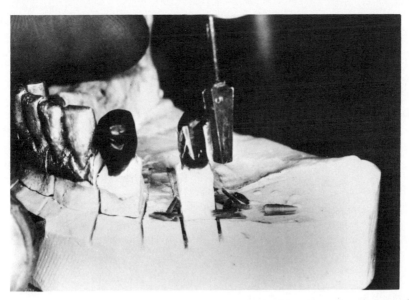

Fig. 24-27. Axial surfaces of wax patterns being prepared to approximate taper before casting and milling.

of the abutments. The average taper is 6 degrees. A Konometer may be used for the same purpose.

Metal sprues are used to remove the finished wax-ups, which are coated with a surface-wetting agent and invested in Beauty-Cast* according to instructions. The castings are bench-cooled, cleaned, and pickled in acid. Individual castings are checked for fit and the margins finished to a high shine. The dies with the copings are placed back into the master model and are now ready for milling.

The master model can be rotated around the milling arm, or the master model can be secured in place and the milling arm rotated around it. In either case, the milling speed for gold should be at least 5,000 rpm. An application of a thin film of oil on the cast coping surface is an advantage during milling. All segments of the milling cast must be removable to allow access for machine millings (Fig. 24-28).

*Whip-Mix Corp., Lexington, Ky.

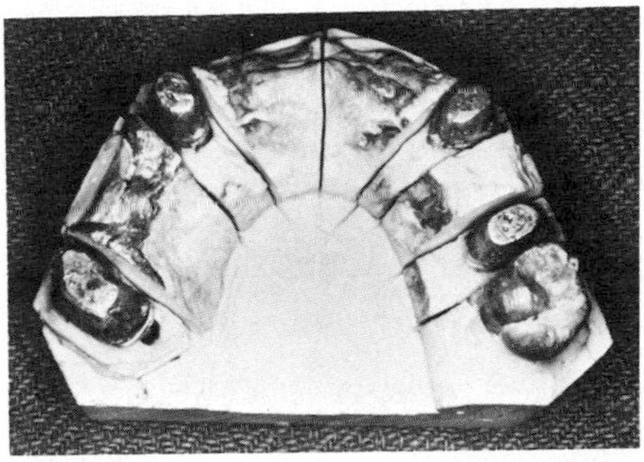

Fig. 24-28. All segments of master cast must be removable to allow access for precision milling.

PREPARATION AND ASSEMBLY OF THE TELESCOPE PROSTHESIS

After the copings are completed and fitted on the abutment teeth (Fig. 24-29), final centric, vertical, and lateral jaw relations are recorded. Several instruments, materials, and techniques are suitable for these procedures. A plaster impression is then taken to record coping-to-gingiva and denture-bearing tissue relationships. The final telescope prosthesis is construct-

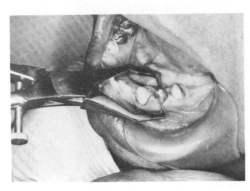

Fig. 24-29. Baade pliers is used to remove tight-fitting copings. Setscrew prevents crimping or scarring the thinly machined "finished" copings.

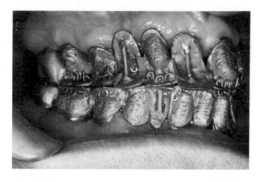

Fig. 24-30. Framework is assembled and tried in mouth.

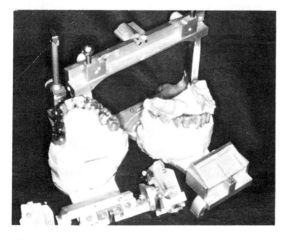

Fig. 24-31. New centric jaw relation is taken, and case is remounted for final refinement of occlusion.

ed on the master cast made from this impression. The telescope crowns, pontics, and framework are waxed and, if required, tried in the mouth so that esthetic and functional relationships may be verified.

Waxing of the telescope crowns is accomplished in the following manner. The milled coping is warmed and coated with a thin layer of separating medium. It is then dipped into molten wax so that the first layers are applied. The remaining wax is added in a conventional manner. The pontics and framework are waxed and designed according to their use for porcelain, acrylic veneers, or full cast crowns.

If denture teeth are used in the final wax-up, a matrix is made so that the framework and denture teeth can be secured after the framework parts are cast and assembled.

After completion of the wax-up the patterns are removed and inspected for smoothness. The castings must be made according to recognized principles of spruing, investing, casting, and bench cooling. A careful inspection of the inside of the telescope castings is a routine procedure. Any bubbles on the inner surface or in line angles could keep the casting from going to place and could damage the milled coping. Type III gold is commonly used.

Now the telescope castings are tested for retention. The ideal force to remove the crown from its coping is between 0.5 and 1 kg. This force is measured with a Kontaktometer spring gage.

When the telescope castings are satisfactory, they are soldered to other parts of the framework and tried in the mouth, and the case is remounted for final occlusal adjustments (Figs. 24-30 and 24-31).

In the porcelain case smaller segments of the entire case are tried in at the biscuit bake stage, and after equilibration, soldering keys are made and the case is soldered when the porcelain baking is complete.

DELIVERY OF FINISHED PROSTHESIS

Cementation is performed after all elements of the telescope prosthesis fit accurately. Petrolatum is placed between the telescope crowns and the copings. Zinc phosphate cement is mixed and placed in the copings, which are then carried to the mouth in the telescope prosthesis and cemented to place. Care must be exercised to avoid entrapment of cement between the coping and telescope crowns.

Postoperative instructions include a warning to the patient that individual teeth may be tender for a short time because of minor tooth movement and cementation. Removal and cleaning techniques are demonstrated to the patient. A duplicate of the telescope prosthesis may be constructed with acrylic resin and worn by the patient whenever modification or repair becomes necessary on the finished prosthesis.

SUGGESTED REFERENCES

1. Essig, C. J.: The American textbook of prosthetic dentistry, Philadelphia, 1896, Lea Brothers & Co.
2. Jorgensen, N. B., and Hayden, J., Jr.: Premedication, local and general anesthesia in general dentistry, Philadelphia, 1967, Lea & Febiger.
3. Körber, K. H.: Konuskronen-Teleskop, Heidelberg, 1971, Dr. Alfred Hüthig Verlag GmbH.
4. Körber, K. H.: The Konometer—a device for the rational preparation of conical crowns, Zahnaerztl. Welt/Rundschau 79(14):595-601, 1970.
5. Krug, R. S., and Markley, M.: Cast restoration with gold-foil-like margins, J. Prosthet. Dent. 22:54-65, July 1969.

GENERAL REFERENCES

Baum, L.: Advanced restorative dentistry: modern materials and techniques, Philadelphia, 1973, W. B. Saunders Co.
Boitel, R. H., and Steiger, A. A.: Precision work for partial dentures, Zurich, 1959, Berichthaus, Buchdruckerei.
Loiselle, R. J., Crum, R. J., Rooney, G. E., Jr., et al.: The physiologic basis for the overlay denture, J. Prosthet. Dent. 28(1):4-12, July 1972.
Miller, P. A.: Complete dentures supported by natural teeth, J. Prosthet. Dent. 8(6):924-928, Nov.-Dec. 1958.
Schweitzer, J. M., Schweitzer, R. D., and Schweitzer, J.: The telescoped complete denture: a research report at the clinical level, J. Prosthet. Dent. 26(4):356-372, Oct. 1971.
Yalisove, L.: Crown and sleeve-coping retainers for removable partial prosthesis, J. Prosthet. Dent. 16(6):1069-1085, Nov.-Dec. 1966.

25

Alumina-reinforced ceramics*

John W. McLean

The advantages of the complete porcelain veneer crown have already been described and it still remains in the foremost rank among dental restorations (Chapter 6).

The main disadvantage of dental porcelain is its fragility. It is well known that sudden fracture may occur in a complete porcelain veneer crown that has insufficient or improper tooth support. Meticulous attention to the preparation of the complete veneer crown has also been emphasized in Chapter 6.

Fractures in dental porcelain originate

*Text by John W. McLean, O.B.E., D.Sc., M.D.S. (London), L.D.S., R.C.S. (England).

from microcracks in the surface (Fig. 25-1). These cracks may be caused during cooling of the porcelain crown, resulting in surface stress. The outside layer or skin of the porcelain will cool more rapidly than the interior. Consequently the skin will be under compression while the interior will contain tensile stresses, since its thermal contraction may be partially prevented by the rigid skin that has solidified. Such a differential change may fracture or rupture the skin to produce minute cracks when the opposing stresses try to neutralize each other in this region. Surface-grinding effects produced by too coarse an abrasive or overheating will also contribute to the pro-

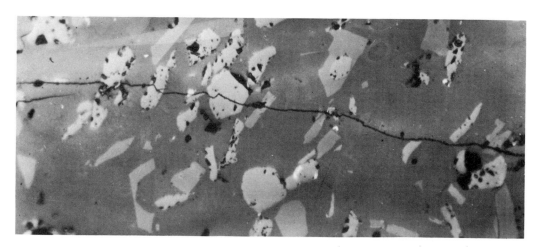

Fig. 25-1. Photomicrograph of fracture path in two-phase system of aluminous dental porcelain reinforced with fused alumina crystals. (Courtesy Warren Spring Laboratory, Stevenage, England.)

duction of microcracks. Fractures in dental porcelain originate from these microcracks at the surface that act as stress concentrators. According to the Griffith crack theory, the deeper the crack, the greater the stress concentration; brittle fracture may occur with almost explosive force.

The bonding of porcelain to metal has largely overcome these problems, but frequently with the sacrifice of esthetic properties. One of the limiting factors in the use of bonded-porcelain crowns is that sufficient tooth tissue must be removed to allow for at least a 1.5 mm space for gold and porcelain. This requirement is not always safely met and particular difficulty may be experienced in younger patients where extensive removal of tooth tissue is biologically undesirable. Although a thin gold veneer may be placed on the palatal surface of the tooth, the labial surface will often present a greater problem since it is here that strength is dominated by esthetic consideration. Many adult teeth do not lend themselves to thick labial veneers. It is obvious that the metal reinforcement places a heavy demand on the technician's skill in obtaining good color values.

ALUMINA-REINFORCED PORCELAINS

To overcome the objections to using metal reinforcement, research has been directed toward formulating higher strength porcelains by use of alumina crystals as the reinforcing phase.[1,2] These aluminous porcelains have recently become available; the esthetics obtainable with them are comparable to a modern vacuum-fired, regular porcelain.

One must clearly understand that the strength of aluminous porcelain, though being nearly double that of regular porcelain, still does not allow the use of these materials on inadequately prepared teeth or where the occlusion contraindicates the use of an all-porcelain restoration. The operator must be aware that he

is still limited by the strength of ceramics in thin section and that aluminous porcelain is offered primarily as a replacement for, and to extend the use of, regular porcelain.

High-fusing regular porcelain is composed of a high potash content feldspar together with a 10% to 15% content of quartz, the latter possibly acting as a strengthener.[3]

The low- and medium-fusion porcelains contain feldspar fluxed by a borosilicate glass, which reduces the firing temperature but at the same time decreases the resistance of the fired body to pyroplastic flow. The regular porcelains may be referred to as glasses, since their free crystalline content is very limited. By contrast, the aluminous porcelains contain up to 50% free crystalline material and can therefore be classed more accurately as porcelains.

FORMULATIONS OF ALUMINOUS PORCELAINS

It has been shown that when crystalline grains of high strength and elasticity were introduced into a glass or porcelain of similar expansion, the strength and elasticity of the mixture, when fired, were found to increase progressively with the proportion of the crystalline phase.[4] The choice of high-strength crystals that can be used satisfactorily in dental porcelain is limited, and research in this field indicated that aluminum oxide (Al_2O_3) is the most promising material for use in complete porcelain-veneer crown powders.[2]

Alumina is the oxide of aluminum commonly extracted from the mineral bauxite, which is mainly a hydrated aluminum oxide. According to normal practice the ore is crushed and ground to -10 mesh and is digested in a concentrated solution of caustic soda. The alumina-bearing liquor recovered from this process is clarified, and the alumina is precipitated in the form of alumina trihydrate crystals, which are then washed and dried without the removal of the chemically combined water. The alumina trihydrate is converted to alumina by calcination, usually in a rotary kiln at a temperature of 1,100° F, which drives off the chemically combined water in the hydrate to form gamma-alumina. Further calcination converts it to alpha-alumina.

For ceramic applications, the calcined alpha-alumina is generally ball-milled and commercially supplied as a fine powder, usually below 10 or 20 μm in size. To obtain suitable alumina crystals for reinforcing dental porcelain, one fuses calcined alumina in an electric arc furnace at approximately 4,000° F, where complete melting of the crystals occurs. On cooling, very large crystals of fused alumina are formed and these are then ground and sized by standard mineralogic techniques.

The fused alumina crystals are then mixed with specially formulated glass powders of matched expansion to form aluminous porcelain. During firing the glass will melt and flow around the alumina crystals. A strong ionic bond is formed between the glass and alumina phase, resulting in an alumina-glass composite. Theoretically, the inclusion of fused alumina crystals into a glass of similar thermal expansion may be considered as a constant-strain system, and the stress in each phase should be proportional to its elasticity. The overall stress applied to the body should lie in value between the stresses in the two phases. If both phases have similar critical strain, the strength of the body will vary with the effective modulus of elasticity, and fracture has an equal chance of starting in either phase. In the absence of thermal expansion differences the fracture passes indiscriminately through the glass or the included crystalline grain (Fig. 25-1). Sometimes the crack deviates at the boundary of a grain, presumably to reach a crack already present in the grain, but in *no case does it avoid a fused alumina crystal.*

Ceramics containing more than 75% alumina are referred to as *high aluminas;* materials below this level are classed as *aluminous porcelains.*

Dental aluminous porcelain contains 45% to 50% by weight of alumina crystals and its strength measured in terms of modulus of rupture (bending strength) can be more than double that of regular porcelain. A typical 50% aluminous dental porcelain is compared in Table 25-1 with a regular dental porcelain.

Aluminous porcelain is used in jacket crown work as a core porcelain to strengthen the overlaying enamel and resist the deepening of surface microcracks. By use of an aluminous porcelain core, the higher modulus of elasticity of this material will stiffen the entire ceramic component and improve the resistance of the jacket crown to torque. The esthetic limitations of the anterior metal-reinforced porcelain crown frequently indicate the use of the aluminous porcelain type. Aluminous porcelain has also been successfully used in dowel crowns and many

Table 25-1. Modulus of rupture of 50% fused alumina content porcelain and a regular medium-fusing feldspathic porcelain of the vacuum type

Material	Modulus of rupture (p.s.i.)			Standard deviation	Variance coefficient (%)
	Average	Low	High		
Aluminous porcelain, 50% alumina	22,458	19,335	25,543	2,387	10.63
Regular porcelain, medium-fusing	11,076	10,079	13,925	1,270	11.47

types of bridges. An alumina-reinforced core porcelain, when used as a palatal backing on a jacket crown, will also increase the impact resistance in the biting area.

Indications for use

Aluminous porcelain crowns should not be constructed on conic preparations or where there is insufficient tooth structure to support the fused porcelain restoration. The preparation must have planes at a right angle to the force of mastication. The aluminous porcelain veneer crown is not recommended as a general replacement for the porcelain-fused-to-metal restoration and is contraindicated in the closed-bite condition where lingual clearance is less then 0.8 mm.

The alumina-reinforced crown is comparable in appearance with a regular vacuum-fired porcelain crown and is more suitable for anterior restorations than are metal-reinforced crowns when appearance is of paramount importance. Clinical experiments with 1,334 alumina-reinforced porcelain-veneer crowns produced a fracture rate of less than 0.5% over a 3½-year trial period.[5] The crowns constructed for these experiments were all reinforced on the palatal surface with aluminous porcelain and the surface was then covered with a sealing glaze. The high strength of the full palatal–backed aluminous porcelain core contributed to this low fracture incidence.

The atypical preparation

In many instances the dentist is faced with the problem of restoring a tooth in which destruction of enamel and dentin by caries or placement of fillings has reduced the area of sound tooth structure to a minimal level. It is in this situation that aluminous porcelain has particular value since the additional strength may provide the balance between fracture and a durable restoration. Fig. 25-2 illustrates a typical situation in which the mesial sur-

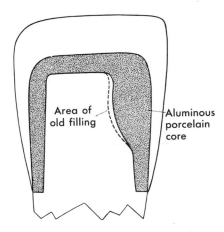

Fig. 25-2. Typical restoration for aluminous porcelain jacket crown, with destruction of tooth dentin; portion restored with core porcelain.

face of the classic outline form of the preparation has been encroached upon by a filling. It is important when preparing the tooth that *maximum cervical support* is provided for the crown and that the area of the old filling not be restored with cement. The maximum bulk of aluminous core porcelain is used to restore this area; its mechanical properties are thereby used to the best advantage. By retaining near parallelism at the cervical third of the rebuilt axial walls, the dentist gives maximum support to the crown in this difficult situation.

Principles of esthetics

Ideally, the ceramist should fabricate a custom-built shade guide of complete porcelain-veneer crowns and use these in conjunction with shade buttons. Such a procedure is suited to the individual dentist or technician. However, the large laboratory owner is generally presented with a specific shade, selected by the dentist from a modern multiblended vacuum-fired tooth shade guide.

The aluminous porcelains were formulated with this situation in mind and a description of the blending of a vacuum-fired shade-guide tooth is most pertinent to the ensuing discussion on aluminous porcelain crown construction.

An examination of a modern multi-blended vacuum-fired denture tooth reveals that it comprises four basic colors (Fig. 25-3). These colors consist of a backing porcelain containing the pin anchorage, a darker dentin color that is carried up into the gingival part of the tooth to create a dense neck area, and the body or dentin porcelain overlaid by a translucent enamel. This enamel porcelain covers the labial and palatal aspects of the incisal edge and overlays the dentin on the entire labial surface. Various concentrated body and surface stains are applied as "effect" masses. These vacuum-fired teeth simulate a natural tooth extremely well.

To duplicate a vacuum-fired shade-guide tooth, one must fire the aluminous porcelain in layers corresponding to the thickness of the shade-guide tooth

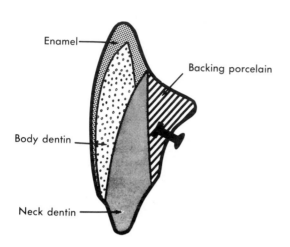

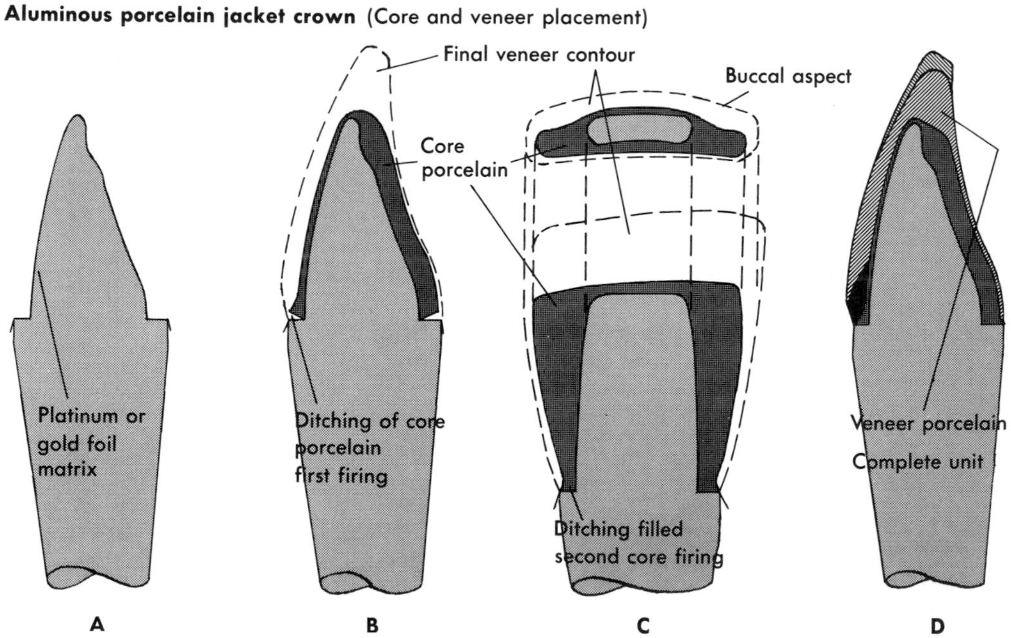

Fig. 25-3. Cross section of multiblended vacuum-fired denture tooth.

Aluminous porcelain jacket crown (Core and veneer placement)

Fig. 25-4. A, Tooth preparation with foil matrix. **B,** First buildup core, "ditched" prior to placement in muffle. **C,** Distribution of core and veneer porcelain for second firing. **D,** Distribution of core porcelain, body veneer porcelain, and enamel veneer porcelain over labial neck dentin.

enamel and dentins (Figs. 25-4 and 25-5). The aluminous core porcelain will correspond to the dense backing porcelain containing the pin anchorage. *The high-strength core must extend to the full contour of the palatal surface and the labial surface is chamfered from the gingival to the incisal so that the core tapers to a thickness of not more than 0.3 mm at the incisal edge of the preparation. Where the total labial thickness is less than 1 mm, the core may be further thinned in this area, always bearing in mind that at least 0.5 mm of dentin and enamel porcelain is required to obtain natural blending and depth of translucency.* It is essential to maintain a 0.5 mm core thickness at the cervical third since this will provide a strong ring reinforcement. The core can be masked with quite a thin section of gingival or neck dentin in this area

and a dense neck area is also beneficial to esthetics.

The gingival or neck dentin porcelain should also be chamfered into the tooth to allow an overlay of body dentin that will establish the main color in the crown. The overlay of enamel porcelain and the incisal translucent will now create a natural enamel effect and provide depth of translucency to the finished crown. One should note that the aluminous dentin porcelains are generally more translucent than the porcelains used for fusing to metal and resultantly the overall finish to the crown will provide more luster and internal light refraction and reflection.

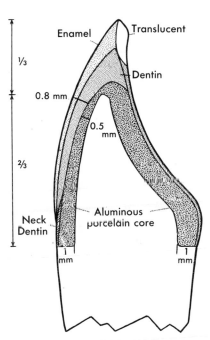

Fig. 25-5. Cross section of aluminous porcelain jacket crown; correct placement of high-strength core porcelain and overlaying veneers of dentin and enamel porcelains.

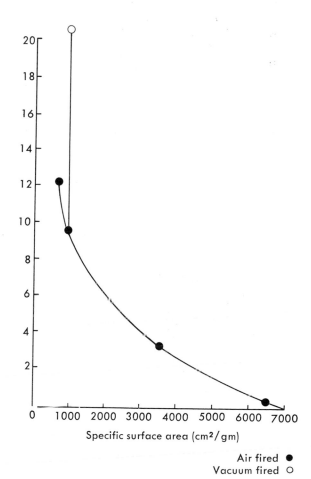

Fig. 25-6. Effect of specific surface (fineness) of alumina on opacity of aluminous core porcelains.

At first sight it may appear that the aluminous core porcelains are opaque, but a study of Fig. 25-6 will reveal that the current powders that fall within a specific surface area of 1,000 to 1,200 cm²/gm do provide quite a high degree of light transmission when vacuum-fired. In this case the 1 mm thick specimens were transmitting over 20% light and resultantly these core porcelains will not present such problems as the opaques used in the bonded porcelains (specific surface area 6,000 cm²/gm) where a background of metal is used.

The most common fault observed with the gold-bonded porcelain crown in the anterior region is caused by "metameric color effects" deriving from the use of opaque backgrounds. Metameric effects are produced by changes in the spectral distribution of the illuminants, that is, daylight to artificial light. These changes cause two apparently similar colors to look different and may be explained by the difference in pigments used to obtain the color; porcelain pigments are different from natural enamel and dentin colors.

Fig. 25-7 illustrates the main problem experienced with the anterior porcelain-fused-to-gold crown. Two critical paths of reflectance are generally present and, if there is an inadequate depth of enamel and dentin porcelains, the opaques will tend to look chalky and bright yellow in reflected light, particularly of the tungsten type. Because of this deficiency, the technician will borrow space as indicated by the dotted line in Fig. 25-7. The crown is now overcontoured and may create gingival problems because of the creation of a cervical stagnation area (CSA). The gingival contour of a porcelain-fused-to-gold crown will therefore present a greater esthetic problem than will the aluminous porcelain crown where no metal background is used. Metameric effects can still be produced with an aluminous porcelain veneer crown and these will generally occur at the incisal third of the preparation when core placement is incorrect and prevents an adequate thickness of overlaying enamel and dentin.

Aluminous porcelain materials* (Table 25-2)

Aluminous porcelain crown powders consist of three main components:
1. A high-strength core porcelain containing as much as 50% fused alumina crystals
2. Dentin
3. Enamel-veneer powders made from glasses containing a high combined alumina content that overlay the high-strength core and give color and translucency to the complete veneer.

Two types of aluminous core porcelains are available.
1. The low-fusing cores, containing 45% by weight of alumina crystals

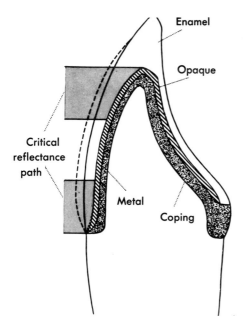

Enamel

Opaque

Critical
reflectance
path

Metal

Coping

Fig. 25-7. Cross section of fused porcelain to gold crown; critical reflectance paths and area of potential overcontouring.

*All references to Aluminous Porcelain are those of Columbus Dental Manufacturing Co., Columbus, Ohio (S.D.T.)

Table 25-2. Aluminous porcelain materials

Materials	Number of colors	Fusing temperature	Use
Low-fusing core	5	1,992° F	Core base for crowns, bridges, etc.
High-fusing core	5	2,012° F	
Dentin	22	1,652° to 1,742° F	Main color component
Enamel	4 Air 3 Vacuum	1,652° to 1,742° F	Air and vacuum versions of enamel colors
Translucent	(AT #1) 2 (AT #2)	1,652° F 1,508° F	Modifiers and correction materials
Modifiers	13	1,652° to 1,742° F	Modifiers for basic color range, mixed with dentin or enamel
Add-on	8	1,472° to 1,508° F	Correcting or adding to the fired crown
High alumina reinforcements	1	Stable up to 2,732° F	Strengtheners and substructures for crowns and bridges

and maturing within the temperature range of 1,850 to 1,922° F

2. High-fusing cores containing 50% alumina crystals that are fired at 2,012° F

The high-fusing core porcelains are stronger but because of their higher alumina content, are more opaque. These materials are better confined to the lingual surfaces. The range of firing will depend on the fusibility of the glass fluxes used as the bonding matrix; these vary from manufacturer to manufacturer. All the materials require similar handling and firing techniques, but to clarify these techniques a description will be given of materials maturing in the 1,922° F range for the low-fusing core, 2,012° F for the high-fusing core, and 1,652° to 1,742° F for the dentins and enamels.

Core material. There are two of these materials, a low-fusing core (LFC) and a high-fusing core (HFC). These core materials are basically the same except for their fusing point. The low-fusing core fuses at 1,922° F, whereas the high-fusing core fuses at 2,012° F. Their advantage lies in the fact that they are extremely stable while the lower fusing enamels and dentins are subsequently being fired. After the core has been fired, the platinum matrix can be stripped from it before the lower fusing dentins and enamels are fired, but this is not advised. The foil

should be stripped as one of the last steps in construction. The core material is very similar in purpose to a metal reinforcement.

Dentin material. This material forms the esthetic body of the crown and is most important in providing proper shade. It fuses at 1,652° to 1,742° F.

Air-fired enamel. This is purely what the name suggests and is used as an *enamel* or *translucent coating* for the crown. It also fuses at 1,652° to 1,742° F.

Vacuum-fired enamel. This material is substituted for air-fired enamel when vacuum firing is being done. It also fuses at 1,652° to 1,742° F.

Translucents. There are two translucents, AT 1 and AT 2, both of which are similar and used in a similar way to the enamels. Where vacuum firing is done, these are replaced by the vacuum-fired enamel as in the case of the enamels. AT 1 fires in the normal range (1,652° to 1,742° F.) of the other overlay materials, whereas AT 2 fires at 1,508° F.

Aluminous porcelains

7 Enamel shades (1,652° to 1,742° F)

Air	Vacuum
AE 1—light gray	VE 4
AE 2—blue gray	VE 5
AE 3—gray	VE 6
AE 4—pink yellow	

2 Translucent shades (AT 1—1,652° F; AT 2—1,508° F)

AT 1—light gray tint
AT 2—warm light gray tint; surface glaze and carrier for stain

22 Dentin shades (1,652° to 1,742° F)

D 5—light yellow	D 6—white yellow
D 7—gray yellow	D 8—dark yellow
D 9—gray yellow	D 10—brown yellow
D 11—light cream	D 12—gray cream
D 13—cream	D 20—white cream
D 21—gray cream	D 22—gray yellow
D 23—yellow	D 24—yellow gray
D 25—cream yellow	D 26—yellow
D 27—dark yellow	D 31—gray yellow
D 32—brown yellow	D 39—gray cream
D 40—gray	D 41—gray

10 Core shades—low-fusing core (LFC) (1,922° F); high-fusing core (HFC) (2,012° F)

LFC 12—light gray	HFC 8—cream
LFC 13—light yellow	HFC 13—light yellow
LFC 25—dark yellow	HFC 25—dark yellow
LFC 41—gray yellow	HFC 41—gray yellow
LFC 50—white	HFC 50—white

9 Add-on shades (1,472° to 1,508° F; shade number corresponds to similar number of dentin porcelain)

AO 5	AO 9
AO 8	AO 20
AO 13	AO 31
AO 23	AO 41
AO 32	

CONSTRUCTION OF THE ALUMINOUS COMPLETE PORCELAIN-VENEER CROWN

Die preparation and the adaptation of the 0.025 mm platinum foil have been previously described. The requirements for constructing an aluminous porcelain crown are identical to the basic methods of constructing a regular vacuum-fired complete porcelain-veneer crown.

TECHNIQUE FOR CONSTRUCTING LOW-FUSING CORE PORCELAIN

The buildup of the core porcelain is best done with the brush technique (Fig. 25-8). A fine sable brush is used. Dip the brush into distilled water and absorb excess moisture on a sponge. The tip of the brush should now have a fine point. The low-fusing aluminous core porcelain is mixed with distilled water on a glass

Table 25-3. Formulas to reproduce New Hue shades, air-fired

Shade	Core	Dentin	Enamel
59	HFC 13 with wash LFC 12	D 20	1—AE 1 1—D 20
60	HFC 13	3—D 23 ½—D 13	4—AE 1 1½—Dentin mix
61	HFC 13	3—D 20 1—D 5	AE 3
62	HFC 13	3—D 20 1½—D 5 1¼—D 23	4—AE 1 1—Dentin mix
65	HFC 25	2—D 23 2—D 5	4—AE 2 1—Dentin mix
66	HFC 25	3—D 23 ½—D 13	4—AE 1 1—Dentin mix
67	HFC 25	3—D 31 ⅛—D 32	4—AE 2 1—Dentin mix
68	HFC 25	3—D 31 ¼—D 32	4—AE 2 1—Dentin mix
69	HFC 41	3—D 8 1—D 9	4—AE 3 1—Dentin mix
77	HFC 25	4—D 41 ½—D 32	4—AE 3 1—Dentin mix
81	HFC 25	2—D 32 1—D 23	4—AE 2
87	HFC 41	3—D 31 1—D 32	4—AE 2 1—Dentin mix

NOTE: These are basic formulas and are not meant to provide exact shade matches. Variations may be obtained by the addition of small amounts of other dentins or stains to the basic formulas. Enamels and translucents may be interchanged or mixed together.

Table 25-4. Formulas to reproduce Bioform shades, air-fired*

Shade	Core	Dentin	Enamel
59	HFC 13 with wash LFC 12	D 20	1—AE 1 1—D 20
62	HFC 13	D 5	4—AE 1 2—D 5
65	HFC 25	D 23	4—AE 1 2—D 23
66	HFC 13 with wash M 2	D 25	4—AE 1 2—D 25
67	HFC 25	6—D 25 $1/_{16}$—M 5	4—AE 1 2—Dentin mix
69	HFC 13	D 10	4—AE 1 2—D 10
77	HFC 13	D 8	4—AE 1 2—D 8
81	HFC 13	3—D 10 1⅛—D 32	4—AE 1 2—Dentin mix

*For vacuum firing, replace the following: AE 1 with VE 4; AE 2 with VE 5; AE 3 with VE 6; AT 1 with VE 4; AT 2 with VE 5. C—core material; D—dentin material; AE—air-fired enamel material; VE—vacuum-fired enamel material.

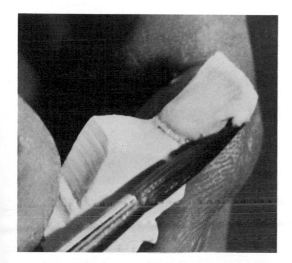

Fig. 25-8. Buildup of porcelain by means of brush technique.

slab to a *thick* and *creamy* consistency. Never use thin mixes since they can cause separation of the alumina and glass powder. The point of the brush may now be gently pushed into the edge of the porcelain mix so that it picks up a small bead of porcelain. The bead is transferred to the platinum matrix and placed in position on the palatal surface. By repeating these movements the ceramist can quickly build up the core layer to an *even thickness* of approximately 0.6 mm over the entire crown. Incremental buildup will reduce the trapping of air and rapid placement of the core porcelain in the exact position required will be achieved. There is no excess material, and one will avoid slumping of the porcelain by periodically absorbing excess moisture with a paper tissue or cloth. Once the initial buildup of the core is complete, the die is vibrated with a porcelain carver handle and the porcelain core is held on the labial side in a folded paper tissue. The tissue may then be folded over the incisal edge to absorb excess water on the palatal surface. Thorough vibration of the aluminous porcelain is essential, since this crystalline ceramic will benefit from meticulous condensation. Even vaccum-firing will not eliminate large entrapped air bubbles.

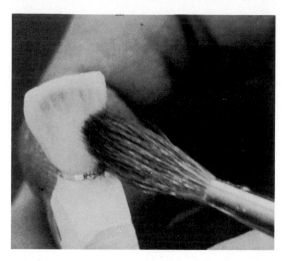

Fig. 25-9. Completed aluminous porcelain core.

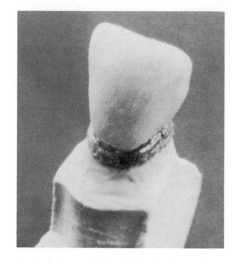

Fig. 25-10. Completed buildup of core porcelain with shoulder "ditched."

The die is reseated in the model, the surface of the core-porcelain slightly moistened, and further porcelain added on by the brush technique (Fig. 25-8). This additional porcelain should cover the entire lingual surface of the preparation and increase the thickness at the labial cervical collar (Fig. 25-7). The lingual porcelain must be built up to the maximum extent of the occlusion (Fig. 25-9) and finally brush-shaped.

CERVICAL RELIEF

Aluminous porcelain has a 40% volume porosity in the powder bed and must shrink on firing like any ceramic material. One of the satisfactory ways of overcoming this shrinkage is to "ditch" the cervical shoulder with a sharp instrument (Fig. 25-10). The clearance of porcelain from this area will allow the main bulk of aluminous porcelain to shrink centrally onto the platinum foil without overdistorting the apron.

It is possible to fire an aluminous porcelain core in one bake, but if a precision fit is required, the two-stage cervical relief technique must be employed.

The core is now ready for its first firing and it is important for the ceramist to have a good knowledge of processes involved in sintering dental porcelain.

VACUUM-FIRING AND AIR-FIRING TECHNIQUES

Much controversy surrounds the methods of firing crowns, arising in the main from an incomplete understanding of the sintering or fusion processes that occur during the firing of a porcelain.

There is generally no difference in the chemical composition of the vacuum-fired or air-fired porcelains and often a manufacturer will prepare both materials from the same glass frit. The only difference between the materials is the particle size of the powders and the amount of pigment, opacifiers, or crystalline material used to obtain the dentin or enamel colors. Vacuum-firing porcelain powders generally have a grain-size distribution of less than 40 μm with the major distribution in the 5 to 10 μm range. For air-fired porcelains, the largest size may be 70 μm or slightly more, and all sizes less than 7 μm are removed. The air-firing porcelain powders therefore have a natural size distribution between 7 and 70 μm.

All porcelain powders reveal a volume porosity in the dry powder bed of 35% to

45% depending on the packing ratio of the powder particles. When these porcelains enter the hot zone of the furnace, each grain will be contacting its neighbor, and furnace atmosphere will be present in the void spaces. The grains of porcelain will lense at their contact points and weld together once the softening point of the glass is reached. The entire ceramic body will start to contract, generally *toward its greatest bulk.* The furnace atmosphere or porosity at the grain boundaries will tend to be swept out through these boundaries and, depending on the time-temperature cycle, this porosity can be almost entirely eliminated. The ideal time-temperature cycles are employed by the industrial ceramist where most of his work must be air-fired.[6] The "green" ware is placed on trays that enter a tunnel kiln and the ceramic ware is gradually moved along the tunnel until it reaches the hot zone of the furnace. This process can often exceed 24 hours. Gases formed in the ceramic can escape; very high densities are obtainable in the fired body.

The logic of this procedure is self-evident, since the sintering or fusion of any porcelain is directed toward eliminating the voids between the powder particles. Furnace atmosphere trapped in these voids can only escape by slow sintering since a rapid rise to the fusion point will merely *seal the surface* and any entrapped air cannot escape. If gas is entrapped in the fired body, it may cause the ceramic to "bloat" or swell.

Dental procedures usually demand a quick-firing technique and violate accepted industrial ceramic practice. Vacuum-firing was introduced to mitigate to a certain extent this situation. Vacuum-firing will reduce the size of porosities in a porcelain body, but it will not eliminate them. Quick-firing can still seal the surface, and the continued use of vacuum from this point is often useless and can be dangerous, since it increases the risk of bloating. Although vacuum-firing techniques were introduced mainly to increase the translucency and homogeneity of dental porcelain, one may also note that, when properly used, vacuum can also assist in the more rapid escape of gases. An appreciation of the sintering processes of ceramics can therefore give a guide to the successful firing of dental porcelain.

If air-firing methods are employed, a very slow maturation period is required to allow the escape of entrapped gas or air bubbles. Such a procedure can produce an extremely dense ceramic.

In the case of vacuum-firing, the above process should ideally still be the same, but the vacuum will assist in the more rapid removal of entrapped gas or furnace atmosphere from the void spaces. Resultantly the firing schedule for a vacuum-processed ceramic can be reduced. Vacuum porcelain powders also possess an additional advantage inasmuch as the powder is finer and the void spaces smaller. Any entrapped bubbles will therefore be smaller and remain more discretely in the fired body. By contrast the coarser air-fired porcelain will reveal larger porosities.

The increasing popularity of the vacuum-fired porcelains is therefore understandable. They can be handled easily and fired more rapidly, and the surface may be ground and repolished more easily. Consistent color and translucency are also obtainable when rapid firing techniques are employed, although there is a limit to the speed of this operation.

However, one must clearly understand that the ceramist can still produce outstanding results with air-fired porcelain, provided that he understands the sintering processes involved in firing porcelain crowns. It is possible to produce air-fired crowns that are indistinguishable from vacuum-processed porcelain; air-firing techniques are still capable of providing the dentist with a restoration of the highest quality.

Aluminous porcelain when fired is a two-phase crystal-glass solid, and its strength will be influenced by the amount of porosity surrounding the fused alumina crystals. If air-firing techniques are used, a *very slow maturation period* is required, thus allowing the gradual escape of entrapped air and gases. The best results will be obtained when a firing schedule of 50° F per minute or less is observed and high densities will be obtained in the fired body. This firing schedule should ideally be used when one vacuum-fires on aluminous core porcelain. However, *once the manufacturer's recommended maximum maturing temperature is reached, the vacuum must be broken.* Continued vacuum-firing of aluminous porcelain at high temperature can produce bloating in the ceramic body. Vacuum should only be used to aid the escape of gases and reduce porosity in the porcelain body while the glass phase is softening and starting to flow around the alumina. Once the glass phase has become viscous, prolonged vacuum will cause this phase to bloat and gross weakening of the porcelain will result.

Aluminous porcelain, when completely sintered, should present an eggshell sheen impervious to the penetration of a water-soluble dye. The cardinal points to bear in mind when firing this new porcelain are the following:

1. Furnace temperature must be at least 400° F below the maximum recommended maturing temperature when the work is introduced into the hot muffle zone: lower temperatures of 400° to 500° F can be even more beneficial in producing a dense ceramic.
2. Raise firing temperature slowly at 50° F per minute.
3. Break vacuum immediately on reaching maximum maturing temperature to prevent bloating.
4. Air-fire work at maximum maturing

temperature for a minimum period of 8 minutes. Longer firing will increase the glaze on the surface and can improve the fired density in aluminous-core porcelains with a 50% alumina content. Periods of up to 30 minutes can be used with absolute safety and there is no risk of spoiling the ceramic. The only precaution required before applying the dentin and enamel porcelain is to *remove any surface glaze on the core with a diamond stone prior to firing the enamel porcelains.*

Aluminous core porcelain—first firing

The core porcelain must be slowly dried in front of the open furnace door for at least 4 minutes. It may then be placed on the firing platform for a further 3 minutes. Modern vacuum furnaces, which employ a pushrod on a vertical slide, are ideal for this procedure (Fig. 25-19). The recommended firing schedule for the 1,922° F core porcelain is as follows:

Drying	(Furnace 1,750° F)
Muffle entrance	4 minutes
Firing platform	3 minutes
Apply vacuum	28 inches
Firing	
Enter hot zone of furnace at 1,750° F	
Raise temperature to 1,922° F. at 50° F per minute	
Switch off vacuum at 1,922° F	
Hold at 1,922° F in air for 5 minutes	
Cooling	
Slow cool to 1,500° F	
Remove work and allow to cool at room temperature	

Aluminous core porcelain—second firing

The platinum apron is reburnished at the gingival shoulder and more core porcelain applied to fill in the ditched area.

The second firing should now follow the exact procedure adopted for the first firing, except for the final period of maturation in air, which should be extended to 8 minutes (Fig. 25-11).

After the core porcelain is cooled, a simple test may be performed to see

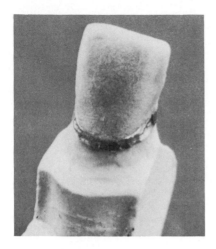

Fig. 25-11. Aluminous core after second firing.

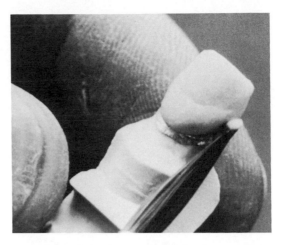

Fig. 25-12. Covering core with body porcelain after second firing.

whether it is fully sintered. A little ink or water-soluble dye is applied to the surface. If the core is not fully sintered, the ink will soak into the pores on the surface and, despite subsequent washing in water, will still be visible. If the core is completely vitrified, the ink may be washed off the surface quite easily and the core porcelain should exhibit an eggshell finish. If there is any doubt over the complete vitrification of the core, it is safer to raise the temperature of the furnace by 20° F. and refire in air for 5 minutes.

A *thin wash of core porcelain must never be used.* Maximum core thickness, particularly on the palatal surface, will provide resistance against torque and improve the thermal shock resistance of the finished crown. If the body of the crown is highly reinforced, the deepening of microcracks on the surface will be resisted by the high-modulus core porcelain.

Application of gingival and body veneer porcelains

An aluminous porcelain veneer powder is selected to match the color of the neck area of the shade-guide tooth. A creamy mix of this powder is applied over the core porcelain, also by use of the brush technique. The porcelain is vibrated and

dried with a paper tissue. The main body or dentin color is then applied on all surfaces of the core porcelain and condensed to position (Fig. 25-12). A more intense color may be introduced over this thin layer of dentin to give a central body effect to the tooth in the gingival third (Fig. 25-5). A study of the shade-guide tooth will reveal the exact position of these colors. The crown is then positioned on the model, and the palatal and labial areas are corrected with the necessary amount of dentin porcelain to obtain full tooth contour. The incisal edge should also be extended by 1 to 1.5 mm to allow for firing shrinkage. It is much easier to cut back a fully contoured crown for the enamel application than to attempt to judge the incisal blend at this stage. The crown may be modeled with a brush or porcelain carver to obtain a smooth finish.

Application of enamel veneer porcelain

The dentin is scalloped with a sharp knife to provide the exact depth and blend of enamel porcelain (Fig. 25-13). Blending of the enamels will be improved if the dentin porcelain is kept moist.

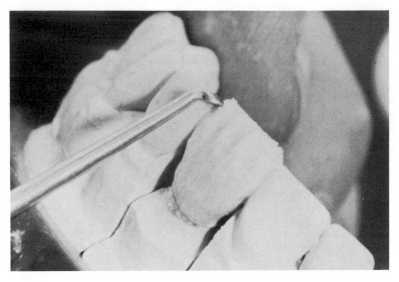

Fig. 25-13. Removal of some dentin porcelain to be covered with enamel porcelain.

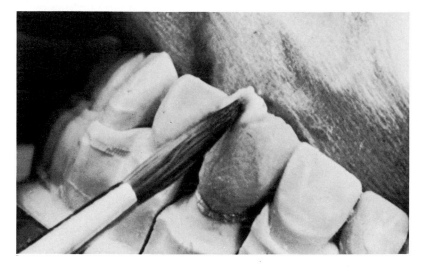

Fig. 25-14. Application of enamel porcelain over incisal dentin body color.

A creamy mix of the enamel porcelain is prepared and applied with a sable's hair brush to the incisal area (Figs. 25-14 and 25-15). The enamel blend may demand complete coverage of the dentin according to the shade and mode of construction of the shade-guide tooth. Excess water is absorbed by vibration and brush-shaping, but care must be taken not to overvibrate and cause slumping of the porcelain.

Final characterization

The incisal area may be greatly improved in esthetics by the judicious use of translucent porcelain combined with concentrated colors. For example, proximal translucence can be improved by removal of a small quantity of enamel porcelain from the mesial and distal surfaces. This porcelain must be removed so that translucent porcelain can be wrapped around the entire proximal surface (Fig.

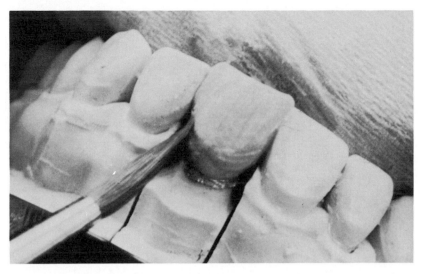

Fig. 25-15. Enamel porcelain applied to incisal edge and blended gingivally over body porcelain.

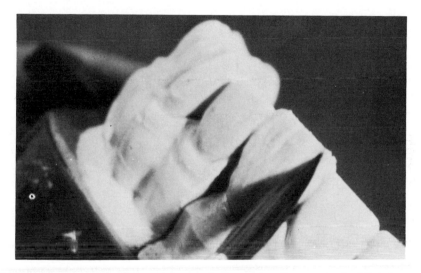

Fig. 25-16. Translucent porcelain applied proximally near incisal third area.

25-16). White or blue stain may be applied over the exposed enamel surface prior to the application of the translucent porcelain, and this will aid the breakup of light and enliven the incisal corners. This stain must be applied in minute quantity and the lightest touch with the brush is necessary to avoid gross effects.

The central areas of the incisal edge may also be scalloped into V shaped grooves and treated similarly (Fig. 25-17). At the bottom of the groove a small quantity of dentin porcelain is laid in, and orange stains are blended in at the incisal end of the groove (Fig. 25-18). Enamel porcelain is then blended over the thin dentin layer to create a beveled area exactly similar to the one for the enamel-dentin blend. If the translucent porcelain is now applied over the incisal grooved

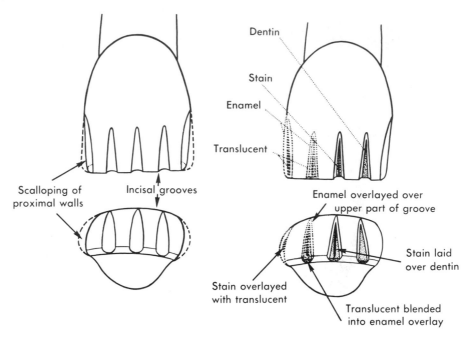

Fig. 25-17. Incisal edge grooved for stains and translucent porcelain.

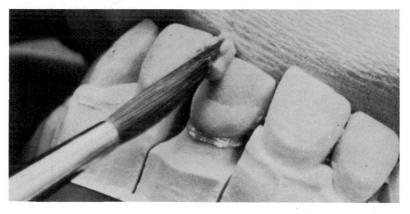

Fig. 25-18. Stain laid in at bottom of groove and covered with enamel porcelain.

area, it will create a three-dimensional effect (Fig. 25-19). The incisal enamel will appear extremely lifelike, and the inlaid concentrated colors will reproduce the effect of enamel cracks or striae.

The importance of beveling the enamel porcelain in the groove line should be emphasized since it will prevent a sharp demarcation line from appearing when the translucent porcelain overlays the entire groove. This translucent porcelain must be used in very small quantity since excess material will create a washout effect.

In some cases a sharp incisal blend of translucence is required; this may be simulated by addition of more translucent porcelain behind the incisal edge.

Subtle use of inlaid concentrated colors (modifiers) and translucent porcelains

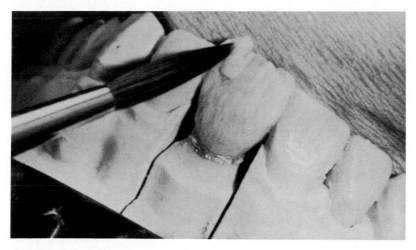

Fig. 25-19. Translucent porcelain applied over grooved area in Fig. 25-18 to complete three-dimensional effect.

will often transform a porcelain crown that otherwise could look quite artificial in the mouth.

ALUMINOUS PORCELAIN INTENSE COLOR MODIFIERS

These modifiers are available in a range of 13 colors and are used in obtaining shades or variations of shades by addition to or by firing over aluminous porcelain.

M	1—Opalescent	M	7—Dark brown
M	2—White/pink	M	8—Pink
M	3—Ivory/cream	M	9—Gray
M	4—Gray/brown	M	10—Blue
M	5—Light orange	M	11—White
M	6—Orange	M	12—Light cream
		M	13—White/white

These intense colors may be mixed with any of the dentins or enamels in the aluminous porcelain range or used undiluted as they are (fusing temperature—1,652° F).

Contact area adjustment

Once the final buildup of the crown is completed, additional translucent and dentin porcelains (1,472° to 1,508° F) may be added to the proximal surfaces to allow

for firing shrinkage and the surface gently smoothed with a large soft brush.

Firing the veneer porcelain
(dentin and enamel)
Biscuit firing for 1,742° F porcelain
Air-firing technique
Drying
Muffle entrance for 4 minutes
Firing platform for 3 minutes
(Furnace at 1,000° to 1,200° F)
Firing
Enter hot zone of furnace at 1,000° F
Raise temperature at 50° F per minute
Hold temperature at 1,650° F for 3 minutes
Vacuum-firing technique
Dry as for air firing
Firing
Enter hot zone of furnace at 1,300° F
Apply vacuum at 20 inches
Raise temperature at 50° F per minute
Break vacuum at 1,650° F
Hold at 1,650° F for 3 minutes

The surface of the crown should now be at a high biscuit stage. Firing aluminous veneer porcelains to a low biscuit is not recommended since most of these materials are made from single-phase glasses that are improved in color and thermal shock resistance by firing to nearly full maturity. If the crown still presents a low biscuit surface, it must be refired for 3 to 4 minutes to increase vitrification.

Grinding and staining

The biscuit-stage aluminous porcelain crown should preferably be ground with diamond stones used exclusively for this work. After any occlusal or contact-area adjustments have been made, the crown may be tried in the mouth. Duplication of the surface forms of the adjoining natural teeth may be achieved by grinding of the aluminous porcelain surface with very fine diamond wheel stones. Smoother areas may be created by use of rubber-bonded carbide wheels, but the surface must be thoroughly cleaned afterward with detergents or an ultrasonic cleaner.

Surface "effect" stains may now be applied and a thin streak of orange stain on a darker dentin color may be applied behind the tip of the incisal edge to produce the slight milkiness present in many natural teeth. Orange or brown stain is also effective when applied on the mesial and distal surfaces, since these colors are highlighted through the enamel surface.

Glazing

It should be emphasized that stressing of a complete porcelain-veneer crown because of thermal shock is severe when a biscuit-fired crown is rapidly introduced into the furnace. Minute thermal cracks can be formed in the glazed surface that are not apparent to the naked eye (Fig. 25-1). Surface weakening caused by these microcracks is therefore built into the crown. At a later stage the crown may fracture in service because of the deepening of these cracks under occlusal loading, and catastrophic failure may occur when the patient is eating nothing harder than bread and butter.

The ceramist must therefore *take the greatest care in preheating his biscuit-stage crown very slowly to ensure that all areas of the crown expand evenly.* The principle of the industrial tunnel kiln is therefore the ideal at which to aim. The crown should be moved stage by stage into the hot zone of the furnace muffle, and simple preheating at the entrance is not sufficient. *A minimum period of 5 minutes should be given to moving the crown into the hot zone, and the firing tray should be inserted at 1-minute intervals.*

All glazing must be accomplished in air and where possible a powerful electric lamp will enable the ceramist to view his glazed surface directly. *The recommended glazing period for the 1,742° F aluminous porcelain is 4 to 4.5 minutes.* However, visual inspection of the surface remains the best method of ensuring that the tooth anatomy has been maintained. The aluminous porcelain dentin and enamel porcelains contain a high content of combined alumina and are resultantly very resistant to slump or pyroplastic flow at their recommended maturing temperature. Rounding of angles and loss of detail are invariably produced by glazing at too high a temperature. It is therefore essential to maintain a constant check on the accuracy of the furnace pyrometer and to bear in mind that, if necessary, a little more time spent on glazing at a lower temperature will ensure brighter colors and greater surface detail. Greenish porcelain is produced by quick-firing at too high a temperature; the glass is overvitrified. In some cases, it may even devitrify, producing flecked areas in the surface.

THE POSTERIOR ALUMINOUS PORCELAIN CROWN

An alumina-reinforced crown may be constructed on the posterior teeth, but it must only be used where at least 1 mm of core porcelain can be used for occlusal protection. To obtain optimum reinforcement, the core porcelain should contain 50% by weight of alumina (high-fusing core) and should cover the entire occlusal and lingual surfaces (Fig. 25-20). Subse-

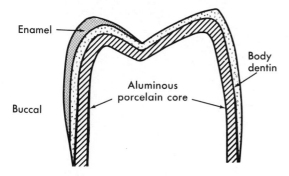

Fig. 25-20. Correct preparation of premolar aluminous porcelain crown.

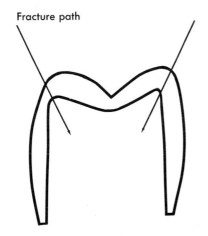

Fig. 25-21. Incorrect preparation of premolar aluminous porcelain crown.

quent firing shrinkage will allow sufficient room for a thin layer of dentin and enamel powders. The buccal surface may be completed with the same technique used for the anterior crown.

The tooth preparation must simulate the original tooth-contour line and present no sharp angles on the occlusal surface (Fig. 25-21). If a thin amount of porcelain is present between the occlusal-axial walls, fracture is almost inevitable.

PREFORMED HIGH-ALUMINA CERAMIC REINFORCEMENTS

High-alumina ceramics used in dentistry generally contain at least 97% pure alumina, and they differ considerably from aluminous porcelain (Table 25-1).

Aluminous porcelain is a mixture of alumina crystals and a glass flux, and during sintering, the glass forms a matrix for the harder and stronger alumina crystals. In the case of high alumina, although small quantities of fluxing agents are used, the main process that occurs during firing is termed "recrystallization."

Many theories exist regarding the exact processes that occur during the firing cycle of high alumina. However, it appears that during firing, the following steps occur. First, welding occurs at points of contact between adjacent oxide particles, giving rise to a lensing effect as normally occurs in sintering processes, that is, partial fusion. Migration of atoms then takes place from one particle to another, resulting in a shift in particle boundaries on recrystallization. During recrystallization, the shift in grain boundaries results in the formation of a closely interlocking crystalline structure of considerable strength, with the improved packing of the particles resulting in shrinkage of the oxide mass (Fig. 25-22). Fluxes such as CaO_2, SiO_2, TiO_2, and MnO_2 bond the structure together and increase diffusion in the alumina itself.

High-alumina ceramics are made from calcined alumina powders that have been mixed with suitable binders and a release agent. The alumina "dough" can then be automatically dry-pressed or extrusion-molded for use as crown or bridge reinforcements (Figs. 25-23, *A*, and 25-26).

The molded articles are then slowly oven-dried and fired at a fusion temperature of up to 3,012° F, with the resulting product being a hard impermeable ceramic of very high strength and chemical resistance (Table 25-6). The fired alumina is considerably stronger than aluminous porcelain and has proved, under clinical tests, to be as strong as current metals (Fig. 25-24).

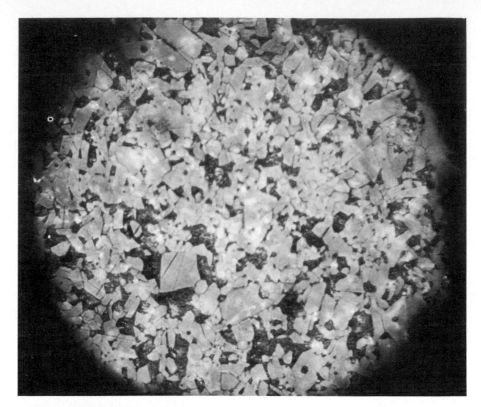

Fig. 25-22. Photomicrograph of recrystallized alumina.

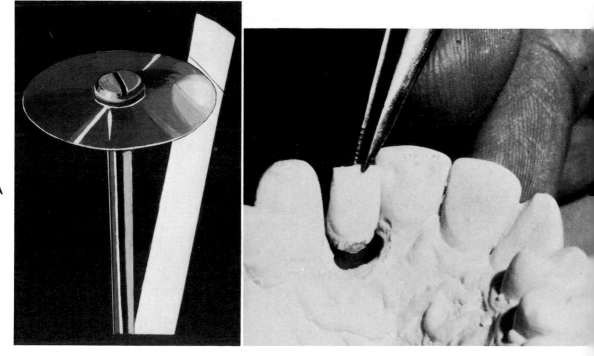

A

Fig. 25-23. A, High-alumina strip is cut with diamond disc. **B,** High-alumina strip to be placed on lingual surface of tooth in Figs. 25-5 and 25-26, for added strength and translucence.

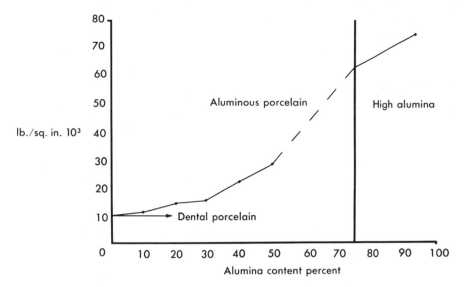

Fig. 25-24. Modulus of rupture of aluminous porcelain and high alumina.

Table 25-5. Preformed high-alumina rods, tubes, and strip*

Type	Number	Length (mm)	Internal diameter (mm)	External diameter (mm)	Uses
Oval tube	T.1	50	1.5 × 2.0	2.5 × 3.0	Dowel-crowns
Oval tube	T.2	50	1.8 × 2.5	2.8 × 2.5	Dowel crown tube pontics
Oval tube	T.3	50	2.0 × 3.0	3.0 × 4.0	Dowel-crown tube pontics
Oval tube	T.4	50	2.0 × 2.5	4.0 × 4.5	Tube pontics
Oval rod	R.1	50		2.8 × 3.5	Bridge connectors
Round rod	R.2	50		1.0	Bridge connectors
Round rod	R.3	50		1.5	Bridge connectors
Curved strip	S.1	50		7.1 × 0.7	Reinforced linguals on jacket and dowel-crowns Reinforcement for cantilever bridges
Dovetail—slotted backing	A.1	50		4.0 × 2.27	Facing on metal substructure

*Cutting and shaping of all high-alumina reinforcements are best done with diamond instruments rotating at not less than 20,000 rpm. Areas where the porcelain buildup will contact the model should be treated with a release agent. (Courtesy Columbus Dental Mfg. Co., Columbus, Ohio.)

High-alumina ceramics are colored to a neutral dentin shade by use of high-temperature resistant pigments such as manganese-alumina pink, vanadium-zircon blue, and praseodymium-zircon yellow. This background of pure color is very re-ceptive to veneering with the more translucent veneer porcelains (Fig. 25-23, *B*). The bonding at the interface between aluminous porcelain and high alumina is of a chemical nature, and an ionic bond between the oxide constituents of both materials is achieved. This can be shown by observation of the fluorescent effect at the interface when examined under ultraviolet light.

High-alumina reinforcements are used to reinforce aluminous complete porcelain crowns and to provide high-strength anchorage systems for bridge pontics, facings, dowel crowns, and all ceramic bridges. High alumina is supplied in the form of reinforcing rods, tubes, dovetail backings, and sheets (Table 25-5).

PALATAL REINFORCED CROWNS
High-alumina curved strip (S.1)

The method of using a curved strip was devised to increase the strength of the complete aluminous porcelain crowns, particularly in the closed-bite situation. Clinical experience has indicated that high-alumina strips used as a palatal reinforcement can provide strength in the critical occluding area and prevent midline or half-moon fractures. The technique is particularly useful on the anterior crown where space limits the use of porcelain-fused-to-gold crowns (Fig. 25-25). The high-alumina curved strip becomes an integral part of the core porcelain and will enable aluminous porcelain crowns to be constructed where all-porcelain restorations would definitely be contraindicated.

Technique

As much as possible of the palatal surface is covered with the sheet without interference with incisal esthetics or lingual contour (Fig. 25-26). The slight curvature of the strip may be orientated in any direction so at to adapt as closely as possible to the palatal form of the preparation. The dentist may wish to bear in mind the curvature of the strip and select a similar-diameter cutting wheel with which to prepare the palatal section of the preparation, to ensure a fully fitting insert without leaving an unreinforced area palatocervically. Objections to using such a preformed reinforcement can be raised regarding the universal application of this technique to all preparations since every tooth will differ in palatal curvature. Clinical experience under laboratory conditions has indicated that at least 70% of all preparations can be fitted with high-alumina sheet reinforcement without interfering with occlusion or esthetics.

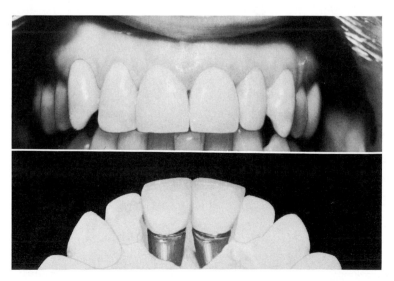

Fig. 25-25. Labial and lingual views of two upper central incisors with aluminous porcelain crowns.

luminous porcelain jacket crown (Alumina sheet reinforcement)

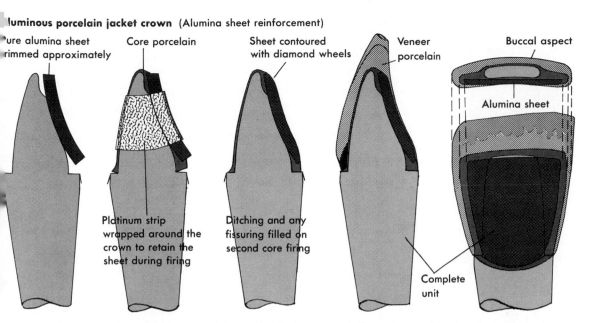

Fig. 25-26. Aluminous porcelain crown built up to full contour with alumina sheet reinforcement on die covered with 0.025 mm platinum matrix.

Table 25-6. High-alumina reinforcement components

Tensile strength	lb/sq. inch	20,000
Compressive strength	lb/sq. inch	250,000
Bending strength	lb/sq. inch	50,000
Impact strength	kg/cm	5.5
Thermal conductivity	at 20° C cal/cm/cm²/sec/°C	0.050
Hardness—Moh scale		9
Coefficient of linear expansion—parts/million/°C	20° to 400° C	6.6
	20° to 600° C	7.2
	20° to 1,000° C	8.2
Porosity	Fuchsine dye penetration	Nil
	Water absorption	Nil
Working temperature, maximum	°C	1,800

The platinum matrix is prepared as for a conventional crown. The alumina strip is applied to the preparation and marked with a pencil to an estimated size and cut off square with a diamond disc. Further shaping is by diamond wheel. Exact contour is not imperative at this stage. A little high-fusing aluminous core porcelain is applied to the palatal area of the preparation and partially condensed by gentle tapping of the model and absorbing with a paper tissue or gauze.

The shaped alumina backing sheet is roughened with a diamond wheel stone, and any contaminant is removed by heating in a furnace. The backing is then positioned with tweezers and settled into the core porcelain until it is firmly against the platinum matrix. When the opposing teeth are positioned, the insert may tilt slightly if there is contact, and it should be pushed into better adaptation at this point. It is left in this position and more porcelain is added around the proximal and incisal edges, with care taken not to trap air under the sheet. The insert is held tightly by finger pressure with a tissue and gently condensed.

At this stage the full core form may be built up, condensed, and relieved at the shoulder, with care taken not to alter the position of the insert. Alternatively the insert may be fired to the matrix first. Whichever method is used, it is important to retain the insert in close contact with the matrix during firing. This may be done by wrapping of a narrow strip of platinum around the complete fabrication, and the ends may be linked by a simple finger-formed tinner's joint. If this is not done, the steam pressure behind the insert during drying may cause the insert to come away from the porcelain or to fall away under its own weight. This stage is fired until complete shrinkage of added core porcelain has occurred (2,012° F).

The shoulder is reburnished and the cervical space is filled, together with any fissuring around the insert. The core porcelain is then given a final firing of at least 8 minutes at 2,012° F.

The edges of the insert are tapered into the core porcelain by contouring with a diamond wheel, and any high points on the occlusion are eased (Fig. 25-26).

The insert should not be thinned to less than half its thickness over a large area, but it has been found reliable to thin a pinpoint area to 0.25 mm. If space permits, it is desirable (although not critical) to cover the insert with core porcelain. It should, however, be finally covered with at least a thin glaze veneer.

The final buildup is of dentin and enamel as described for the aluminous porcelain crown (Fig. 25-26).

SELECTED REFERENCES

1. McLean, J. W.: A higher strength porcelain for crown and bridge work, Br. Dent. J. **119**:268, 1965.
2. McLean, J. W., and Hughes, T. H.: The reinforcement of dental porcelain with ceramic oxides, Br. Dent. J. **119**:251, 1965.
3. Genin, L. G.: Effect of quartz on the strength of porcelain, Glass and Ceram. (Moscow) **15**:35, 1958.
4. Binns, D. B.: Some physical properties of two-phase crystal-glass solids. In Stewart, G. H., editor: Science of ceramics, New York, 1962, Academic Press, Inc., vol. 1.
5. McLean, J. W.: The development of ceramic oxide reinforced dental porcelains with an appraisal of their physical and clinical properties, MDS thesis, University of London, 1966.
6. Adriaasen, J. A. T.: Personal communication, 1966.

GENERAL REFERENCES

Austin, C. R., Schofield, H. Z., and Haldy, N. L. Alumina in whiteware, J. Am. Ceram. Soc. **29**:341, 1946.
Batchelor, R. W., and Dinsdale, A.: Some physical properties of porcelain bodies containing corundum, Trans. Seventh Int. Ceramics Cong., London, 1960, p. 31.
Blodgett, W. E.: High strength alumina porcelains, Ceram. Bull. **40**:74, 1961.
Brecker, S. C.: Crowns, Philadelphia, 1961, W. B. Saunders Co.
Brecker, S. C.: Clinical procedures in occlusal rehabilitation, Philadelphia, 1966, W. B. Saunders Co.
Fonvielle, F. P., and Semmelman, J. O.: Int. Assoc. Dent. Res., 1967.
Hasselman, D. P. H., and Fulrath, R. M.: Proposed fracture theory of a dispersion-strengthened glass matrix, J. Am. Ceram. Soc. **49**:68, 1966.
Johnston, J. F., Mumford, G., and Dykema, R. W.: Modern practice in dental ceramics, Philadelphia, 1967, W. B. Saunders Co.
Martinelli, N.: Dental laboratory technology, St. Louis, 1970, The C. V. Mosby Co.
McLean, J. W.: A higher strength porcelain for crown and bridge work, Br. Dent. J. **119**: 268, 1965.
McLean, J. W.: The alumina tube post crown, Br. Dent. J. **123**:87, 1967.
McLean, J. W.: High alumina ceramics for bridge pontic construction, Br. Dent. J. **123**:571, 1967.
McLean, J. W.: The science and art of dental ceramics, Louisiana State Univ. Monographs I and II, 1974, and Monographs III and IV, 1976.
Tylman, S. D.: Theory and practice of crown and bridge prosthodontics, ed. 5, St. Louis, 1965, The C. V. Mosby Co.
Vines, R. F., Semmelman, J. O., Lee, P. W., and Fonvielle, F. D.: Mechanisms involved in securing dense, vitrified ceramics from preshaped partly crystalline bodies, J. Am. Ceram. Soc. **41**:304, 1958.

26

Dental restorations using ceramics fired to gold alloy castings

Stanley D. Tylman

A metallurgical development by Granger[1] gave accurate iridioplatinum castings of individual crowns and complete reinforced fixed partial structures. Granger modified the stress bar or truss by designing ferrule-shaped copings for the pontic section of the truss (Fig. 26-1) for fixed partial dentures.

A complete description of the Granger reinforced porcelain bridges has been given in previous editions of this textbook. Discussions of the Micro-Bond palladium-platinum alloy types of porcelain bridges are also found in the previous editions. Although both the Granger castings and the platinum alloy types of Micro-Bond are satisfactory from the standpoint of utility and esthetics, the comparatively high cost of materials and the time involved in their construction, plus the need for unusually skillful technicians to perform the necessary work, make it necessary to confine the discussion here to the more generally used present-day ceramic-metal types of bridges (Fig. 26-2) employing the gold alloy.

The science of metallurgy of precious metals has advanced greatly in the last decade, as has the knowledge and application of the high-temperature refractory casting investments. This has enabled the dentist to obtain accurately fitting cast metal structures that support the fused porcelain components of a ceramic-metal fixed partial prosthesis. The coefficients of expansion and contraction of the alloys and porcelains have been balanced and the molecular bond obtainable today between metal and porcelain has modified the necessity of basic mechanical retention between the two. A combination of chemical, mechanical, and van der Waals phenomena provides retention for porcelain to current porcelain-fused-to-metal restorations.

With a properly designed structure of metal, the present special gold alloys bonded molecularly to porcelain are sufficiently strong to meet the requirements to which the structure will be subjected. These alloys are comparable to the type IIIC and type IV casting gold alloys generally used in fixed partial denture construction.

PORCELAIN FUSED TO METAL

Among the list of gold alloys that were first available for commercial laboratory use were Ney-Oro P16, with Thermalite porcelain, 1750° F[2]; Micro-Bond High Life with Micro-Bond porcelain[3]; and Jelenko and Aderer golds used with Ceramco porcelains.[4] The physical properties of these metals were listed in the sixth edition.

Manufacturers have improved these properties so that the strength of the metals presently available is ample for long-span bridges as well as individual

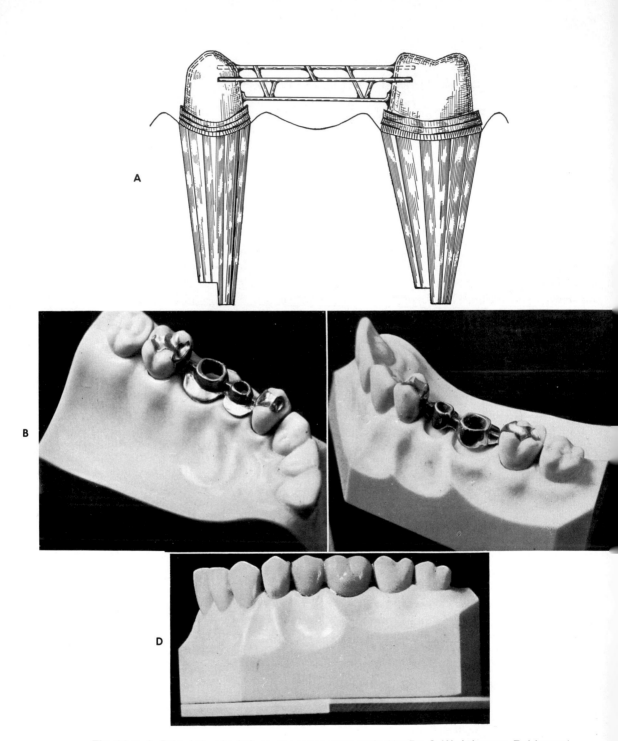

Fig. 26-1. A, Principle of reinforcement recommended by Dr. C. W. Johnson. **B,** Lingual view of cast iridioplatinum structure soldered to two retainers. **C,** Occlusal view of model shown in **B. D,** Buccal view of finished bridge.

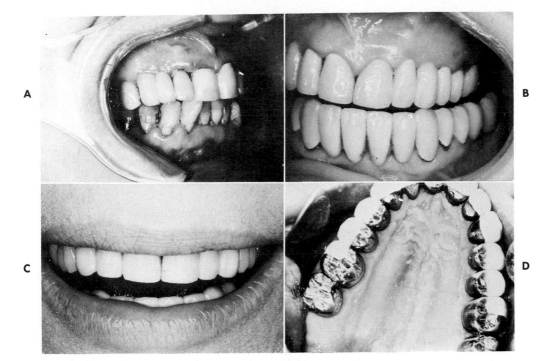

Fig. 26-2. A, Patient with advanced caries and periodontal disease prior to treatment. Despite recalls and hygienic instructions, this case will enjoy limited success. **B,** Patient in **A** shown after endodontic, periodontic, and restorative rehabilitation. Porcelain-fused-to-metal crowns were used as restorative units. Lateral excursions of mandible require additional attention to develop satisfactory occlusal pattern. Tissue response to porcelain-fused-to-metal restorations can be classified as fair to poor in this instance because of patient's oral hygiene. Note buildup of debris in lower anterior quadrant of mouth. **C,** Reestablishment of more esthetic and physiologically acceptable occlusal plane frequently results in improved mental hygiene and personality of patient. **D,** Occlusolingual view of patient in **A.** Lingual stamp cusps remain in gold to facilitate occlusal modification before and after insertion. Terminal molar is a complete gold crown to maintain vertical dimension (posterior vertical stabilization).

crowns. This is made possible by the hardening mechanisms that are used after the casting procedures. Obviously, the higher fusing metals employed in porcelain-fused-to-metal restorations require specifically designed investments. The manufacturer's instruction for their use should be meticulously followed during investing, burning out, and casting.

The New Hue and Bioform shade guides (Table 26-1) are two of the shade guides commonly used by the dentist to select shades for patients. Vita Porcelain shade guides are also rapidly increasing in popularity. Initially the shades of porcelain fused to metal lacked the vitality necessary for esthetics, but improvement in technique and ceramics have increased the vitality of the shades to the point that these restorations are second only to complete gold crowns in the number of teeth restored in fixed prosthodontics. However, the technique requires careful attention to certain details of preparation and procedures to obtain maximum benefits.

Table 26-1. New Hue and Bioform shade guides

| Shade | Porcelain | | Opaque | |
	Gingival	Incisal	Gingival	Incisal
		Trubyte New Hue vitality scale		
60	60N	(2)91 + (1)60N	G	H
61	61N	(1)90 + (1)WP	(1)D + (1)A	(1)H + (1)A
62	62BN	90	G	H
65	65BN	(2)91 + 65BN	(1)F + (1)G	H
66	66BN	(2)90 + (1)66BN	(1)D + (1)G	H
67	67BN	(2)91 + (1)67BN	D	H
68	68N	(2)91 + (1)68N	(1)D + (1)G	H
69	69BN	(2)92 + (1)69BN	(1)D + (1)H	H
77	77BN	(2)92 + (1)77BN	(1)F + (1)H	H
78	78N	(2)92 + (1)78N	F	H
81	81BN	(2)92 + (1)81BN	F	H
87	87BN	92	F	H
		Trubyte Bioform (vacuum) shades		
59*	59*	(1)59 + (1)95	(2)G + (1)A	(2)G + (1)A
60	60B	96	F	(1)H + (2)A
62	62BN	(3)90 + (1)62BN	(2)G + (1)H	H
64	64B	(2)91 + (1)Trans.	D	H
65	65BN	(3)91 + (1)65BN	(1)F + (1)G	H
66	66BN	91	(1)G + (1)D	H
67	67BN	(3)91 + (1)67BN	D	H
68	68B	(3)91 + (1)Trans.	(1)D + (1)G	H
69	69BN	(2)92 + (1)69BN	(2)G + (1)H	H
70	70B	(3)91 + (1)70B	F	H
77	77BN	(2)92 + (1)77BN	(1)F + (1)H	H
81	81BN	(3)93 + (1)81BN	F	H
82	44	(1)92 + (1)Ging. Bl.	F	(1)F + (1)H

TOOTH PREPARATION

The tooth preparation is discussed in Chapter 6 under veneer crowns. The preparation is similar to that of a Hollenback crown, that is, a shoulder on the labial aspect, and a shoulder or chamfer on the lingual aspect. Beveled labial and buccal with rounded shoulders are now considered a more satisfactory preparation for porcelain-fused-to-metal restorations.[5] Removable dies made with hard stone (Fig. 26-3) and so forth are a necessity. This procedure has been described in Chapter 10. As with all veneered cast-gold crown preparations, a sufficient

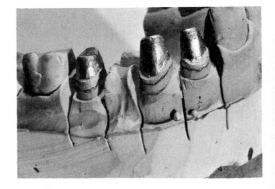

Fig. 26-3. Preparation for fixed prosthesis with exaggerated labial and buccal gingival bevels.

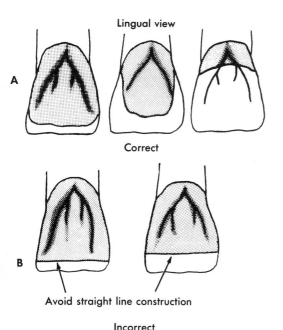

Lingual view

A

Correct

B

Avoid straight line construction

Incorrect

Fig. 26-4. A, Correct lingual design of casting. **B,** Incorrect design. (Courtesy J. M. Ney Co., Bloomfield, Conn.)

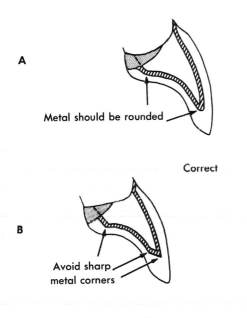

A

Metal should be rounded

Correct

B

Avoid sharp metal corners

Incorrect

Fig. 26-5. A, Correct proximal, incisal, and gingival design. **B,** Incorrect design. (Courtesy J. M. Ney Co., Bloomfield, Conn.)

amount of tooth structure must be removed to leave adequate labial or buccal space for the gold and porcelain veneer.

FIXED PROSTHESIS CONSTRUCTION
Wax-metal design

During the waxing and finishing of the cast metal, the labial aspect is given special shape (Figs. 26-4 and 26-5). Straight line construction and sharp metal corners are to be avoided or fracture will occur. The junction of metal and porcelain should *not* be placed in stress-bearing areas, that is, where the mandibular incisor strikes the lingual surface of the maxillary incisors (Fig. 26-6). The farther away the striking areas of functional occlusion are from these junctions, the less likely the fracture of the porcelain. Try-ins of porcelain-fused-to-metal crowns prior to glazing are desired when they are in strategic occlusal relationships. The metal design in Fig. 26-7 may be adequate for mandibular incisors and some maxillary incisors, but the junction of metal and porcelain of this design may be improper for a maxillary canine during functional disocclusion. Fig. 26-8 is usu-

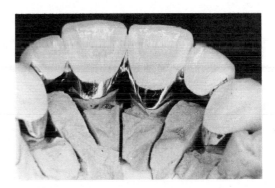

Fig. 26-6. Lingual view of maxillary six-unit porcelain-fused-to-metal fixed prosthesis where junction of porcelain and metal is not within striking range of mandibular teeth. Note design of lateral pontics (Stein type of design).

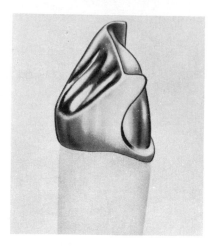

Fig. 26-7. Ney-Oro type of crown having entire incisal portion of porcelain. (Courtesy J. M. Ney Co., Bloomfield, Conn.)

ally the design of choice for canines and short-bite cases because of the superior strength resulting from this metal-porcelain design.

The advent of superior golds and improved porcelains made possible restorations with a natural appearance, adequate strength, and acceptable tissue compatibility needed for fixed prostheses. Careful adherence to these advanced techniques (Fig. 26-8, *F-H*) enhances the construction of restorations having acceptable esthetics (Fig. 26-9) and service. The discussion of these advancements includes three parts: (1) metal phase, (2) porcelain phase, and (3) troubleshooting phase (listing some of the most common errors and describing their cause and solution).

Metal phase

The importance of the design and construction of the metal substructure cannot be overemphasized. It is important not only from the standpoint of strength but also from its effect on the esthetic result of the final restorations. This is especially true with the newer porcelains, with which more innovative approaches are employed for achieving shades of a more vital and natural appearance. The color

is concentrated in the undercoat and covered with a layer of more translucent porcelain. This will effect a more reliable duplication of the natural dentition.

Because of the strong influence on the final shade by the undercoat, uniformity of thickness of the body porcelain becomes extremely important. Position and design of the metal substructure (Fig. 26-8) greatly determine the thickness and contour of the final restoration. Bulk can be reduced and the original morphology of the teeth more accurately duplicated.

The following are some general rules to remember when constructing the metal work.

Pontics. Pontics should be designed and constructed according to the principles listed for abutments, that is, uniform distribution of porcelain surrounding the metal substructure. There are specific points of importance that direct the application of porcelain to the pontic substructure, but none of these is as important as the uniform thickness of porcelain and the position of the substructure in relation to the crest of the edentulous ridge and the areas to be subjected to occlusal stress (Fig. 26-10). An additional consideration is the embrasure area. The pontic must have sufficient bulk for strength but

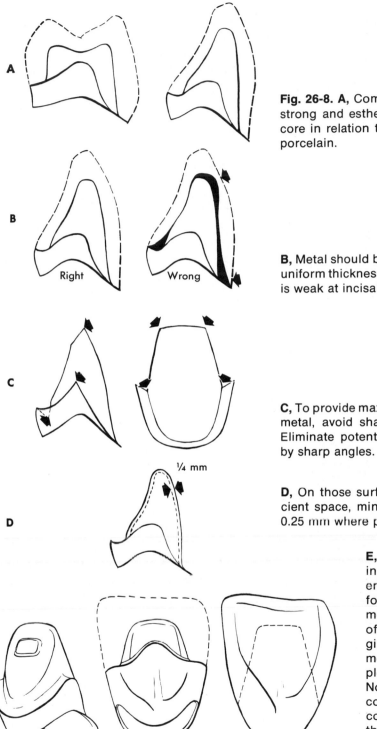

Fig. 26-8. A, Complete porcelain coverage is strong and esthetic; correct shape of metal core in relation to thickness and contour of porcelain.

B, Metal should be constructed to provide for uniform thickness of porcelain. Labial surface is weak at incisal and gingival areas.

C, To provide maximum fusion of porcelain to metal, avoid sharp corners and undercuts. Eliminate potential cleavage points created by sharp angles.

D, On those surfaces where there is insufficient space, minimum thickness of metal is 0.25 mm where porcelain is to be applied.

E, Some solutions for those instances when there is not enough room for metal and for porcelain: *left,* island of metal in lingual incisal area of incisal occlusion; *center,* gingival half covered with metal on lingual; *right,* complete porcelain coverage. Note that full porcelain coverage, or as nearly full coverage as possible, makes the strongest restoration. (**A** to **E,** Courtesy J. M. Ney Co., Bloomfield, Conn.)

Continued.

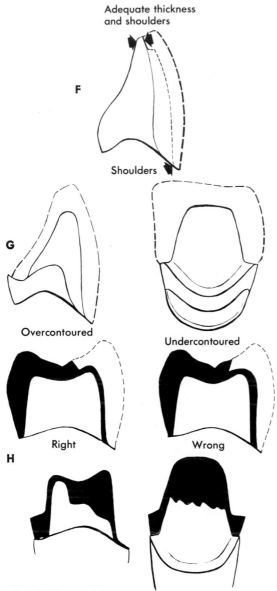

Fig. 26-8, cont'd.
F, Two important considerations in veneer types of crowns: (1) incisal or occlusal metal edge should be heavy enough to resist burnishing; (2) there should be incisal and gingival shoulder to support porcelain.
G, Metal should always be shaped and contoured to provide harmonious blend with porcelain at finish lines. Right or slightly obtuse angle of metal at porcelain-metal junction is most desirable contour.
H, Broken or badly decayed abutments should be restored to normal contours. (Courtesy Dr. R. Vining and Howmet Co.)

also have adequate embrasure area to be cleansible and create a climate for supportive tissue health (Figs. 26-9, *B*, and 26-11).

Connectors. There are a number of important design principles relating to multiple unit connectors that must be adhered to if the maximum in esthetics and in strength of a bridge is to be achieved (Fig. 26-11). When an irregular arrangement is desired, one may need to modify the guidelines presented in Fig. 26-11.

Spruing

1. Use large sprues, preferaby straight 10-gage sprues.
2. Sprue bridge on model, waxing one sprue to each unit. Join sprues together with additional wax. This serves as added support when the bridge is removed from the model.
3. If a reservoir sprue is used, the reservoir must be not more than $1/16$ inch from the unit in order to properly "feed" the casting during the cooling and shrinkage period. If a unit has more mass than the reservoir, thicken the reservoir so that its mass will be greater than the unit it feeds. If reservoirs are close together, join them with a little wax.
4. The total length of the sprue from the button to each unit should be ¼ inch. In spans of considerable length or curvature, the button need not be round but may follow the general curvature of the span being sprued.
5. Sprue units so that the abutment openings are facing up to avoid trapping air during investment procedure.
6. Sprue posterior pontics into the heaviest cusp. Sprue anterior veneers at the incisal edge of the thick lingual wax and thin labial wax.
7. The sprued bridge should be waxed on the crucible former to allow ¼ inch of investment over the pattern. This allows for escape of gas from

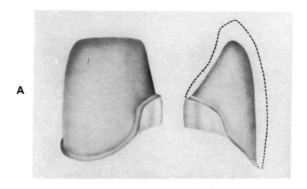

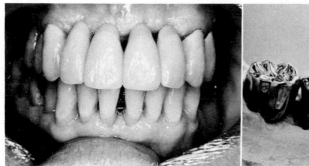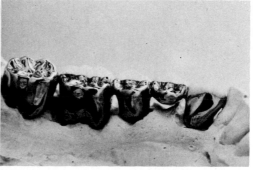

Fig. 26-9. A, Casting with heavy linguoproximal coping used with complete porcelain coverage of crown. **B,** Six-unit maxillary bridge placed for a patient with advanced periodontal condition. Note cervical stain used to characterize radicular portion of pontics. Position and extent of embrasure area depends on hygienic dictates and lip line of patient. **C,** Mandibular posterior porcelain-fused-to-metal crown. Note porcelain veneer is placed from one half to one third down buccal inclined plane. This allows for stamp cusp of maxillary arch to contact metal, a position that facilitates further occlusal adjustment after cementation of restoration. **(A,** Courtesy Dr. R. Vining and Howmet Co.; **B,** courtesy Charles Bagley Porter, New Orleans.)

the mold when the metal is cast.

8. Wax out all right angles, which may fracture and be incorporated into the molten metal.

Investing and burnout

1. Line casting ring with one layer of asbestos, and brush the entire surface with melted wax, securing the asbestos to the ring.

2. Mix the special investment used with porcelain fused to metals to the manufacturer's suggested water-liquid ratio.

3. There is approximately 14 to 15 ml of water-liquid mixture combined with 100 gm of investment. Mix for 20 seconds with vacuum equipment.

4. Fill the investment ring to avoid damage to the pattern and trapping air.

5. The investment is allowed to set for 60 minutes before burnout. Hygroscopic procedures are preferred by some operators. Manufacturer's recommendations should be closely followed.

6. Place ring in furnace at room temperature, and bring the furnace temperature to 1,300° F and soak for 90 minutes.

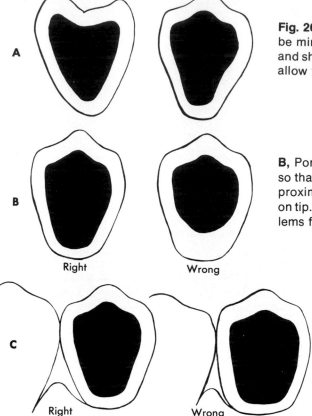

Fig. 26-10. A, Pontic should be contoured to be miniature of finished unit's size, location, and shade to ensure consistency; they should allow for 1 to 1.5 mm thickness of porcelain.

B, Pontics should be long enough gingivally so that when undercoat is applied there is approximately 1 mm space for body porcelain on tip. Shorter pontic will create shading problems for ceramist.

C, Pontic tips should be narrow enough mesiodistally to maintain normal tooth width and to avoid broad, bulky appearance. This will also provide open interdental space, allowing ease of cleaning and affording fewer opportunities for periodontal involvement. (Courtesy Dr. R. Vining and Howmet Co.)

Casting

1. Equipment—a single-orifice tip for gas-oxygen, for example, Micro torch WG-8.
2. Fuel—gas-oxygen.
3. Flame—use a reducing flame with a 1¼-inch inner cone and an 8- to 9-inch entire cone length.
4. Melting—heat alloy without flux in regular unlined Vitallium crucible. Use a new crucible and identify it so that it will be reserved only for porcelain-fused-to-metal alloys. As the alloy becomes molten, it is first shiny and then a dark film forms over the surface. The alloy should be further heated until the melt becomes clean, bright, and very fluid in appearance. Dark green glasses help in seeing this change. Cast the alloy into the mold and allow it to bench-cool until it reaches handling temperature.
5. The ring should be placed in the casting machine so that the units to be cast are trailing the direction of the arm in spinning (Fig. 26-12).
6. Knock off gross investment and sandblast to remove remaining material. Leave the redness of the casting alone since it will disappear, and then quench. The time lapse is usually 5 minutes. Set sandblast air pressure at 30 pounds or less. Sand or glass beads may be used.

Soldering

1. Surfaces to be joined must be smooth, clean, and free of oxides. The metal surfaces should be slightly separated for maximum accuracy.
2. Invest units in special high-heat all-

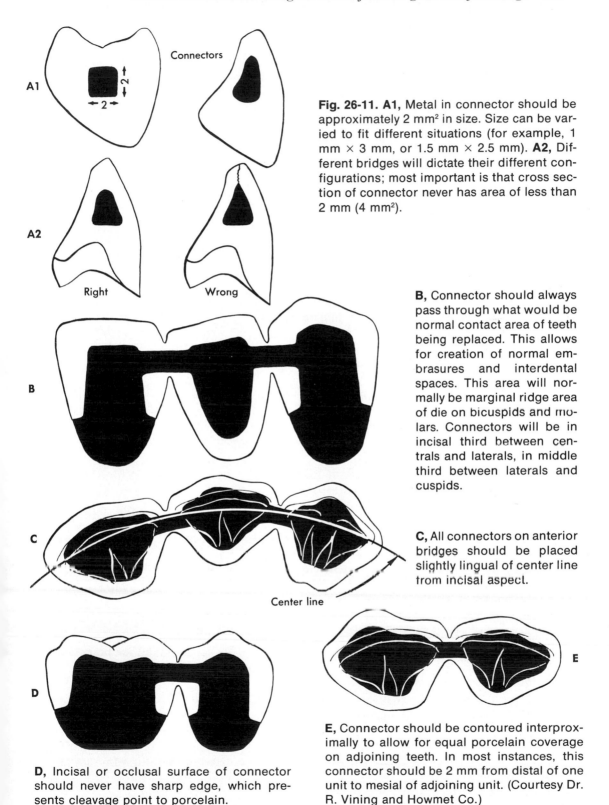

Fig. 26-11. A1, Metal in connector should be approximately 2 mm² in size. Size can be varied to fit different situations (for example, 1 mm × 3 mm, or 1.5 mm × 2.5 mm). **A2,** Different bridges will dictate their different configurations; most important is that cross section of connector never has area of less than 2 mm (4 mm²).

B, Connector should always pass through what would be normal contact area of teeth being replaced. This allows for creation of normal embrasures and interdental spaces. This area will normally be marginal ridge area of die on bicuspids and molars. Connectors will be in incisal third between centrals and laterals, in middle third between laterals and cuspids.

C, All connectors on anterior bridges should be placed slightly lingual of center line from incisal aspect.

D, Incisal or occlusal surface of connector should never have sharp edge, which presents cleavage point to porcelain.

E, Connector should be contoured interproximally to allow for equal porcelain coverage on adjoining teeth. In most instances, this connector should be 2 mm from distal of one unit to mesial of adjoining unit. (Courtesy Dr. R. Vining and Howmet Co.)

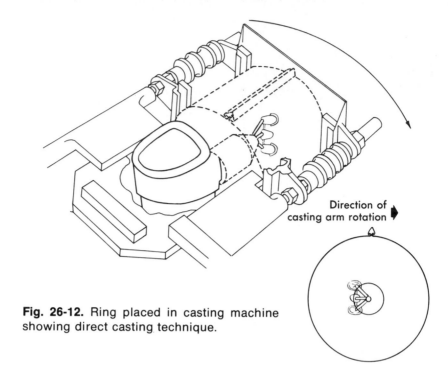

Fig. 26-12. Ring placed in casting machine showing direct casting technique.

Direction of casting arm rotation

purpose soldering investment. Currently deoxidizing phosphate-bound soldering investment (30-minute set) is used.

3. Boil off wax and heat model to dry.
4. Apply soldering flux to areas to be soldered if necessary. The soldered joints will be stronger without the addition of flux.
5. Use a gas-oxygen soldering torch with reducing flame for the soldering operation.
6. Heat the investment until the metal becomes cherry red, apply slightly fluxed porcelain-gold solder to areas to be joined, and apply the flame to the solder. Again dark green glasses help in seeing color changes. When the solder flows freely, remove the flame immediately and allow the entire cast to bench cool.

Alternate method. Some technicians place the entire invested assembly in the porcelain oven after the porcelain has been covered with a thin layer of white wax and heat to the manufacturer's specifications. The solder is placed next to the fluxed metal areas to be joined, and the soldered joint is made as if it were sweated on.

The cast is removed from the oven as soon as the solder has freely flowed, uniting the areas. Some porcelain furnaces have a window through which the technician can observe this critical step. Post-soldering technique is used for this method.

Lastly, the soldered joint with porcelain fused to metal is a relatively weak joint when compared to the all-cast rigid joint when properly cast.

Preparation of metal for porcelain application

1. Grinding and cleaning
   a. Rough grind with hard mounted stone all surfaces of the casting to which porcelain is to be applied. Assorted stones are excellent for this operation. Some technicians prefer aluminum oxide stones or vitrified stones.

b. Clean the metal in ultrasonic cleaner or wash thoroughly with detergent and stiff brush.

c. Rinse metal well in clean water.

2. Degassing the metal

a. Dry metal thoroughly. Avoid handling with fingers.

b. Insert into furnace at 1,200° F and raise furnace to temperature specified by the manufacturer.

c. Hold at specified temperature of 1,920° F for 5 to 7 minutes, remove metal, and cool on bench.

d. Restoration is now ready for porcelain application.

Formerly, bonding agents were used and their application took place prior to, or during, degassing procedures as described above. Most technicians do *not* feel the need for bonding agents either to ensure retention of veneer or to increase esthetics, for example, Britcote.

Porcelain phase in general

There are these steps of porcelain addition:

1. *Opaque (undercoat) layer.* Opaque layers supply the intensity of color needed to create a more lifelike appearance by duplicating the effect of nature where the dentin color reflects through a layer of enamel. This opacity makes it possible to block or mask out the metal with a very thin coat.

2. *Body porcelain.* The body porcelains are formulated to be compatible with the equivalent undercoat shade and help create the same effect.

3. *Incisal porcelain.* Incisal porcelain usually is supplied in two degrees of translucency: light and dark.

4. *Color modifiers.* These porcelains are for modification of basic shades. They are supplied in gray, pink, orange, yellow, peach, etc. If a technician resorts to routine use of color modifiers, characterizing porcelains and add-on porcelains, the technique of porcelain manipulation needs review and further standardization. Various manufacturers give specific directions, which should be closely adhered to for obtaining satisfactory results. As mentioned previously, the advent of semiprecious, nonprecious, and near-precious metals has added a new dimension to porcelain-fused-to-metal alloys. New metals may require deviations from traditional methods of fabrication. Research is presently sparse. Time and basic research could reveal exciting techniques that might make these restorations available to a larger percentage of the populace.

5. *Glazing*

a. Most porcelain used with this technique glazes naturally and does not require the use of special glazing agents. Vacuum is not required.

b. The purpose of the glaze bake is to form a paper-thin film of glaze on the porcelain surface that will not absorb fluids or odors and will ensure satisfactory tissue tolerance. The glaze places the body porcelain under compression.

c. The glaze bake should not be used to smooth down roughly finished porcelain. The heavy glass formation that results from this incorrect practice causes a loss of sharpness and definition, a burnout of color, and severe stresses in the ceramic material.

d. Always bear in mind that the shine of a glaze increases when the tooth or bridge is wet; so fire your glaze bake accordingly. Avoid overglazing and the glassy "false-tooth" appearance that accompanies it.

e. Porcelains will usually glaze at or near 1,800° F. However, do not rely on pyrometer indications alone when firing. Develop the habit of examining the degree of vitrification visually.

TECHNIQUE FOR PORCELAIN APPLICATION IN DETAIL

One method is presented below for orientation to the regimental porcelain manipulation. Current porcelains and techniques of manipulation vary as to the manufacturer's directions and customized approaches of technicians. In addition, the advent of semiprecious and nonprecious metals have modified traditional porcelain manipulation and casting procedures. The diversity that results suggests that only an orientation to porcelain-fused-to-metal techniques is possible. The metals and porcelain may be different, but the basic procedures remain the same.

Opaque porcelain

Application. The selected opaque porcelain is mixed with distilled water to a light creamlike consistency and brushed onto the metal casting. One application is generally sufficient, since most opaques have excellent hiding power.

Air-firing. The work is dried carefully in front of the muffle and slowly inserted into the muffle. The temperature is raised 100° a minute to approximately 1,750° F and held for 2 minutes. The work is removed from the furnace and allowed to cool slowly under a glass cover.

Vacuum-firing. Vacuum-firing is optional, but if used, follow these suggested steps: After the opaque porcelain is dried in front of the muffle, the work is inserted into the furnace at the temperature of 1,200° F, where it is held for 1 or 2 minutes. Turn on vacuum at 1,200° to 1,750° F and release the vacuum to air-fire opaque to 1,850° F. Twenty-five inches of vacuum is normally used to raise the temperature to 1,850° F at the

rate of 100° a minute. It is then removed at approximately 1,850° from the furnace and allowed to cool under a Pyrex glass cover. An eggshell finish is desirable.

Any gray areas that appear after cooling are too thinly covered with opaque. Additional opaque is applied where it is required, and the firing schedule is repeated. Areas with shrinkage cracks were dried too rapidly before firing. If metal is exposed, reapply opaque and refire; otherwise, merely smooth with a clean mounted stone.

First bake (biscuit)

Preparation

1. Place the opaqued castings back on the model, and any copings that did not seat properly relieve with diamond points.
2. Soak the stone model in water to prevent it from absorbing water from the porcelain while it is being applied.
3. The porcelain placed over the edentulous areas beneath pontics must have a smooth surface and must separate easily from the model. Place a piece of damp tissue paper over the pontic area after the porcelain has been built up. This tissue can be easily removed or will burn out in firing.
4. If model is not mounted on a metal articulator, set a steel bur into model with plaster. Stroking the shank of the bur with a serrated tool will provide the required vibration for flowing and condensing of the porcelain.
5. Spatulate the selected porcelain thoroughly on the glass slab until every particle is wet and the mix has a creamy consistency.

Porcelain application

1. Build up the bridge with the gingival porcelain; vibrate and pack as tightly as possible.
2. Bevel the tips and apply the incisal shade blend.
3. Now carve the anatomic form of

each tooth, and separate the teeth from each other by slicing through the porcelain between them to the opaque. Fine-grain porcelain does not require this approach. This permits the teeth to shrink in firing without shrinkage cracks appearing between adjacent teeth. Next, shape the embrasures. Finally, add sufficient porcelain to the contact areas to compensate for shrinkage during firing, and the work is ready for the furnace. Shrinkage can reach 20%.

Air-firing procedure for add-on
1. Dry the work carefully in front of the muffle, starting at 1,200° F and allowing the furnace temperature to cool to 1,000° F.
2. After drying, insert slowly and wait for a few minutes until the furnace temperature again reaches 1,200° F. This will burn out organic matter such as tissue and lint.
3. Raise the temperature 100° a minute until 1,650° F is reached. Hold 2 minutes for a bake. Remove from the furnace and cool under a Pyrex glass.
4. After recontouring, if additional porcelain is needed, repeat the firing cycle as described above.
5. A surface glaze may be obtained by firing to 1,650° F.

Vacuum-firing
1. Dry the work carefully in front of the muffle, starting at a furnace temperature of 1,200° F.
2. After the drying, insert slowly and wait for a few minutes until the furnace temperature reaches 1,200° F again. This will burn out organic matter such as tissue and lint.
3. Apply a minimum of 25 inches of vacuum at 1,200° F and raise the temperature 100° a minute until 1,775° F is reached. Remove from furnace and cool under a Pyrex glass after releasing the vacuum. Increasing the vacuum intensifies the color.

4. After recontouring, if porcelain is needed, repeat the firing cycle after addition.
5. A surface glaze may be obtained by refiring to 1,800° F. A vacuum is unnecessary on glaze bake.

Second bake in detail
Preparation
1. Fit the crown copings back on their dies.
2. Check the bite and grind the porcelain into proper occlusion where necessary.
3. Shape the anatomic contours, embrasures, saddle areas, etc.
4. Clean the bridge thoroughly with a brush and follow with immersion in the ultrasonic cleaner. It is essential that grinding residue be removed before additional porcelain is applied. If diamond wheels have been used, be careful not to leave metal smears on the porcelain. Residues from grinding stones may produce black specks or bubbles. If rubber wheels have been used, any residue not removed will discolor the porcelain with a green stain after firing.

Porcelain application
1. Add porcelain to complete the anatomic form, and, if necessary, add it to the occlusal surface, contact points, and saddle areas.
2. Fire as for the first bake.

Clean-up
1. Reseat the bridge on the model, and check the bite, saddle areas, and contours. Be sure that the dies seat properly. Remove any porcelain from the inside of the copings.
2. If the case is large and fuses unevenly because of unequal proximity to hot muffle walls, it is helpful to refinish the porcelain to produce a smooth surface on the biscuit bake. The texture is then more uniform and the color is easier to see.

3. Clean the work in the ultrasonic cleaner, and it is ready for the try-in or finishing.

Finishing

Preparation. If the bridge has been tried in, wash it thoroughly with a bristle brush, and follow with about 15 minutes' cleaning in the ultrasonic cleaner. When major corrections in color or anatomic form are required after the try-in, a third bake will be necessary.

Porcelain application. It is desirable to fire the third time at the lowest possible firing temperature. Apply stain where required.

Final firing. Heat the case to 1,775° F. It is unnecessary to return vacuum-fired porcelain to the furnace after spot-grinding. Any spot-grinding done after glazing is usually refined. Fit the case back on the model, and the work is completed.

Stains. Stains are color concentrates that are finely ground and designed to mature with the porcelain. These are versatile materials and may be used in any or all of the porcelain additions. Stains should be mixed with Steele's Liquid Medium. They will serve best when they are always available, premixed with Liquid Medium, and spaced neatly on a glass slab, which is covered when not in use.

Fused porcelain can appear more natural if some of the many characteristic stains found in the mouth are reproduced.

Reliability and reproducibility are not confined to the ceramist; these qualifications are the ultimate responsibility of the dentist and, perhaps most important of all, to the reasonable satisfaction of the patient. The dentist will find the final fitting pleasant, and the patient will find the restoration esthetic, durable, and relatively trouble-free. The durability (years) of most stains is indeterminate at this time.

Troubleshooting

Metal phase

1. Incomplete castings
   a. Copings are waxed too thin, less than 0.3 mm.
   b. Casting temperature was not hot enough. This temperature is usually just out of visual range and that is the reason why dark green glasses are suggested.
   c. More than ¼ inch of investment is above highest part of pattern.
   d. Spruing is faulty.
2. Porosity
   a. Shrink pot voids—sprues are too long or too narrow a gage; sprues should be ¼ inch long and 10-gage.
   b. Pinpoint porosity—casting temperature was either too hot or too cold.
   c. Gas porosity—there is incomplete burnout or too much investment over patterns. Investment covering pattern should be ¼ inch thick.
   d. Button is too small to properly feed casting as it solidifies.
   e. Contamination—remelting spills and using a crucible that has been used for other metals or in which flux has been used are some of the possible sources of contamination. A new crucible should be labeled and used for porcelain-fused-to-metal castings only. Casting flux should rarely be used.
3. Cracked molds
   a. Placing mold in burnout furnace may be too soon. (Invested case should set 60 minutes before burnout.)
   b. If invested case is allowed to set in the open overnight or longer, it should be soaked in a bowl of water for 10 minutes before placing in furnace, or placed under a rubber mixing bowl overnight.

Porcelain phase

1. Small check marks may appear in the fired opaque layer.
   a. Undercoat applied may be too heavy or puddled. Units can be used, but on future cases care should be exercised to achieve a thin uniform application.
   b. There may be insufficient dry out before insertion into muffle.
2. Metal shows through undercoat. Undercoat is applied too thin; paint another thin coat and refire.
3. Voids in porcelain at juncture of incisal and body porcelain. Body porcelain is too dry; moisten body porcelain with water so that it will properly accept addition of incisal porcelain.
4. A checking or tearing of porcelain particularly at interproximals may appear, depending on grain size.
   a. There are no interproximal slices, or they are not deep enough.
   b. An unusually large mass of porcelain may appear in a given area. Metal framework should be constructed to provide for a uniform coverage of porcelain.
5. Checking of porcelain may appear, especially in the final biscuit bake. Porcelain may not be dried out thoroughly before introduction into the muffle. If check lines do not open up, many times this problem can be corrected by refiring of the units.
6. Milky appearance to porcelain on second or later firings.
   a. Not thoroughly cleaned after grinding; all grinding dust must be removed.
   b. All traces of detergent or soap are not thoroughly rinsed off.
   c. Vacuum is not sufficient; 27 inches are recommended.
   d. Vacuum is not turned on at 1,200° F.
7. Black streaks and smudges, particularly in interproximals and at porcelain-metal juncture. Metal contamination of porcelain either from dragging metal grindings up onto porcelain or from diamond disc. If case is kept wet with water when grinding is done with the diamond disc, the chance of contamination is greatly reduced.
8. Small voids on surface of glazed units. Surface is not properly filled with porcelain before glaze firing. It can be corrected by filling with a thin mix of half body shade and half add-on and then fired to manufacturer's specifications without vacuum.

There is agreement on the basic principles of the design of the structure and the technical steps of investing, burnout, and casting of most manufacturers' gold alloys. It is also generally agreed that another fundamental requirement for successful fusion of porcelain to a cast gold alloy is the strength of the bond between the metal and porcelain, which would not separate. The nature of this bond has been the subject of much discussion. Was it a chemical or a mechanical bond? Shell and Nielsen stated that the "dental porcelain to dental gold bond, if properly made, was primarily one of interatomic bonding. The total bond had a shear resistance of about 10,000-13,000 pcs.; about one-third of this resistance appeared to be due to the van der Waals forces of wetting, and two-thirds appeared to be due to chemical bonding, perhaps a mixture of ionic, covalent, and metallic bonding. A mechanical bond did not play an important role in the bond strength proper. Roughening per se did not add to the resistance to the shear forces at the bond."[6]

SUMMARY

The use of porcelain-fused-to-metal restorations has been a valuable addition to dentistry. Superior esthetics with additional strength has been desired by the dentist for many years. Improved porcelain and metallurgical refinements will further enhance these restorative procedures.

SELECTED REFERENCES

1. Granger, E. R.: Platinum-iridium castings; a new concept of the dental casting process, J.A.D.A. **27**:1718, 1940.
2. Ney-Oro P-16, Thermalite Porcelain Manual, Hartford, Conn., 1968, The J. M. Ney Co.
3. Micro-Bond high life porcelain technic, Chicago, 1967, Austenal Co.
4. Ceramco basic porcelain manual, Woodside, N.Y., 1963, Ceramco, Inc.
5. Shillingburg, H. T., Hobo, S., and Fisher, D. W.: Preparation design and margin distortion in porcelain-fused-to-metal restorations, J. Prosthet. Dent. **29**:276-284, 1973.
6. Shell, J. S., and Nielsen, J. P.: Study of the bond between gold alloys and porcelain, J. Dent. Res. **41**:1424, 1962.

GENERAL REFERENCES

Argue, J. E.: The problem of tooth color, J.A.D.A. **24**:1341, 1937.

Baker, C. R.: A porcelain-faced crown, J. Prosthet. Dent. **18**:1-9, 1967.

Bastian, C. C.: The individual unit porcelain bridge, J.A.D.A. **29**:1369, 1942.

Bazola, F. N., and Malone, W. F.: A customized shade guide for vacuum-fired porcelain-gold combination crowns, J.A.D.A. **74**(1):114, 1967.

Bentman, D.: Avoiding the "metal-sag" with porcelain-fused-to-metal bridgework, Cereb. Palsy Rev. **1**:9-12, 1966.

Borom, M. P., and Pask, J. A.: Role of adherence oxides in the development of chemical bonding at glass-metal interfaces, J. Am. Ceram. Soc. **49**:1-6, 1966.

Brecker, S. C.: Porcelain baked to gold—a new medium in prosthodontics, J. Prosthet. Dent. **6**:801-810, 1956.

Brecker, S. C.: Improved porcelain fused to gold bridge, Dent. Clin. North Am., pp. 163-173, March 1959.

Bühlmann, H.: [Porcelain—occlusion after the wax-up technic], Zahntechnik (Zur.) **32**(3):245-257, May-June 1974.

Carlsson, B., and Lindholm, R.: [Metal-bonded porcelain—a new alternative in crown and bridge technic], Svensk Tandlak. Tidskr. **59**(6):343-349, 1966.

Clark, E. B.: An analysis of tooth color, J.A.D.A. **18**:2093, 1931.

Clark, E. B.: The color problem in dentistry, Dent. Dig. **37**:499, 1931.

Clark, E. B.: Tooth color selection, J.A.D.A. **20**:1065, 1933.

Clark, E. B.: Manipulation of dental porcelain, J.A.D.A. **22**:33, 1935.

Cohen, R.: Improved esthetics and greater strength using porcelain fused to metal crowns and bridges, N.Y. J. Dent. **30**:168, 1960.

Conod, H.: Etude sur la statique de la couronne jaquette, Rev. Mensuelle Suisse d'Odontol. **47**:485-529, 1937.

Cosgrove, D. J.: A treatment for damaged anterior teeth associated with bruxism, Aust. Dent. J. **19**(5):320-321, Oct. 1974.

Cowger, G. T., and Woycheshin, F. F.: Gold plating to enhance the appearance of porcelain-faced crowns, J. Prosthet. Dent. **11**:925, 1961.

Custer, F., Asgar, K., and Peyton, F. A.: The effect of certain variables in the bond strength of porcelain fused to gold, Int. Abstr. Dent. Res. **40**:94, 1962.

Dahl, B. L.: Some biological considerations in crown and bridge prosthetics, J. Oral Rehabil. **1**(3):245-254, July 1974.

Dérand, T.: Residual stresses in porcelain crowns, Odontol. Revy **25**(3):289-296, 1974.

Dérand, T.: Ultimate strength of porcelain crowns, Odontol. Revy **25**(4):393-402, 1974.

Dunworth, F. D.: Porcelain fused to gold, J. Prosthet. Dent. **8**:635, 1958.

Dupont, R.: Ceramo-metallic restorations, Int. Dent. J. **18**:288, 1968.

Dykema, R. W., Johnston, J. F., and Cunningham, D. M.: The veneered gold crown, Dent. Clin. North Am., pp. 653-669, Nov. 1958.

Ewing, J. E., and Bentman, D.: Porcelain-veneered full-crown restorations made with cadmium patterns, J. Prosthet. Dent. **18**:140, 1967.

Fairhurst, C. W., and Leinfelder, K. F.: Heat treating porcelain enameled restorations, J. Prosthet. Dent. **16**:554-556, 1966.

Farah, J. W., and Craig, R. G.: Distribution of stresses in porcelain-fused-to-metal and porcelain jacket crowns, J. Dent. Res. **54**(2):255-261, March-April 1975.

Gage, J. P.: Anterior porcelain crowns in general practice, Br. Dent. J. **138**(7):256-261, 1 April 1975.

Garofalo, F.: Fundamentals of creep and creep rupture in metals, Macmillan Series in Materials Science, New York, 1965, The Macmillan Co.

Gettleman, L., Freedman, G., Shaw, B., Goldin, J., and Soremark, R.: Studies on a new dental casting gold alloy, J. Dent. Res. **45**(3):595-601, 1967.

Hagen, W. H. B.: Combination gold and porcelain crown, J. Prosthet. Dent. **10**:325, 1960.

Haggard, C. B.: Clinical aspects of porcelain bonded to gold, Rev. Dent. Liban. **15**:15-19, Oct. 1965.

Hama, M., and Inaba, S.: [Studies on the baking of the mixed porcelain affixed to porcelain tooth], Odontology (Tokyo) **53**:256-261, 1965.

Harter, J.: Indication and contraindication for ceramic-metallic combinations in reconstruction unit, Rev. Franc. Odontostomat. 9:834 (corrections, p. 1151), 1962. (Fr.)

Hoffman, E. J.: How to utilize porcelain fused to gold as a crown and bridge material, Dent. Clin. North Am., pp. 57-64, 1965.

Howard, W. W.: Porcelain fused to gold for class IV inlays, J. Prosthet. Dent. 13:761, 1963.

Howell, R. A.: Gold/porcelain anterior crowns, Brit. Dent. J. 111:118, 1961.

Howell, R. A.: Gold/porcelain bridge work, Br. Dent. J. 116:80-82, 1964.

Johnston, J. F., Dykema, R. W., Mumford, G., and Phillips, R. W.: Construction and assembly of porcelain veneer gold crowns and pontics, J. Prosthet. Dent. 12:1125-1137, 1962.

Jones, D. W., and Wilson, H. J.: Porosity in dental ceramics, Br. Dent. J. 138(1):16-21, 7 Jan. 1975.

Kaaber, S.: Dental metal-ceramics: a survey of the development of the enamelling technique in dentistry, Odontol. Tidskr. 75:317-340, 1967.

Kato, Y., Ogura, H., Ishigaki, M., Wakabayashi, Y., and Kagawa, H.: [Statistical investigation of fixed partial dentures], Aichi Gakuin J. Dent. Sci. 12(1):6-17, June 1974.

King, B. W., Tripp, H. P., and Duckworth, W. H.: Nature of adherence of porcelain enamels to metals, J. Am. Ceram. Soc. 42:504-525, 1959.

Knap, F. J., and Ryge, G.: Study of bond strength of dental porcelain fused to metal, J. Dent. Res. 45:1047-1051, 1966.

Kondo, H.: [Key points in the preparation of abutment for the baked porcelain jacket crown], J. Jpn. Dent. Assoc. 27(8):793-797, 1974.

Kreutzmann, H. A.: [Shell ceramics], Zahntechnik (Berlin) 15(3):96-99, March 1974; 15(4):138-141, April 1974; 15(7):295-299, July 1974.

Kurer, P. F.: Letter: "Anterior porcelain crowns in general practice," Br. Dent. J. 138(10):381-382, 20 May 1975.

Lakermange, R., and Gonon, P.: Bridges in reinforced porcelain, J. Am. Dent. Club Paris 2:1, 1934.

Lautenschlager, E. P., Greener, E. H., and Elkington, W. E.: Microprobe analyses of gold-porcelain bonding, J. Dent. Res. 48:1206, 1969.

Lavine, M. H., and Custer, F.: Variables affecting the strength of bond between porcelain and gold, J. Dent. Res. 45:32-36, 1966.

Leibowitch, R.: Porcelain baked on precious metal alloy, Rev. Franc. Odontostomat. 9:825, 1962. (Fr.)

Leinfelder, K. F., et al.: Heat treatment of alloys to be used for the fused porcelain technique: additional data, J. Dent. Res. 43:927, 1964.

Leinfelder, K. F., Fairhurst, C. W., O'Brien, W. J., and Ryge, G.: Evolution of gases from high fusing gold alloys, J. Dent. Res. 45:1154, 1966.

Leinfelder, K. F., O'Brien, W. J., Ryge, G., and Fair-hurst, C. W.: Hardening of high fusing gold alloys, J. Dent. Res. 45:392, 1966.

Leinfelder, K. F., Servais, W. J., and O'Brien, W. J.: Mechanical properties of high-fusing gold alloys, J. Prosthet. Dent. 21:523-528, 1969.

Leone, E. F., and Fairhurst, C. W.: Bond strength and mechanical properties of dental porcelain enamels, J. Prosthet. Dent. 18:155,1967.

Lyons, D. M., Cowger, G. T., Woycheshin, F. F., and Miller, C. B.: Porcelain fused to gold—evaluation and esthetics, J. Prosthet. Dent. 10:319-324, 1960.

Marra, L. M.: An historical review of full coverage of the natural dentition, N.Y. State Dent. J. 36(3): 147-151, March 1970.

Mattox, D. M.: Influence of oxygen on adherence of gold films to oxide substrates, J. Appl. Phys. 37:3613-3615, 1966.

Meadows, T. R.: Clinical comparison of cast gold crowns with acrylic and with fused porcelain veneer facings, J.A.D.A. 66:772, 1963.

Medwedeff, F. M.: Porcelain fused to gold: fixed partial dentures, J. Prosthet. Dent. 18:46-53, 1967.

Mintz, V. W., Caputo, A. A., and Belting, C. M.: Inherent structural defects of porcelain-fused-to-gold restorations: a preliminary report, J. Prosthet. Dent. 32(5):544-550, Nov. 1974.

Moffa, J. P., and Jenkins, W. A.: Status report on base-metal crown and bridge alloys, J.A.D.A. 89(3):652-655, Sept. 1974.

Morrison, K. N., and Warnick, M. E.: Investment compounded specifically for ceramic procedures, J. Dent. Res. 38:762, 1959 (abstr.)

Morse, F. F. E.: Porcelain fused to metal; comparisons of the air-fired and vacuum-fired porcelain jacket crowns and porcelain fused to precious metal, Dent. Pract. 13:99, 1962.

Mumford, G.: The porcelain fused to metal restorations, Dent. Clin. North Am., pp. 241-249, March 1965.

Mumford, G., and Ridge, A.: Dental porcelain, Dent. Clin. North Am. 15(1):33-42, Jan. 1971.

Mylin, W. K.: Present status of porcelain fused to metal restorations, J. Kentucky Dent. Assoc. 14:152, 1962.

Nally, J. N.: Chemicophysical analysis and mechanical tests of the ceramometallic complex, Int. Dent. J. 18(2):309-325, 1968.

Nally, J. N., Meyer, J. M., and Monnier, D.: Topographic distribution of certain elements of alloy and porcelain at the level of the ceramic-metallic bond, Schweiz. Monatsschr. Zahnheilkd. 78(9): 868-878, 1968.

O'Brien, W. J.: Significant developments in dental materials, Connecticut Dent. J. 26:5, 1968.

O'Brien, W. J., Kring, J. E., and Ryge, G.: Heat treatment of alloys to be used for the fused porcelain technique, J. Prosthet. Dent. 14:955-960, 1964.

O'Brien, W. J., and Ryge, G.: Relation between molecular force calculations and observed strength of enamel-metal interfaces, J. Am. Ceram. Soc. **47**:5-8, 1964.

Pop-Nikolov, D.: [Elaboration of an exact porcelain jacket crown and our first clinical experiences], Vojnosanit. Pregl. **31**(4):256-258, July-Aug. 1974 (with Engl. abstr.).

Pruden, H. H.: Solder connections with porcelain fused to gold, J. Prosthet. Dent. **22**:679, 1969.

Ryge, G.: Current American research on porcelain-fused-to-metal restorations, Int. Dent. J. **15**:385-392, 1965.

Schiffer, R.: Soldering technique for high-fusing gold in the porcelain, J. Prosthet. Dent. **22**:4, 1969.

Schmeissner, H.: [The prosthetic therapy of deeply fractured teeth], Dtsch. Zahnaerztl. Z. **29**(9):815-818, Sept. 1974.

Schnell, R. J., Mumford, G., and Phillips, R. W.: An evaluation of phosphate bonded investments used with a high fusing gold alloy, J. Prosthet. Dent. **13**:324, 1963.

Semmelman, J. O.: Fusion of porcelain to metal, Conference for Teachers of Dental Materials, Dec. 1961.

Serova, G. A., Inozemtseva, A. A., and Bikbau, N. S.: [Structure and optic properties of dental porcelain], Stomatologiia (Moskva) **54**(1):48-51, Jan.-Feb. 1975.

Shelby, D. S.: Practical considerations and design of porcelain fused to metal, J. Prosthet. Dent. **12**:542, 1962.

Shell, J. S., and Nielsen, J. P.: Study of the bond between gold alloys and porcelain, J. Dent. Res. **41**:1424, 1962.

Shell, J. S., and Nielsen, J. P.: The strength and nature of the porcelain-to-gold bond. Paper presented before the Dental Materials Group of the International Association for Dental Research Meeting, St. Louis, March 1962.

Sherring-Lucas, G. M.: Bonded porcelain to gold; Degudent-Swiss Vita VMK technique, Dent. Techn. **19**(11):98-103, 1966.

Silver, M., and Klein, G.: Precision attachments in conjunction with cast platinum-porcelain restorations, Dent. Dig. **62**:296, 1956.

Silver, M., Klein, G., and Howard, M. C.: Platinum-

porcelain restorations, J. Prosthet. Dent. **6**:695, 1956.

Silver, M., Howard, M. C., and Klein, G.: Porcelain bonded to a cast metal understructure, J. Prosthet. Dent. **11**:132, 1961.

Silver, M., Klein, G., and Howard, M. C.: An evaluation and comparison of porcelains fused to cast metals, J. Prosthet. Dent. **10**:1055-1064, 1960.

Smith, B. B.: Considerations in the current use of porcelain to gold, Int. Dent. J. **18**:280, 1968.

Straussberg, G., Katz, G., and Kuwata, M.: Design of gold supporting structures for fused porcelain restorations, J. Prosthet. Dent. **16**(5):928-936, 1966.

Suzuki, S.: [Dynamic studies on porcelain fused to gold crown of upper central incisor with three-dimensional photoelastic experiments] (author's transl.), Odontology (Tokyo) **62**(4):585-624, Oct. 1974.

Swartz, M. L., and Phillips, R. W.: A study of adaptation of veneers to cast gold crowns, J. Prosthet. Dent. **7**:817, 1957.

Toreskog, S.: Metal-bound porcelain—an addition to crown and bridge prosthetics, Sverige Tandlakarforb. Tidn. **59**(11):495-499, 1967.

Tuccillo, J. J., and Nielsen, J. P.: Creep and sag properties of a porcelain-gold alloy, J. Dent. Res. **46**(3):579-583, 1967.

Vickery, R. C., and Badinelli, L. A.: Nature of attachment forces in porcelain-gold systems, J. Dent. Res. **47**:683-689, Sept.-Oct. 1968.

Vining, R., and Lust, J.: Micro-Bond presentation: symposium on trends in dental laboratory activities, Walter Reed Hospital, Washington, D. C., 1963.

Warnick, M. E.: Use of porcelain-fused-to-gold in the restoration of fractured young permanent anterior teeth, J. Dent. Child. **29**:3, 1962.

Weinberg, L. A.: A new design for porcelain-fused-to-metal prostheses, J. Prosthet. Dent. **17**(2):178-194, 1967.

Wenzel, W.: [Use of Felserit as a dental model in ceramics], Zahntechnik (Berlin) **15**(2):56-57, Feb. 1974.

Woolson, A. H.: Restorations made of porcelain baked on gold, J. Prosthet. Dent. **5**:65, 1955.

Yamada, S.: Metal-cast dental porcelain, J. Jpn. Dent. Assoc. **19**:111, 1966.

27

Use of acrylic resins in crowns and fixed partial dentures; early use of synthetic resins

Alfred C. Long, William F. P. Malone, and Stanley D. Tylman

The use of synthetic resins in dentistry is not new, but their application to the construction of crowns and bridges is of comparatively recent date. A search of the dental literature, however, discloses that as early as 1938 an article by Selbach[1] was published in which construction of crowns made of synthetic resins is described. The resins employed were made available in four colors—yellow, white, light gray, and dark gray.

EARLY USE OF SYNTHETIC RESINS FOR CROWNS

Synthetic resins for crowns were first demonstrated and used in this country in May 1940, by Wilson.[2] A search of the dental literature discloses an article by Weder,[3] published in Europe in January 1940, describing and illustrating in detail the use of a synthetic resinous plastic material for the construction of individual crowns.

Because the early resins used for this purpose were not suitable nor specifically designed for use in small dental restorations, the results were not entirely satisfactory. Also, many failures were attributable to the fact that the polymer particles that were used in crowns and fixed partial dentures were of too large a mesh, resulting in a product that was coarse and granular in appearance. Dur-

ing the intervening years, manufacturers have developed acrylic resins specially suited for making small restorations.

Not only has a fineness of particle size been developed but also hues have been made available that make it possible for the dentist to match the color of the natural teeth with the same degree of exactness as it is possible to do with the fired porcelain restorations.

Since the acrylic veneer crown has become generally used, it is well at this time to consider the factors that are essential to the successful use of this material. The acrylic resins are not a panacea—they have their limitations as well as their advantages. The acrylic resin crown is not intended to supplant the glazed porcelain-veneer crown, but it should be used where indicated and not where contraindicated.

TYPES OF SYNTHETIC RESINS

The dental synthetic resins fall into one of the following types: phenolic, urea, polystyrene, cellulose, vinyl, the methyl methacrylates, and many types of copolymers. These resins and their copolymers appear to be well suited for the smaller types of restorations.

The methyl methacrylate synthetic resins belong to the thermal plastic group as distinguished from those that are thermal setting, such as the phenol formaldehyde types. There is also the autopolymerizing or self-curing group.

DESIRABLE PHYSICAL PROPERTIES OF RESINS

A synthetic resin, to be suitable for dental purposes, should have (1) toughness (impact strength), (2) flexural strength, (3) tensile strength, (4) permanency, (5) a low cold flow, (6) high resistance to water and solvents, (7) a minimum of dimensional change, (8) high relative hardness, (9) moldability, and, finally, (10) adaptability to a simple technique employing inexpensive equipment. Although there is no single type of synthetic resin that possesses all these desirable qualities to the optimal degree, the acrylic resins possess these qualities to a degree to make them the material of choice for many dental purposes.

MONOMER AND POLYMER

The acrylic resins for crowns and bridges are generally available in the powder and liquid form. The powder, or polymer, is the polymerized form of the liquid monomer. In use, the powder and liquid are mixed in the approximate proportions of 3 to 1 by volume, or 65 to 35 parts by weight, polymer to monomer. This mixture, when permitted to stand in a closed jar, gradually changes to a doughy consistency. The change or the process by which the liquid monomer is converted into the solid polymer is known as polymerization, which is hastened by the application of heat, ultraviolet light, or oxidizing agents. The method that employs heat is generally used by dentists in the processing or polymerization of the resin. In a mixture of monomer and polymer, it is important that not too much of the liquid monomer be used, but only enough so that all the polymer particles are wetted. The greater the amount of monomer used, the greater will be the total shrinkage of the object

molded; in fact, if monomer alone were used, the volumetric shrinkage of an object would be approximately 21%. Moreover, since the monomer is a clear liquid, it polymerizes into a clear, transparent polymer; hence, excessive use of the monomer may modify the color of the processed resin.

The physical properties of acrylic resin, which are of special interest to the dentist, relate to (1) dimensional changes, (2) water imbibition or adsorption, (3) color permanency, (4) flexural strength, (5) relative hardness, and (6) cold flow.

Methods of mixing monomer and polymer

Several methods can be used to mix the monomer and the polymer and place the mixture in the mold or tooth.

First method. In the first method, the one most generally used for small restoration, the liquid and the powder in proper proportions are placed in a jar and thoroughly mixed for several minutes with a glass rod. The cover is then screwed tightly on the jar, where the mixture is permitted to remain for a given length of time, whereupon it reaches a soft, doughlike consistency. In this state, it is suitable for packing in the mold. If a sufficient amount of the monomer has been used, the surface of every particle of the polymer has been penetrated by the monomer. The depth of penetration or dispersion of the monomer in the polymer depends on both the amount of liquid used and the time allowed for its penetration into the particles. When packed in a mold and subjected to heat and pressure, the monomer polymerizes and the entire mixture then becomes one solid mass. If an insufficient amount of monomer is used, and if insufficient pressure and heat are applied, it is probable that some of the polymer particles will not be molecularly welded into one solid piece. Hence, care must be exercised that (1) the proper proportions of powder and liquid are used, (2) a sufficient length of time be allowed for the polymer particles to be thoroughly wetted, and (3) the mass be mixed thoroughly, so that a uniform distribution of the coloring ingredients shall be obtained and all the gross and microscopic air spaces be eliminated within the mass.

Second method. There is a second method of mixing monomer and polymer for the construction of crowns and bridges. In this method, a small amount of the powder is first placed on a glass slab. To this, monomer is added drop by drop from a medicine dropper in an amount sufficient to saturate the polymer. The saturated mass, which has a granular appearance, is immediately taken up with the tip of a spatula, and placed in the mold. While in this granular state, the mass is vibrated and settled into place. More is added until the crown or bridge is filled to its proper form. When two or more colors are employed, a separate pile is made of each powder, saturated with monomer, and each applied where indicated.

If there is an excess of the liquid, it may be absorbed by the addition of dry powder to the small pile. Although this method seems to have certain advantages, it cannot be used with all the acrylics on the market today. It is primarily intended for those acrylic powders, the grain size of which is 100 mesh or finer. This method is not suitable for the powders that are coarser, because the finished prosthesis would have a definite granular appearance.

Third method. The third method of mixing monomer and polymer may be called the "dry-pack technique." The polymer is sprinkled dry into the crown mold. First the gingival color is applied and then the incisal, also in dry powder form. When a sufficient amount has been used to develop the contour of the restoration, monomer is added drop by drop from a medicine dropper, until the mass is sat-

urated. The metal flask containing the mold is now vibrated or tapped on the workbench, so that the moistened particles of the mass gravitate to the deepest portions of the mold. Sufficient monomer is added to slightly oversaturate the mass. The excess liquid is absorbed by sprinkling on additional dry powder. This process of alternately adding powder and liquid is continued until the proper contour is developed. Here again there exists the danger that the coloring ingredients settle to the lower portion of the mold, resulting in poor color distribution.

Fourth method. A fourth method, sometimes used to veneer cast metal crowns, combines the polymer moistened with a special monomer and applied in small increments to the metal (Pyroplast). It is cured directly, exposed to 275° F for 8 minutes after each laminated application. The metal is first covered with an opaque layer and cured for 8 minutes. Then the gingival and the incisal colors are applied and blended, followed by curing each lamination. A special type of curing oven is used, which controls the desired temperature and correct distance at which the restoration is maintained. When fully processed, the veneer is finished and polished. The popularity of this approach has increased greatly in the past decade.

Closure of flask

After the mold has been filled or, better still, slightly overfilled by one of the first three methods just described, a piece of moistened cellophane is placed over the lower half of the flask, covering the exposed acrylic resin. Trial closure is made. On separating the two halves of the flask, more material is added if needed. Then another trial closure is made, but at no time during the trial are the two halves of the flask brought into complete contact; a space of 1 mm is maintained by means of shims, which are removed at the time that final closure of the flask is made before processing. Thereafter, the case may

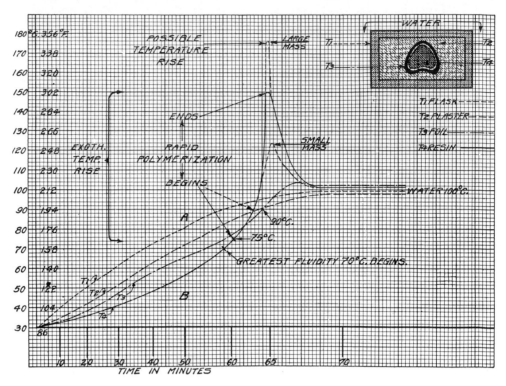

Fig. 27-1. Time-temperature chart explaining certain phenomena in high-heat method of polymerizing methyl methacrylate resin.

be processed by either the slowly rising high-heat technique or the constant low-heat technique. The following discussion does not apply to the autopolymerizing type of resins.

METHODS OF PROCESSING
High-heat method of processing

First, the high-heat or boiling water method will be considered. Certain phenomena have been observed during the processing of the acrylic resins, particularly during the time that polymerization takes place. A study of the chart in Fig. 27-1 will help to explain them. This chart indicates the use of boiling water for the processing. It is apparent that there exists a definite time-temperature relationship in this procedure. Since resins react quickly to higher temperatures, it is advisable to start the processing of the

crown or bridge at a relatively low temperature. The temperature reading on this chart begins at 30° C (86° F).

When the water has reached this temperature, the two halves of the flask are placed in a press and closed to within 1 mm of complete closure. The flask held within the press is now submerged in the water, and heat is applied gradually so that there is an approximate temperature rise of 1° C (1.8° F) per minute. The dotted line A, also designated by *T1*, indicates the temperature of the water bath.

Processing temperature curves. Note that in 10 minutes the temperature of the water will be 40° C (104° F); in 20 minutes, 50° C (122° F); and so on. This is continued until the boiling point of water is reached, 100° C (212° F). Note that the broken line *T1*, representing the temperature rise of the water and the flask, continues in a curved line, rising in proportion to the increase in temperature and lapse of time.

Immediately below is the line designated as *T2*, representing the plaster investment material enclosed within the metal flask. This line also has a relatively proportional rise, but there is an initial lag because the investment is a relatively poor conductor of heat as compared to the metal flask, and, also, the investment is not in direct contact with the surrounding water.

The bottom, solid line, *T4*, represents the resin enclosed within the tin-foiled, plaster-filled flask. It is observed that while the temperature of the resin mass also rises in proportion to the other curves during the first 40 or 50 minutes, there is a considerable initial lag in its relation to line *T1*, the temperature of the water.

In approximately 60 minutes, the temperature of the resin has risen to 70° C (158° F). This is the starting point of its greatest fluidity range, which extends approximately to 90° C (194° F). More will be said later regarding this fluidity range. Possibly a better term to explain the condition of the mass would be "plasticity," since the mixture does not revert to a fluid but merely becomes a softer mass.

Exothermic reaction—heat of reaction. During the next few minutes an interesting phenomenon manifests itself. Between 70° and 75° C (158° and 168° F), the resin temperature curve *T4* takes a sharp upturn, indicating an increase in temperature which is not caused by externally transmitted heat. During the next few minutes, this temperature rise is very rapid, reaching its maximum at approximately 150° C (302° F). From this point it drops rapidly, and shortly the resin reaches the water temperature level of 100° C (212° F). This heat of reaction, also referred to as exothermic temperature rise, takes place during the time when the greatest amount and the most rapid polymerization occurs. According

to Harold Vernon and to Willard Bartoe, chief physicist of Rhom and Haas Company, who assisted in the preparation of this chart, approximately 95% of the polymerization occurs during this short interval of time. As the volume of the polymerized mass is increased, the peak of the exothermic curve may rise to 175° C (379° F), or higher.

Where tinfoil is used as a lining agent in the mold, the line *T3* indicates the temperature of the tinfoil. It will be observed that where the acrylic line *T4* bends upward, it crosses *T3* at about 80° C (176° F). This causes the higher temperature of the acrylic resin to raise the temperature of the tinfoil above 100° C (212° F), but only for a short time, for it quickly returns to the boiling point of water at the same time that the polymerized acrylic does. One may determine the temperature of the flask, investment, foil, and acrylic resin, at any given point, on the chart by dropping a vertical line. Such a line *A-B* at the 50-minute point indicates that when the flask is 80° C (176° F), the investment is 72° C (161° F), the tin foil 66° C (150° F), and the acrylic resin 56° C (132° F).

The data shown in the chart prompt the question, "When does polymerization begin and when is it completed?" It is known that only a slight degree of polymerization occurs before 75° C (167° F) is reached. At 75° C (167° F) polymerization develops rapidly, and in approximately 10 minutes, 95% of it is completed. The total time elapsed from room temperature, 30° C (86° F), to this stage of polymerization is approximately 70 minutes. For safety's sake, it is recommended that an additional 30 to 60 minutes be allowed in boiling water to complete the polymerization, depending on the volume of resin in the mold.

When to close flask. The question may be raised, "Is complete closure of the two halves of the flask advisable before heat is applied; if not, what is the temperature

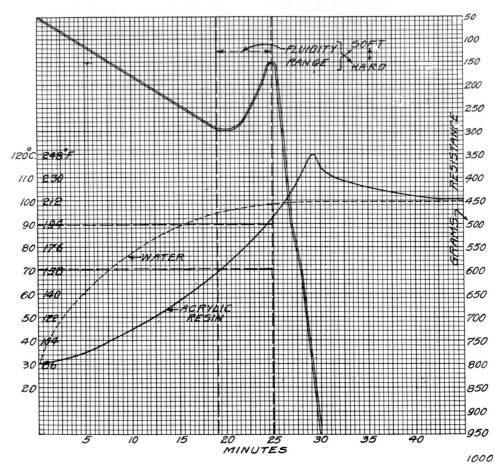

Fig. 27-2. Chart indicates why complete closure of flask should be made during certain temperature ranges.

best suited for complete closure of the flask?" It is known that a thermal expansion of the acrylic resin occurs in the range extending from the initial temperature of 30° C (86° F), to 70° C (158° F) and also that an excess of material in the mold is recommended during this time-temperature interval. The complete closure of the flask should be made when the acrylic material is between 70° and 90° C (158° to 194° F), when the acrylic mass assumes its greatest state of plasticity. It is preferable to make the closure nearer 70° C (158° F) rather than the 90° C (194° F) temperature.

Plasticity curve. The chart in Fig. 27-2

shows the plasticity curve of the acrylic material during processing. It indicates in grams the resistance of the material to displacement under a load. Of the two lower curves, commencing at 30° C (86° F), the bottom dotted-line curve represents the reaction of the acrylic resin, and the middle broken-line curve represents the temperature rise of the heating medium, water. The upper double-line curve indicates the increased resistance of the acrylic material to displacement as the temperature of the acrylic resin is raised. This increase in resistance to displacement is characterized first by a gradual hardening of the mass, in this instance during the first 20 minutes or until the acrylic resin reaches the threshold of the plasticity range at a temperate of 70° C (158° F).

Note that, at this point, the downward path of the curve stops at a resistance of 300 grams and then reverses itself during the next 8 minutes, indicating a reduced resistance to displacement, or a gradual softening of the acrylic material until it reaches 90° C (194° F), or a point of resistance of 150 grams. The curve then drops sharply so that within 5 minutes it reaches a resistance of nearly 1,000 grams. Notice that this approaches the crest of the exothermic curve; this may help to explain why complete closure of the flask is recommended during the short interval of time when the temperature of the acrylic material lies in the 70° to 90° C (158° to 194° F) range.

Elastic memory—skeletal molecular framework. During range of greatest plasticity and period of polymerization, a skeletal framework of molecules, or so-called elastic memory, is created; this is determined by the shape of the mold in which the restoration is processed. This skeletal molecular structure is permanent and is characteristic of each individual restoration. Any effort or technique that subsequently disturbs or displaces this molecular structure will set up internal stresses, which ultimately result in a distortion and misfit of the appliance, because the stressed molecular structure is constantly striving to resume its normal, original form.

Linear shrinkage of acrylic resin. It is impossible to eliminate entirely the shrinkage that occurs during the processing of acrylic resins. Linear shrinkage may vary from 0.47% to 0.56%, or an average of 0.53%, as shown by Sweeney,[4] at the Bureau of Standards. The use of the injector type of flask to force additional material into the hot mold while the enclosed polymerized resin is still soft, in an effort to eliminate this shrinkage, introduces stresses within the prosthesis. Shrinkage occurs only after polymerization of the resin has taken place; hence, any displacement of the polymerized resin by a forcing of additional material into the mold will result in setting up stresses. These are later released at mouth temperature resulting in a variation in the fit of the prosthesis.

When shrinkage occurs, it is not uniform throughout the molded object, because of variations in its size, shape, and cross-section areas.

Porosity. One of the annoying problems associated with acrylic resins is that of porosity. Porosity usually occurs in thick specimens containing a large volume of material, but it is sometimes a defect present in the less bulky restorations also.

As shown in the time-temperature curve (Fig. 27-1), when the acrylic resins reach the 70° to 90° C (158° to 194° F) range, the temperature rises precipitously within a short period of time, that is, in a few minutes. When a large amount of acrylic resin is involved, polymerization, even though rapid, starts from the outer surface and progresses inwardly. When the temperature on the outer surface exceeds 100.3° C and some free monomer remains within the center of the mass, it is possible for the monomer to be volatilized, and the gas so formed is trapped within the polemized mass. It has been found that as the volume of the acrylic resin increases, the time of processing should be lengthened and continued at a lower temperature.

During the initial stages of polymerization, or before complete dispersion of the monomer and polymer has taken place, high temperatures may also cause the monomer to be volatilized and produce bubbles.

To control and reduce the excessive exothermic rise during the polymerization of acrylic resins, several time-temperature schedules have been recommended.

Low-heat method of processing

A second method of processing has been suggested, in which the temperature of the water is brought to 160° to 165° F and kept at this temperature range for a relatively long period of time. Recommendations* that offer three possible methods have been made[5]:

Method 1. (1) Immerse flask in room temperature water. (2) Adjust heat so that water will boil in from 1 to 3 hours (depending on the bulk of resin). (3) Boil 15 minutes.

Method 2. (1) Immerse flask in water at 160° F, and hold at constant temperature for 1½ hours. (2) Increase to boiling temperature and boil 30 minutes.

Method 3. (1) Immerse flask in water at 160° F constant temperature. (2) Hold for 9 hours.

By the low, constant temperature method, polymerization occurs and the exothermic curve is flattened out; thus the possibility of gas and bubble formation is reduced.

Autopolymerization method (self-curing)

The autopolymerizing or self-curing types of resins that have been developed do not depend on heat to initiate the process of their polymerization. Extensive research has been done to determine the best methods for their use and also to compare their physical properties with those processed by methods employing heat.

This method, used more in operative than in prosthetic dentistry, is the brush technique.[6,7] The method is sometimes used to replace broken facings when it is impossible to do so with porcelain. To employ this method, self-curing resin powder and monomer are placed in separate dappen dishes. A fine-pointed camel's or sable's hair brush is moistened in the monomer and then touched to the

*Developed by Harold Vernon, Vernon-Benshoff Co., Inc., Albany, N.Y.

dry powder. By capillary attraction a bead of wet powder attaches itself to the brush tip. This is then carried to the cavity and placed where desired. After 20 to 30 seconds when initial set has occurred, another bead is added. This procedure is continued until the mass is built up to the desired contour, whereupon it is covered with cocoa butter and permitted to polymerize for 15 to 20 minutes. At the expiration of this time it is trimmed to final contour with special burs and discs, after which it is ready for its final polish then, or at a later sitting.

This type of resin is self-curing and is activated by a catalyst to induce polymerization. The catalysts are of the benzoyl peroxide or of the paratoluene sulfinic acid types.

DISADVANTAGES OF POROSITY

Porosity has several definite disadvantages. (1) It weakens the structure in its resistance to forces. (2) The tiny bubbles produce a dispersion of light, which changes or modifies the color of the acrylic resin material. In clear acrylic material, this produces a milky or cloudy appearance in the finished prosthesis similar to that caused by exposure of the resin to water during processing. (3) The pores offer lodging places for bacteria and debris. (4) Pores are irritating to soft tissues.

DIMENSIONAL CHANGES CAUSED BY MOISTURE

When an acrylic appliance has been processed, there is still further opportunity for dimensional change after it is placed in the mouth. Although some acrylic resins have a water absorption factor of less than 0.5% by weight, others, on immersion in water, may show an absorption of almost 3%. The amount of water that an acrylic resin absorbs is quite important clinically. The work done at the Bureau of Standards[4] (Fig. 27-3) shows that acrylic-resin dentures stabilized at a

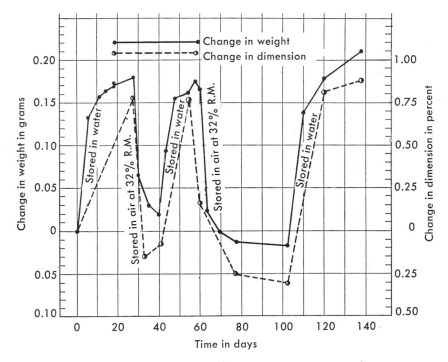

Fig. 27-3. Effect of water on acrylic resin denture at 37° C. (Courtesy U. S. Bureau of Standards; from Sweeney, W. T.: J.A.D.A. **26:**1963, 1939.)

constant relative humidity of 32% when placed in water, expanded approximately 0.8% within a period of 27 days. It was further noted that acrylic dentures that expanded on immersion in water shrank when they were removed and exposed to the air to dry, and frequently shrank to less than their original dimensions. Slight dimensional changes occurring in complete dentures may be tolerated and compensated for by the resilient mucosa. They do not present the same degree of difficulties and dangers present in complete veneer crowns when the prostheses are in direct contact with hard and unyielding tooth tissue. Even a small fractional dimensional change of a cemented crown, from a dry to a saturated condition, may be sufficient to cause the failure of the restoration at the marginal cement joint. This reaction of the resin to moisture suggests that crowns made of acrylic resins should be immersed in water until they reach "saturation expansion," after

which they are dried before being cemented.

No doubt a technique may be developed wherein the shrinkage incident to the processing of the material can be balanced by the subsequent expansion from water absorption together with the use of a stone die material having a sufficient hygroscopic expansion.

BIOLOGIC COMPATIBILITY OF ACRYLIC RESINS

Clinically, the acrylic restorations have proved themselves to be biologically compatible if the tooth has been properly prepared and if the restoration itself conforms to the same physiologic and mechanical requirement of the standard types of gold and porcelain restorations. Apparently, the absorption of water by the acrylic material does not react harmfully on the contiguous soft tissues. One of the objectionable features noted is a slight tendency of the material to become stained. This, however, may be the result of improper oral hygiene.

The acrylic resins are not resistant to abrasion when they are opposed by ground porcelain surfaces or by natural teeth whose surfaces are not smooth and rounded. Our observation has been that an acrylic tooth in contact with another acrylic prosthesis, in the presence of saliva, does not undergo any mechanical abrasion but it does flow.

COLD FLOW OF RESINS

The behavior of an acrylic resin in the mouth and under applied force has a decided influence upon its application and upon the design of the prosthesis in which it is used. The suitability of the acrylic resin for use in crowns and bridges has been questioned on the basis of its hardness, that is, whether there is sufficient resistance of the material to penetration, abrasion, or cold flow.

The work of Peyton and Mann[8] indicated that even though an elastic recovery occurs after the removal of the load from the resin, this recovery is not complete, inasmuch as a permanent distortion remains. This finding of Peyton is based upon the application of a static load of 3,550 pounds per square inch for 7 days continuously. It would be interesting to know what, if any, would be the permanent distortion of this material if loads comparable to the forces of occlusion were applied intermittently over a similar period of time. The question is raised whether such permanent deformation is cumulative under these conditions.

Clinical experience indicates that the acrylic resins possess the necessary toughness or resistance to impact force, provided that there exists a sufficient bulk of material and that no shearing planes are effective.

No attempt is made here to discuss the chemistry or detailed physical properties of the various types of synthetic resins, since this information may be found in texts on this subject.[9] One must remember that the profession is dealing with a comparatively new material applied to new uses. That the synthetic resins have their limitations is readily admitted by those studying their physical properties and clinical applications. The correct approach is not an effort to replace all other dental materials with it, but to determine by scientific study and clinical observation its rightful uses and limitations in dental practice.

INDICATIONS FOR ACRYLIC CROWNS

One of the prime indications for the use of the acrylic-veneer crown is in very young patients.[9] There are instances, for example, in which the upper anterior central incisor has been fractured, or in which proximal decay has reached a point requiring the placement of a complete coronal restoration. In such patients the pulp chamber is usually large and the pulp would be endangered if a typical shoulder type of preparation were made for such a young patient in order to place a fired porcelain-veneer crown. It is much better in such circumstances to use an acrylic-veneer crown, which does not require the removal of all the enamel nor the preparation of a gingival shoulder in the dentin. An acrylic crown would in this instance be the restoration of choice.

Occasionally, it is found that in closebite patients the acrylic-veneer is preferable to the porcelain-veneer crown. In those mouths in which the teeth are of the opalescent dentin type, the so-called dentinogenesis imperfecta, it has been found that the acrylic-veneer crown has served much better than the glazed porcelain type.

Where the bonded, porcelain-veneer crown has failed over a cast gold core in combination with a bridge, it has been found that the acrylic type is less likely to fracture than one made of porcelain.

The second indication for acrylic resins in crowns is found in their use as a veneer for the cast gold crown. This type of veneer crown may be used in individual restorations or in crowns used as bridge retainers. Although the ground-in porcelain-facing type of crown may be used in most cases, there are times when the acrylic veneer possesses certain advantages over the fired porcelain veneer. Experience has shown that should a patient wear through the gold incisal protection, a porcelain veneer will snap out of the casting, whereas one made of acrylic veneer is elastic and flows under stress and will not break out of the casting. There are other conditions of unusual contour or occlusal relationship that have been more effectively met by the use of acrylic rather than glazed porcelain crowns.

Because the acrylic resins have a greater resilience than glazed porcelain, it is found that they are better able to absorb shock; for this reason acrylic crowns can be used successfully in very thin layers where porcelain could not be used (for example, in some adolescents). Consequently, in those instances in which a temporary protection is desired for the tooth of a child and a shoulderless type of crown is indicated, it should be made of acrylic resin rather than of glazed porcelain.

Where temporary, corrective, or esthetic veneers are desired for public entertainers, these also may be made of synthetic resins.

ACRYLIC RESIN VENEER CROWNS: EFFECT OF TOOTH PREPARATION ON CROWN FABRICATION AND FUTURE PERIODONTAL HEALTH*

Acrylic resin veneers (or any of the tooth-colored veneering materials) are placed on cast metal crowns for esthetic purposes only. Many veneered crowns that meet the requirements of fit and oc-

---

*Summary by Alfred C. Long, Professor of Dentistry, The Ohio State University College of Dentistry.

clusion fail as restorations because they are not acceptable to the periodontium. They are not acceptable because they are oversized and improperly contoured, particularly on the veneered surface. As a general rule, unless the tooth is malposed, periodontally involved, or in contact with the clasp of a removable partial denture, the closer a veneered metal crown duplicates the size and shape of the original tooth, the more acceptable it is to the periodontium. Improper tooth selection and inadequate reduction of the tooth surfaces to be veneered seem the most likely causes of oversized and overcontoured veneered metal crowns. All veneering materials require a certain thickness to esthetically mask the underlying metal, and the space for whatever thickness is necessary must be obtained during tooth preparation if overcontouring the veneer is to be avoided. Although any tooth can be reduced enough to assure the necessary space, not all teeth can be successfully reduced because the end result with some teeth will be permanent pulp damage or exposure or insufficient tooth structure remaining to support the restoration. Therefore, not all teeth are suitable or can be successfully prepared for veneered crowns.[10]

To ensure adequate space for acrylic resin veneers on teeth that can be successfully reduced, two areas are most critical during tooth reduction; both are on the veneered surface or surfaces. First is the cervical finishing line, which must be a shoulder *at least* 0.8 mm wide if the veneer is to extend apically to the free margin of the gingival tissues and also be thick enough in that area to mask the underlying metal without overcontouring (Figs. 27-4 to 27-6). If a wider shoulder can be successfully prepared, by all means do so. The shoulder must also extend onto the proximal surfaces if the veneer is to extend on to these surfaces (Figs. 27-7 to 27-9). The second critical area is the incisal or occlusal third of the

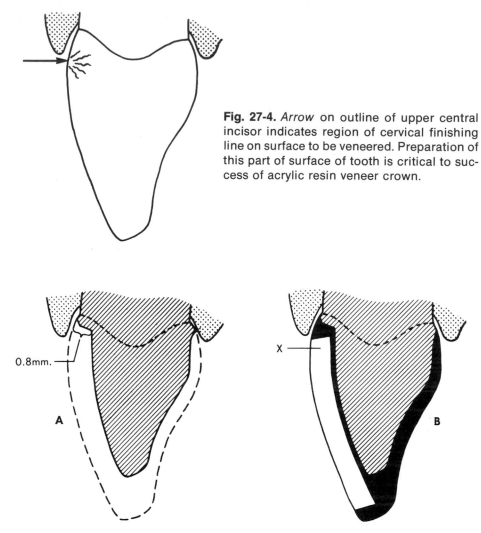

Fig. 27-4. *Arrow* on outline of upper central incisor indicates region of cervical finishing line on surface to be veneered. Preparation of this part of surface of tooth is critical to success of acrylic resin veneer crown.

0.8mm.

A

X

B

Fig. 27-5. Properly prepared tooth. **A,** *Dotted line,* Contour of original tooth. Cervical finishing line on surfaces to be veneered must be a shoulder, at least 0.8 mm wide. **B,** Acrylic resin veneer crown on tooth; 0.8 mm shoulder permits acrylic resin veneer to extend apically to free margin of gingival tissues and to be thick enough at X to effectively mask underlying metal without being overcontoured.

veneered surface. Most surfaces to be veneered have some vertical convexity and should have a similar convexity after preparation if the veneer is to have adequate thickness in these areas while the original tooth size and shape in the restoration are being duplicated (Figs. 29-2, 29-3, 27-10, and 27-11). Too often, the prepared tooth surface from the shoulder to the incisal or occlusal is flat, whereas the original surface had some convexity. This practice usually results in inadequate veneer thickness at the incisal or occlusal third of the veneer (Figs. 27-12 and 27-13). When preparing posterior teeth, one can use the intercuspal distance as a guide (Fig. 27-14). After preparation the distance between corres-

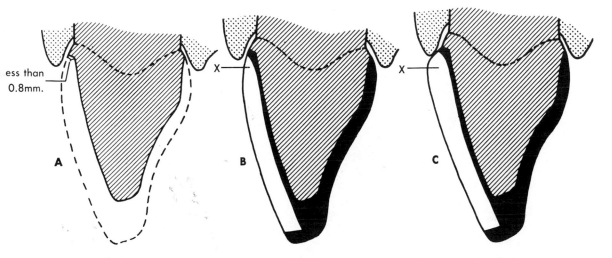

Fig. 27-6. Improperly prepared tooth. **A,** Cervical shoulder on this preparation is less than 0.8 mm wide. **B,** Inadequate shoulder width permits acrylic resin veneer to extend apically to free margin of gingival tissues, but veneer is too thin at X to effectively mask underlying metal. **C,** Veneer on this crown is overcontoured at X to mask metal. Resultant restoration does not duplicate size and shape of original tooth, as shown by *dotted line* in **A.**

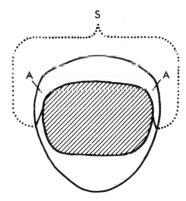

Fig. 27-7. Cross section through improperly prepared central incisor shown at level of proximal shoulder, *S.* Shoulder narrows or disappears as it approaches and extends onto proximal surfaces, *A.*

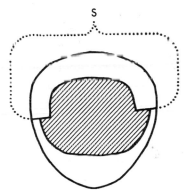

Fig. 27-8. Cross section through properly prepared central incisor shown at level of proximal shoulder, *S.* Entire shoulder must have adequate width to ensure veneer thickness.

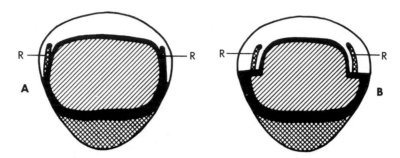

Fig. 27-9. Cross sections through two prepared upper central incisors and their acrylic resin veneered crowns shown at level of retentive loops, *R.* **A,** Inadequate proximal shoulder preparation has made proper positioning of retentive loops impossible. It is unlikely that loops in this position give adequate retention to veneer, and it is likely that veneer will not effectively mask them. **B,** Adequate proximal shoulder preparation permits proper positioning of retentive loops, *R.*

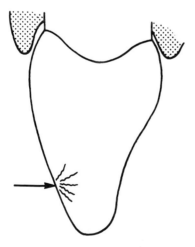

Fig. 27-10. *Arrow* indicates other critical part of preparation of labial surface of tooth to be veneered. Adequate tooth reduction in incisal third of labial surface is vital to success of acrylic resin veneer crown.

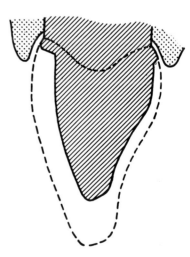

Fig. 27-11. Properly prepared tooth. Natural undercuts must be removed during preparation, but original tooth form or convexity, *dotted line*, is simulated in contour of preparation.

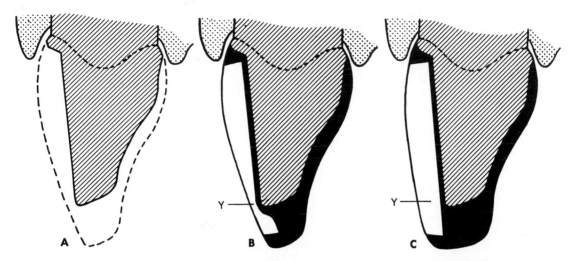

Fig. 27-12. Effect of inadequate preparation. **A,** Labial surface of preparation is too straight from shoulder to incisal edge. Adequate cervical shoulder has been prepared, but labial surface does not simulate form of original tooth. **B,** This error in preparation results in veneer being too thin at *Y* to effectively mask underlying metal. **C,** Alternative is overcontouring of veneer at *Y*. Resultant restoration does not duplicate size and shape of original tooth.

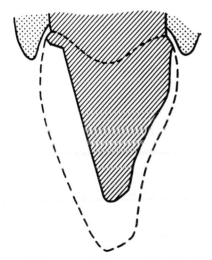

Fig. 27-13. Improperly prepared tooth. Flat labial surface in this preparation poses no problem in obtaining adequate veneer thickness at any point, but overreduction of middle and cervical thirds has weakened retention and resistance form and may have injured or exposed pulp.

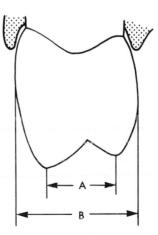

Fig. 27-14. Distance between cusp tips is less than overall width of posterior teeth. *A,* Buccolingual intercuspal measurement; *B,* greatest buccolingual crown measurement. *A* is one half to two thirds of *B* on approximately 80% of all posterior teeth.

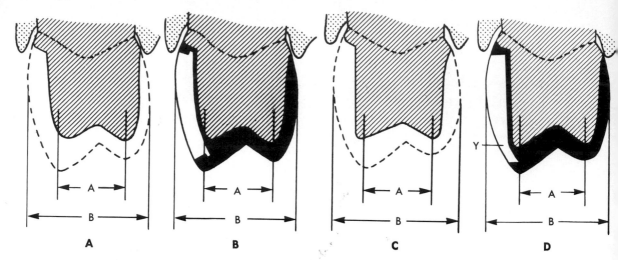

A   B   C   D

Fig. 27-15. Comparison of effects of properly and improperly prepared teeth. **A,** Properly prepared tooth (*A,* original buccolingual intercuspal distance; *B,* greatest original buccolingual crown width). Note that curvature of surface to be veneered closely follows original curvature of tooth *(dotted line),* and that intercuspal measurement of preparation is less than intercuspal measurement before preparation at *A.* **B,** Properly prepared tooth is covered by acrylic resin veneer crown that has adequate veneer thickness throughout. Note that dimensions at *A* and *B* have been duplicated in restoration. **C,** Improperly prepared tooth. Note that surface to be veneered is flat and that intercuspal measurment on preparation is greater than it was originally at *A.* **D,** Improperly prepared tooth is covered by acrylic resin veneer crown that does not have adequate veneer thickness at *Y,* because distances (*A* and *B*) are duplicated in restoration.

ponding buccal and lingual cusps should be the same as or less than it was before preparation (Figs. 27-15 and 27-16).

The principles of tooth preparation for clasped veneered crowns are the same as for crowns that are not to be clasped. However, it is necessary to remember that the shape and size of a crown to be clasped usually differ to some degree from those of the original tooth. The difference and the degree are determined by the design of the removable partial denture and by its path of insertion (Fig. 27-17). Only when these factors become known, after a preliminary survey of the diagnostic cast, is it possible to estimate the amount and location of tooth reduction necessary to ensure adequate veneer thickness. Tooth reduction sufficient for a

veneered crown that is not to be clasped *may* or *may not* be sufficient for one that is to be clasped (Figs. 27-18 and 27-19).

Veneered crowns closely resembling original tooth shape and size cannot be used on every tooth, since some teeth cannot be successfully prepared and since a change from original tooth shape and size is indicated for some veneered crowns. However, many oversized, over-contoured, veneered crowns, which neither look like teeth nor are in harmony with the periodontium, could have been avoided if the critical areas of the preparation had been altered.

Repair of crowns with synthetic resins

Acrylic resins may be used with satisfaction to replace a fractured, detached

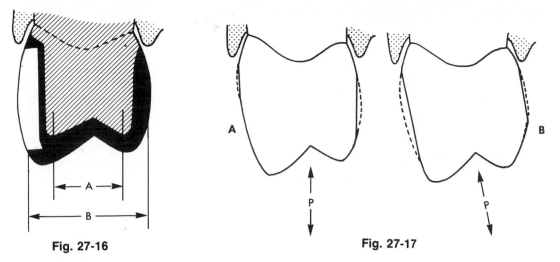

Fig. 27-16   **Fig. 27-17**

Fig. 27-16. Improperly prepared tooth. *A,* Original buccolingual intercuspal distance; *B,* greatest original buccolingual crown width. Note general overcontouring of restoration necessary to obtain adequate thickness of resin veneer and metal thickness and increased size of occlusal table; both changes resulted because insufficient tooth structure was removed from occlusal third of vertical walls of tooth and because intercuspal distance after preparation was greater than it was originally, *A.*

Fig. 27-17. Potential crown outlines are changed on identical tooth contours when indicated path of insertion, *P,* of removable partial denture is changed. **A,** Potential crown outline, as determined by path of insertion, *P,* varies only slightly from original tooth outline. **B,** Potential crown outline, as determined by path of insertion, *P,* varies considerably from original tooth outline, particularly on surface to be veneered. *Dotted lines,* Original tooth outline in **A** and in **B.**

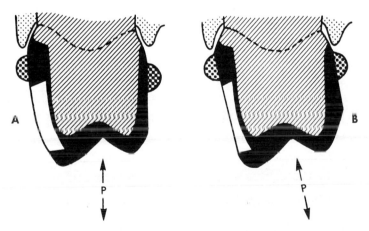

Fig. 27-18. Effect of changing path of insertion of removable partial denture on form of crown. Tooth has been properly prepared for veneer crown that is not to be clasped, but it has been restored with veneer crowns that are designed for clasping. Path of insertion, *P,* of removable partial denture is different on two drawings. **A,** Preparation is acceptable for this clasped crown since shape and size of this crown, as determined by path of insertion, *P,* still permit adequate veneer thickness. **B,** Identical preparation is not acceptable for this crown, since shape and size of this crown, as determined by different path of insertion, *P,* do not permit adequate veneer thickness.

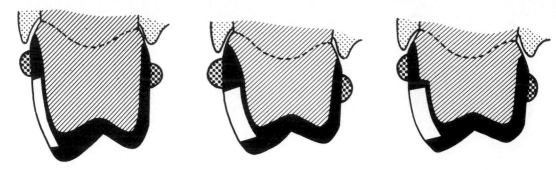

Fig. 27-19. Chamfer type of preparations are covered by acrylic resin veneer crowns that are retainers for clasps. *Left,* Retention and resistance forms have been maintained, but veneer thickness is inadequate. *Center,* There is adequate veneer thickness, but convergence of buccal and lingual walls of preparation toward occlusal surface has weakened retention and resistance forms. *Right,* Retention and resistance forms have been maintained, and there is adequate veneer thickness because of modification in preparation of buccal surface of tooth (note combination shoulder and chamfer on buccal surface of preparation).

dowel type of crown. When such a fracture occurs and it is not deemed advisable to remove the dowel from the canal, the remaining portion is removed from the root face and a crown is contoured in ivory-colored wax, after which it is removed from the protruding portion of the dowel and prepared for investment in a crown flask.

A half-inch length of wire of the same diameter as the dowel remaining in the tooth is inserted into the opening in the base of the wax crown. After the crown has been processed and removed from the investment, a pair of flat-nosed pliers is heated slightly. With this the wire extending from the base of the crown is grasped, and with a slight rotary motion it is withdrawn from the crown, leaving an opening that will fit the dowel extension still remaining in the natural tooth. The acrylic crown is then finished, polished, and cemented directly over the dowel.

Repair of facings

The acrylic resins have also proved very valuable in replacing fractured porcelain facings on pontics and crowns; these may be either of the long pin facing type or of the patented replaceable types. If the acrylic resins serve no other purpose than as a satisfactory material for repairing fractures, they deserve a place among dental materials. The fourth method, previously mentioned, of applying and curing the resin by open exposure to 275° F is useful in repairing restorations not permanently attached to the teeth.

DISADVANTAGES OF ACRYLIC CROWNS

Opposed to the advantages mentioned above are certain disadvantages in the use of synthetic resins for crowns and bridges. Under certain conditions of pressure, the resins exhibit qualities of flow that may have serious end results. In individual restorations it has been observed that in the course of time well-rounded and well-placed contact areas frequently lose their convexities and become flat surfaces.

The property of flow in resins, though advantageous under cetain conditions, as in the case of an acrylic veneer facing, may prove harmful if the flow of the material in a crown is sufficient to break the

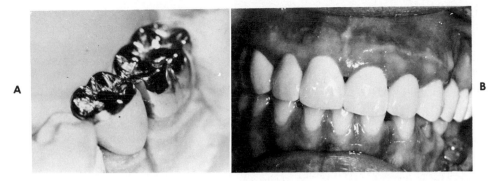

Fig. 27-20. A, Caution must be exercised in protecting mandibular stamp cusps with metal. If this junction of acrylic resin and metal is placed on occlusal surface, facing will be displaced or excessively worn. It should be a rare occasion to place acrylic facings on mandibular molars. **B,** Full maxillary fixed prosthesis seated after 3 months of wearing treatment restoration. Development of optimal esthetics and establishment of adequate interproximal embrasures is facilitated. Acrylic veneers were used to facilitate occlusal modification and prevent an inordinate number of fractures from vigorous occupation of patient.

mechanical union at the gingival margins. Likewise, unless an acrylic crown has been saturated to its maximum expansion before being cemented, it will absorb an additional amount of water in the mouth, causing a dimensional change and breaking the existing union. Therefore, great caution (Fig. 27-20) must be used in the clinical application of this material. Just what the relationship is between the hardness of the synthetic resins and the amount of wear that restorations made of these materials undergo is still being investigated. Whether actual attrition takes place or whether the loss of cusp height is the result of the displacement of the material because of flow should be determined by further investigation.

EARLY USE OF SYNTHETIC RESINS IN FIXED PARTIAL DENTURES

The first recorded use of synthetic resins for the construction of bridges is found in the literature as early as 1931; these were constructed by Geier[11] in Europe at that time. Because the resins were not so highly developed as they are

today nor available in the desired hues, the use of synthetic resin bridges did not make much progress until a more suitable type of acrylic resin was presented to the profession by the manufacturers in this country. The development of the acrylic bridge and its increased use parallels that of the acrylic-veneer crown.

INDICATIONS FOR ACRYLIC FIXED PARTIAL DENTURES

Acrylic bridges are indicated in those places where esthetics are desirable anteriorly and occlusal relationships are difficult to develop posteriorly. In the past, the fired porcelain bridge, reinforced with a metal truss, was the restoration of choice. This type of prosthesis, however, is very exacting in its technique and usually it is relatively expensive. The acrylic bridge meets the requirements of esthetics and at the same time it is economical to construct. Moreover, whereas the fired porcelain bridge requires manipulative skill above that possessed by the average dentist, the acrylic resin bridge is relatively simple to construct.

Also, the acrylic bridge may be used at times where even the fired porcelain bridge is contraindicated. Its main advantage and use today is as a temporary structure while the permanent structure is being fabricated. It is also useful as a splint in periodontal treatment.

Advantages of acrylic fixed restorations

The advantages of the synthetic resin type of bridge[12] are the following.

"(1) It is esthetic to a high degree. The observation has been made and the nature of the material is such that it harmonizes and blends with the natural teeth better than any material at our disposal today. (2) The technic of constructing an acrylic bridge is relatively simple as compared to that required for making a glazed porcelain bridge which is reinforced with an iridioplatinum truss. (3) The time required for its construction is less than that necessary for other types of bridges, particularly the glazed porcelain bridge. (4) It is relatively inexpensive to make. (5) Reports in the literature, and clinical evidence, seem to substantiate the belief that the acrylic resin is biologically compatible to the oral tissues. (6) Properly processed methyl methacrylate is impermeable to bacteria, although the resin does not inhibit the growth of bacteria. (7) The acrylic bridge is relatively durable. (8) It possesses a high impact strength. (9) It is light in weight. (10) It is easy to finish and polish. (11) Additional material may be added to it without remaking the entire structure. (12) If manufactured facings or crowns of acrylic resin are used, the color and contour of the bridge may be predetermined before the completion of the entire bridge."*

Disadvantages of acrylic fixed partial dentures

There have been noted, however, certain limitations and disadvantages:

(1) The acrylic resin is likely to be porous if it is not properly manipulated and processed. (2) If the restoration is placed under continuous pressure or subjected to intermittent pressure, it flows. This results in the loss of the contour, as well as its proximal contact areas. (3) Restorations made of acrylic resin have sometimes become discolored in the mouth.

*From Salisbury, G. B.: Modern trends in dental acrylics, Dent. Dig. **51**:196, 1945.

Although many explanations have been offered for this discoloration, the fact remains that occasionally it still occurs. (4) In the event of the failure of a pontic, it is almost inevitable that the entire restoration must be removed in order to make the repair. (5) It abrades easily. (6) There is the annoyance for those people who chew gum habitually of having the chewing gum stick to the restoration.[12]

In consideration of the above advantages and disadvantages it is evident that the acrylic bridge is not a panacea and that its use as an anterior restoration should be the exception rather than the general rule. The standard type of bridge using the acrylic facing with the cast gold occlusal portion is still the restoration of choice in most cases in the posterior quadrants for developing an occlusal relationship.

Types of acrylic fixed partial dentures

Three types of bridges may be constructed in which the acrylic resins are employed. The first type of acrylic bridge is made entirely of the acrylic resin. Its primary use today is that of a temporary restoration. No metal is used either in the retainers or in the pontics of the restoration. Such a bridge is indicated in the anterior region of the mouth and is usually limited to a short-span restoration. Because no metal is used, the two retainers are usually acrylic-veneer crowns. These types of bridges are used mainly for provisional bridges in conjunction with periodontal stabilization.

The second type of acrylic restoration is that which employs metal retainers in the abutment teeth. These may be complete or partial cast veneer crowns. The pontics are constructed in a manner similar to the regular type of fixed bridge except that instead of using a long pin porcelain facing, the porcelain part is replaced with acrylic resin. One must specially prepare and design the gold portion of the pontic to afford sufficient mechanical retention and protection against displacement of the resin. This type of acrylic bridge has proved quite satisfactory to date. See Chapter 10.

The third type of acrylic restoration is one in which the pontic is constructed entirely of acrylic resin but it is supported by an internal metal truss. With this type of bridge the standard cast retainers may be used or the ferrule type of castings may be made to go over the abutment teeth; these subsequently are covered entirely with the acrylic resin, with metal vertical stops on the ferrules.

Types of abutment preparations

The preparation of teeth for three-quarter retainers and complete shoulder crowns has been fully described in previous chapters, and no further discussion of these is undertaken here. The metal reinforcing truss, however, needs further consideration.

Use of metal trusses. The metal truss gives rigidity to the bridge, and at the same time it furnishes the necessary supporting strength to the acrylic pontic to withstand the forces of mastication. Therefore the metal part must be made of an alloy that possesses the necessary strength with minimum bulk. Pure gold and pure platinum are not suitable for this purpose; either type C or clasp metal gold alloys (type D) or one of the chrome-cobalt types may be employed.

To obtain the maximum strength from a given amount of metal in the truss, various shapes and designs have been developed for this purpose.

Types of metal trusses. Earlier, pieces of round wire extending from one retainer to the other were used; later, square wire was used. It was found, however, that wire alone did not afford the necessary amount of resistance to torsional or pressure forces.

The next development was the use of the T- and the Y-shaped metal bars, the same type as was used for early fired porcelain bridges. Although this shape of the truss bar was an improvement over the round or square bar, it still did not furnish the required amount of support for the resin.

Many other types of trusses were subsequently developed—some using cross pieces of heavy wrought wire placed at the center of each pontic; others using a cast metal structure.

The advantage of the cast type of truss over the wrought-wire type lies in the fact that the extent and shape of the truss may be easily shaped in wax to meet any existing conditions irrespective of tissue irregularity or contour. Also the truss may be so positioned and shaped that it gives a saucerlike support to the pontic against the forces of compression and tension. A cast truss may also be reinforced and made thicker in those areas where greater forces will be exerted on the bridge.

Purpose of metal trusses. The question has been raised whether the incorporation of a metal within an acrylic restoration creates cleavage planes and areas of highly localized stress within the resin. To what degree these exist has not been definitely established; however, the characteristic properties of flow and elasticity that the acrylic resins exhibit are a definite handicap to their use in bridge restorations. A properly designed metal truss in an acrylic bridge has enabled it to withstand the forces of mastication to a limited degree.

A metal truss is always attached to the metal retainers in the abutment teeth. As previously stated, these may be either the complete cast crowns, the three-quarter crowns, or intracoronal retainers. At times the ferrule or thimble types of retainers are used, usually with the shoulder type of tooth preparation; these are covered entirely with the resin in the finished bridge.

Use of opaque resin. Where metal structures are used in conjunction with acrylic resins, it is necessary to cover the metal with an opaque resin to prevent the color of the metal from showing through in the finished bridge.

CONCLUSION

Because the dental profession has a better understanding of the limitations as well as the advantages of this type of material in bridge prosthesis, the acrylic bridges as constructed today and the conditions under which they are used make it possible for the acrylic restorations to serve satisfactorily for longer periods of time under certain selected conditions.

SELECTED REFERENCES

1. Selbach, F. W.: Crowns and bridges of artificial resin, Zahnärztl. Rundschau **26:**1, 1091, 1938.
2. Wilson, W. E.: Casting of plastic inlays and crowns, Dent. Dig. **46:**202, 1940.
3. Weder, K.: Crowns, dowel teeth and bridges made of synthetic resins, Zahnärztl. Rundschau **49:**3, 1940.
4. Sweeney, W. T.: Denture base material: acrylic resin, J.A.D.A. **26:**1963, 1939.
5. Vernonite Workbench: Low-heat technic processing, Pittsburgh, Pa., 1945, Vernon-Benshoff Co., Inc., vol. 2, p. 1; vol. 4, p. 1.
6. Peyton, F. A.: Self-curing resins for direct inlay, J. Michigan Dent. Soc. **32:**32, 1950.
7. Nealon, F. H.: Acrylic restorations: operative non-pressure procedure, N.Y. J. Dent. **22:**201, 1952.
8. Peyton, F. A., and Mann, W. R.: Acrylic and acrylic-styrene resins: their properties in relation to their uses as restorative materials, J.A.D.A. **29:**1852, 1942.
9. Tylman, S. D., and Peyton, F. A.: Acrylic and other synthetic resins used in dentistry, Philadelphia, 1946, J. B. Lippincott Co.
10. Long, A. C.: Acrylic resin veneer crowns: the effect of tooth preparation on crown fabrication and future periodontal health, J. Prosthet. Dent. **14:**370, 1968.
11. Geier, W.: Experiences with Hekodent and Rockodenta-colloid as crown and bridge material in patients, Dtsche. Zahnärztl. Wochenschr. **13:**191, 1931.
12. Salisbury, G.: Modern trends in dental acrylics, Dent. Dig. **51:**196, 1945.

GENERAL REFERENCES

Adams, C.: Properties and uses of cold curing acrylic in prosthetics, Iowa Dent. J. **42:**20, 1956.
Alvares, L. C., and Paulo, S.: Radiopacity of acrylic resins, Oral Surg. **22:**318-324, 1966.
American Dental Association Specification No. 13 for Self-Curing Repair Resins (first revision approved December, 1958, effective Jan. 1, 1959), J.A.D.A. **58:**136, 1959.
Atkinson, H. F., and Grant, A. A.: Pressure changes in polymerizing polymethyl methacrylate, J. Dent. Res. **44:**1040, 1965.
Buonocore, M. G.: Report on a resin composition capable of bonding to human dentin surfaces, J. Dent. Res. **35:**846, 1956.
Bowen, R. L.: Use of epoxy resins in restorative materials, J. Dent. Res. **35:**360, 1956.
Bergman, B. O.: Test denture for masticatory studies, Dent. Abstr. **6:**678, 1961.
Bergman, B. O.: Studies on the permeability of acrylic facing material in gold crowns, a laboratory investigation using Na^{22}, Acta Odontol. Scand. **19:**297, 1961.
Blatterfein, L.: Planning and contouring of acrylic resin veneer crowns for partial denture clasping, J. Prosthet. Dent. **6:**386, 1956.
Brown, R. E.: Full gold-acrylic veneer crown, Roy. Can. Dent. Corps Q. **1:**11, 1960.
Caul, H. J., and Sweeney, W. T.: Relationship between residual monomer and some properties of self-curing dental resins, J.A.D.A. **53:**60, 1956.
Cornell, J. A., and Powers, C. M.: Effect of varying peroxide and polymer on the rate and degree of polymerization of polymethyl methacrylate slurries, J. Dent. Res. **38:**606, 1959.
Cornell, J. A., Stone, K., and Ellis, S.: Tensile strengths of modified methyl methacrylates and various rates of loading, J. Dent. Res. **34:**740, 1955 (abstr.).
Cornell, J. A., Jordan, J. S., Ellis, S., and Rose, E. E.: Method of comparative wear resistance of various materials used for artificial teeth, J.A.D.A. **54:**608, 1957.
Crone, F. L., and Bloch, P.: Penetration of C^{14}-labelled methyl-methacrylate into the dentine, Acta Odontol. Scand. **16:**247, 1958.
Ehrlich, A.: Erosion of acrylic resin restorations, J.A.D.A. **59:**543, 1959.
Fiasconaro, J. E., and Sherman, H.: Sealing properties of acrylics, N.Y. Dent. J. **18:**189, 1952.
FitzRoy, D. C., Swartz, M. L., and Phillips, R. W.: Physical properties of selected dental resins, part II, J. Prosthet. Dent. **13:**1108, 1963.
Frankel, H. J.: Uses of autopolymerizing acrylic resins in fixed partial prosthesis, J. Prosthet. Dent. **8:**1003, 1958.
Franks, A. S. T.: Clinical appraisal of acrylic tooth wear, Dent. Pract. Dent. Rec. **12:**149, 1962.
Goodfriend, D. J.: Practical analysis of occlusal procedures, J. Prosthet. Dent. **16:**557-571, 1966.
Hall, R. W.: Retention for cast gold acrylic veneer crowns, Roy. Can. Dent. Corps Q. **1:**15, 1960.
Hedegard, B.: Cold polymerizing resins: a clinical

and histological study, Acta Odontol. Scand. **13**(suppl. 17):13, 1955.

Hedegard, B.: Evaluation of materials for anterior bridges with special reference to acrylic resins, Int. Dent. J. **12**:33, 1962.

Hirsch, L., and Weinreb, M. M.: Marginal fit of direct acrylic restorations, J.A.D.A. **56**:13, 1958.

Issa, H.: Marginal leakage in crowns with acrylic resin facings, J. Prosthet. Dent. **19**:281, 1968.

Kafalias, M. C., Swartz, M. L., and Phillips, R. W.: Physical properties of selected dental resins, part I, J. Prosthet. Dent. **13**:1087, 1963.

Klaffenbach, A. O.: Anterior fixed bridge prosthesis including acrylic resins, J. South. Calif. Dent. Assoc. **13**:19, 1940.

Klaffenbach, A. O.: Anterior fixed bridge prosthesis including acrylic resins, J.A.D.A. **34**:670, 1947.

Kramer, I. R. H.: Development of characteristic changes in the dental pulp following the use of resins containing methacrylic acid, J. Dent. Res. **34**:782, 1955 (abstr.).

Kramer, I. R. H.: Reaction of the pulp to self polymerizing resins, Br. Dent. J. **101**:378, 1956.

Krikos, A.: Self-curing resins in constructing patterns for small castings, J. Prosthet. Dent. **20**: 235-238, 1968.

Lamstein, A., and Blechman, H.: Marginal seepage around acrylic resin veneers in gold crowns, J. Prosthet. Dent. **6**:706, 1956.

Langeland, K.: Pulp reactions to resin cements, Acta Odontol. Scand. **13**:239, 1956.

Langeland, K.: Pulp reactions to resin cements, Dent. Abstr. **2**:660, 1957.

Lastra, M. J.: Comparative study of acrylic and porcelain jacket crowns, Dent. Abstr. **2**:76, 1957.

Levy, R. I.: Acrylic inlays, crowns and bridges, Philadelphia, 1950, Lea & Febiger.

McCune, R. J., Phillips, R. W., and Swartz, M. L.: A study of a new resin veneering material, J. South. Calif. Dent. Assoc. 36(12):496, 1968.

McLoud, J. W.: Some physical properties of a new cross-linked plastic filling material, Br. Dent. J. **110**:375, 1961.

Manning, J. E.: Guide to use of acrylic resin filling materials, Int. Dent. J. **8**:48, 1958.

Martins, E. A., Peyton, F. A., and Kingery, R. H.: Properties of custom-made plastic teeth formed by different techniques, J. Prosthet. Dent. **12**: 1059, 1962.

Miller, T. H.: Allergies to acrylic resins, Iowa Dent. Bull. **40**:285, 1954.

Muller, O., and Maeglin, B.: Histological changes in the pulp of teeth filled with self-polymerizing resins, Int. Dent. J. **4**:167, 1953.

Myerson, R. L.: Use of porcelain and plastic teeth in opposing complete dentures, J. Prosthet. Dent. **7**:625, 1957.

Myerson, R. L.: Effect of cross-linking on mechanical damping and stiffness of methacrylates, Int. Abstr. Dent. Res. **40**:89, 1962 (abstr.).

Nealon, F. H.: Acrylic restorations; operative nonpressure procedure, J. Prosthet. Dent. **2**:512-518, 1959.

Ohashi, M.: Observations on the generating mechanism of internal porosity in polymerization of methyl methacrylate resin for dental use, J. Nihon Univ. School Dent. **4**:1, 1961.

Peyton, F. A., and Craig, R. G.: Restorative dental materials, ed. 4, St. Louis, 1971, The C. V. Mosby Co.

Peyton, F. A.: Various developments in dental plastics, Minneapolis Dist. Dent. J. **38**:69, 1954.

Peyton, F. A., and Craig, R. G.: Current evaluation of plastics in crown and bridge prosthesis, J. Prosthet. Dent. **13**:743, 1963.

Phillips, R. W.: Newer restorative resins, J. Indiana Dent. Assoc. **42**:151-152, 1967.

Pine, B.: Pontics for gold-acrylic resin fixed partial dentures, J. Prosthet. Dent. **12**:347, 1962.

Roche, H. A. P.: Assessment of the values of porcelain versus methylmethacrylate in jacket crown and bridgework, Br. Dent. J. **87**:23, 1949.

Rose, E. E., Lal, J., and Green, R.: Effects of peroxide, amine and hydroquinone in varying concentrations on the polymerization rate of polymethyl methacrylate slurries, J.A.D.A. **56**:375, 1958.

Rose, E. E., Lal, J., Green, R., and Cornell, J. A.: Direct filling resin materials; coefficient of thermal expansion and water sorption of polymethyl methacrylate, J. Dent. Res. **34**:589-596, 1955.

Ryge, G., and Foley, D. E.: Effect of dry heat processing on the physical properties of acrylic crowns, J.A.D.A. **66**:672, 1963.

Sausen, R. E., Armstrong, W. D., and Simon, W. J.: Penetration of radiocalcium at margins of acrylic restorations made by compression and noncompression technics, J.A.D.A. **47**:636, 1953.

Schwartz, J. R.: The acrylic plastics in dentistry, Brooklyn, N.Y., 1950, Dental Items of Interest Publishing Co., Inc.

Schwartz, N. L.: Processing acrylic resin veneers using sectional cores, J. Prosthet. Dent. **10**:330, 1960.

Selberg, A.: Acrylic veneers and bridgework, Tennessee Dent. Assoc. **29**:28, 1949.

Seltzer, S.: Penetration of microorganisms between the tooth and direct resin fillings, J.A.D.A. **51**:560, 1955.

Sim, J.: Allergic reaction to denture base material, J. Can. Dent. Assoc. **24**:292, 1958.

Skinner, E. W., and Jones, P. M.: Dimensional stability of self curing denture base acrylic resins, J.A.D.A. **51**:426, 1955.

Slack, F. A.: Notes on dentures, jackets, crowns and bridges, J.A.D.A. **32**:1112, 1945.

Slack, F. A., Jr.: Experiments in directional polymerization, Dent. Dig. **63:**356, 1957.

Slack, F. A., Jr., Sweeney, W. T., McParland, P. V., and Miller, I. F.: Use of acrylics for crowns, bridges and inlays, Pennsylvania Dent. J. **12:**115, 1945.

Soremark, R., and Bergman, B.: Studies on the permeability of acrylic facing material in gold crowns; a laboratory investigation using Na²², Acta Odont. Scand. **19:**297, 1961.

Terry, I. A., and Harrington, J. H.: Abrasion tests on acrylics, J.A.D.A. **65:**377, 1962.

Vernon, H. M.: Glossary of terms used in plastic arts, J. Prosthet. Dent. **8:**1055, 1958.

Vieira, D. F., and Phillips, R. W.: Influence of certain variables on the abrasion of acrylic resin veneering materials, J. Prosthet. Dent. **12:**720, 1962.

Waerhaug, J., and Löe, H.: Tissue reaction to self-curing acrylic resin implants, Dent. Pract. Dent. Rec. **8:**234, 1958.

Waerhaug, J., and Zander, H. A.: Reaction of gingival tissues to self-curing acrylic restoration, J.A.D.A. **54:**760, 1957.

Yamamoto, T.: Self-curing acrylic pattern used in indirect technic for casting full crowns, Dent. Abstr. **7:**515, 1962.

28

Gnathologic procedures using the Denar Model D5A and pantograph*

David L. Koth, Niles F. Guichet, and Robert Pinkerton

The Denar Model D5A articulator is a precision mandibular movement simulator, a mechanical equivalent of the lower half of the head. The articulator has total capability to reproduce all mandibular movements or jaw positions recorded by any chew-in technique, checkbite, or the more sophisticated method employing a pantograph. The ability of this articulator to accurately reproduce the patient's mandibular movements is limited only by the accuracy of the record to which it is adjusted. The Denar D5A articulator reduces the diagnostic recordings and resultant movements produced by the articulator to numeric values. This permits the instrument to be reprogrammed for treatment function. The specifications thus established accurately define the parameters within which the restoration is to be constructed in order to eliminate eccentric interferences (Fig. 28-1).

ANTERIOR AND POSTERIOR CONTROL AREAS

Dental articulators are conventionally constructed to be reasonable facsimiles of their anatomic counterparts because this construction provides the most convenient means of producing the desired movements. In the application of an articulator to the fabrication of occlusal restorations, the articulator is programmed to produce a motion that is a determinant of the occlusal anatomy being developed. The motion produced by the instrument is dictated by the settings of its posterior or condylar controls and its anterior or incisal guide control.

In practical application, tremendous clinical significance of these control areas

*This chapter is based on the lecture notes, published material, and illustrations of Niles Guichet, D.D.S. (Instructor, University of California Postgraduate School of Dentistry, Anaheim, California), which he used when presenting his concepts and specific procedures for occlusal treatment with Denar Model D4A articulator and pantograph and which he prepared in collaboration with Robert J. Pinkerton, B.S., D.D.S., Anaheim, California. Currently the Model D5A has been marketed by the Denar Corp. David L. Koth, D.D.S., M.S. (Director, Fixed Prosthetics, Medical College of Georgia, Augusta, Georgia) has further modified the chapter since the sixth edition to present the newly introduced model.

Instrumentation and procedures involved in gnathology may at first seem complicated and difficult, but it has been the experience of many teachers that third- and fourth-year dental students have successfully used the hinge-axis face-bow and the adjustable articulator in dental school clinics, provided that the basic principles of gnathology were taught to them understandably and that these principles were integrated early in their preclinical, technical, and biologic courses. The use of the pantograph with a more refined adjustable articulator brings dental prosthodontics the opportunity to advance another step. (S.D.T. and W.F.P.M.)

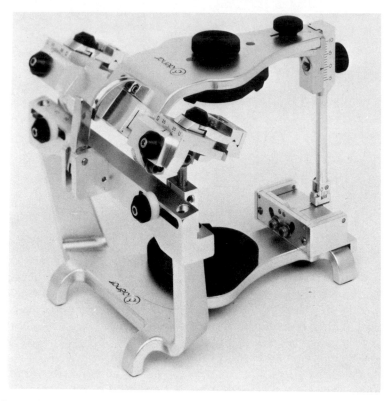

Fig. 28-1. Denar D5A articulator. Note adjustments and scales. (Courtesy Denar Corp., Anaheim Calif.)

is found in their capacity to be precisely readjusted after the diagnosis, so the instrument will produce a motion that facilitates the efficient accomplishment of the prime objective, fabricating the desired occlusion. The ability of the motion programmed in the articulator to be interpreted in calibrated control areas and expressed in numeric values permits the same instrument or another instrument in a remote location to be programmed subsequently without the expenditure of additional time and expense. This is clinically significant in that it encourages the treatment sequence to be accomplished according to the dentist's or patient's desires rather than by instrument limitations.

In the use of an articulator to facilitate the fabrication of the desired occlusion, there are three general areas of consideration.

1. *The posterior-control areas (the condylar controls).* These control areas are adjusted in consideration of the patient's temporomandibular joint characteristics, which are identified with the aid of a pantograph or alternate condylar movement recording means such as chew-in techniques or checkbite methods.

2. *The anterior-control area (the incisal guide).* This control area is of equal importance to the posterior-control area. In existing occlusions, it is adjusted in consideration of the vertical overbite and horizontal overjet relation of the anterior teeth. In edentulous mouths the overbite and overjet position of the anterior teeth is established by phonetic and esthetic measurements.

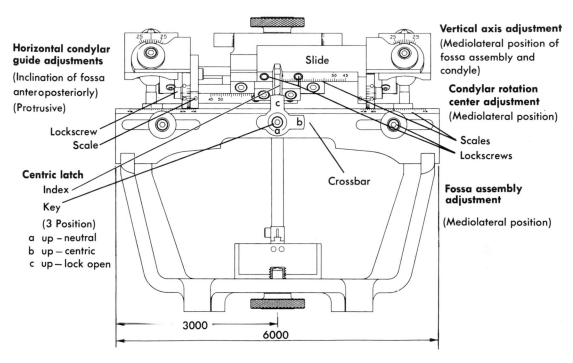

**Centric latch;
Vertical axis (mediolateral position of fossa assembly and
condyle) protrusive**

**Horizontal condylar
guide adjustments**

(Inclination of fossa
anteroposteriorly)

(Protrusive)

Lockscrew
Scale

Centric latch

Index

Key

(3 Position)
a up – neutral
b up – centric
c up – lock open

Slide

Crossbar

Vertical axis adjustment
(Mediolateral position of
fossa assembly and
condyle)

**Condylar rotation
center adjustment**
(Mediolateral position)

Scales
Lockscrews

**Fossa assembly
adjustment**

(Mediolateral position)

3000

6000

Fig. 28-2. Rear view of Fig. 28-1. (Courtesy Denar Corp., Anaheim, Calif.)

3. *The centric-occlusal position of the mounted casts in proper orientation to the control areas.* This is the most important of the three general areas of consideration. Accurate orientation of the mandibular cast to the maxillary cast at the cenric occlusal position is of paramount importance and is often the most difficult and most time-consuming accomplishment of these three areas of consideration in occlusal treatments. Here the dentist must rely on his knowledge of neuromuscular physiology, hinge-axis theory, and equilibration, checkbite, and laboratory technique.

ARTICULATOR CALIBRATIONS

In the diagosis, the articulator is used to measure temporomandibular joint char-

acteristics. *In treatment,* it is used to establish the specifications or measurements to which the restoration is to be constructed. In any measuring procedure, the measurement is made in relation to an initial reference or starting position. In the measurement of the anatomic determinants of occlusion, the initial references are the *horizontal reference plane* and the *midsagittal reference plane.* These initial reference planes established on the patient are also identified on the articulator, the mechanical equivalent of the lower half of the head.

Horizontal reference plane

The horizontal reference plane of the articulator is the horizontal plane that intersects the centers of rotation in the

Component terminology

Anterior controls

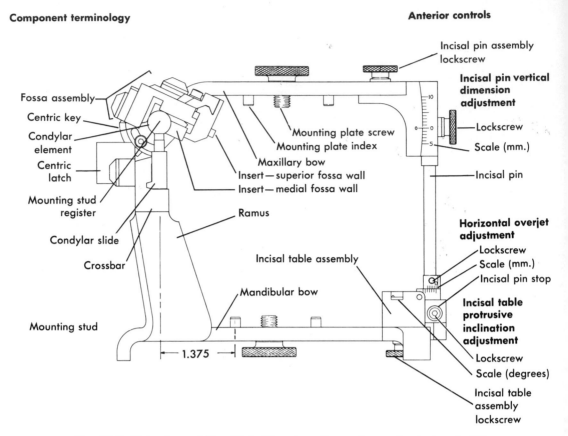

Fig. 28-3. Side view of Fig. 28-1. (Courtesy Denar Corp., Anaheim, Calif.)

condylar elements and is parallel to the upper and lower bows of the articulator.

Midsagittal reference plane

The midsagittal reference plane of the articulator is the vertical plane that passes anteroposteriorly through the middle of the articulator.

The diagnostic data registered by the mandibular movement record are interpreted in the calibrated control adjustments of the articulator and expressed in numeric values of millimeters and degrees. These numeric expressions are in relation to specific positions or planes of reference, which can be precisely relocated.

POSTERIOR CONTROL AREA

Vertical axes of rotation (Fig. 28-2): Expressed in millimeters from the midsagittal plane.

Horizontal condylar path (Fig. 28-3): Expressed in degrees from the horizontal reference plane.

Immediate sideshift (Fig. 28-4): Expressed in millimeters from the centric position of the mandible.

Progressive sideshift (Fig. 28-4): Expressed in degrees from the sagittal plane that passes through the point at which the progressive sideshift begins.

Sagittal displacements of the rotating condyle (Fig. 28-4): Backward or forward; expressed in degrees from the coronal plane; rear wall of fossa adjustment. Up or down; expressed in degrees from the horizontal plane; top wall of fossa adjustment.

ANTERIOR CONTROL AREA

Vertical dimension of the incisal pin (Fig. 28-3): Expressed in millimeters of opening or closing of the articulator in the area of the incisor teeth. In the Denar D5A articulator, this dimension is read directly on the incisal pin. This calibration was computed on the basis of the average anatomic dimensions of a skull as described by Bonwill being transferred to the articulator so that the plane of occlusion of the anterior teeth would be coinciden-

Sideshift adjustments

Sagittal displacements of
rotating condyle adjustment

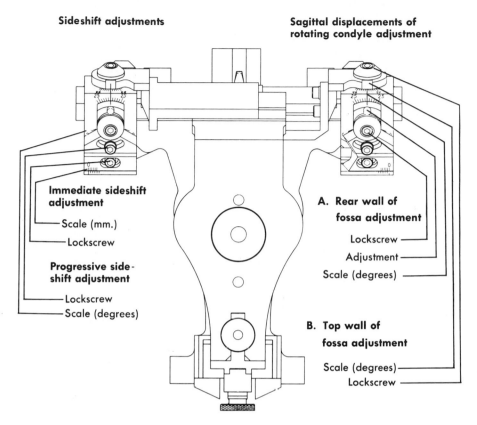

**Immediate sideshift
adjustment**

— Scale (mm.)

— Lockscrew

**Progressive side-
shift adjustment**

— Lockscrew

— Scale (degrees)

**A. Rear wall of
fossa adjustment**

Lockscrew —

Adjustment —

Scale (degrees) —

**B. Top wall of
fossa adjustment**

Scale (degrees)—

Lockscrew —

Fig. 28-4. Top view of Fig. 28-1. (Courtesy Denar Corp., Anaheim, Calif.)

tal to the midhorizontal plane of the articulator. The scale is calibrated in 1 mm increments.

Horizontal overjet adjustment (Fig. 28-3): Expressed in millimeters from the transverse vertical or coronal plane that passes through the labioincisal angle of the mandibular anterior teeth. The vernier scale is calibrated in increments of 0.2 mm.

Incisal table, protrusive, and lateral wing adjustments (Fig. 28-3): Expressed in degrees from the horizontal plane. The scales are calibrated in 5 degree increments.

POSTERIOR CONTROL ADJUSTMENTS

The vertical axes can be adjusted mediolaterally from 45 to 75 mm mediolaterally as measured from the midsagittal reference plane. The scales for this adjustment are calibrated in 1 mm increments.

In locating the mediolateral position of

the vertical axes, one must adjust the fossa assemblies first. To do this, one must loosen the fossa assembly slide-lock screws (Fig. 28-2). After the adjustment, the mediolateral position of the fossa can be maintained by gentle tightening of only one of the lock screws provided on each slide. (Two screws are provided because in some positions one of the screws on the upper slide will be behind the centric-latch index.) The mediolateral position of the condylar elements is subsequently adjusted to a position 1 to 2 mm lateral to the fossa elements by loosening of the condylar—rotation centric—adjustment lock screw. The upper member of the articulator is then brought to rest on the lower member and the correct mediolateral orientation of the respective members is accomplished by engagement of the centric latch in the centric position. The thumb is then used to push the condylar element medially until it engages the medial wall of the fossa; the locknut is secured. It is important that the immediate sideshift adjustment be set to zero when this adjustment is made.

HORIZONTAL CONDYLAR GUIDE ADJUSTMENT: ANTEROPOSTERIOR ANGLE OF THE EMINENTIA PROTRUSIVE

The anterior position inclination of the superior fossa wall or fossa assembly can be adjusted from 0 to 60 degrees from the horizontal or horizontal reference plane by loosening of the horizontal condylar guide lock screw. The scale for this adjustment is calibrated in 5-degree increments (Figs. 28-2 and 28-26).

Immediate-sideshift adjustment

Fig. 28-4 illustrates the superior view of the maxillary assembly detailing the immediate-sideshift adjustments. The medial fossa wall can be displaced medially by loosening of the immediate-sideshift adjustment lock screw.

The amount of the displacement and the amount of immediate sideshift allowed is indicated on the vernier scale. The adjustment is set to zero when the apex of the reference mark is indexed to the most lateral mark on the upper scale. The lines on the upper scale marked with the numeral are 1 mm apart. The lines on the lower scale identified with the reference mark are 0.8 mm apart. Consequently, when the medial fossa wall is displaced medially 0.2 mm to allow a 0.2 mm immediate sideshift, the second pair of lines will line up indicating the 0.2 mm displacement. As the medial fossa wall is displaced more medially, each successive pair of lines that registers indicate an additional 0.2 mm displacement

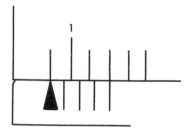

Fig. 28-5. Vernier scale. (Courtesy Denar Corp., Anaheim, Calif.)

of the medial fossa wall or immediate sideshift permitted. Fig. 28-5 illustrates this scale with the 0.2 mm increments on the lower scale marked.

Progressive-sideshift adjustment

Fig. 28-4 illustrates a superior view of a fossa assembly detailing the progressive-sideshift adjustment. The medial fossa wall can be set at any pitch from 0 to 30 degrees to the sagittal plane by loosening of the progressive-sideshift lock screw. This permits the mandibular member of the articulator to move progressively laterally as the traveling condyle functions along the medial wall of the fossa (Fig. 28-28).

Sagittal displacement of the rotating condyle; backward and forward rear-wall adjustment

Fig. 28-4 illustrates a superior view of a fossa assembly detailing the rear-wall adjustment. The posterior fossa wall can be inclined anteriorly or posteriorly 30 degrees from the coronal plane by loosening of the rear-wall adjustment lock screw. The degree of anterior inclination of the rear wall is indicated on the lateral portion of the scale. The degree of medial inclination of the rear wall is indicated on the medial portion of the scale. The scale is calibrated in 5-degree increments (Fig. 28-29).

Lateral condylar path adjustment; lateral adjustment; orbiting path adjustment

As a mandibular lateral excursive movement is made, the traveling condyle moves downward, forward, and inward and orbits around the opposite or rotating condyle (sometimes referred to as the "working condyle" because it is on the working side). The path the orbiting condyle travels along the superior fossa wall will be different from the path it travels when a straight protrusive excursive movement is made. In almost all cases, the anteroposterior inclination of this path to the horizontal plane is equal to or greater than the path traveled in the protrusive excursive movement. The horizontal condylar path adjustment is used to establish this orbiting path on the articulator. Sometimes one horizontal condylar adjustment will establish the correct anteroposterior angle of the eminentia for both the protrusive condylar path and the orbiting path. If it does not, the shallower path is used in routine clinical treatments. (This will be the protrusive path with very rare exceptions.) If the correct angle of the eminentia for both the protrusive path and orbiting path is not established at one horizontal condylar inclination setting and it is desired to accurately reproduce mandibular movement, the anteroposterior angle of the eminentia should be set to the steeper path (generally the orbiting path), and then the correct inclination of the shallower path should be established by custom-grinding of the inferior surface of the superior fossa wall.

The superior and medial fossa wall inserts are available in various anatomic curvatures. They are available in nylon for continuous usage and in acrylic. The acrylic inserts are available to facilitate custom modification of these inserts by grinding and the addition of cold-cure acrylic in those cases in which it is necessary to allow the instrument to produce a movement that will enable the pantograph to accurately track the recorded lines. The superior wall inserts are interchangeable, right and left. The medial wall inserts are provided in right- and left-hand sets. A complete stock of other inserts is available.

Custom-grinding inserts

This procedure is generally done only when the articulator is being adjusted to a pantographic recording and it is desired that the styli accurately track the recorded lines in all their detail when this cannot be accomplished simply by selection of the proper fossa inserts and by use of the articulator adjustments. Final inserts are selected and the articulator is adjusted to produce the desired movement permitting the styli to track the recorded lines; additional stock must be removed from the inserts in selected areas. These selected areas on the inserts are identified with the aid of carbon paper. Carbon paper is inserted between the condyle and the insert to be modified, and the articulator is moved in a limited excursion where it fails to produce the desired movement. This marks the area of the insert to be modified. The insert is then ground with a Fastcut stone or vulcanite cutter having a ⅜-inch radius. The procedure is repeated until sufficient stock is removed from the fossa-insert so that the instrument will produce the desired movement. When the inserts are removed from the articulator, a sharp instrument is used to identify them with the patient's name or number and whether they are right or left so that they can be filed for future reference.

ANTERIOR CONTROL ADJUSTMENTS
Vertical dimension of incisal pin; incisal pin adjustment

The incisal pin assembly can be removed from the articulator without changing the vertical dimension of the incisal pin assembly, by loosening of the incisal pin assembly lock screw (Fig. 28-3). Loosening the incisal pin vertical dimension adjustment lock screw permits the vertical dimension of the incisal pin to be increased 10 mm or decreased 5 mm. The scale is calibrated in millimeters in the area of the incisor teeth. Note that the two washers on the incisal pin lock screw have matching concave convex surfaces that should always face toward each other.

Horizontal overjet adjustment; long centric adjustment

In order to adjust to the horizontal overjet of anterior teeth or to provide for horizontal movement in the articulator to specify an area of centric for complete denture construction, one can retract the foot of the incisal pin from the inclines of the incisal table by loosening the lock screw (Fig. 28-3). The foot of the incisal pin rests on the incisal pin stop.

Protrusive inclination of the incisal table; angle of the incisal table anteroposteriorly; anterior vertical overbite adjustment

Loosening the incisal table protrusive inclination permits the incisal table to be inclined upward from 0 to 60 degrees to the horizontal plane anteroposteriorly. This inclination is read on the scale calibrated in 5-degree increments.

Lateral wings of the incisal table; angle of the incisal table mediolaterally

By loosening the lock screws on the anterior surface of the incisal table, one can incline the lateral wings of the incisal table up to an angle of 45 degrees to that member of the incisal table that inclines anteroposteriorly. The adjustable incisal table is replaceable with a custom incisal platform of acrylic, which can be easily modified for special requirements.

INITIAL REFERENCE

In any measuring procedure, the measurement is made in relation to an initial reference or starting position. In the measurements of the posterior anatomic determinants of occlusion, the initial references are the horizontal reference plane and the midsagittal plane.

Horizontal reference plane

The horizontal reference plane is a plane established on the face of the patient by an anterior reference point and two posterior reference points from which measurements of the posterior anatomic determinants of occlusion are made. The three reference points that locate the horizontal reference plane are arbitrarily established. However, once the measurements are made, the reference points cannot be changed if the measurements are to remain valid.

Anterior reference point

The anterior reference point is a point on the face at some fixed dimension above the incisal edges of the maxillary anterior teeth that will position the plane of occlusion in the middle of the articulator vertically when the maxillary cast is transferred to the articulator in relation to this reference point. The anterior reference point is located in relation to the fixed immovable inner canthus of the eye so it can be permanently recorded and precisely relocated. This reference point is efficiently located with a 43 mm notch fixed in the Denar Reference Plane Locator.

Posterior reference points

The posterior reference points are two points located one on each side of the face in the area of the terminal hinge axis. These points will be registered by the pantograph and transferred to the horizontal axis of the articulator. The specific influence the location of the terminal hinge or horizontal axis has on mandibular movement is in a motion that occurs about that axis, that is, the opening arc and arc of closure of the mandibular teeth (sagittal plane rotation).*

In fabricating occlusions, the only functional use of an articulator is when it functions in accord with its control areas and is used as a gage or shearing device in determining the exact shape of the occlusal surfaces. This only occurs when the incisal pin is on the incisal table. In these functional uses, arcs of rotational movement that occur about the horizontal axis are slight and occur only in *eccentric* positions. These arcs are so imperceptibly influenced by the precise location of the horizontal axis that exactness in its location is of no clinical significance.

The only time rotational movement about the horizontal axis can be of sufficient magnitude to be clinically significant is when insufficient consideration given to the precise location of the horizontal axis could cause an error in the occlusion. This could only occur (1) when the mandibular cast is transferred to the articulator by means of a centric record taken at an increased vertical dimension and then by rotational movement about the horizontal axis the correct vertical dimension is restored, or (2) by a significant change in the vertical dimension on the articulator. EXAMPLE: Assume a situation in which the mandibular teeth were disoccluded from the maxillary teeth along an opening arc that occurred by rotational movement about the terminal hinge axis (horizontal) and a centric record taken at an increased vertical dimension. If this centric record were then used to transfer the mandibular cast to an articulator in which the relation of the maxillary cast to the horizontal axis of

the instrument did not coincide with the relation of the maxillary teeth to the terminal hinge axis of the patient, when the mandibular teeth are reoccluded to the correct vertical dimension by rotational movement about the horizontal axis of the articulator, they would follow a different arc or path of closure than they traveled in the disoccluding arc. Consequently, they would not return to their original starting position. An error would be introduced in the *centric* occlusal position that could be of clinical importance.

If the mandibular cast is going to be transferred to the articulator by means of a centric record taken at an increased vertical dimension, the posterior reference point must coincide with the terminal hinge axis of the patient and precise hinge-axis location is necessary in order to avoid the possibility of this error. In this manner the arc of opening on the patient and the arc of closing on the articulator will coincide and the centric occlusal position will be *theoretically* accurate. Alternately, however, if simultaneous even contacting and indexing of the teeth occur at the correct vertical dimension with the condyles in terminal hinge position, the most accurate way of transferring the mandibular cast to the articulator is by occluding it with the maxillary cast. In this case, rotational movement about the horizontal axis must be of insufficient magnitude for precise hinge-axis location to be of any clinical significance. Posterior reference points selected by average anatomic measurements are indicated because precise hinge-axis location offers no advantage.

Summary

The manner in which the mandibular cast is transferred to the articulator is the specific determinant of the method employed to locate the posterior reference points.

RULE: If the mandibular cast is to be

---

*A sagittal plane rotation of the mandible is a rotational movement of the mandible in which each point within the mandible stays within its own respective sagittal plane and rotates about an axis (horizontal) perpendicular to that plane.

transferred to the articulator by means of a centric relation record taken at an increased vertical dimension, or if the vertical dimension is going to be changed on the articulator, the posterior reference points must be precisely located. (Fig. 28-13).

RULE: If the mandibular cast is to be transferred to the articulator by means of a centric relation record taken at the correct vertical dimension, the posterior reference points may be selected by average anatomic measurement.

NOTE: In extensive reconstruction procedures where the restoration is to be seated in the mouth and subsequently remounted in the articulator by means of a centric relation record taken at an increased vertical dimension for final occlusal correction prior to cementation, precise hinge-axis location is always indicated. However, in the diagnostic mounting of study casts or in minor restorative procedures, the mandibular cast is sometimes transferred to the articulator at a minimal vertical opening without precise hinge-axis location. In these instances the possible introduction of errors is subsequently eliminated when the restoration is seated in the mouth.

REFERENCE PLANE LOCATION
(Figs. 28-6 to 28-9)

When one uses the average anatomic measurements in locating the horizontal reference plane, the reference plane location aids can be used to advantage. These consist of:

1. Reference plane locator
2. Reference plane marker
3. 43 mm notch to locate anterior reference point
4. Hole to locate posterior reference point

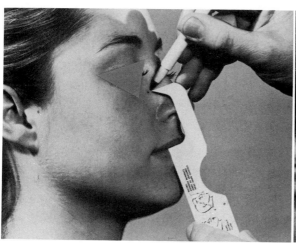

Fig. 28-6

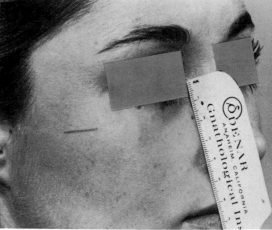

Fig. 28-7

Fig. 28-6. Locate anterior reference point by indexing notch against incisal edge of maxillary anterior tooth or, preferably, lower lip line. (Courtesy Denar Corp., Anaheim, Calif.)

Fig. 28-7. Record relation of anterior reference to fixed immovable inner canthus of eye so that anterior reference point may be precisely relocated if necessary. RULE: If mandibular cast is to be transferred to articulator by means of centric record taken at correct vertical dimension, locate posterior reference points by average anatomic measurement. (Courtesy Denar Corp., Anaheim, Calif.)

5. Millimeter scale
6. Hole to index to reference-plane support rod

CLUTCH CONSTRUCTION (REGISTRATION TRAY)

To locate the hinge axis or perform a pantographic survey, one needs a pair of clutches* to index the hinge axis locator or pantograph to the dental arches. Denar provides two clutch formers, a dentulous clutch former and an edentulous clutch former to facilitate the efficient fabrication of clutches. The dentulous clutch former is used for all clutch fabrication except for the totally edentulous patient.

---

*Such clutches are sometimes called registration trays. (S.D.T.)

Dentulous patient

An ideal clutch is one that is very thin over the tops of the cusps but thick for rigidity in the central sections without soft-tissue impingement. The impressions made by the teeth should be very slight with little or no detail but positive enough to provide accurate indexing to the teeth. With a little experience, this can be accomplished routinely.

The clutch former is a template mechanism that locates two acrylic clutch frames (Fig. 28-10) in proper position for construction of clutches directly in the mouth. A spacer is used to relocate the lower or upper clutch frame distally to accommodate class II or class III arch relations. When the lower clutch frame is repositioned distally with the spacer to accommodate extreme class II arch relations, the clutch die is pulled to its most distal position and the opening that oc-

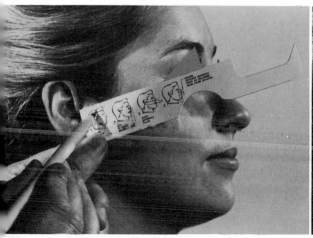
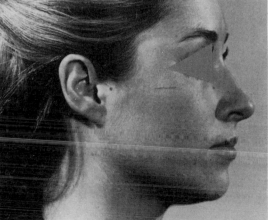

Fig. 28-8   **Fig. 28-9**

Fig. 28-8. Position reference plane locator forward from middle of upper margin of external auditory meatus to outer canthus of eye and mark posterior reference points through hole provided in reference plane locator. Align reference plane locator between anterior and posterior reference points on right side of patient just out of contact with patient's face so as not to displace skin; scribe reference plane on right side of patient's face. (Courtesy Denar Corp., Anaheim, Calif.)

Fig. 28-9. Initial references, posterior reference points, and horizontal plane of reference scribed on patient's face. (Courtesy Denar Corp., Anaheim, Calif.)

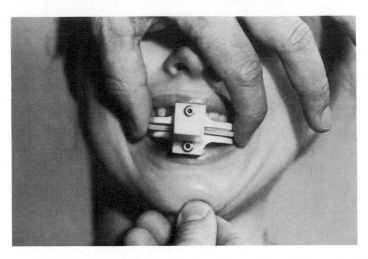

Fig. 28-10. Clutch former in patient's mouth. (Courtesy Denar Corp., Anaheim, Calif.)

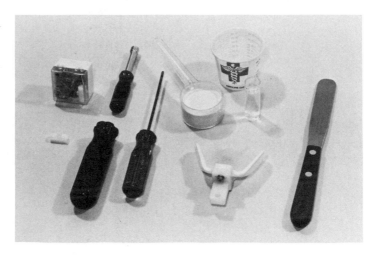

Fig. 28-11. Equipment and material needed for clutch construction. (Courtesy Denar Corp., Anaheim, Calif.)

curs anteriorly between the clutch frames is occluded with utility wax to prevent the bonding together of the upper and lower clutches. Anteriorly the clutch frame has a precision index to which an anterior crossbar assembly can be precisely located. Laterally it has retentive side arms to which cold-cure acrylic will bond. To accommodate wide arches, one may reshape these side arms. Interposed between the clutch frames is the rubber clutch die, which prevents the cold-cure

acrylic of the upper and lower clutches from bonding to each other during clutch fabrication. On the inferior surface of the clutch die, a center bearing screw is supported in the correct location for incorporation by the cold-cure acrylic into the mandibular clutch. On its superior surface is a form over which is cast the area in the maxillary clutch, which the center bearing screw will glide in when the patient executes mandibular movements. This form, cast in the maxillary clutch,

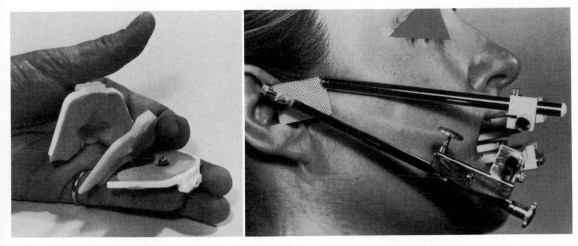

Fig. 28-12   **Fig. 28-13**

Fig. 28-12. Disassembled clutch former. (Courtesy Denar Corp., Anaheim, Calif.)
Fig. 28-13. Stylus against microdot pattern in hinge-axis analyzer. (Courtesy Denar
Corp., Anaheim, Calif.)

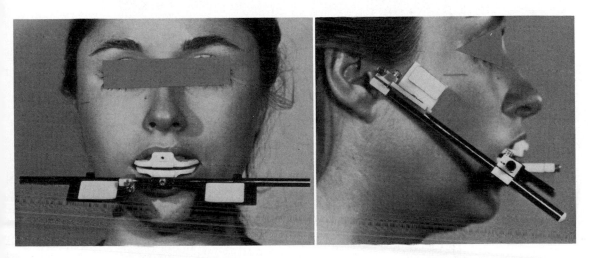

Fig. 28-14   **Fig. 28-15**

Fig. 28-14. Clutches checked in patient's mouth for stability. (Courtesy Denar Corp.,
Anaheim, Calif.)
Fig. 28-15. Reference plane supports rod clamp parallel to reference plane scribed on
patient's face. Posterior reference pins are horizontal and lightly touch posterior
reference points marked on patient's skin. (Courtesy Denar Corp., Anaheim, Calif.)

subconsciously encourages (propriocep-
tively programs) patient cooperation in
executing directed excursive movements
(Fig. 28-11). Three fourths of a vial of
monomer will produce the correct amount

of acrylic resin to fabricate clutches.
Slightly more than half the mix is used to
fabricate the upper clutch. Immerse the
loaded clutch former in hot water to
hasten cure. Allow the acrylic resin to set

beyond the tacky stage to a tough consistency that resists displacement.

While supporting the clutch former in the intermaxillary space with the left hand, guide the patient in terminal hinge closure to obtain desired impressions of teeth. Immediately remove the clutch former from the mouth. When the acrylic has set to a very tough consistency, return the clutch former to the mouth for final cure and maximum accuracy.

Disassemble the clutch former (Fig. 28-12). Check the clutches in the mouth

for stability (Figs. 28-13 and 28-14). Adjust center bearing screw height so that there is a 1 mm clearance between clutches when the mandible is in the terminal hinge position. IMPORTANT: In attaching anterior crossbar assemblies of the pantograph or face-bow to the clutch, always completely index the crossbar assembly and the clutch before inserting the screw. This will support the projecting nozzle on the clutch index and prevent its breakage when the screw is inserted. Always use a screw length that

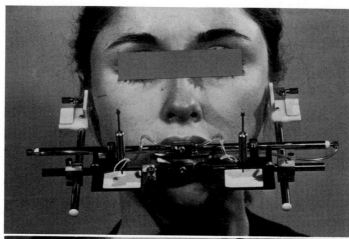

Fig. 28-16

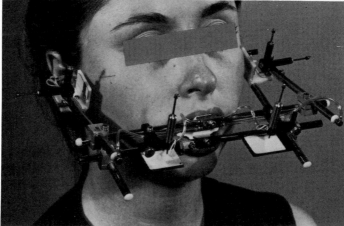

Fig. 28-17

Fig. 28-16. Anterior recorder assembly attached to mandibular clutch. (Courtesy Denar Corp., Anaheim, Calif.)

Fig. 28-17. Assembled Denar pantograph prior to attachment of control valve to pantograph manifold. (Courtesy Denar Corp., Anaheim, Calif.)

gives full-length thread engagement to the clutch, and do not overtighten so as not to strip plastic threads in clutch.

DENAR PANTOGRAPH

The Denar pantograph is a precision mandibular movement recording instrument (Figs. 28-15 to 28-17). It provides the dentist with an accurate, simple, and fast means of recording mandibular movement and jaw positions. Pneumatically powered from the dental air syringe, a push-button controlled device auto-matically and simultaneously lifts all styli upon the dentist's command (Fig. 28-18). This enables the dentist to obtain a total recording of the patient's mandibular movements and to discriminate between erratic abnormal jaw movements and pure peripheral movements in a practical efficient manner. Additionally, the pantograph permits each record and procedural step to be double-checked for accuracy before one proceeds to the next step. To ensure accuracy, the styli are depressed and their relation to the scribings

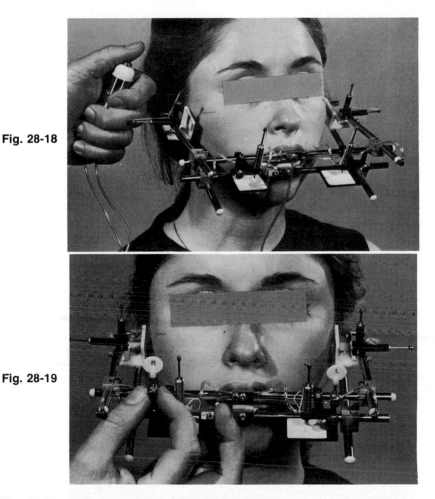

Fig. 28-18

Fig. 28-19

Fig. 28-18. Stylus control valve connected to pantograph manifold; when lever is depressed, styli are held in retracted position. (Courtesy Denar Corp., Anaheim, Calif.)
Fig. 28-19. Patient in centric relation; heated pins are placed in wax wells and are secured. (Courtesy Denar Corp., Anaheim, Calif.)

is confirmed as the patient maintains centric relation (Fig. 28-19). The centric pins are heated and placed into the wax walls and secured.

Although there are many reasons for the simplicity and ease of operation of the Denar pantograph, one of the most important is the ease of clutch construction.

One-step transfer

The Denar pantograph, unlike original research instruments, can be transferred directly to the articulator, eliminating the necessity of additional procedural steps employing a mounting stand.

Systems approach

The design of the Denar clutch former, pantograph, and D5A articulator reflects the systems approach to the solution of problems that heretofore prevented the reduction of sophisticated researches to practical application. Engineered into the system's design are features that produce results or conveniences automatically. For example, the center bearing screw of the lower clutch will always be in correct relation to the center bearing screw area of the upper clutch. The crossbars of the

pantograph will be properly aligned on the patient's face. The pantograph and articulator design are compatible. The pantograph transfers directly to the articulator. The pantograph is constructed to complement the articulator and the side arms of the pantograph do not crisscross. This allows the upper member of the articulator along with the attached upper members of the pantograph to be lifted easily from their lower counterparts for convenient change or modification of fossa guide inserts. Additionally, since all scribers are constant to the upper assembly, the record tables and recorded lines are constant to the lower assembly and condyles. This allows easy interpretation of the recording. The resultant savings in time and accuracy are of extreme significance to a practicing dentist.

Transferring the pantograph to the Denar D5A articulator

The posterior reference pins are screwed all the way in and the telescoping mounting axis is expanded to index over the tips of the posterior reference pins (Fig. 28-20). The number on the scale indicates the position to which the

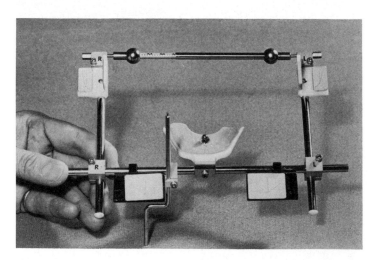

Fig. 28-20. Transfer of pantograph to Denar articulator. (Courtesy Denar Corp., Anaheim, Calif.)

vertical axes are adjusted to accept the pantograph. The vertical axes are adjusted to this position.

The articulator is prepared to receive the pantograph by the anteroposterior angle of the eminentia being set to 25 to 30 degrees. The progressive sideshift is set to 5 degrees. All other adjustments, including the vertical dimension of the incisal pin and the incisal table adjustments, are set to zero. Mounting studs are positioned in the holes provided in the lateral aspects of the condylar elements.

The recorder is transferred to the articulator by the posterior reference pins, which are indexed in the holes provided in the lateral extremities of the mounting studs (Fig. 28-21). The reference plane support rod is allowed to rest on the surface bearing the articulator. A mounting stand is constructed by attachment of the recorder to the lower mounting plate with dental stone. A manufactured mounting stand is also available.

The upper member of the articulator is positioned on the lower and engaged in

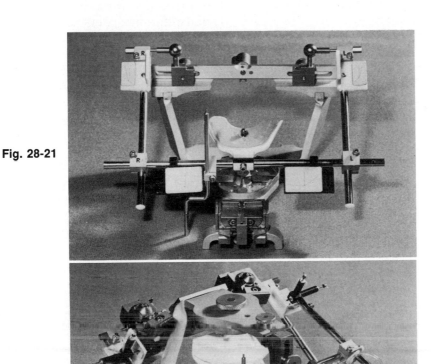

Fig. 28-21

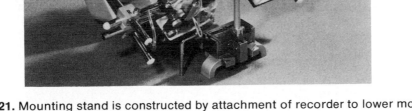

Fig. 28-22

Fig. 28-21. Mounting stand is constructed by attachment of recorder to lower mounting plate with dental stone.

Fig. 28-22. Study cast secured in maxillary clutch for mounting. (Courtesy Denar Corp., Anaheim, Calif.)

the lock-open position with the centric latch. An elastic may be used to ensure positive seating of the condyles in their respective fossa. The right and left centric pins are accurately located in their respective guide tubes in exactly the same orientation they had when the wax chilled about them. The scriber is then oriented to the recorder by the centric pins, which are indexed in the impressions they made in the hard inlay wax in the wax wells on the recorder. The maxillary clutch is allowed to rest on the center bearing screw in the lower clutch prior to securing of the maxillary clutch to the upper mounting ring.

When the scriber is transferred to the articulator, a cast may or may not be placed in the maxillary clutch for mounting (Fig. 28-22). In almost all cases, clutches are constructed and the pantographic record is obtained prior to tooth preparation. Generally a study cast—or, if sufficient unprepared teeth remain for accurate orientation of the cast in the clutch, a working cast—is transferred to the articulator simultaneously with the pantograph. If extensive tooth preparation is to be performed, it is recommended that the pantographic record be obtained prior to tooth preparation and subsequently, after the teeth are prepared, the working cast be transferred to the articulator with a face-bow.

If a maxillary cast is to be transferred to the articulator simultaneously with the pantograph, the cast is accurately indexed in the upper clutch and secured with sticky wax. If the cast does not seal accurately in the clutch, it may be necessary to remove the maxillary clutch from the scriber and trim away excess acrylic with a vulcanite bur or a Fastcut stone.

If the dentist elects not to transfer the maxillary cast to the articulator at this time but will transfer only the pantograph to the articulator to diagnose temporomandibular joint characteristics, he will subsequently transfer the maxillary cast

to the articulator by means of a face-bow. In this case additional retention of the upper clutch should be achieved by adaption of additional cold-cure acrylic retentive modules to the superior surface of the clutch.

Fig. 28-23 illustrates a study cast transferred to the articulator simultaneously with the pantograph and secured to the maxillary bow with dental stone. The mounting studs, which may interfere with the adjustment of the posterior walls, must be removed. Support the hinge-axis reference pin and loosen the hinge-axis pin support. Retract the posterior reference pins and remove the hinge-axis pin support. The mounting studs can then be removed. Remove the centric pins and the reference plane support rod. Retract the styli. Open the articulator and turn the centric latch to the neutral position.

The maxillary bow with attached scriber assembly can be removed from the mandibular bow for convenient modification of the fossa inserts if desired (Fig. 28-24). Diagnosing temporomandibular joint characteristics by setting the articulator to the pantographic record is described on p. 692.

FACE-BOW TRANSFER

A dental face-bow is used to transfer the relationship of the dental structures (maxillary cast) to a mechanical equivalent of the lower half of the head (dental articulator) in the same relation to posterior-control areas (fossa-condylar region) as the dental structures of the patient. The Denar Pantograph also functions as a face-bow and can be used to accomplish this procedure (see Fig. 28-20).

Posterior reference points are established, and a clutch, edentulous clutch, or bite fork is indexed to the maxillary teeth or arch. The face-bow is then attached to one of the aforementioned devices and adjusted so as to register the location of

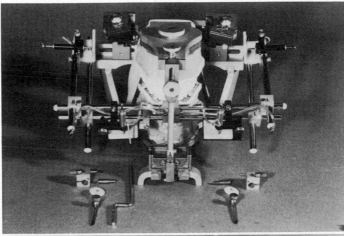

Fig. 28-23

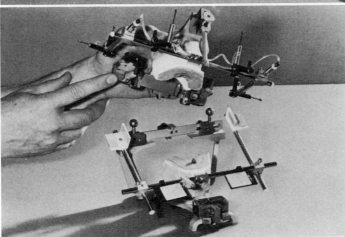

Fig. 28-24

Fig. 28-23. Components removed from articulator-pantograph assembly to facilitate adjustment procedure. (Courtesy Denar Corp., Anaheim, Calif.)

Fig. 28-24. Maxillary bow with attached scriber assembly removed from mandibular bow for modification of fossa insertion, if desired. (Courtesy Denar Corp., Anaheim, Calif.)

the maxillary arch to the posterior reference points and horizontal reference plane. Subsequently the face-bow is used to transfer this relationship to the dental articulator. When a bite fork is used to register to the maxillary teeth, a thin layer of low-fusing impression compound is attached to its superior surface. The compound is flamed to a dead soft consistency and then tempered in a water bath. The bite fork is then carefully and lightly indexed to the maxillary teeth so as not to displace mobile teeth, and the compound

is allowed to cool. The objective is to achieve slight impressions of cusp tips only, without penetration of the compound. The dental cast should then be tried in the bite fork registration to confirm accurate seating.

An anterior crossbar assembly is secured to the bite fork, and the assembly is brought to the mouth and indexed to the maxillary teeth. The patient is instructed to maintain the position of this assembly with a thumb.

Orient the face-bow side arms so that

the posterior reference pins are horizontal and lightly touch the posterior reference points on the patient's face. The posterior reference pins should be completely screwed into their housings when this is done. Secure the side-arm clamps as tightly as possible. Adjust the reference plane support rod clamp parallel to the reference plane scribed on the patient's face.

Insert the reference plane support rod in the reference plane support rod clamp, approaching it from its inferior surface. Index the reference plane locator on the reference plane support rod in the hole provided. With the reference plane locator resting on its support rod, adjust the position of the reference plane support rod up or down and, by line of sight, accurately orient the reference plane locator coincidental to the horizontal reference plane on the patient's face by the posterior reference pins and the anterior reference point. Secure the reference plane support rod in its clamp with the offset in the rod to the left. The posterior reference pins are retracted into their housing so as not to scratch the patient's face on removal. One can now remove the face-bow record from the mouth and use it to accurately relate a maxillary cast in an articulator.

The telescoping mounting axis is extended to index over the tips of the hinge-axis pins. The calibrated scale indicates the position to which the vertical axes of rotation of the articulator are adjusted in order to accept the recorder.

The vertical axes of the articulator are adjusted to this dimension. Be sure to adjust the mediolateral location of the fossa elements first. Mounting studs are indexed in the lateral aspects of the condylar elements.

The face-bow can now be indexed to the articulator by indexing of the posterior reference pins in the holes provided in the mounting studs. The maxillary cast is secured to the bite fork with a rubber band or sticky wax. If the maxillary cast is heavy and causes deflection of the face-bow, the bite fork should be supported with a maxillary cast support.

The centric latch can be used to hold the articulator in the lock-open position to facilitate laboratory procedures in securing the maxillary cast to the mounting plate. Care should be taken in closing the articulator after the mounting stone has been added to ensure that the condylar elements maintain contact with the superior and rear fossa walls.

Adapt a small piece of wax to the anterior margin of the mounting plate prior to mounting to it. This will provide a key way after mounting into which a plaster knife can be inserted to facilitate easy removal of the mounting stone.

ADJUSTING THE D5A ARTICULATOR TO THE PANTOGRAPHIC RECORD

When the pantograph is transferred to the articulator, if the articulator is adjusted to duplicate exactly the temporomandibular joint characteristics of the patient, it will accurately describe the protrusive, orbiting, and rotating condylar paths of the patient and the styli will track the recorded lines. Conversely, if the articulator is adjusted so that the styli accurately track the recorded lines, the temporomandibular joints characteristic of the patient will be simulated in the fossa-condylar control elements of the articulator. Furthermore, these characteristics will have been reduced to a numeric value of millimeters or degrees expressed on the calibrated adjustment scales of the articulator.

Depending on the dentist's objectives, the articulator may be adjusted so the styli (1) accurately follow the lines, or (2) follow a path relative to the lines. Generally speaking, most accurate reproduction of the patient's mandibular movement can be accomplished most efficiently by selection of the appropriate fossa inserts or by custom modification of

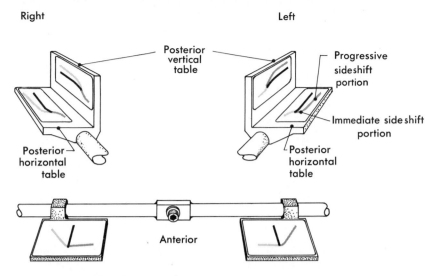

Right   Left

Posterior
vertical
table

Progressive
sideshift
portion

Immediate side shift
portion

Posterior
horizontal
table

Posterior
horizontal
table

Anterior

Fig. 28-25. Correlation of pantographic tracings to excursive movements.

these inserts. Fig. 28-25 is a diagrammatic illustration of the pantographic recording tables. The black lines reflect the characteristics of the protrusive condylar path (character and anteroposterior inclination of the eminentia). The shorter light lines reflect the characteristics of the rotating condylar path (sagittal displacements of the rotating condyle—the horizontal table reflects backward-forward displacements, the vertical table reflects up-down displacements). The longer light lines reflect the characteristics of the orbiting condylar path (the vertical table reflects the character and anteroposterior inclination of the eminentia; the horizontal table registers timing of the sideshift—immediate and progressive).

When adjusting the D5A to pantographic writings, the operator should be thoroughly familiar with the significance of each line in the tracings and which characteristic of the temporomandibular articulation it most graphically reflects. When studying Fig. 28-25, remember that the styli are fixed to the maxilla and fossae and that the record tables move with the mandible and condyles. The operator should also be thoroughly familiar with

the location of the articulator adjustments that control the mechanical equivalents of these temporomandibular joint characteristics and with the location of the corresponding lock screws and scales of these adjustments.

When setting an articulator to pantographic scribings, the operator should know whether it will be to his advantage or disadvantage to have the articulator accurately reproduce mandibular movement (styli follow the lines) when the articulator is being used in its treatment function to define the occlusal anatomy of a restoration under construction. If it is not to his advantage to have the articulator reproduce mandibular movement, he should know where the stylus should be set relative to the line to have the instrument produce the movements that will dictate the desired occlusal form. This knowledge will permit the operator to set the articulator to the scribings with the minimal expenditure of time and effort so it will produce a movement that will permit the least potential for error.

In adjusting an articulator to pantographic tracings, the operator must manipulate the articulator in a manner to

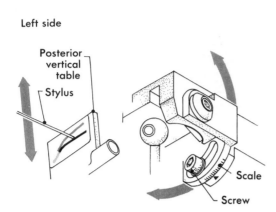

Fig. 28-26. Setting anteroposterior angle of eminentia or protrusive path adjustment (protrusive excursion illustrated).

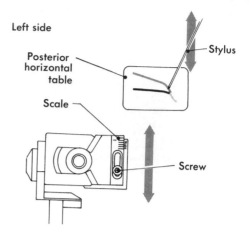

Fig. 28-27. Setting immediate sideshift on medial fossa wall adjustment (right lateral excursion illustrated).

maintain positive contact of the condyles against the appropriate fossa-bearing surfaces. With a little experience the operator will soon develop the best hand grasps of the instrument to accomplish this most conveniently.

The recommended technique to employ in adjusting an articulator to pantographic scribings is to move the articulator in a test excursive movement in the appropriate direction while observing the movement of the styli relative to the line to which it is being adjusted. If a modification of the temporomandibular joint characteristic of the articulator is indicated, this adjustment is made and another test excursion is executed. This procedure is repeated until the desired setting is achieved.

SEQUENCE OF ADJUSTMENTS

1. *Protrusive:* The articulator is manipulated so that all vertical styli track the protrusive lines. One adjusts the protrusive condylar path by setting the posterior horizontal styli relative to the black line in Fig. 28-26.
2. *Immediate sideshift:* The outer line on the horizontal record table is inspected to determine its character and the appropriate medial fossa wall is selected or the visually determined amount of immediate sideshift is introduced into the instrument

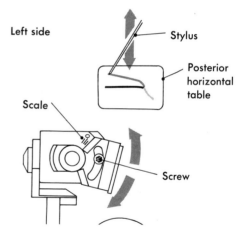

Fig. 28-28. Setting progressive sideshift on medial fossa wall adjustment (right lateral excursion illustrated).

for trial. The articulator is manipulated in the appropriate lateral excursive movement, and the immediate sideshift is timed by adjustment of the posterior vertical styli relative to the immediate-sideshift portion of the outer line on the posterior horizontal table, as illustrated in Fig. 28-27.
3. *Progressive sideshift:* The articulator is manipulated in the appropriate lateral excursive movement and the progressive sideshift is adjusted by a setting of the posterior vertical styli relative to the outer line on the posterior horizontal table, as illustrated in Fig. 28-28.

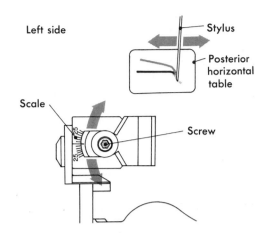

Fig. 28-29. Setting rear wall on forward and backward displacement of rotating condyle adjustment (right lateral excursion illustrated).

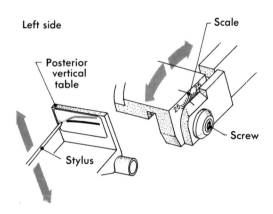

Fig. 28-30. Setting top wall on upward and downward displacement of rotating condyle adjustment (left lateral excursion illustrated).

4. *Rear-wall adjustment (anteroposterior inclination of rotating path):* The articulator is manipulated in the appropriate lateral excursive movement and the rear wall is adjusted by a setting of the posterior vertical styli relative to the short line on the posterior horizontal record table, as illustrated in Fig. 28-29.

5. *Vertical axis adjustment (mediolateral location of fossa condylar elements):* After the rear wall adjustment is made, the anterior vertical styli will most often accurately trace the anterior gothic arch tracings. If the styli do not track the medial legs of the tracings accurately, the articulator is manipulated in the appropriate lateral excursive movement and the vertical axes are adjusted until the styli track the medial leg of the anterior tracing. Moving the vertical axes medially relocates the medial leg of the anterior tracing more anteriorly relative to the styli, and vice versa.

6. *Orbiting path:* The articulator is manipulated in the appropriate excursive movement and the anteroposterior angle of the eminentia is adjusted by a setting of the posterior horizontal styli relative to the long upper (light) line on the posterior vertical record table, as illustrated in Fig. 28-26.

7. *Top wall adjustment (upward-downward inclination of rotating path):* The articulator is manipulated in the appropriate lateral excursive movement and the mediolateral inclination of the superior fossa wall is adjusted by a setting of the posterior horizontal stylus relative to the short (light) line on the vertical record table, as illustrated in Fig. 28-30.

RECIPROCAL INFLUENCE OF ADJUSTMENT

Reciprocal means "expression of mutual influence or relation." When the pantograph is assembled, although the styli will move in and out of their respective cylinders, they all have certain fixed relations to each other. Therefore when an articulator is adjusted to move one stylus relative to a line, that adjustment may have a mutual or reciprocal influence on other styli relative to their recorded lines. The listed sequence of settings takes into consideration the reciprocal influence of adjustments and sets forth the recommended sequence for most efficient adjustment of an articulator to pantographic scribings. However, an understanding of the reciprocal influence of adjustments is an aid in setting the articulator. These reciprocal influences can be categorized into three classes: (1) protrusive (right and left); (2) horizontal (settings 2-3-4-5); and (3) orbiting-rotating (settings 6-7).

Protrusive. When one adjusts the protrusive path, an adjustment of one side of the articulator will have a reciprocal influence on the horizontal stylus on the opposite side of the instrument. Therefore the location of both horizontal styli should be given consideration when adjusting the protrusive paths.

Horizontal. The vertical styli tracings reflect the translations and rotations of the mandible in the horizontal plane. All vertical styli are fixed relative to each other, and an adjustment of any one stylus has a reciprocal effect on the other three. It is important that settings 2, 3, 4, and 5 be done in that sequence.

Orbiting-rotating. The setting of the stylus to the orbiting path has a reciprocal influence on the position of the opposite horizontal styli relative to the rotating line. Therefore the location of both horizontal styli should be given consideration when one adjusts the orbiting condylar path (setting 6) and the opposing rotating condylar path (setting 7).

CHECKBITE PROCEDURE

The checkbite procedure is employed to register the relation of the mandibular dental structures of the patient to the maxillary structures by means of an interocclusal or checkbite record. The checkbite record is subsequently used to accurately locate the mandibular cast in the articulation at the recorded position. Checkbite records can be used to register centric and eccentric mandibular positions at any vertical dimension.

Transfer the maxillary cast to the articulator by registering the relation of the maxillary structures of the patient to the initial references with a face-bow. Subsequently this record is used to accurately locate the maxillary cast in the articulator for mounting. Transfer the mandibular cast to the articulator by occluding it with the maxillary cast, checkbite procedure, or a combination of the two.

In the transfer of the mandibular cast to the articulator, if the mandibular cast can be occluded accurately in the most intercusped position, the most accurate way to transfer the mandibular cast to the articulator is by occlusion of it with the maxillary cast. However, if deflective contacts

exist, these must either be removed by grinding so that the cast can be accurately oriented in the desired most intercusped position or the centric relation record must be taken at an increased vertical dimension by checkbite procedure.

A combination of occluding casts and checkbite registration is employed when there is an absence of deflective contacts but there is insufficient interocclusal contacts to establish stability or accurate orientation of casts to each other. This condition is frequently established after partial mouth-tooth preparation and equilibration of the unprepared teeth.

There are many satisfactory recording agents such as waxes and bite-registration pastes, and many techniques with which these agents can be employed to advantage in checkbite registration. However, there is no universal method that proves optimal in all situations. Therefore the dentist must be knowledgeable in the anatomy of the related structures, in neuromuscle physiology, and in the physical properties of dental materials that determine checkbite accuracy. This will enable him to effect a method of choice as varying situations present themselves.

It is not within the scope of this chapter to present an exhaustive discourse on checkbite procedure. However, one recommended procedure that affects the basic principle of checkbite technique is presented. Variations of this technique can be employed as circumstances dictate. The following basic principles should always be employed in any checkbite technique:

1. The checkbite record should be obtained as close to the vertical dimension at which the restoration is to be constructed as possible.
2. The recording medium interposed between the teeth should be of a dead soft consistency as the mandible is brought to the desired position so as to prevent deflection of the

mandible or mobile teeth, or the programming of muscle function.

Technique

The following technique can be used to register the mandibular position at the correct vertical dimension or at an increased vertical dimension. It can be used to register centric or eccentric positions. Described will be the registration of the centric relation position of the mandible at the minimal increase of vertical dimension that will result in lack of posterior tooth contact.

Fabricate an occlusal programmer by softening a small piece of base plate wax in a water bath to a soft consistency and adapt it over several teeth in the anterior segment of the mouth. Manipulate the mandible into centric relation and gently guide the patient in terminal hinge closure lightly tapping the soft wax. Establish a broad simultaneous contact of several mandibular teeth with the wax. The wax is then removed from the mouth and chilled in tap water. The thickness of wax used should be the minimum to effect posterior disocclusion.

Apply a small amount of denture adhesive cream to the wax (occlusal programmer) in the area that adapts to the lingual surfaces of the maxillary anterior teeth. Reposition the occlusal programmer in the mouth by reindexing it to the maxillary teeth. This occlusal programmer thus establishes a predetermined stop to vertical closure with the condyles in centric relation and with an absence of contacting deflective inclines by group functioning of teeth in the anterior segment of the mouth where the occluding pressures are the least. The occlusal programmer reprograms muscle function so as to eliminate resistance to terminal hinge closure previously programmed by deflective contacts, and the dentist can now more easily manipulate the mandible in repeated terminal hinge closure in accomplishing the checkbite record.

Similar occlusal programmers can be fabricated in eccentric position to facilitate obtaining eccentric checkbite records.

Suitable checkbite recording medium is placed on the mandibular posterior teeth area and the mandible is guided in terminal hinge closure. The checkbite recording medium is allowed to harden without the patient executing a biting pressure. Block out deep fissures, grooves, and undercuts on the teeth and cavity preparations by wiping petroleum jelly over the teeth with the index finger before a zinc oxide–eugenol paste material is used for checkbite registration.

Occlusal programmers can be constructed to index the mandible in protrusive, rigid lateral, and left lateral mandibular positions to facilitate obtaining of checkbite records of these mandibular positions.

Maximum accuracy can be ensured if the fossa-condylar settings are adjusted to the patient's temporomandibular joint characteristic prior to the time the mandibular cast is transferred to the articulator. This procedure should always be followed when casts on which restorations are to be constructed are transferred to the articulator. If the temporomandibular joint characteristics are unknown when the mandibular cast is transferred to the articulator, the anteroposterior angle of the eminentia should be set to 25 to 30 degrees and the progressive sideshift adjustments are set to 5 to 10 degrees. All other adjustments are set to zero.

The articulator is inverted, and the mandibular cast is accurately oriented to the mandibular cast by means of the interocclusal checkbite record. The mandibular cast is secured to the mounting plate with dental stone.

Eccentric checkbite technique

The anteroposterior angle of the eminentia and the progressive sideshift adjustment of the articulator can be set to eccentric checkbites.

Protrusive adjustment. The incisal pin assembly is removed from the articulator. Set the progressive sideshift adjustment to its maximum setting and set all other adjustments to zero including the angle of the eminentia. Place the protrusive checkbite record (not the occlusal programmer) on the mandibular cast. Relate the maxillary bow of the articulator to the mandibular by carefully seating the maxillary cast in the checkbite record. Stabilize the casts in the checkbite record by lightly pressing on the top of the articulator. Note that the condylar elements are displaced away from the posterior, medial, and superior walls of the fossa. Increase the anteroposterior angle of the eminentia until the superior wall of the fossa contacts the condylar element. Lock the fossa in this position and repeat on the opposite side.

Progressive sideshift adjustment. Place the lateral checkbite record on the mandibular cast. Relate the maxillary bow of the articulator to the mandibular bow by carefully seating the maxillary cast in the checkbite record. Stabilize the casts in the checkbite, applying slight pressure to the top of the articulator. Note that the medial fossa wall does not contact the condylar element. Decrease the progressive side shift adjustment from its maximum setting until the medial fossa wall contacts the condylar element. Lock the medial fossa wall in this position and repeat on the opposite side.

GENERAL REFERENCES

Arstad, T.: Capsular ligaments of the temporomandibular joint and the retrusion facets of the dentition in relationship to mandibular movements, Am. Equilibration Soc. Compend. **4**:24, 1960 (abstr.).

Atwood, D. A.: A critique of research of the posterior limit of the mandibular position, J. Prosthet. Dent. **20**:21, 1968.

Atwood, D. A.: A critique of research of the rest position of the mandible, J. Prosthet. Dent. **16**:848, 1966.

Aull, A. E.: Condylar determinants of occlusal patterns, J. Prosthet. Dent. **15**:826-846, 1965.

Avery, J. K., and Rapp, R.: Investigation of the mechanism of neural impulse transmission in human teeth, Oral Surg. **12**:190, 1959.

Baer, P. N.: Analysis of physiologic rest position, centric relation, centric occlusion, J. Periodont. **27**:181, 1956.

Ballard, C. F.: Consideration of the physiological background of mandibular posture and movement, Trans. Br. Soc. Study Orthodont., pp. 117, 126, 1955.

Baraban, D. J.: Establishing centric relation and vertical dimension in occlusal rehabilitation, J. Prosthet. Dent. **12**:1157, 1962.

Beck, H. O.: Jaw registrations and articulators, J.A.D.A. **73**:863, 1966.

Beck, H. O., and Morrison, W. E.: Method for reproduction of movements of the mandible; research progress report, J. Prosthet. Dent. **12**:873, 1962.

Bell, D. H.: Sagittal balance of the mandible, J.A.D.A. **64**:486-495, 1962.

Bennett, G. T.: The kinematic geometry of the small movements of the mandible, Br. Dent. J. **45**:228, 1924.

Bennett, N. G.: Contribution to the study of the movements of the mandible, J. Prosthet. Dent. **8**:41, 1958.

Bergman, S. A.: Importance of temporomandibular joint roentgenograms in mouth rehabilitation, N.Y. Dent. J. **20**:103, 1954.

Berman, M. H.: Accurate interocclusal records, J. Prosthet. Dent. **10**:620, 1960.

Berry, D. C.: Constancy of the rest position of the mandible, Dent. Pract. Dent. Rec. **10**:129, 1960.

Berry, H. M., Jr., and Hoffmann, F. A.: Cineradiographic observations of temporomandibular joint function, J. Prosthet. Dent. **9**:21, 1959.

Beyron, H. L.: Characteristics of functionally optimal occlusion and principles of occlusal rehabilitation, J.A.D.A. **48**:648, 1954.

Bolender, C. L.: Significance of vertical dimension in prosthetic dentistry, J. Prosthet. Dent. **6**:177, 1956.

Boos, R. H.: Maxillomandibular relations, occlusion, and the temporomandibular joint, Dent. Clin. North Am., pp. 19-35, March 1962.

Boos, R. H.: Vertical, centric and functional dimensions recorded by gnathodynamics, J.A.D.A. **59**:682, 1959.

Borgh, O., and Posselt, U.: Hinge axis registration: experiments on the articulator, Odont. Revy **7**:214, 1956; J. Prosthet. Dent. **8**:35-40, 1958.

Boucher, C. O.: Maxillomandibular relations and records, Trans. Am. Dent. Soc. Europe **68**:8, 1962 (abstr.).

Boucher, C. O.: Occlusion in prosthodontics, J. Prosthet. Dent. **3**:633-656, 1953.

Boucher, L. J.: Limiting factors in posterior movements of mandibular condyles, J. Prosthet. Dent. **11**:23-25, 1961.

Boucher, L. J.: Anatomy of the temporomandibular joint as it pertains to centric relation, J. Prosthet. Dent. **12**:464 (disc. pp. 473-475), 1962.

Boucher, L. J., and Jacoby, J.: Posterior border movements of the human mandible, J. Prosthet. Dent. **11**:836, 1961.

Boyd, J. B., Jr.: Relationship between occlusion, occlusal equilibration and crown and bridgework and partial denture prosthesis, Alum. Bull. Indiana Univ. School Dent., pp. 4-7, 36-38, Aug. 1959.

Brodie, A. G.: The three arcs of mandibular movement as they affect wear of the teeth, Lecture presented before the University of Illinois Orthodontic Alumni Meeting, Chicago, March 1968.

Brotman, D. N.: Hinge axis, J. Prosthet. Dent. **10**: 436, 631, 636, 1960.

Chestner, S. B.: Considerations in the prescription of occlusal rehabilitation, J.A.D.A. **55**:790, 1957.

Christensen, F. T.: Effect of incisal guidance on cusp angulation in prosthetic occlusion, J. Prosthet. Dent. **11**:48, 1961.

Christiansen, R. L.: Rationale of the face bow in maxillary cast mounting, J. Prosthet. Dent. **9**:388, 1959.

Cohen, R.: More on the Bennett movement, J. Prosthet. Dent. **9**:788, 1959.

Cohen, R.: Hinge axis and its practical application in the determination of centric relation, J. Prosthet. Dent. **10**:248, 1960.

Cohn, L. A.: Integrating treatment procedures in occluso-rehabilitation, J. Prosthet. Dent. **7**:511, 1957.

Cohn, L. A.: Two techniques for interocclusal records, J. Prosthet. Dent. **13**:438, 1963.

Cooper, H., Jr.: Bridge construction; functional occlusion in bridgework, J. Michigan Dent. Assoc. **40**:296, 1958.

Courtade, G. L.: Foreword to symposium on occlusal rehabilitation, Dent. Clin. North Am., pp. 575-576, Nov. 1963.

D'Amico, A.: The canine teeth—normal functional relation of the natural teeth of man, J. South. Calif. Dent. Assoc. **26**:1, 49, 127, 175, 194, 239, 1958.

D'Amico, A.: Application of the concept of the functional relation of the canine teeth, J. South. Calif. Dent. Assoc. **27**:39, 1959.

D'Amico, A.: Functional occlusion of the natural teeth of man, J. Prosthet. Dent. **11**:899, 1961.

Decker, J. C.: Traumatic deafness as result of retrusion of condyles of mandible, Ann. Otol. Rhinol. Laryngol. **34**:519, 1925.

Derksen, A. A., and Van Haeringen, W.: Protrusive movement in articulators, J. Dent. Res. **37**:127, 1958.

DiSalvo, N. A.: Neuromuscular mechanisms involved in mandibular movement and posture, Am. J. Orthodontics **47**:330, 1961.

Dixon, A. D.: Structure and functional significance of the intra-articular disc of the human temporomandibular joint, Oral Surg. **15**:48, 1962.

Duncan, E. T., and Williams, S. T.: Evaluation of rest position as a guide in prosthetic treatment, J. Prosthet. Dent. **10**:643, 1960.

Edwards, L. F.: Some anatomic facts and fancies relative to the masticatory apparatus, J. Prosthet. Dent. **5**:825, 1955.

el-Aramany, M. A., George, W. A., and Scott, R. H.: Evaluation of the needle point tracing as a method for determining centric relation, J. Prosthet. Dent. **15**:1043, 1965.

Foster, T. D.: Use of the face-bow in making permanent study casts, J. Prosthet. Dent. **9**:717, 1959.

Fountain, H. W.: Seating the condyles for centric relation records, J. Prosthet. Dent. **11**:1050, 1961.

Franks, A. S. T.: Observations on the rest position of the mandible, J. Dent. Res. **39**:1098, 1960.

Freese, A. S.: Myofascial trigger mechanism in temporomandibular joint and allied disturbances, Oral Surg. **14**:933, 1961.

Garnick, J., and Ramfjord, S. P.: Rest position; an electromyographic and clinical investigation, J. Prosthet. Dent. **12**:895, 1962.

Gehl, D. H.: Vertical dimension, jaw relation records and occlusion, Dent. Clin. North Am., pp. 321-332, July 1960.

Glickman, I.: Occlusion and the periodontium, J. Dent. Res. **46**:53, 1967.

Goodfriend, D. J.: Practical analysis of occlusal procedures, J. Prosthet. Dent. **16**:557-571, 1966.

Gottsegen, R.: Centric relation; the periodontist's viewpoint, J. Prosthet. Dent. **16**:1034-1038, 1966.

Graf, H., and Zander, H. A.: Tooth contact patterns in mastication, J. Prosthet. Dent. **13**:1055-1066, 1963.

Granger, E. R.: Functional relations of the stomatognathic system, J.A.D.A. **48**:638, 1954.

Granger, E. R.: Functional concepts of dentistry, Illinois Dent. J. **25**:226, 1956.

Granger, E. R.: Prosthetic relations of the temporomandibular joint, North-West Dent. **38**:117, 1959.

Granger, E. R.: Clinical significance of the hinge axis mounting, Dent. Clin. North Am., p. 205, March 1959.

Granger, E. R.: Establishment of occlusion: the articulator and the patient, Dent. Clin. North Am., p. 527, Nov. 1962.

Granger, E. R.: Method of recording functional relations, J. South. Calif. Dent. Assoc. **27**:381, 1959.

Granger, E. R.: Practical procedures in oral rehabilitation, Philadelphia, 1962, J. B. Lippincott Co.

Granger, E. R.: Temporomandibular joint in prosthodontics, J. Prosthet. Dent. **10**:239, 1960.

Griffin, C. J., and Sharpe, C. J.: Distribution of elastic tissue in the human temporomandibular meniscus especially in respect to "compression" areas, Australian Dent. J. **7**:72, 1962.

Guichet, N. F.: Procedures for occlusal treatment, Anaheim, California, 1969, Denar Corp.

Gysi, A.: Practical application of research results in denture construction (mandibular movements), George Wood Clapp, Collaborator, J.A.D.A. **16:** 199, 1929.

Hankey, G. T., and Nash, D. F. E.: Temporomandibular disorders, the result of trauma, malocclusion and muscular imbalance, Am. Equilibration Soc. Compend. **4:**86, 1960.

Hickey, J. C., Allison, M. L., Woelfel, J. B., Boucher, C. O., and Stacy, R. W.: Mandibular movements in three dimensions, J. Prosthet. Dent. **13:**72-92, 1963.

Huffman, R. W., Regenos, J. W., and Taylor, R. R.: Principles of occlusion, laboratory and clinical teaching manual (Ohio State University), Columbus, Ohio, 1969, Huffman & Regenos Press.

Hughes, G. A., and Regli, C. P.: What is centric relation, J. Prosthet. Dent. **11:**16-22, 1961.

Hurst, W. W.: Vertical dimension and its correlation with lip length and interocclusal distance, J.A.D.A. **64:**496, 1962.

Isaacson, D.: Clinical study of the Bennett movement, J. Prosthet. Dent. **8:**64, 1958.

Jacobsen, A. M.: Function analysis of temporomandibular joint disturbances, J. South. Calif. Dent. Assoc. **30:**35, 1962.

Jankelson, B.: Physiology of human dental occlusion, J.A.D.A. **50:**671, 1955.

Jankelson, B.: Considerations of occlusion in fixed partial dentures, Dent. Clin. North Am., p. 187, March 1959.

Jankelson, B.: Dental occlusion and the temporomandibular joint, Dent. Clin. North Am., pp. 51-62, March 1962.

Jankelson, B.: A technique for obtaining optimum functional relationship for the natural dentition, Dent. Clin. North Am., pp. 131-141, March 1960.

Jarabak, J. R.: Electromyographic analysis of muscular and temporomandibular joint disturbances due to imbalance in occlusion, Angle Orthodontist **26:**170, 1956.

Jerge, C. R.: The neurologic mechanism underlying cyclic jaw movements, J. Prosthet. Dent. **14:**667-681, 1964.

Jerge, C. R.: Temporomandibular joints and centric relation, Pennsylvania Dent. J. **61:**5, 12, 1957.

Kapur, K. K., and Yurkstas, A. A.: Evaluation of centric relation records obtained by various techniques, J. Prosthet. Dent. **7:**770, 1957.

Kawamura, Y.: Neuromuscular mechanisms of jaw and tongue movement, J.A.D.A. **62:**545, 1961.

Kazis, H., and Kazis, A. J.: Complete mouth rehabilitation, N.Y. J. Dent. **28:**199, 1958.

Kazis, H., and Kazis, A. J.: Complete mouth rehabilitation through fixed partial denture prosthodontics, J. Prosthet. Dent. **10:**296-303, 1960.

Kingery, R. H.: Maxillomandibular relationship of centric relation, J. Prosthet. Dent. **9:**922, 1959.

Koski, K.: Axis of the opening movement of the mandible, J. Prosthet. Dent. **12:**888, 1962.

Krajicek, D. D., Jones, P. M., Radzyminski, S. F., et al.: Clinical and electromyographic study of mandibular rest position, J. Prosthet. Dent. **11:**826, 1961.

Kurth, L. E.: Methods of obtaining vertical dimension and centric relation; a practical evaluation of various methods, J.A.D.A. **59:**669, 1959.

Kurth, L. E.: From mouth to articulator; static jaw relations, J.A.D.A. **64:**517, 1962.

Kyes, F. M.: Temporomandibular joint disorders, J.A.D.A. **59:**1137, 1959.

Lauritzen, A. G., and Bodner, G. H.: Variations in location of arbitrary and true hinge axis points, J. South. Calif. Dent. Assoc. **29:**10, 1961; J. Prosthet. Dent. **11:**224, 1961.

Lauritzen, A. G., and Wolford, L. W.: Hinge axis location on an experimental basis, J. South. Calif. Dent. Assoc. **29:**354, 1961: J. Prosthet. Dent. **11:** 1059, 1961.

La Vere, A. M.: Lateral interocclusal positional records, J. Prosthet. Dent. **19:**350, 1968.

Leff, A.: Gnathodynamics of four mandibular positions, J. Prosthet. Dent. **16:**844, 1966.

Lieb, D. E.: Generated path in fixed denture prosthesis, Minneapolis Dist. Dent. J. **46:**25, 1962.

Lindblom, G.: Anatomy and function of the temporomandibular joint, Acta Odont. Scand. **17** (supp. 28):7, 1960.

Linkow, L. I.: Oral rehabilitation technique utilizing copper band impressions, J. Prosthet. Dent. **11:**716, 1961.

Lipke, D., and Posselt, U.: Functional anatomy of the temporomandibular joint, Am. Equilibration Soc. Compend. **4:**73, 1960.

Lipke, D. P.: Hinge axis and its value, Bull. Greater Milwaukee Dent. Assoc. **25:**197, 1959.

Logan, L. R.: Electromyographic investigation of the occlusal position of the mandible as determined by a hinge axis method, J. South. Calif. Dent. Assoc. **30:**133, 1962.

Lucia, V. O.: Centric relation—theory and practice, J. Prosthet. Dent. **10:**849, 1960.

Lucia, V. O.: Gnathological concept of articulation, Dent. Clin. North Am., pp. 183-197, March 1962.

McCollum, B. B.: A research report; basic text for the postgraduate course in gnathology, South Pasadena, Calif., 1955, The Scientific Press.

McCollum, B. B.: Mandibular hinge axis and a method of locating it, J. Prosthet. Dent. **10:**428, 1960.

MacQueen, D.: Is an early cuspid rise essential to periodontal health?, J. West. Soc. Periodont. **6:**76, 1958.

Mann, A. W., and Pankey, L. D.: Oral rehabilitation:

part I, use of the P-M instrument in treatment planning and in restoring the lower posterior teeth; part II, reconstruction of the upper teeth using a functional generated path technique, J. Prosthet. Dent. **10**:135-162, 1960.

Marevskaya, A. P.: Development of proprioceptive reflexes in the muscles of mastication, Dent. Abstr. **4**:30, 1959.

Mazur, B.: Construction of plastic registration trays, J. Prosthet. Dent. **16**:904, 1966.

Messerman, T.: A means for studying mandibular movements, J. Prosthet. Dent. **17**:36-43, 1967.

Meyer, F. S.: Generated path technique in reconstruction dentistry, II: fixed partial dentures, J. Prosthet. Dent. **9**:432, 1959.

Moller, E.: The chewing apparatus; an electromyographic study of the action of the muscles of mastication and its correlation to facial morphology, Acta Physiol. Scand. **69**(suppl.):280-281, 1966.

Morgan, D. H.: Diagnosis of temporomandibular joint problems, J. South. Calif. Dent. Assoc. **33**:523, 1965.

Moulton, G. H.: Centric occlusion and the freeway space, J. Prosthet. Dent. **7**:209, 1957.

Moulton, G. H.: Importance of centric occlusion in diagnosis and treatment planning, J. Prosthet. Dent. **10**:921, 1960.

Moyers, R. E.: Some physiologic considerations of centric and other jaw relations, J. Prosthet. Dent. **6**:183, 1956.

Murphy, W. M.: Rest position of the mandible, J. Prosthet. Dent. **17**:329, 1967.

Nevakari, K.: Analysis of the mandibular movement from rest to occlusal position; a roentgenographic-cephalometric investigation, Acta Odont. Scand. **14**(suppl. 19):9, 1956.

Niswonger, M. E.: The rest position of the mandible and centric relation, J.A.D.A. **21**:1572, 1934.

Nuttall, E. B.: The principles of obtaining occlusion in occlusal rehabilitation, J. Prosthet. Dent. **13**:699, 1963.

Osborne, J.: Mandibular-maxillary relationships in oral rehabilitation, Int. Dent. J. **16**:308-405, 1966.

Oursland, L. E., and Carlson, R. D.: Study of the horizontal axis of rotation of the mandible, J. South. Calif. Dent. Assoc. **26**:212, 1958.

Parsons, M. T., and Boucher, L. J.: The bilaminar zone of the meniscus, J. Dent. Res. **45**:59-61, 1966.

Perry, H. T.: The temporomandibular joint, Am. J. Orthodont. **52**:399-400, 1966.

Phillips, R. W.: Report of the Committee on Scientific Investigation of the American Academy of Restorative Dentistry, J. Prosthet. Dent. **19**:416, 1968.

Posselt, U.: Hinge opening axis of the mandible, Acta Odont. Scand. **14**:49, 1956.

Posselt, U.: Movement areas of the mandible, J. Prosthet. Dent. **7**:375-385, 1957.

Posselt, U.: The physiology of occlusion, Philadelphia, 1962, F. A. Davis Co.

Posselt, U.: Under what circumstances should the mandible be placed in terminal hinge position in occlusal adjustment or restorative procedures? J. West Soc. Periodont. **5**:5, 1957.

Posselt, U.: An analyzer for mandibular positions, J. Prosthet. Dent. **7**:368, 1957.

Posselt, U.: Range of movement of the mandible, J.A.D.A. **56**:10, 1958.

Posselt, U., and Addiego, B. J.: Gnatho-thesiometric study of various mandibular positions in individuals with normal and abnormal function of the temporomandibular joints, Odont. Revy **9**:1, 1958.

Posselt, U., and Nevstedt, P.: Registration of the condyle path inclination by intraoral wax records—its practical value, J. Prosthet. Dent. **11**:43, 1961.

Posslet, U., and others: The split cast technique, Odont. Revy **13**:270, 1962.

Posselt, U., and Franzen, G.: Registration of the condyle path inclination by intraoral wax records; variations in three instruments, J. Prosthet. Dent. **10**:441, 1960 (reprint).

Posselt, U., and Thilander, B.: Influence of the innervation of the temporomandibular joint capsule on mandibular border movements, Acta Odont. Scand. **23**:601-613, 1965.

Ptack, H.: Temporomandibular joint and its importance to the prosthodontist, J. Can. Dent. Assoc. **26**:341, 1960.

Pyott, J. E., and Schaeffer, A.: Centric relation and vertical dimension by cephalometric roentgenograms, J. Prosthet. Dent. **4**:35, 1954.

Ramfjord, S. P.: Bruxism, a clinical and electromyographic study, J.A.D.A. **62**:21, 1961.

Ramfjord, S. P.: The significance of recent research on occlusion for the teaching and practice of dentistry, J. Prosthet. Dent. **16**:96-105, 1966.

Ramfjord, S. P., and Ash, M.: Occlusion and rehabilitation, Philadelphia, 1966, W. B. Saunders Co.

Ricketts, R. M.: Details of occlusion, Pacific Palisades, Calif., 1966, Dome, Inc.

Ricketts, R. M.: Occlusion—the medium of dentistry, J. Prosthet. Dent. **21**:39, 1969.

Rivalut, M. A., and Tabet, G. A.: Factors determining the movements and positions of the mandible, Int. Dent. J. **11**:217, 1961.

Roberts, M.: Comparison of the rest vertical dimension of the face as determined clinically and electromyographically, Am. J. Orthodontics **45**:872, 1959.

Ross, J. H.: Dentist's responsibilities in temporomandibular joint disturbances, J. Florida Dent. Soc. **32**:17, 1961.

Saizar, P.: Retrusive movement of the mandible, Actualités Odontostomat. **16**:187, 1962.

Sandquist, U.: Some remarks on the background to certain proprioceptive muscle reflexes with special regard to their occurrence in the jaw muscles, Acta Odont. Scand. **18**:331, 1960.

Schei, O., Waerhaug, J., Lovdal, A., and Arno, A.: Tooth mobility and alveolar bone resorption as a function of occlusal stress and oral hygiene, Acta Odont. Scand. **17**:61, 1959.

Schier, M. B. A.: Temporomandibular joint roentgenography; controlled erect technics, J.A.D.A. **65**:456, 1962.

Schuyler, C. H.: Considerations of occlusion in fixed partial dentures, Dent. Clin. North Am., pp. 175-185, March 1959.

Schweitzer, J. M.: Conservative approach to oral rehabilitation, J. Prosthet. Dent. **11**:119, 1961.

Schweitzer, J. M.: Masticatory function in man; mandibular repositioning, J. Prosthet. Dent. **12**:262, 1962.

Shanahan, T. E. J., and Leff, A.: Mandibular and articulator movements: part VIII, physiologic and mechanical concepts of occlusion, J. Prosthet. Dent. **16**:62-72, 1966.

Sheppard, I.: Effect of hinge axis clutches on condyle position, J. Prosthet. Dent. **8**:260, 1958.

Sheppard, I. M.: Bracing position, centric occlusion, and centric relation, J. Prosthet. Dent. **9**:11, 1959.

Sheppard, I. M.: Closing masticatory strokes, J. Prosthet. Dent. **9**:946, 1959.

Sheppard, I. M.: Anteroposterior and posteroanterior movements of the mandible and condylar centricity during function, J. Prosthet. Dent. **12**:86, 1962.

Shore, N. A.: Symptomatology of temporomandibular joint dysfunction, J. New Jersey Dent. Soc. **31**:10, 1959.

Shore, N. A.: Treatment of temporomandibular joint dysfunction, J. Prosthet. Dent. **10**:366, 1960.

Shore, N. A.: Interpretations of temporomandibular joint roentgenograms, Am. Equilibration Soc. Compend. **4**:152, 1960.

Shpuntoff, H., and Shpuntoff, W.: Study of physiologic rest position and centric position by electromyography, J. Prosthet. Dent. **6**:621, 1956.

Sicher, H.: Changing concepts of the supporting dental structures, Oral Surg. **12**:31, 1959.

Sicher, H.: Temporomandibular articulation; concepts and misconceptions, Oral Surg. **20**:281, 1962.

Stallard, H.: Physiology of chewing, J. Dist. Columbia Dent. Soc. **34**:9, 1959.

Stallard, H., and Stuart, C. E.: Eliminating tooth guidance in natural dentitions, J. Prosthet. Dent. **11**:474, 1961.

Stansbery, C. J.: Functional position checkbite technique, J.A.D.A. **16**:421, 1929.

Storey, A. T.: Physiology of a changing vertical dimension, J. Prosthet. Dent. **12**:912, 1962.

Stuart, C. E.: Why dental restoration should have cusps, J. South. Calif. Dent. Assoc. **27**:198, 1959.

Stuart, C. E., and Stallard, H.: Diagnosis and treatment of occlusal relations of the teeth, Texas Dent. J. **75**:430, 1957.

Swenson, H. M.: Complete mouth reconstruction or destruction? J.A.D.A. **65**:345, 1962.

Thilander, B.: Innervation of the temporo-mandibular joint capsule in man; an anatomic investigation and a neurophysiologic study of the perception of mandibular position, Trans. Roy. Schools Dent. Stockholm Umea, no. 7, pp. 9-67, 1961.

Trapozzano, V. R., and Lazzari, J. B.: Study of hinge axis determination, J. Prosthet. Dent. **11**:858, 1961.

Trapozzano, V. R., and Lazzari, J. B.: The physiology of the terminal rotation position of the condyles in the temporomandibular joint, J. Prosthet. Dent. **17**:122-133, 1967.

Uccellani, E. L.: Use of a muscle relaxant as an aid in obtaining centric registration, J. Prosthet. Dent. **10**:92, 1960.

Vaughan, H. C.: Occlusion and the mandibular articulation, Dent. Clin. North Am., pp. 37-50, March 1962.

Weinberg, L. A.: Physiologic objectives of reconstruction techniques, J. Prosthet. Dent. **10**:711, 1960.

Weinberg, L. A.: Evaluation of the face-bow mounting, J. Prosthet. Dent. **11**:32, 1961.

Weinberg, L. A.: An evaluation of basic articulators and their concepts, J. Prosthet. Dent. **13**:622, 1963.

Weinberg, L. A.: An evaluation of basic articulators and their concepts: part II, arbitrary, positional, semiadjustable articulators, J. Prosthet. Dent. **13**:645, 1963.

Wester, L. H.: Occlusion in the fixed bridge, Texas Dent. J. **76**:172, 1958.

Wing, G.: Temporomandibular joint and general dental practice, Australian Dent. J. **6**:94, 1961.

Woelfel, J. B., Hickey, J. C., Stacy, R. W., and Rinear, L.: Electromyographic analysis of jaw movements, J. Prosthet. Dent. **10**:688-697, 1960.

Zimring, M. J.: Gnathology; an introduction, Dent. Students' Mag. **46**(2):131-187, 1967.

Zola, A.: Morphologic limiting factors in the temporomandibular joint, J. Prosthet. Dent. **13**:732-740, 1963.

Zola, A., and Rothschild, E. A.: Condyle positions in unimpeded jaw movements, J. Prosthet. Dent. **11**:873, 1961.

29

Color: principles, selection, and reproduction in crowns and fixed prosthodontics—materials, equipment, and application

Stanley D. Tylman

PRINCIPLES AND THEORIES

Every dentist strives toward the ideal in facial art when he replaces lost teeth with crowns or fixed prosthodontics. Although the requirements of function and comfort are important in a restoration, one cannot minimize the fact that the esthetic values are also extremely desirable. Psychologically, the esthetic factors are of considerable consequence because of the reactions they produce in the individual. Many patients who have avoided social contacts because of the appearance of their dentures, either natural or artificial, have returned to their normal social and business relationships after rehabilitation of their mouths through prosthodontics.

Normal facial expression, correct occlusion, and proper mastication are frequently concomitant with and dependent on the restoration of the esthetic factors.

Art, or more specifically facial art, has been defined in many ways. As it applies to fixed prosthodontics, it possesses certain fundamentals whose objectives are to restore lost form, function, and appearance, without, at the same time, disclosing the presence of restorations or the means used in the attainment of those objectives.

The concept and the development of the esthetics of teeth have found some unusual methods of expression. The use of war paint and cosmetics was common practice throughout the ages; the placing of jewels in ears and rings in the nose is likewise known and recorded. Even the mutilation of different parts of the body was believed to contribute something to the esthetic qualities of the individual; as witness the flat heads of some Indian tribes, the bound feet of Chinese women, and the coloring, filing, or even knocking out of teeth by many of the African tribes. From this primitive and grotesque idea of facial art, the concept has gradually passed through a process of evolution to a higher plane and to a better appreciation of the fundamentals of true facial art.

FUNDAMENTALS OF FACIAL ART

First among these fundamentals may be listed harmony, as expressed through likeness in contour and color of the eyes, hair, skin, and teeth and also the harmony of texture, direction of axes, etc.; second is the interest as created by sufficient variety in shape, color, texture, and contours. Then there is the fundamental of proportion, the proportion of form and size of the teeth themselves, the dentures

703

as a whole, and the relationships that exist between the forms of the teeth, the face, and the head. The fundamentals of balance, both symmetric and asymmetric, are found in the occlusion. The fundamental of exactness, as related to restorative dentistry, applies to the restoration of the correct anatomy, position, and dental relationships.

Another fundamental of facial art is an understanding of the light factors, both artificial and natural, and the physical changes that they produce in the color effects, and the subjective, physiologic variations or contrasts developed in each individual. The last important fundamental is that of color. This involves not only its composition and analysis, but also the relevance of these factors to the restoration of esthetic values in dentistry.

Fundamentals of color (hue)

In order to select and reproduce colors in porcelain restorations, either crowns, bridges, or inlays, it is essential that the dentist be familiar with the theory, classification, and phenomena of color. Although it is true that some men are possessed of an inherent sense of color harmony, the majority may acquire this faculty only by intense study and experimentation.

A knowledge of color may be gained in two general ways: one is by observation and association, that is, a person may by constant contact with objects of beauty and color acquire an intuitive color sense. This method, however, is a slow process and uncertain in its creative esthetic possibility. The other way is to study the theory, application, and phenomena of color and light. This will acquaint the student with the laws and principles of color, which, once understood, enable him to perceive, match, and reproduce the color effect of natural teeth with confidence and success. The fascination of the work increases as progress is made.

Color defined. The term "color," as or-

dinarily applied, is the sensation or impression produced by the number and character of light rays striking the retina. The effect of light is the result of light waves, just as the effect of sound is the result of sound vibrations striking the eardrum. It is impossible to tabulate directions for using color without an understanding of the physical laws of light, which explain some of the color phenomena with which the dentist must contend in prosthetic restorations.

Physical laws of light and color. If the texture and composition of all objects were so similar that all the rays of light would be reflected from the object to the eye, everything would be white. Since this is not so, one must conclude that various objects differ both in texture and composition to such a degree that they absorb certain rays and reflect others. These different rays travel at varying speeds through substances. One may demonstrate this fact by passing a single ray of white light through a prism, which will break up the white light into a brilliant strip of a variety of colors, among which are a pure blue, a pure red, and a pure green, with the intermediary gradations. This is known as the spectrum (Plate 2).

If an object absorbs all the color rays except blue, which it thus reflects, it is designated as a blue object or has a blue effect.

Substances through which one can see other objects clearly are called *transparent,* but those through which vision is impossible are designated as *opaque.* When a substance transmits some light but not enough for vision, it is *translucent.* When a beam of light strikes a smooth body lying in its path, a large part of the light that falls upon it from one direction is sent off in some other direction by *reflection.* If the surface of the object is rough, the light that falls upon it is scattered in all directions and gives *diffused reflection.* Some of the light in-

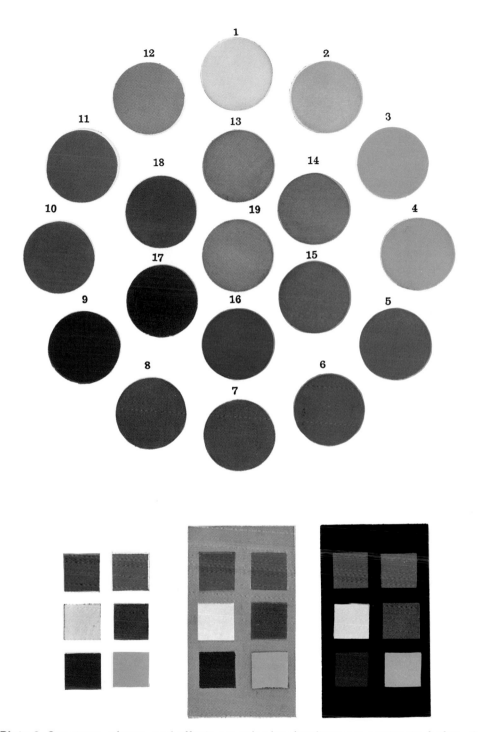

Plate 2. Spectrum, **above,** and effects on color by simultaneous contrasts, **below. 1,** Yellow; **2,** yellow green; **3,** green; **4,** blue green; **5,** blue; **6,** blue violet; **7,** violet; **8,** red violet; **9,** red; **10,** red orange; **11,** orange; **12,** yellow orange; **13,** gray yellow; **14,** gray green; **15,** gray blue; **16,** gray violet; **17,** gray red; **18,** gray orange; **19,** neutral gray.

cident upon the object will sometimes penetrate it; the rays that pass through it are said to be *transmitted*. This process of transmission is always accompanied by some loss of light; light that is lost in this way is said to be *absorbed*. When all the rays are absorbed, the object is *opaque*.[1]

Any classification of colors is arbitrary to a certain degree[2] (Plate 2). Certain groups will dispute whether the primary colors are red, yellow, and blue, or red, green, and violet-blue. The first group is classified according to pigments, whereas the other is classified according to lights. The dentist is not interested so much in a color system that attempts to establish one particular classification as he is in a method whereby he more easily can select porcelains of certain colors or combinations of colors and by their proper manipulation reproduce the color *effects* found in the natural teeth.

The problem does not deal with the various pigments alone; if it did, there would be very little difficulty inasmuch as porcelains are available in various colors, shades, and tints. The colors at the dentist's disposal possess certain qualities, which, if utilized, enable him more nearly to simulate nature.

Color constants. Just as a certain musical sound or a combination of sounds may produce an agreeable or a disagreeable sensation, so also may a certain color or a certain combination of colors produce analogous effects. Every color or hue has three qualities called color constants: (1) color tone, or the quality by which, for example, bluish red differs from orange-red; (2) color luminosity (chroma), by which, for example, light red differs from dark red; (3) color purity (value), by which, for example, a pure or spectral red differs from a broken or grayish-red (Webster); (4) brilliance; and (5) saturation. To the dentist it is of importance to know that the most luminous colors or hues are yellow first, and orange next, whereas the least luminous are blue

and violet (see lower portion of Plate 2). Teeth, therefore, that have a predominance of gray and dark brown present a lifeless appearance, whereas those predominating in yellow or orange appear vital and translucent. In one the rays are mostly absorbed; in the other they are transmitted and reflected. By the addition of certain hues to others, the luminosity or translucency can be increased or decreased. The addition of red or brown to yellow increases its luminosity; similarly, its removal decreases it. The removal of a pulp, no doubt, has some effect on the luminosity of a tooth. Since yellow and orange possess this highly desired characteristic of luminosity, these hues should be used as the foundation for most inlays and crowns.

Next in importance to yellow with its red modifications is the blue hue. This may vary in shade toward the variations with red or toward the greenish tints. It has its importance in the incisal and the occlusal regions. The tints of greenish hue are the more luminous inasmuch as green is a combination of blue with yellow. Although green is rarely used as a pure color, except for staining purposes, its addition to grays of a bluish tendency tends to intensify the grays. Brown made more brilliant by the addition of yellow is indicated as a base color for either inlays or crowns for older patients or those with stained teeth. Whenever it is desired to dull a color, such as yellow, the slight addition of gray will accomplish the result. Certain colors known as advancing colors have a feeling of warmth about them, whereas others called the receding colors have a cold, bleak reaction. Who has not, at one time or another, studied a painting and felt that something was lacking? The slight addition of a color would change the entire effect; the following is an example of this.

A picture depicts an evening scene on the shores of a bay. Projecting out into the water, on a small promontory, squats a fisherman's hut. The artist beautifully portrays fleecy clouds floating in the moonlit sky, the trees nodding in the evening breezes, and tied to the pier a small boat riding the undulating waves. Everything seems to lend to the scene an atmosphere of peace and calm, and yet something is lacking. One dip of the brush, a few strokes, and an inanimate scene is transformed into one radiating with life; it is simple; the dark windows of the hut are painted with orange color. At once there is life in the hut, life in the picture. This helps to explain why yellow and orange are referred to as "warm colors."

Again, it is noticed upon viewing distant mountain ranges that the general effect is one of a bluish haze. The outline of the mountains is visible, but there is no definite differentiation of color until one comes nearer, when not only the different colors, but also the various tones of colors can be distinguished. These phenomena are more noticeable if there is no sunshine.

Color contrast and harmony. In addition to the effect produced by adding one color to another, there is the effect produced by contrasting one color with another. If red, yellow, and blue are used as the basis for the color scheme, three secondary colors are obtained by combining two of these primary colors. Red and yellow produce orange; yellow and blue produce green, whereas blue and red produce violet. The secondary colors likewise may be combined to form tertiary combinations, and these may again form others. With such a variety of colors to contend with, it is reasonable to suppose that certain combinations will harmonize whereas others will clash.

The interest of the dentist is mainly in those colors that harmonize. Color harmony may be of two kinds, harmony of analogy and of contrast. This phase of the color problem is also of special importance to the complete-denture prosthetist, who must harmonize the artificial dentures with the predominating colors of each patient. When there are two tones of one color, such as orange and red, there is harmony of analogy because there is a common ingredient in both, that is, red. However, it is possible to have harmony with neither color having a common ingredient. This is a harmony of contrast exemplified by the colors of red and green, red being a primary and green a combination of the other two primaries, yellow and blue. Another factor of importance to the dentist is the type of light available and the effect of the different colored lights on color selection and reproduction. A light may come from a concentrated source, as from a focused lamp, or it may come from a large luminous body, such as the sun. The former type of light will cast a sharp, well-defined shadow of an object, whereas the latter type of light, such as daylight, will cast a shadow of an indefinite, fading outline. This may explain some of the phenomena that confront a dentist in his practice. A porcelain inlay viewed in daylight always looks better than under a focused light, because with the latter the shadows are sharper.

Effect of light on color. In addition to the intensity of the light, it is advisable to determine the *color* of the *light used* at the time a color is selected. Normal daylight varies in its hue, depending on the time of day. The early morning rays are of a pinkish tint; the sun at high noon sends white rays; whereas near the horizon it emits rays of an orange-red hue. A cloudy day usually casts purplish rays. The light from a skylight is bluish white, whereas that from an electric arc varies from white to bluish white and violet. An incandescent lamp of normal brilliancy gives yellow light, but, when the voltage is low, it turns orange.

In selecting colors, therefore, the type of light and the time of day must be taken into account. There is also a change in the color effect when the rays of one color fall upon another. This fact should call attention to the influence that the color of the curtains and walls may have on color determination and selection.

Simultaneous contrast. Another effect that must be taken into consideration during color selection is that obtained by simultaneous contrast (Plate 2). As will be observed, some colors show to better advantage on a black background; others show better on a gray, whereas all look good on white. The juxtaposition of black has the effect of intensifying the luminosity of the colors; gray subdues and neutralizes them; whereas white deepens their tone. The practical value of this principle is evident when one determines the tone of a basic color in a natural tooth.

Color in natural teeth

The next consideration is the color value found in natural teeth. It is essential that a thorough study of the predominating colors be made before any attempt is made at matching with shade guides. The color of natural teeth is not uniformly of a single hue or purity value. Even in the same individual there exists a strong difference of intensity not only between the different teeth, but even in the same tooth, where there is a variation of tint, shade, or intensity. It is of utmost importance to be able to discern color *pigmentation* and color *effect,* as well as their mutual interdependence. Although it is true that the pigment of a tooth determines its basic color, there are other factors involved: the thickness and density of dentin; the thickness and distribution of enamel; the pulp size and proximity to labial surface; environment darkness, depth of oral cavity, the color and mobility of the lips; abrasion; stains; external surface texture and contour; position in arch; intensity and color of light falling upon the tooth.

Upon careful study of natural teeth one is able to distinguish the following basic colors; yellow, orange, and yellows with a greenish or a brownish tinge; in the

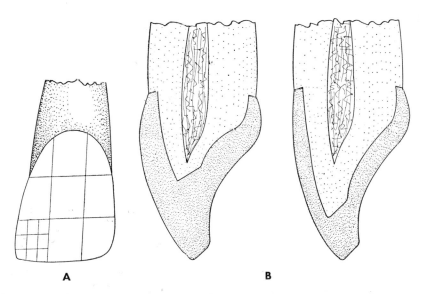

Fig. 29-1. A, Chart to indicate selection of color and its intensity and distribution. **B,** Although correct lines of body and enamels are same, color effect will be different because of variation in thickness of labial surfaces of porcelain.

enamel or overlying colors there may be blue or gray with a mirage effect toward the yellow. The color of the incisal enamel is not attributable to pigmentation so much as it is to the reaction of a translucent substance to light, subject to the laws of physics.

Selection of color for prosthetic restorations

Color distribution in teeth. The first consideration in the selection of colors is the variation of hues in the various sections of the tooth. The gingival third is usually some tone of orange or yellow; the incisal third is either a blue or a gray; whereas the middle section may be an overlapping of both colors. The distribution of these colors is not always uniform; at least the color effects are not. Thus one is advised to draw a diagram of the tooth (Fig. 29-1, A) and divide it into squares, noting how far the gingival color extends incisally on the labial and on the labioproximal line angles; this record will assist one later when applying the porcelain.

Determination of color. A difficulty usually encountered in color perception is the interference from surrounding colors. To eliminate this influence, a piece of neutral gray paper with an opening cut in it should be placed over the teeth. The colors may then be more accurately determined. Many dentists have had failures in the selection of colors for inlays because they determined the shade in the same manner that they make a selection for a complete porcelain crown or a denture, that is, from a standard tooth guide without first determining the basic and the overlying colors. Others have had difficulty because they selected a basic color and proceeded to bake the inlay with the one color. This will usually result in partial success only, because the color of a natural tooth varies from the gingival to the incisal areas. It is well to remember also that in different locations on the labial or buccal surface the thickness of the enamel varies. In other words, a labial inlay in the gingival region would be simulated by a thin *overlying* color of blue or yellowish gray and a *deep layer* of basic color. Inasmuch as dentin is slightly translucent and its surface, microscopically, is not smooth (Fig. 9-1), the underlying porcelain color must present an unglazed surface of the same characteristic texture. Similarly, a labial inlay in the incisal half of a tooth could have a thinner but more intense layer of basic color with a thicker overlying enamel color. Again, a similar inlay in a bicuspid would need an intensified enamel-colored porcelain, inasmuch as the enamel in a natural bicuspid is very thick in the occlusal half.

For the same reasons, when selecting colors for a jacket crown, one needs to determine the basic hue and its distribution and intensity of tone. This latter condition can be determined through a study of the effects produced by firing of porcelains of certain hues in varying thicknesses. To illustrate: look through one sheet of amber-colored glass; it has a certain hue, a certain luminosity. By superimposing another similar sheet of glass and looking through both, one will see that the hue remains pure but its effect is a deeper tone; a third sheet will further accentuate the effect. The same is true of porcelains. The basic hue may be correct, but, unless it is applied and fired in the proper thickness, the depth of the hue will not harmonize with the tooth. As a rule, it is necessary to intensify the basic hue of a porcelain-veneer crown. The dentin of a natural tooth has normal fullness, which gives the effect of a certain luminosity. Were it possible to set the finished porcelain crown without interposing cement, the object would be to reproduce the natural tone of the basic hue; as it is, the cement not only excludes the color of the dentin, but it also absorbs much of the transmitted light striking the crown.

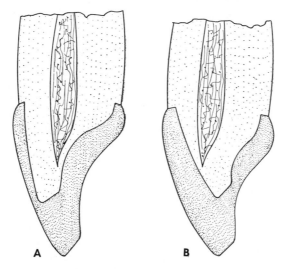

Fig. 29-2. Cement color will show through crown **A**; thick layer of porcelain on crown **B** will produce different color effect.

Effect of tooth preparation on color. The gingivoincisal length of the tooth preparation in relation to the gingivoincisal length of the finished crown also has an influence on color selection and reproduction (Fig. 29-2, *B*).

Effect of light on color. Frequently the dentist determines and selects the proper color but does not analyze the effect of light upon it. If the tooth has an irregular or a marked surface, it may influence the dentist in selecting a porcelain of a darker shade. It is well in selecting colors to view the tooth from all angles in order to study the reflection of light, the influence of the lips in excluding light, the position of the lips in repose and in laughter. It is necessary to obtain a close view, as well as one several feet distant. If there exists any doubt as to the proper color to use or the proper thickness of the various colors, veneer shade guides of several combinations and thicknesses should be constructed. These, when fired and tabulated, will prove of great help for subsequent doubtful cases. Such an individualized, custom-made shade guide will prove extremely valuable not only in the selection and reproduction of tooth colors

in the complete porcelain-veneer crown, but even more so in color determination for porcelain-fused-to-metal crowns. They can be constructed quickly and, in time, constitute a valuable color guide.

Enamel color. It is doubtful whether enamel possesses any color pigment. Even in those cases in which it appears quite blue or gray, upon illumination from the lingual aspect, it is found to be quite translucent, even bordering on transparency. The depth of the oral cavity and the width of the lip line have an important bearing on the incisal color effect. It is probable that the size, arrangement, and shape of the enamel rods may also have some bearing on the color effect.

REPRODUCING COLORS IN PORCELAIN

The dentist should not only have an understanding of color and be able to recognize its various qualities, but should also be able to reproduce the needed color in porcelain. As stated previously, colors are produced by various mesmeric pigmented porcelains or by superimposition of one pigmented layer of porcelain upon another. By increasing or decreasing the thickness of different layers, one may produce various effects with two pigments. If the overlying layer is too thin, it becomes translucent to a degree that the basic color reflection destroys the effect of the enamel color; if the basic color is too deep, it also may affect the desired color scheme.

For reproduction of the desired color in inlays, several ways have been suggested and used. Some dentists apply the various shades in layers; others build the inlay in sections; some mix their colors before applying; whereas still others use one basic color and control the desired shade by the color of cement used. The layer method is preferable. By its use the location and amount can be accurately controlled and the natural gradations of hue obtained. Each tone will maintain its individuality, and yet they all will blend harmoniously.

Influence of cement on color

The influence of cement on the color of porcelain is greater in the inlay than in the crown. When light is incident upon the surface of an inlay, its angle of reflection may permit its transmission. Should the direction be such as to encounter cement, a shadow results. A transparent cement would help solve to a degree this difficulty; recent efforts along this line are encouraging, but they are still in the experimental stages.

Although the color of cement influences that of the crown, its effect is not very pronounced, except when the labial wall of porcelain is too thin or too thick (Fig. 29-2). The reproduction of colors in the porcelain-veneer (jacket) crown is dependent on several factors. One of the important ones is a correct tooth preparation (Fig. 29-3); another is the proper dis-

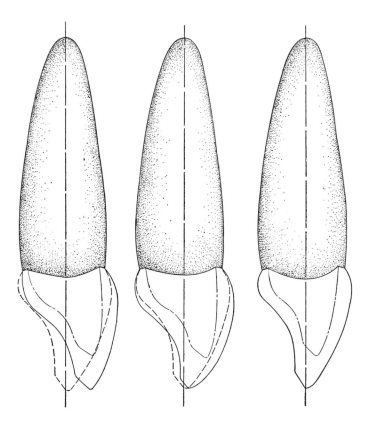

Fig. 29-3. Crowns on left were built too far labially because of improper preparation of teeth; crown on right, labial contour in proper alignment with proximating teeth.

tribution of the basic and the overlying porcelains, generally known as the gingival or body colors and the incisal or enamel colors.

Distribution of porcelain

In addition to correct distribution of colors, the thicknesses of the two pigmented porcelains must be in proper proportion. The natural tooth color effects are usually reproduced in a crown: first, by placement of a layer of the predominating body color porcelain in the gingival third; and second, by restoration of the incisal third usually in one color, the enamel. These two colors, one extending incisally and the other gingivally, overlap each other in the middle third of the tooth and give the desired blended color effect of a natural tooth (Fig. 29-4, A). When it is necessary to shorten the incisal length of a finished crown, the shaded color effect area appears to locate itself incisally.

Surface texture of porcelain

The texture of the porcelain surface influences the shade of a porcelain-veneer (jacket) crown. Given two crowns of identical hues, distribution, and degree of firing, it is a simple matter to deepen the hue value of one by placing grooves or facets in its labial surface; this may be done with stones or a diamond point and by refiring of the restoration.

Position and shape of tooth

A tooth in the anterior part of the mouth appears lighter than one in the bicuspid or molar region, because of the angle of the reflected light. The degree of mesiodistal convexity also influences the color effect.

There are times when three colors of porcelain are used, in which event the distribution may be made as shown in Fig. 29-4, B. The intermediate zone consists of a mixture of the gingival and incisal porcelains.

Use of stains and stained porcelain

In a crown having the correct basic gingival and incisal colors, the color of the facing or the artificial tooth may be modified in two ways: first, by the use of stains; second, by the use of stained porcelain. The former is a true mineral stain, whereas the latter is porcelain of a modified composition and a lower fusing range than that with which the crown was built, except that a pigment has been

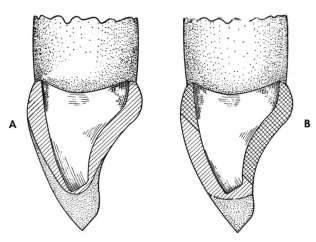

Fig. 29-4. A, Usual distribution of body and enamel-colored porcelain. **B,** Three colors of porcelain may be distributed as shown.

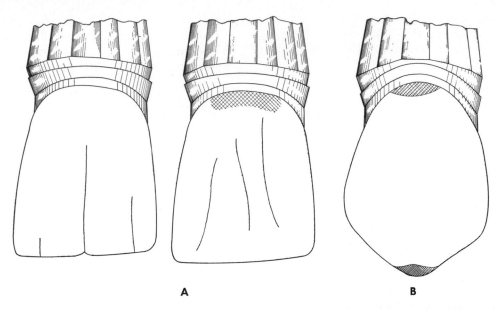

Fig. 29-5. A, Enamel checks and fissures simulated by use of stains or stained porcelain. **B,** Enamel defects and stains simulated by use of stained or translucent porcelain.

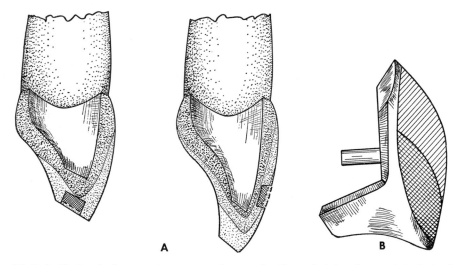

Fig. 29-6. A, Method of preparing crowns for application of stained porcelain to incisal or labial surfaces. **B,** Method used to change or modify shade of a porcelain pontic.

added to it to give the desired depth of stain. The judicious use of stains or stained porcelains will result in artistic effects not attainable in any other manner. Teeth may be darkened or lightened; labioenamel checks, cervical stains (Fig. 29-5, *A*), or incisal stains may also be effectively reproduced (Fig. 29-5, *B*). The pale bluish effect may also be obtained by the proper application of stains at the incisal surface (Fig. 29-5, *B*).

Although similar results may be obtained by use of stained porcelain, certain preliminary procedures are necessary.

To reproduce an enamel check, one scratches a pencil line of the desired length and depth on the labial surface of the crown or facing with a diamond point. The scratch is filled with a small amount of lower-fusing stained porcelain, the excess being carefully brushed away, and the added porcelain is fired to a glaze.

To reproduce a dark stained surface frequently seen along the incisal edge of the anterior teeth, one first cuts a groove mesiodistally into the incisal surface of the porcelain crown to the desired width and to a depth of about 0.25 mm. This is filled with the stained porcelain of the desired color and glazed (Fig. 29-6, *A*). For a more natural effect, stained porcelain is usually covered with a thin layer of the incisal colored porcelain; after glazing, the effect is more natural since the stain appears embedded in dentin rather than being superficially applied.

The use of mineral stains is contraindicated on the incisal edge or on those surfaces that may be exposed to attrition; in such locations mineral stains are worn away in a relatively short time.

If neither mineral stains nor the stained porcelains are available for modifying or changing the color of a facing or crown, the labial surface is ground down until only a basic layer of porcelain remains. With this as a foundation, new porcelains, usually of a lower fusing range but of the proper basic and incisal colors, are applied and fused; in this way a new color is developed in the facing or crown (Fig. 29-6, *B*).

Restoring glazed surface

Whenever it is necessary to grind a facing or a porcelain crown to alter its contour, it is imperative that the surface be reglazed in order that its true color effect be restored and that a hygienic surface be assured.

A glaze may be restored to a ground porcelain surface in one of three ways: First, the facing or crown, having been thoroughly cleansed, may be replaced in the muffle and brought to a glaze temperature. The danger of such a procedure lies in the possibility of the porcelain restoration rounding its margins, thus losing its fit. Furthermore, by subjection of a facing or crown to a second glazing temperature, the color of the porcelain is likely to be diluted.

A second method for restoring the glaze surface of a porcelain crown consists of the application of a thin layer of porcelain, which will glaze at a lower temperature than the crown or facing, thus eliminating the possibility of rounded edges or color changes.

The third method usually employed is the application of dental glazes. Whereas the lower-fusing porcelain used in the second method is of the same color as the facing or the crown, dental glazes are transparent and colorless. A dental glaze also fuses at a lower temperature than the porcelain surface to which it is applied. Although a glaze is used as a thin film and without any effect on the color, low-fusing porcelain must usually be applied in bulk and hence may alter the shade of the facing or crowns. To be satisfactory, a dental glaze must have approximately the same coefficient of expansion and contraction as the porcelain to which it is applied; otherwise the surface will appear crazed upon cooling.

In every instance in which a crown surface is to be reglazed by any one of the three methods, certain precautions must be taken: first, that the surface is absolutely clean of all debris; second, that the surface has been first polished smooth; and third, that all the little pores and openings in the porcelain crown or facing first have been filled with compatible dry porcelain powder or glaze before the final glazing is done.

Grinding porcelain. One precaution should be observed in grinding porcelain with an abrasive stone; contamination of the porcelain with grinding debris should be avoided. This may be done by use of only new, clean stones for the grinding. When the grinding is performed dry, it should be done under a blast of compressed air so that all loose particles may be immediately blown clear of the porcelain. The other and better method of avoiding contamination is to hold the porcelain and the stone under water while grinding. "Grinding semiwet" will produce a paste consisting of particles of porcelain, abrasive crystals, and the bonding material of the stone; once this paste works into the pores of the porcelain, it is almost impossible to remove it, except in an ultrasonic cleaning device.

Glazing technique. Several manufactured glazes are available to the dental profession. Each is satisfactory, provided that the instructions of the manufacturer are carefully observed.[3]

Additional methods of altering the contour or the color of teeth, together with additional techniques for reglazing, may be found in the standard texts.[4,5]

Usually it is simpler to match the correct color in manufactured bridge facings than in crowns built up entirely from porcelain powders. Manufactured bridge facings that correspond to the colors found in the shade guides of the manufacturer are available. When using such facings, the dentist need only be able to recognize the basic gingival and incisal predominating colors in the natural teeth and to relate them correctly with the colors in the shade guide. If this is accurately done, very little color difficulty should be experienced. Certain precautions, however, must be observed relative to the backing, soldering, or cementing of the facings; if disregarded, a color modification may occur to alter the original selection of the facing.

When manufactured teeth are used, either for crown or bridge restorations, their selection should be correct from the standpoint not only of color but also of size and form. A size should be selected that requires very little grinding or modification for its use; the form should correspond with the characteristic type of the arch and face of the patient.

The technique and procedures involved in the application and firing of porcelain are discussed more fully in Chapter 25, which deals with the construction of porcelain-veneer crowns.

At this time attention is called to the relationship that exists between optical illusions and restorative dentistry, whether it be a single porcelain-veneer crown or a unit of a fixed partial denture. Blancheri[6] offers the following excellent observations and illustrations in explaining this relationship:

Visual perception is the response of the eye to the following factors:
1. Light
2. Movement
3. Outline form
4. Surface form
5. Color

The eye is, first of all, sensitive to light but tires (fatigues) very rapidly to continued stimulus. Light reflection is of importance but is more properly discussed under surface form.

Sensitivity to movement of an object is next in order but is of little significance in this discussion.

The eye is very sensitive to outline form. This is easily understood by remembering how easily a silhouette is recognized. Surely each of us has had the experience of watching a carnival artist cut out black paper silhouettes which were immediately recognized. The value of this principle was understood by military authorities in the recent conflict when thousands of airplane pilots and observers were trained to recognize aircraft by silhouette alone. This is a principle which has been relatively neglected in dentistry and yet is particularly true regarding teeth, as perception of outline form is differentiation of very unlike things: that is, the tooth, relatively white in color, surrounded gingivally by the gingival tissue, interproximally by the dark and usually stained interproximal contacts, and incisally by the shadow of the oral cavity. This shadow is very important in talking and smiling. It silhouettes the incisal edges.

The eye is understandably less sensitive to surface form of teeth as it involves the delicacy of binocular perspective of minute variations. However,

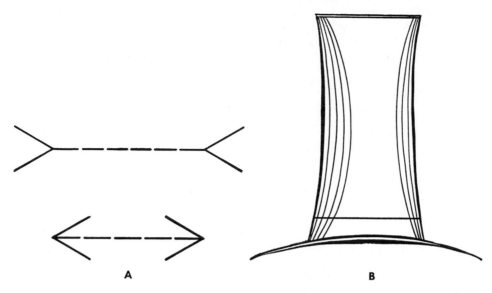

Fig. 29-7. A, Both horizontal lines are same length. **B,** Brim of hat is as wide as hat is tall. (Courtesy R. L. Blancheri.)

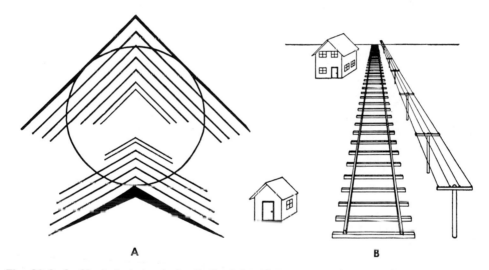

Fig. 29-8. A, Circle is true circle. **B,** Both houses are exactly same size. (Courtesy R. L. Blancheri.)

surface form must not be disregarded as it is easily controlled and is responsible for light reflection. Control of light reflection is one of our most valuable tools, especially when enamel offers such an excellent reflecting surface.

Finally, the eye is less sensitive to color than is commonly supposed, particularly to the infinite and minute color variations found in teeth. This is stated, not to minimize the importance of correctly matching shades, but instead to emphasize other relatively neglected factors. It must also be remembered in selecting shades that the eye fatigues very rapidly to color stimulus. First impressions are more accurate. It is much better to compare shade samples with teeth in five-second glances than to compare steadily for sixty or even thirty seconds.

Not only is the eye sensitive to stimuli but it is also susceptible to trickery. We are well aware of the

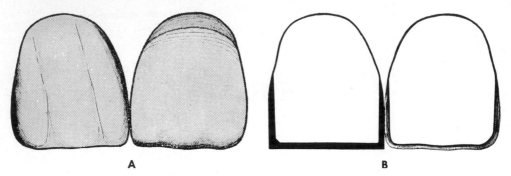

Fig. 29-9. A, Both teeth are same width and length. **B,** Careful contouring of partial veneer preparation minimizes objectionable display of gold. (Courtesy R. L. Blancheri.)

trickery practiced by the sleight-of-hand artist; we are less aware of the trickery of lines and angles. [This is demonstrated in Figs. 29-7 to 29-9.]

The main principles to be learned from these examples [Figs. 29-7 to 29-9] are that vertical lines accent height—horizontal lines accent width—shadows add depth—angles influence the lines they intersect. Also remember that curved surfaces are softer, more pleasing than harsh angles.

In applying these principles to everyday dental problems, let us first consider the problem of restoring a missing central where the space is wider, narrower, or longer than the remaining central. If the space is wider [Fig. 29-10] a very practical solution is to use a replacement wide enough to fill the space. The porcelain is kept as thick labio-lingually as possible and the contact point is kept as far lingually as possible. On the labial surface, we will mentally superimpose the labial outline form of the remaining central and by grinding the mesial and distal surfaces (mostly on the distal surface) we will taper the facing from the contact area to the superimposed labial outline form. The new mesial and distal surfaces formed by grinding should be glazed and stained to lend depth. By greying these edges they appear indistinct and fade away. Also, remembering that darker shades appear smaller and lighter shades appear larger, it would be wise to use a shade slightly darker than the natural central. At the time of grinding the mesial and distal surfaces to shape the new outline form, the labial surface form of the remaining central is closely copied, with particular attention being paid to duplicating any ridges and depressions that will reflect light. It is not the presence of these ridges and grooves per se that gives individual character to a tooth; it is the individual pattern of light reflection that determines tooth character.

To reverse the application, let us assume the same missing tooth but with a space narrower than the

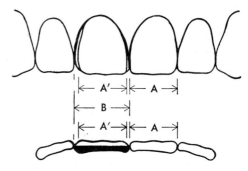

Fig. 29-10. A, Width of remaining central incisor. **A',** Superimposed pattern of remaining central incisor. **B,** Space originally available. (Courtesy R. L. Blancheri.)

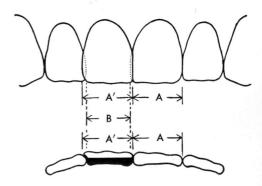

Fig. 29-11. A, Final width of remaining central incisor. **A',** Superimposed pattern of remaining central incisor. **B,** Space to be filled (total width of porcelain). (Courtesy R. L. Blancheri.)

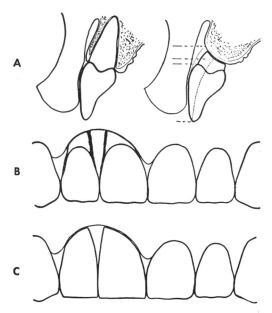

Fig. 29-12. Excessive resorption of ridge necessitating longer crown or facing. Normal outline form superimposed. Cementoenamel line is adapted. (Courtesy R. L. Blancheri.)

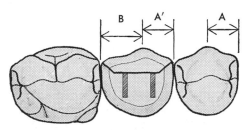

Fig. 29-13. A, Width of first bicuspid from mesial surface to height of buccal contour. **A',** Width of pontic from mesial surface to height of buccal contour. **B,** Width of distal half of pontic (wider than mesial half). (Courtesy R. L. Blancheri.)

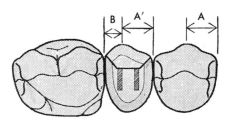

Fig. 29-14. A, Width of first bicuspid from mesial surface to height of buccal contour. **A',** Width of pontic from mesial surface to height of buccal contour. **B,** Width of distal half of pontic (narrower than mesial half). (Courtesy R. L. Blancheri.)

remaining central [Fig. 29-11]. First the remaining tooth may be narrowed by slightly reducing the mesial surface. A facing wider than the space is chosen and the labial outline form and surface form of the remaining central is duplicated as nearly as possible, again keeping in mind factors of light reflection. The mesial and distal surfaces are then ground from the lingual labially, taking care to not alter the labial outline, until the facing fits the space, resorting to overlapping if necessary.

Where excessive ridge resorption presents the problem of requiring a facing much longer than the tooth to be matched [Fig. 29-12, *A*], it is again desirable to superimpose the outline form of the remaining central and grind in a very definite cementoenamel junction line [Fig. 29-12, *B*]. Again copy the surface form as closely as possible, also keeping in mind the correct position in the arch. The root position may then be sloped back to contact the ridge [Fig. 29-12, *A*], glazed and stained a yellowish color to simulate an area of gingival recession. A faint deepening of the color toward the apex of the root form, as well as a definite demarcation line at the cemento-enamel junction, heightens the illusion. I prefer this method to the addition of any type of pink stain or material in an attempt to match gum tissue.

The same principles are applied to restoring bicuspids except that, instead of superimposing the labial outline form, the portion of the buccal surface between the mesio-buccal line angle and the buccal height of contour is copied [Figs. 29-13 and 29-14].

Let us assume an upper right second bicuspid is missing and the space is wider than the first bicuspid [Fig. 29-13]. A replacement is chosen which is wide enough to fill the entire space and by grinding the distal half of the buccal surface, the height of buccal contour is moved mesially until the mesial half of the buccal surface approximates that of the first bicuspid.

Assuming the same missing tooth but with a space too narrow for a full pontic, the same principle is applied [Fig. 29-14]. A pontic is chosen and ground so the buccal form from the mesio-buccal angle to the height of buccal contour approximates that of the first bicuspid. This leaves the distal half much narrower than the mesial half but, inasmuch as this distal plane is not visible during average mouth movements, the total effect is very favorable.

These basic applications can be altered to suit practically any variation found in the mouth.*

---

*From Blancheri, R. L.: Optical illusions and cosmetic grinding, Rev. de Assoc. Dent. Mexicana 8:103, 1950.

SELECTED REFERENCES

1. Crew, H.: General physics, ed. 3, New York, 1918, The Macmillan Co., chap. 12.
2. Snow, B. E., and Froehlich, H. B.: The theory and practice of color, Chicago, 1920, The Prang Co., p. 20.
3. Columbus Dental Mfg. Co.: The art of staining and glazing artificial teeth, Columbus, Ohio, 1936.
4. Peyton, F. A., and Craig, R. G.: Restorative dental materials, ed. 4, St. Louis, 1971, The C. V. Mosby Co.
5. Skinner, E. W., and Phillips, R. W.: The science of dental materials, Philadelphia, 1967, W. B. Saunders Co.
6. Blancheri, R. L.: Optical illusions and cosmetic grinding, Rev. de Assoc. Dent. Mexicana 8:103, 1950.

GENERAL REFERENCES

Berger, C. C.: Control of color of crowns for pulpless anterior teeth, J. Prosthet. Dent. 19(1):58-59, 1968.
Contino, R.: Personal communication, 1976.
Gill, J. R.: Color selection—its distribution and interpretation, J.A.D.A. 40:539, 1950.
Heilbrun, G.: Problem of taking shades, Illinois Dent. J. 31:249, 1962.
Katz, S. R.: Aesthetics in ceramics, J. Can. Dent. Assoc. 32(4):224-230, 1966.
Pilkington, E. L.: Natural effects in porcelain, J.A.D.A. 17:1290, 1930.
Pincus, C. L.: Esthetic variations in jacket crowns involving periodontal and other deformities, N.Y. J. Dent. 24:132, 1954.
Preston, J. D.: Color in fixed prosthodontics, monograph, Wadsworth Hospital Center, Los Angeles, Calif., 1973.
Saklad, M. J.: Esthetic factors in selection of tooth form and color, Dent. Clin. North Am., pp. 231-252, March 1959.
Sproull, R. C.: Color matching in dentistry. Part I. The three-dimensional nature of color. Part II. Practical applications of the organization of color, J. Prosthet. Dent. 29(4):416-424; 29(5):556-566, 1973.
Tashjian, H. H.: Color problem in jacket crowns, J.A.D.A. 50:193, 1955.
Thomas, J. E., Lacroix, R., and Villemot, J.: Color in ceramics, Ann. Odontostomat. 24(5):209-214, 1967.
Weinberg, L. A.: Esthetics and the gingivae in full coverage, J. Prosthet. Dent. 10:737, 1960.
Wheeler, R. C.: Complete crown form and the periodontium, J. Prosthet. Dent. 11:722, 1961.
Yock, D. H.: Porcelain jacket veneer crown preparation, Iowa Dent. J. 43:267, 1957.

Index